Contents

ACCIDENT & EMERGENCY

THEORY INTO PRACTICE | SECOND EDITION

Edited by

Brian Dolan MSc(Oxon) MSc(Nurs) RMN RGN

Director of Service Improvement and Patient Flow, Canterbury District Health Board, Christchurch, New Zealand
Director, Dolan & Holt Consultancy Ltd, Stratford upon Avon, Warwickshire, UK
Vice Chair, RCN Emergency Care Association

Lynda Holt MA RGN EN DipHS

Managing Director, Dolan & Holt Consultancy Ltd, Stratford upon Avon, Warwickshire, UK
Formerly Chair, RCN Emergency Care Association

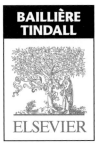

BAILLIÈRE TINDALL

ELSEVIER

EDINBURGH LONDON NEW YORK OXFORD PHILADELPHIA ST LOUIS SYDNEY TORONTO 2008

BAILLIÈRE
TINDALL
ELSEVIER

© 2008 Elsevier Limited. All rights reserved.

Second edition 2008

ISBN 978-0-7020-2684-3

British Library Cataloguing in Publication Data
A catalogue record for this book is available from the British Library

Library of Congress Cataloging in Publication Data
A catalog record for this book is available from the Library of Congress

Note
Medical knowledge is constantly changing. Standard safety precautions must be followed, but as new research and clinical experience broaden our knowledge, changes in treatment and drug therapy may become necessary or appropriate. Readers are advised to check the most current product information provided by the manufacturer of each drug to be administered to verify the recommended dose, the method and duration of administration, and contraindications. It is the responsibility of the practitioner, relying on experience and knowledge of the patient, to determine dosages and the best treatment for each individual patient. Neither the Publisher nor the author assumes any liability for any injury and/or damage to persons or property arising from this publication.

The Publisher

ELSEVIER
your source for books,
journals and multimedia
in the health sciences
www.elsevierhealth.com

Working together to grow
libraries in developing countries
www.elsevier.com | www.bookaid.org | www.sabre.org
ELSEVIER   BOOK AID International   Sabre Foundation

The publisher's policy is to use **paper manufactured from sustainable forests**

II

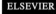

Printed in China

Contributors

Brian Boag FFEN BSc(Critical Care) RGN RMN PGCHE PGDE
Principal Lecturer, School of Nursing and Midwifery, University of Cumbria, Carlisle

Sheelagh Brewer BA MIPD
Senior Employment Relations Adviser, Royal College of Nursing, London

Michael Brown MSc BSc(Hons) PGCE RGN RNLD
Consultant Nurse/Teaching Fellow, NHS Lothian/Napier University, Edinburgh

Elaine Cole MSc BSc PgDip(Ed) RGN
Lecturer Practitioner, Emergency Care Barts and the London NHS Trust/City University, London

Andrew Cook BSc(Hons) RGN
Policy & Practice Manager (Independent Healthcare) Healthcare Commission, London

Judy Davies MA SRN DipN
Formerly Senior Nurse, Emergency Department, Norfolk and Norwich Hospital, UK

Mary Dawood MSc BSc(Hons) RGN
Consultant Nurse, Emergency Department, St Mary's Hospital, London

Orla Devereux RGN RM DipMgt
Clinical Nurse Manager, Emergency Department, Mayo General Hospital, Castlebar, Ireland

Brian Dolan MSc(Oxon) MSc(Nurs) RMN RGN
Director of Service Improvement and Patient Flow, Canterbury District Health Board, Christchurch, New Zealand
Director, Dolan Holt Consultancy Ltd, Stratford upon Avon, Warwickshire, UK
Vice Chair, RCN Emergency Care Association

Charlotte Douglas BSc RGN
Clinical Nurse Educator, Emergency Department, Christchurch Hospital, New Zealand

Julie Flaherty MA BSc(Hons) DPPN RSCN RGN ENB HA Cert Ed
Children's Unscheduled Care Nurse Consultant, Hope Hospital, Salford

Paula (Polly) Grainger MN(Clinical) RN
Associate Clinical Nurse Manager, Emergency Department, Christchurch New Zealand

Elspeth Hair RMN RGN
Formerly Associate Director BankAide, NHS Lanarkshire, Scotland

Lynda Holt MA RGN EN DipHS
Managing Director, Dolan & Holt Consultancy Ltd, Stratford upon Avon, Warwickshire, UK, Formerly Chair, RCN Emergency Care Association

Kirsty Jack RMN
Senior Tutor General Services Association/CFMA Manager, NHS Lothian/ Department of Workforce and Organisational Development, Royal Edinburgh Hospital

Gary J Jones CBE RN FRCN FFNF
Managing Director Health Care Training & Development Services Ltd, Grays, Essex

Heather Josland BN RN PGCert
Nursing Lecturer, School of Nursing, Christchurch Polytechnic Instititute of Technology, (CPIT), Christchurch, New Zealand

Tim Kilner BN(Hons) RN SRP PGCE DipIMC RCSEd
Head of Education and Development, Gloucestershire Ambulance Service NHS Trust

Antonia Lynch MSc RGN
Consultant Nurse Emergency Department, Barts and the London NHS Trust, London

Janet Marsden MSc BSc(Hons) RGN OND MIMgt
Senior Lecturer, Manchester Metropolitan University, Manchester

Donna McGeary BSc(Hons) RGN Dip Child Nursing
Sister, Emergency Department, Belfast City Hospital

Nicola Meeres Barrister BA(Hons) DipHE
Course Director, Dolan & Holt Consultancy Ltd, Stratford upon Avon, Warwickshire

Barbara L Neades MPhil BN RMN RGN RNT
Senior Lecturer / Senior Nurse, Napier University Edinburgh / West Lothian Healthcare NHS Trust, St. Johns Hospital, Livingston, West Lothian

Mike Paynter RGN RN REMT
Nurse Practitioner, Urgent Treatment Centre, Bridgwater Community Hospital, Bridgwater, Somerset

Dr Stewart Piper PhD MSc PG Dip Ed RGN
Senior Lecturer, Homerton School of Health Studies, Peterborough

Tanya Reynolds MSc BSc RGN
Consultant Nurse Emergency Department, Homerton University Hospital NHS Foundation Trust, London

Marion Richardson BD(Hons) RN DipN Cert Ed RNT
Senior Lecturer, Programme Leader, Department of Nursing and Midwifery, University of Hertfordshire, UK

Karen Lesley Sanders MA RGN RNT Cert Ed
Senior Lecturer, London South Bank University, London

Valerie Small MSc RGN RNT
Advanced Nurse Practitioner, Emergency Department, St James' Hospital, Dublin, Ireland

Margaret Sowney MSc BSc(Hons) RNT RGN RNLD
Lecturer, School of Nursing, University of Ulster, Londonderry, Northern Ireland

Emma Tippins MSc RN
Matron Emergency Care, Heatherwood and Wexham Park Hospitals NHS Trust Wexham Park Hospital, Slough, Berkshire

Anita Tyler MSc BN RGN RSCN
Nurse Practitioner, Paediatric Emergency Unit, University Hospital of Wales, Cardiff

Jamie Walthall LLB(Hons) BSc DipN RGN
Formerly Resuscitation Services Manager, Royal Berkshire Hospital, Reading

Barbara Warncken ARRC MA BSc(Hons) RMN RGN
Staff Nurse, Ex-services Mental Welfare Association (Combat Stress), Tyrwhitt House, Leatherhead, Surrey

Rosie Wilkinson BSc(Hons) RGN OND RCNT RNT CHRN(US), Dip Ethics
Independent Nurse Consultant, Senior Nurse, Hyperbaric Medicine, Diving Diseases Research Centre, Plymouth

Preface

While emergency nursing may simply be a practice, its practice is far from simple. In the few years since the first edition of this book was published in 2000, the practice of emergency nursing has become ever more complex and challenging. That noted, it remains as it always has and hopefully always will be, a practice that has people at its centre. While the roles and titles may differ, whether as clinicians or patients, the human interaction that is at the heart of care remains a constant.

While acknowledging the humanity and compassion that is central to good care, Accident and Emergency: Theory into Practice reflects changes in clinical practice since the last edition. It retains the eight-part format it had in the last edition, so, following the Introduction are Trauma Management; Trauma Care; Psychological Dimensions; Emergency Care; Practice Issues in Emergency Care; and Professional Issues in Emergency Care.

One of the more subtle but important changes adopted throughout the book, is replacement of Accident & Emergency (A&E) by Emergency Department (ED). In part this reflects a move away from the tautology of A&E as a term but also because increasingly ED is the shorthand that being adopted world-wide in emergency care.

This edition, has a dedicated chapter looking at the unique needs of people with learning disabilities and we are very proud of its inclusion. Likewise, three excellent chapters from emergency nurses in New Zealand as well as two equally excellent chapters from the Republic of Ireland are indicative of the first edition's broad international appeal.

The internationally respected educationist, Michael Oakshott once wrote that 'education is a conversation between the generations'. To that extent, Accident and Emergency: Theory into Practice seeks to continue that conversation across the generations of emergency nurses by giving voice to experts across the field of emergency care to share their knowledge, wisdom and passion for emergency care. The first edition of this book was not the start of this conversation nor will this edition complete it. What they will share in common, however, is to strengthen and amplify that conversation and thus, hopefully make it both more interesting and important than ever. It is a conversation that is far from simple in practice but one that we believe remains a crucial endeavour.

Brian Dolan and Lynda Holt
Stratford upon Avon, 2007

Introduction: Nursing in emergency care

Gary Jones CBE

CHAPTER CONTENTS

Emergency nursing is dynamic, complex and progressive. It is about providing an immediate nursing response to meet the full spectrum of human need. To understand emergency nursing, and indeed emergency nurses themselves, it is necessary to review the history of the speciality, to consider patient attendance and to show how changing attitudes influence the service provided. In addition, this chapter will consider key reports which have shaped the organization and delivery of ED care and trends will be identified.

THE COMING OF CASUALTY

Like the emergency service itself, emergency nursing has developed from the casualty departments of the old voluntary hospitals and workhouses. In England, until the time of the dissolution of the monasteries in the Middle Ages, medicine, nursing and welfare were traditionally in the hands of the church. Between then and the 18th century there was no urge to build hospitals for the sick or to establish nursing orders. The main reason for this apparent lack of interest was that no more effective care could be given in a hospital than could be given at home by relatives and friends.

As medicine developed and a new spirit of philanthropy emerged, the initiative for founding charity hospitals became a reality. By 1825, 154 charity hospitals had been built in England (Baly 1973). These hospitals, which became the voluntary hospitals in the 19th century, received funding from public subscription. Admission was often by a ticket system and the employer made a contribution to the hospital for his employees. Within these voluntary hospitals, the out-patients department provided care for casual attenders. This service, which was often provided free of charge, allowed doctors to select patients who were 'interesting' and were of use to their developing speciality. Nurses resembled domestic workers and were few in number.

Although the outpatient service provided for both the patient's as well as the doctor's needs, it was unpopular with the newly emerging general practitioner (GP). The GPs felt the outpatient system was unfair competition, and many patients with primary health care problems attended the outpatients department rather than seeking health care from them. Because of these complaints, it was agreed that a patient should only be seen at hospital if referred by a GP; however, this system could be bypassed in an emergency. The 'casualty' could be seen as a casual attender in the newly established casualty departments.

FROM CASUALTY TO ACCIDENT AND EMERGENCY

Casualty comes from the word 'casual'. Although not an inspiring term, it is still in use today despite the introduction of the term 'accident and emergency' nearly 50 years ago. The Platt Report (Standing Medical Advisory Committee 1962) recommended the change of title in a deliberate attempt to discourage casual attenders and recommended that casualty departments should change in function. Primary care to casual attenders, it suggested, should be secondary to the provision of a 24-hour ED service. The major responsibility was to provide care for serious accident and medical and surgical emergencies. The report further recommended that this new service should be appropriately staffed and equipped and a named consultant identified. A Health Service Accreditation working group (1997) has developed agreed service principles for an ED service which stress quality standards of care (Box I.1).

PATIENT ATTENDANCE

Although the Platt Report (Standing Medical Advisory Committee 1962) identified that the major responsibility of the ED should be to provide care for serious emergencies, it also recognized that the secondary or subsidiary function was still to provide care for casual attenders. Perhaps because of this, the public's perception of the ED service did not change and, consequently, today the public continue to use the service for both emergency and primary health care needs.

The National Audit Office (1992a,b) and Audit Commission (1996) reports highlighted the continued increase in new attenders. In England, there was an increase from 9.2 million patients in 1979 to 11.2 million in 1990/91. By 2005/6, this figure had

---

Box I.1   Service principles for an accident and emergency service

A first class service that will always deliver to the highest standards

- Patients are entitled to the highest possible standards from their ED
- Minor injuries units are expected to provide the same level of relevant standards as ED services and contemporary standards of best practice
- Pre-hospital care will be constantly developed to provide a system that meets the highest expectations and contemporary standards of best practice
- Every ED will be organized to receive patients of all types and severity and should always be open
- Clinical audit shall be developed to ensure the professional assessment of clinical treatment and the effectiveness and efficiency of services
- Staff shall be appropriately trained, qualified and experienced, with staffing levels that reflect the work patterns of the department

A service that is part of hospital–wide provision

- Hospitals with an ED will give priority to emergency cases over non-urgent cases for admission
- Where possible, acute management of a single episode of care will be managed on one hospital site
- Appropriate hospital facilities must be on site to support the ED
- Treatment shall be coordinated with other specialities and integrated to form a single service

A service that puts patients first

- Service provision will ensure equity for all sections of the population, not least in respect of access to services
- The service should be provided in a manner which is sympathetic to the individual's privacy, dignity and religious and cultural beliefs
- Patients and, where appropriate, relatives, friends or siginificant others (with the patient's consent) will be kept informed of clinical progress and prognosis
- Where the consent of a patient is required for treatment or participation in research, patients will be given the choice of whether to participate, with the potential benefits and any possible attendant risks clearly explained

risen to 17.7 million per year (Department of Health 2006a). In Scotland, in the 10 years from 1982 to 1992 there was an increase of 230 000 new patient attenders (National Audit Office 1992b). The reports identified that patients attend ED emergency with a wide variety and range of illnesses and injuries. Only a small proportion, less than 0.5%, are seriously ill or severely injured (Audit Commission 1996).

Chambers and Johnson (1986) indicated that while factors such as age, sex, social class, geographical location and availability of GP services are likely to influence attendance, their effects are largely unknown. Walsh (1990a), in his study of 2000 adults aged 16–60, found attendance to be predominantly from the young male group. He also noted a correlation between lower socioeconomic status and attendance. Travelling distance to the department is another major factor which influences ED attendance (Fone et al. 2006, Afilalo et al. 2004).

The primary care research project at King's College Hospital (Department of General Practice and Primary Care/Department of Accident & Emergency Medicine 1991) found that the most common reason patients gave for attending the ED was a problem with access to their GP, and nearly one-third of patients considered that their problem was not appropriate to general practice. Studies of primary care accessibility found that the perception of accessibility influences the choice of services in an emergency and that people without a car are more likely than others to perceive that the nearest major emergency department is too far away (Farmer et al. 2004). The Audit Commission (2001) found that while some patients are acutely ill or injured and need immediate life-saving treatment, many more require urgent care and others are not seriously ill and may not require any treatment at all.

Appropriateness of attendance

Over the last 30 years, the appropriateness of attendance to an ED has been debated both formally and informally, with many departments actively seeking to discourage patients who, in the opinion of the staff, are 'inappropriate attenders' (Richards et al. 1979, Dale et al. 1992, Derlet & Young 1997, Gribben 2003). Perceived inaccessibility of primary care providers is among the leading reasons for non-urgent use of emergency departments (Afilalo et al. 2004). Calnan (1984) interviewed patients in their own homes following an ED attendance: 62 had made no attempt to contact their general practitioner, and of those who did, a third were unsuccessful. The study concluded that most people who go directly to hospital do so because of the circumstances in which they find themselves. Geographical location, peer pressure and perceived urgency of the condition were all factors in the decision (Fone et al. 2006).

Walsh (1990b), using a medical definition of 'appropriate attendance', found that of those patients in his study who were allocated one of the two categories 'appropriate' or 'inappropriate', 27.5% were considered inappropriate. He also found that the majority of the patients considered inappropriate were suffering from non-traumatic conditions and were much more likely to require medication. While recognizing that the term 'inappropriate attender' is not acceptable, it is important to differentiate between those patients who attend the ED suffering with a primary health care problem and those who are suffering with an ED problem. A patient suffering with a primary health care problem requires the expertise of the GP and a nurse with skills in primary care. The ED patient requires care that can only be given by ED medical and nursing specialists.

RESPONDING TO THE DEMAND AND PREPARING THE EMERGENCY SERVICES FOR THE FUTURE

In response to the continued increase in patient attendances and waiting times a number of initiatives have been developed in an attempt to decrease the use of emergency departments and simultaneously improve emergency care access to the public. At the same time the term 'accident' has been challenged by many emergency care personnel. They argue that few of the incidents seen in emergency care are real accidents; most incidents are preventable using steps such as taking care when driving, health and safety standards etc., and therefore the term accident is misleading.

Over the last 10 years the emergency care environment has dramatically changed. Once the domain of the emergency departments, emergency care and in particular emergency nursing are now provided via the telephone (NHS Direct, NHS 24), in nurse-led minor injury units (within current emergency departments or specific centres within the community setting) and in numerous community walk-in centres. This change in how patients access emergency care has altered the pattern of work for many emergency departments and has dramatically altered emergency nursing.

Numerous publications have been produced over the last 10–15 years that have put in place the foundations of current recommendations. Developing Emergency Services in the Community (NHS Executive 1997) was the foundation stone of emergency care outside the hospital and was directly responsible for the setting up of emergency telephone helplines (NHS Direct, NHS 24). In addition this work recommended the mapping of emergency services, research into how people's consultation behaviour occurs in emergencies and many issues around first aid training/provision. More recently the NHS Plan (2000), The Audit Commission review (2001), the ED modernization programme and the publication of Reforming Emergency Care (2001) have all altered the way emergency services are provided.

The NHS Plan (Department of Health 2000) effectively promised to eliminate ED overcrowding, more commonly known as trolley waits, by the end of 2004. The development of Reforming Emergency Care (Department of Health 2001) led to the transformation of emergency department patient flow in England (National Audit Office 2004), so much so that since 2005, most emergency departments in England now see, treat and discharge/admit 98% of patients within four hours. While concerns remain about how 'real' the performance improvement is (BMA 2007), few would wish to return to the days of serious ED overcrowding where one- and two-day waits in the emergency department for inpatient beds were not unknown. While the improvements reflect whole system improvements that are measured in ED, the guiding principles are of Reforming Emergency Care (Box I.2).

PROVIDING EMERGENCY NURSING

Emergency nursing while being patient-driven is also directly affected by national, regional and local initiatives. Several national documents published in recent years are having, and will continue to have, dramatic effects on the way nursing is practised (Clinical Standards Advisory Group 1995, 1996, 2001, Department of Health 1997, 2001, 2006b). A Vision for the Future (Department of Health 1993)

provides, as its title suggests, a vision for nursing and a framework for action. Providing the reader with five key areas and 12 targets, it indicates that the participation of nurses will improve the general health and life expectancy of the whole population. This statement, coming so closely after the publication of The Health of the Nation (Department of Health 1992), encourages emergency nurses to develop the health promotion and accident prevention aspects of their role. Challenging the Boundaries (RCN A&E Association 1994) set out the role, boundaries and targets for the future. More recently the NHS Plan (Department of Health 2000) sets out the Government's plan to give the people of England a health service fit for the 21st century. For nurses the plan provides a range of actions to be undertaken, including the Chief Nursing Officer's 10 key roles for nurses, many of which are specifically relevant to emergency nursing.

Emergency nursing in whatever setting should be directed to providing a quality care service meeting the patient's needs. Wilkinson (1991) highlighted the plight of an 85-year-old lady and her husband when admitted to an emergency department. The lady, incontinent and suffering from a fractured neck of femur, lay on a trolley for 6 hours. During this time she did not receive pressure area care and later developed a sacral sore. Wilkinson asked:

> If we cannot give care such as this woman needed, when she needed it, what can we do? What is the point of 'high tech' medicine if the essentials somehow get forgotten or neglected along the way? How can a six-hour wait in an accident and emergency department be justified? Is this an indicator of a 'high-quality service'?

Emergency nursing has developed considerably since the days of the casualty departments in the old voluntary hospitals and workhouses. Gradually, as nurses worked in the speciality, they began to develop knowledge and skills beyond their general training. In 1972, the Accident & Emergency Nursing Forum (now the RCN Emergency Care Association) was established within the Royal College of Nursing (RCN). In 1975, the Accident & Emergency Nursing Course was developed. Various emergency nursing courses which stem from that first course are now available in many universities. More recently the development of the RCN Faculty of Emergency Nursing is due to transform the way emergency nurses develop their career pathways and link their competency to patient needs.

Box I.2 Principles of reforming emergency care

- The service is to be designed around the patients
- It is to be consistent no matter where the patient attends
- The patient to be treated by the professional with the best skills to meet their needs
- Information to be transferable within the NHS
- There should be no delays in the care process
- There should be clear consistent measurable standards

2002 was a particularly important year for emergency nursing. Not only was it the 30th anniversary of the RCN Accident & Emergency Nursing Association, it was also 40 years since the speciality of Accident & Emergency came into existence.

Emergency nursing and the role of the emergency nurse have been influenced, and in many instances directed, by patient needs/demands. It is somewhat ironic that the casualty departments of the pre-1962 era were developed because of pressure from GPs not wanting to lose patient attendances, yet now a number of patients either attend the emergency department or use other emergency care services (NHS Direct, minor injury units, walk-in centres) as a direct result of GP mistrust or of not being included on a GP list (Walsh 1990b).

In an attempt to identify and clarify the current position of emergency nursing, the then RCN A&E Nursing Association in 1994 set out its beliefs with regard to emergency nursing in a document called 'Challenging the Boundaries' (RCN 1994). The Association believed the patient must be the main focus of attention and that care must be provided within a collegiate relationship between health care professionals. The Association identified the emergency department as the interface between primary and secondary care and believed the service should be seen as part of the community and not simply as a department within a hospital. It believed that certain aspects of the current service, such as minor injury and emergency primary health care, could be provided by nurse-run clinics within the community. Reflecting on the current Reforming Emergency Care document (Department of Health 2001), much of the Association's previous work is reflected in this publication.

Challenging the Boundaries (RCN 1994) argued that the emergency nurse should be seen as the leader in the initiation and coordination of patient care. She acts as a focus for the coordination and delivery of multidisciplinary care and delivers that care in partnership with the patient and significant others. In addition the work of developing the Faculty of Emergency Nursing led to a refinement of a definition of emergency nursing (Endacott et al. 1999);

> The provision of immediate nursing care to people who have defined their problem(s) as an emergency or where nursing intervention may prevent an emergency arising.
>
> The emergency nurse accepts, without prior warning, any person of any age requiring health care, with undifferentiated and undiagnosed problems originating from social, psychological, physical, spiritual or cultural factors.

The RCN A&E Nursing Association (1994) also recognized the difference between the emergency nurse and the emergency nurse specialist, often titled now as either a Clinical Nurse Specialist or an Emergency Nurse Practitioner (ENP). The ENP prescribes and initiates appropriate interventions, monitors, refers or discharges. The ENP also takes autonomous decisions with, or on behalf of, the patient, and acts as advocate to maximize health potential and promote continuity of care. To achieve this, the nurse must have an appropriate education and competency must be continually assessed.

Pamela Kidd (Assistant Professor, University of Kentucky, USA), in her address to the International A&E conference in New South Wales in 1993, argued that emergency nurses look beyond the physiological and anatomical problems to the complexities of the patient's needs and to the reason behind the incident or problem. They look at the social and environmental factors and the ongoing care of the patient. The emergency nurse realizes that her care is not isolated but is the beginning of what can be a very lengthy process for the patient, relatives and friends.

Models/frameworks to assist in providing emergency nursing care

In whatever setting the emergency nurse works it is essential that a structured approach be undertaken in the care of the patient. A model of nursing is simply a framework that provides a structure to nursing care. Numerous models of nursing are available and the debate continues as to which one, if any, is suitable not only for emergency care but also for nursing practice generally. Chalmers (1990) defines a model of nursing as a set of formulated ideas about the practice of nursing in which the nature of people is central. She argues that nursing models provide a much needed alternative knowledge base from which nurses can practise in an informed way. Melia (1990) opposes this view and considers that not only has the development and use of nursing not had a positive influence upon nursing practice, but that this trend has served to limit the development of nursing. She considers it is a phase that nursing is going through which has had little effect on care. Kenny (1993) believes that while nursing models are relevant to the nursing profession, they have not always been seen as relevant to individual nurses and consumers of health care. He argues that nurses still need a set of explicit concepts to guide their practice; however, instead of being seen as a restrictive straightjacket, models should inform and nurse.

Ali (1990) introduced three distinct models to nurses working in an emergency department, over a 12-week period. These models were Orem (1980), Roper and the Human Needs model (Roper et al. 1983). Ali found that Orem and Roper were less suitable than the Human Needs model and that the department's philosophy could be placed easily within the needs framework. She also found that by using a model of nursing within the emergency care setting, it helped to develop the relationships between emergency nurses and their patients and relatives. It provided the foundation for quick, concise and accurate patient assessment and made joint care planning and evaluation possible.

Walsh and Kent (2001) argue that any profession must have well-established theoretical foundations and that a model of nursing provides this for accident and emergency. Walsh and Kent believe that the model used in ED should be based on the concept of self-care and favours Orem as a model that should be considered. They believe that Orem's (1980) view of nursing, moving from a wholly compensatory phase to a partly compensatory phase and on to a final educational developmental stage, is appropriate for ED. They suggest that Orem (1980) encourages nurses to anticipate potential problems and to include the family circumstances in care planning and that, by providing a concise and relevant assessment model from which a care plan can be derived, nurses will avoid the sort of pitfalls that are all too familiar in ED.

Jones's (1990) care structure is based on a process of care which allows the nurse to return to looking at the patient and acting on the basis of professional judgement. The process comprises a model of nursing, a triage system, a problem-oriented approach encompassing passing assessment, problem identification, goals, intervention and evaluation, and the necessary documentation. Jones (1990) believes that practice-based models are more acceptable to emergency nurses and that such models can provide the framework for organized nursing assessment, planning, intervention and evaluation. He believes it is impossible to ignore the medical model, as a great deal of nursing care is based on restoring normal anatomical and physiological activity, but argues that a nursing model provides a better framework for holistic care (Box I.3). His Components of Life model (Jones 1990) is based on an analysis of practice and represents what actually exists. The Components of Life model is not conceived from an idea in the same way as a theory-based model, but takes into account more than one model of nursing; nevertheless, he believes it is a model in its own right.

> **Box I.3 The value of a model of nursing in ED**
>
> - It provides a structure to nursing care
> - It provides a framework for holistic care
> - It makes the patient a person
> - It allows for social as well as physical problems to be addressed
> - It provides health promotion and envirnomental safety oppourtunities
> - It develops a partnership between the nursing staff and the patient and relatives
> - It is the foundation for quick, concise and accurate patient assessment, intervention and evaluation
> - It allows for joint care planning
> - It provides for an organized and structured documentation system
> - It ensures that all staff are moving in the same direction
> - It prevents aspects of care being missed

In 2001/2, development of the Jones Dependency Tool (JDT) enabled the Components of Life model to be slightly restructured but not lose its simplicity of use. Now under the title Jones Components of Life Framework (Jones 2002) the original seven identified components are now six (linking environmental safety with health and social needs) and continue to be easily memorized and lend themselves to simple documentation (Fig. I.1). Working through each component, the nurse is able to build up a picture of the patient's problems and intervene in a logical manner. The communication component encourages the nurse to assess the patient's consciousness level, human behavioural state and physiological senses and to identify any complaint of pain. This component also links up with one of the model's four universal goals (Box I.4), which is the establishment of a partnership with the patient and the relatives and friends.

Dependency

There are both immediate and longer-term benefits linked with measuring patient dependency in the emergency department.

Direct patient care

- Individual patients can be allocated the most appropriately skilled nurse to provide their care (competency). At present the allocation of nurses and health care assistants to individual patients is not clearly defined. With the launch of the Faculty of Emergency Nursing core and specific

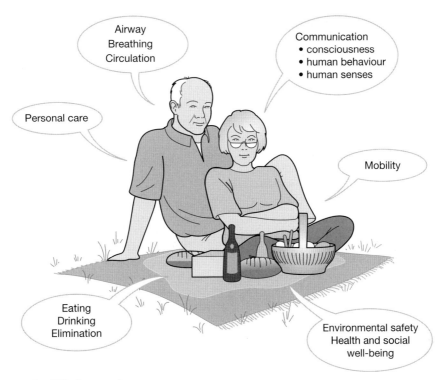

Figure I.1 Components of Life Framework

Communication: humans are social beings who through communication and relationship with others achieve much of their quality of life. Partnership is developed through communication and information is shared. Human behaviour communicates much of the person's attitude, moods, religious beliefs, sexual identit y and emotions. The physiological senses are also important in the establishment of good communications.

Airway, breathing and circulation: oxygen is vital to life. To ensure normal tissue activity, a clear airway, normal respiratory function and adequate circulation is essential.

Mobility: the ability to move enables the individual to engage in work and play. It provides the individual with independence and social well being.

Personal care: the ability to maintain personal care allows the individual to retain good hygiene and reduce the risk of ill health through infection.

Eating, Drinking and Elimination: health is maintained by the adequate intake of food and water. Through normal digestive and metabolic activities the body is able to function normally and eliminate waste.

Environmental safety, Health and social well-being: individual's require a safe environment and the recognition of self-care to maintain health. Depending on the individuals work, lifestyle and attitude, the degree of risk will vary. Individuals have a desire to remain in good health. Economic as well as social circumstances have a bearing on the individual's ability to maintain health. A balance often has to be achieved between the wish to remain healthy and social activities that can put health at risk. Social well-being is very individual but for many will include good health, mobility, the ability to communicate and interrelate with others, rest, a stable living environment and financial well-being.

competency levels have been established. Linking the competency of the nurse to individual patient dependency will ensure the patient's nursing care needs are met.

- Individual component headings can be used to identify specific risks to the patient where preventive action can be taken. Example – a patient demonstrating a risk to self or others would require extra attention/intervention. Changes in pulse rate, respiratory rate and oxygen saturation are key indicators of an improvement or deterioration in a patient's dependency (Alcock et al. 2002, Crouch & Williams 2001).

- The tool can be linked with standards based on both the JDT component headings and the individual statements that make up each component. By linking the JDT and locally established standards of care the overall care of all patients should improve.

- Individual component headings link with the component headings for the framework (model) allowing for a structured assessment, intervention

---

> **Box I.4 The four universal goals for ED nurses**
>
> - To establish a partnership with the patient/relatives
> - To achieve a level of independence in the patient appropriate to his condition or injury and by so doing, assist him to restore health and maintain quality of life
> - To enable the individual to avoid ill-health or injury through self-care, health education and environmental safety
> - To ensure that the patient received optimum effectiveness from medically prescribed treatment

and evaluation of patient care with records following the same format.

Department/workload

- The use of the JDT to review patient allocation to specific areas of the department/correct use of key areas such as the resuscitation room. Unpublished work by McClelland (2002) demonstrated how the JDT was used to identify the dependency of patients allocated to the resuscitation room and how many patients could have been allocated more appropriately.
- A clear picture of the workload at any given time can be obtained and this can be used to trigger actions to reduce the workload when it reaches an agreed threshold. By agreeing a threshold level of dependency within the department everyone within the hospital (including non-clinical staff) will be able to appreciate the current workload and take appropriate action. Example – agreed threshold level is 30. This could be made up of 10 totally dependent patients, 15 high-dependency patients or 30 moderate-dependency patients. Clearly a mix of all three will be present. Low-dependency patients do not influence the score.
- Planning nursing and other staff establishments and skill mix based on a more accurate picture of nursing workload over an agreed period.

The main purpose of such a tool is therefore threefold

1. It can be used to ensure that the patient is allocated to a nurse with the relevant competencies to provide the care required.
2. It can provide a dependency rating across the department that can be calculated and actions taken if the threshold level is reached.

3. It can be used to determine nursing numbers and with dependency/competency factors can determine skill mix.

The tool is in two sections; section A provides six key component headings with each one having three ratings of dependency, ranging from total dependence to total independence (Boxes I.5 and I.6). On arrival and subsequently throughout the stay in the ED, this section provides the dependency score of the patient. Based on the dependency score a number of actions can be implemented, for instance:

1. The nurse allocated to the patient should have the relevant competencies to provide care for the patients' dependency.
2. The dependency rating across the department at any given time can be calculated and actions taken if a threshold level is reached.

Section B reflects the nursing workload that the patient dependency creates and is generated by each of the four dependency scores. Under each dependency heading is a number of nursing interventions – direct and indirect (Box I.6). These interventions reflect both direct and indirect nursing time. This section can be used to determine nursing numbers and with dependency/competency factors can determine skill mix (Crouch et al. 2000, Jones 2002).

THE NURSE/PATIENT RELATIONSHIP

Communication, one of the key components in the Jones Components of Life Framework (JCLF), and the establishment of a partnership with the patient and significant others, one of the four universal goals of the JCLF, are essential parts of emergency nursing care. Unless a partnership is formed, it will be difficult for the individual to appreciate the process of care and the need for self-care guidance. The Patient's Charter (Department of Health 1991a, 1996) identified the need for a named, qualified nurse to be responsible for the patient's nursing care. This charter standard was designed to create a better partnership between the patient/significant other and the nurse.

The development of the named nurse standard presented some problems within emergency care. These problems mainly stemmed from the confusion between methods of delivering care and the purpose of the named nurse standard. Crinson (1995) notes that many of the principles underpinning The Patient's Charter and The Health of the Nation (Department of Health 1992) had support among senior nursing staff, but these organizational

Box I.5 Jones Dependency Model Section A

Choose one box (3, 2, 1) from each component (one or more factors in the box is sufficient to receive the allocation). Place each rating in the rating column. Then add the rating scores to give an overall JDT dependency score.

Component	3	2	1	Rating
Communication	• Complete impairment due to either loss of one or more senses • Pain being at the higher range of the visual analogue scale • Unresponsive • Language barrier • Extensive behavioural problems	• Impairment or potential for impairment of one or more senses • Pain at the mid range of the visual analogue scale • Responding only to verbal/pain stimulation • Difficulty due to language barrier • Anxious/tearful/ distressed	• Able to communicate through all senses • Pain at the lower range of the visual analogue scale • Alert • No language barrier • Cooperative/relaxed	
ABC	• Cardiac/Respiratory Arrest (or risk of arrest) • Complete impairment of ABC or shock	• Risk of impairment to airway breathing or circulation (potential for shock due to condition)	• No ABC problems • Minor wounds	
Mobility	• Total immobility	• Partial mobility loss • Patient requires trolley/ wheelchair	• Fully mobile • Minor limb problem	
Eating, drinking, elimination and personal care	• Total loss of bowel/ bladder function and/or hyperemesis • Total loss of independent self-care	• Partial loss of bowel/ bladder function and/or vomiting • Partial loss of independent self-care	• Normal bowel/bladder control. No vomiting • Able to maintain independent self-care	
Environmental safety, health and social needs	• Demonstrates danger to self or others • Appears to require extensive social support	• Appears unable to fully understand risks • Appears to require some social support	• Shows total ability to fully understand risks • Does not appear to require social support	

Total JDT rating =

6–7	=Low dependency	Overall score=0	
8–12	=Moderate dependency	Overall score=1	
13–15	=High dependency	Overall score=2	
16–18	=Total dependency	Overall score=3	Dependency score=

Glossary of terms

Complete impairment = complete loss

Impairment = some degree of loss

Senses = any one of the five especially sight, hearing, touch

Language barrier = inability to speak or because of different language to nurse

Behavioural problems = psychological or drug related

Total loss = total inability to control own functions (may be ongoing)

Social support = co-ordination of – relatives/environment/service provision

Shock = hypovolaemic, cardiogenic, obstructive, distributive requiring immediate intervention

Partial mobility loss = has some ability to move limbs but may require help with sitting/standing

Box I.6   Jones Dependency Tool Section B

Once the dependency score has been obtained in section A , section B should reflect the nursing workload

(D) = direct care, (I) = indirect care. Individual patients will vary in the workload generated but in most cases one or more activities in each component section will be required.

Patient Dependency 3 = Total dependency
Patients requiring total nursing care and a one-one input.

Patient Dependency 2 = High dependency
Patients who require a high level of nursing intervention but less than that required by a totally dependent patient.

Patient Dependency 1 = Moderate dependency
Patients who require moderate levels of nursing intervention and are encouraged to become independent.

Patient Dependency 0 = Low dependency
Patients who require a minimal level of nursing intervention and are virtually self-caring. May require some first aid at triage.

Component	Total dependency 3	High dependency 2	Moderate dependency 1	Low dependency 0
Communication	• Nurse present at all times (one -one) (D/I) • Constant attention due to behavioural problems/need for psychological support (D) • Constant support/ frequent contact with relatives (I) • May require analgesia IM/IV	• Constant observation (but not requiring one-one) (D/I) • Frequent attention due to behavioural problems/need for psychological support (D) • Frequent support/ contact of relatives/friends due to severity/ death of patient (I) • May require analgesia IM/IV	• Nurse available in calling distance (D/I) • Reassurance/ psychological support (D) • May require relatives to be informed/ explanation (I) • May require analgesia IM/IV	• Nurse available in the department (D/I) • Reassurance (D)
ABC	• Frequent (15 minutes) vital signs (D) • Constant airway/ breathing attention (D) • Resuscitation (D) • Rapid IV fluids (D) • Extensive or time consuming interventions/tests (D/I)	• Vital signs 1/2–1 hourly (D) • Observation/ intervention with airway/breathing (oxygen administration) (D) • Frequent IV fluids (D) • Require various blood tests (D/I)	• Vital signs 2–4 hourly (D) • IV fluids (D)	• Vital signs once only (D)
Mobility	• Frequent pressure area care (D) • Constant elimination support (D) • Extensive or time consuming interventions/tests (D/I)	• Pressure area care 1–2 hours (D) • Require X-rays/ scans (D/I)	• Pressure area care 4/6 hourly (D)	• Nil specific

Eating, drinking, elimination and personal care	• Requires constant attention to care	• Assistance with bedpans/urinals (D)	• Assistance with toiletry/commode/ walking to toilet (D)	• Nil specific
Environmental safety, health and social needs	• Constant attention due to behavioural problems (D) • If discharged will require complex discharge arrangements involving more than one service provider (I) • Admission planning (I) • Will require escorting to wards/ departments (D) • Extensive time consuming health promotion/self-care advice required (D)	• Frequent attention due to behavioural problems (D) • If discharged will require complex discharge arrangements involving more than one service provider (I) • May require admission planning (I) • Will require escorting to wards/ departments (D) • More extensive health promotion/ self care advice required (D)	• May require some discharge planning linked with one service provider (I) • May require admission planning (I) • May require escorting to wards/departments (D) • Requires some health promotion/self-care guidance (D)	• Discharge planning is uncomplicated (I) • Some health promotion/self-care may be required (D)

developments had less impact on the quality of care in emergency care than intended, essentially because of a failure to provide sufficient resources. Jones (1993a,b) indicates that the named nurse in emergency care is the nurse allocated to a patient and that this can be achieved irrespective of the method used to deliver care. If primary nursing is the method used within the emergency department, then the primary nurse and the named nurse are one and the same. If team nursing is in use then either the team leader or other nurses within the team can be identified as the named nurse. With patient allocation, a given number of patients can be allocated to each named nurse. The number of patients will vary depending on the patients' dependency. In the community setting the ENP or nurse providing health care via the telephone are clearly the named nurses. The triage nurse may be the most appropriate person to be the named nurse for patients arriving and waiting to be seen by the doctor or nurse practitioner.

While it is appreciated that continuity is important, and the way initial assessment in emergency care is changing, it is also unrealistic in many departments for the same nurse to follow the patient through all stages of care. When a change of named nurse does occur, the patient as well as the relative/friends must be informed. It is the principle of the patients knowing which nurse is looking after them that is important.

While both the patient and the nurse have a joint responsibility for establishing the partnership, it is the nurse who has the prime responsibility for achieving a good working relationship with the patient. The nurse must attempt to prevent her own attitude or prejudices damaging the establishment of the partnership, and thereby causing a breakdown in communication. Stockbridge (1993) states that if the nurse has negative perceptions of the patient, her own non-verbal communication will cause the patient to behave in such a way that the nurse's perceptions are confirmed. The patient may be labelled as difficult.

Wright (1991) and Kent & McDowell (2004) identify that most complaints from relatives of sudden-death victims involve basic communication skills. Many patients complain of doctors not sitting down, not using eye contact and only spending a brief time with them. Listening and having the ability to react appropriately to the patient's problems require the nurse to have a working knowledge of social, psychological, physical, spiritual and cultural factors that can cause problems with communication and with the development of a partnership. The nurse must understand that altered body image, mental health, drugs, alcohol and many other factors will often create barriers to good communication.

Anxiety-provoking factors, such as fear of the unknown, personal arrangements, possible complications and treatments, can also lead to poor communication (Walsh & Kent 2001). Wright (1986) indicates that due to the breakdown in the individual's coping mechanisms, the nurse may no longer be seen as a person who can help, but rather an obstacle preventing that individual getting what he wants. Through formal emergency nursing education, the nurse may learn to overcome many of these problems and develop skills to ensure that the nurse/patient relationship is maintained.

WAITING TIMES

While the causes of long waiting times are complex and no two departments have exactly the same set of problems, many factors are within their control. For instance, re-attendance rates vary from less than 1 to over 54. The Audit Commission (1996) suggests ways in which re-attendances can be reduced (Box I.7). Its recommendations have also been echoed in Reforming Emergency Care (Department of Health 2001) and other reports (Department of Health 2006b,c, National Audit Office 2004, Audit Commission 2001).

Box I.7 Ways to reduce planned ED attendances

- Ensuring more patients are seen by experienced ED doctors the first time they attend. Uncertainty by junior doctors about diagnosis or treatment can lead to more investigations and more return visits
- Requiring SHOs to consult a middle or senior grade doctor, if one is present in the department, before booking clinical appointments for patients
- Ensuring all re-attenders are seen by a senior doctor or nurse
- Asking GPs or practice nurses to assess the quality and outcomes of treatment provided rather than arranging return ED attendances for these to be monitored
- Improving knowledge of facilities offered by GP practices, e.g. for removal of sutures and renewal of dressings, both through personal contact and by making a directory available
- Periodic audit of reasons for re-attendance to ensure that all are justified clinically or by the need to assess outcomes and the quality of care. This audit may require better information systems
- Agreeing protocols with other specialities for deciding who should be seen in which clinics
- Discontinuing minor operations which could be performed more appropriately elsewhere

---

Emergency nurse practitioners are often introduced in the belief that waiting times will be instantly reduced. Waiting times are a constant source of irritation to patients and staff alike. Introducing nurse practitioners may reduce the waiting times, but whether they are present or not, Dolan (1998) argues, patients have a right to be kept informed about what is going on. While a nurse practitioner service can reduce overall waiting times, for some patients their individual overall time in the department may increase because of the service provided. Many emergency nurse practitioners identify the need for health education and safety awareness instruction and thereby increase the overall time the patient spends in the department. The emphasis must be on improved care rather than the conveyor-belt approach (Iankova 2006, Mason et al. 2005).

SPECIFIC AREAS OF EMERGENCY NURSING

Sudden death

About 1 in 400 ED patients either die while in ED or are brought in dead and, as Purves and Edwards (2005) note, caring for people whose relatives have died suddenly and unexpectedly is one of the most difficult and challenging events to which health care professionals must respond. Recommendations by the British Association of Accident & Emergency Medicine and The Royal College of Nursing (1995) to the Chief Nursing Officer and Chief Medical Officer at the Department of Health aim to improve the care of the relatives and friends of sudden-death victims. As well as providing guidance on the design of sitting rooms and visiting rooms, the recommendations also explore methods of educating staff and supporting relatives during this crucial time. Dealing with sudden death in ED is described in detail in Chapter 13.

Children

Nationally, one-quarter of all ED patients are under 16. The Children Act (Department of Health 1989) and the work of the RCN Children in ED Special Interest Group have had major effects on the way children are cared for in the ED environment. The Clinical Standards Advisory Group (1995) has stated that every hospital with an ED should have on-site paediatricians and the Department of Health (1991b) set a target that each ED seeing children should have at least one registered sick children's nurse on duty 24 hours a day and this has also been supported by the Royal College of Paediatrics and Child Health (1999).

While the target is still not being met (Playfor 2001), (RCPCH 2007), more departments are now employing registered sick children's nurses and many departments have, by creating children's areas, responded to the needs of the child. (See Part 4, 'Life Continuum'.)

Trauma care

The nurse's role in the care of the trauma patient has grown considerably. Scott (1990) recognized that in the front line of an ED, the ability to perform the tasks needed to save life when time is of the essence is as essential for nurses as it is for ambulance personnel and doctors. The publication of the Royal College of Surgeons of England's (1988) Report on the Management of Patients with Injuries stimulated interest in the care of trauma patients. Within 2 years of its publication, two trauma nursing courses had been established within the UK. Both courses were developed by nurses for nurses. The Advanced Trauma Nursing Course is provided jointly by the Royal College of Nursing and the College of Surgeons of England. The Trauma Nursing Core Course is a bought package from the United States and is provided by Trauma Nursing Ltd (www.traumanursing.org).

There is a long-standing recommendation that hospitals should have a trauma team (Campling et al. 1989). Paynter (1993) believes that the philosophy of trauma nursing is spreading and indicates that as more ED trauma-trained nurses return to their individual departments, the procedure for assessing and managing critically injured patients is improving. O'Mahony (2005) goes further, suggesting that nurses are ideally placed to ensure that the environments in which they work are adequately structured to deal with trauma patients. (See Part 1, Trauma Management, and Part 2, Trauma Care.)

THE FACULTY OF EMERGENCY NURSING

For a number of years the development of a Faculty of Emergency Nursing (FEN) took place within the structure of the Royal College of Nursing but it became an independent body in 2006. The Faculty approach was adopted, in part, in direct response to the ongoing tendency to develop generic 'critical care' courses. In some ways, these courses detract from the speciality of emergency nursing and fail to recognize the uniqueness and diversity of emergency nursing practice (Crouch & Jones 1997). The lack of consensus on terms such as specialist/advanced practice, inadequate career structure, proliferation of courses, lack of standardization, no core standards of practice and no effective competency framework were many of the reasons for developing a faculty.

The Faculty of Emergency Nursing is defined as:

> 'A body of nurses committed to improving patient care through the setting and maintaining of standards for practice and the facilitation of lifelong learning and career progression through education, research and leadership within the specialism'.

The Faculty of Emergency Nursing is structured around an integrated clinical competency and career framework, which provides recognition of clinical competency against competency standards through accreditation and submission of an extended CV (Windle et al. 2004). The standards have been developed by emergency nurses for emergency nurses across both core and specific areas of emergency care and can be found on the internet at http://www.facultyofemergencynursing.org/

A Faculty-concentric model has been developed encompassing core and specific competencies to which nurses will map themselves and through the development of a personal portfolio will be accredited for professional practice.

The Faculty provides

- the career and competency framework
- a framework for peer review and accreditation
- links with higher education institutions
- research and scholarship
- a national and international voice for emergency nursing

FEN offers members a range of benefits which include:

- a clear pathway for career development
- a mechanism for developing and recording competence using FEN's core and specific competency framework
- access to role models/peer review
- the opportunity to evidencing achievement through portfolio
- linking experience from practice, CPD activity and academic achievement

The purpose of the Faculty is to produce the 'gold standard' for education and development of ED nurses. The standard will be promoted throughout the UK to ensure that each ED nurse has the opportunity to advance his or her career in a structured way (Fig I.2). It is hoped that the Faculty will provide the opportunity to advance the speciality and provide a career structure for ED nursing.

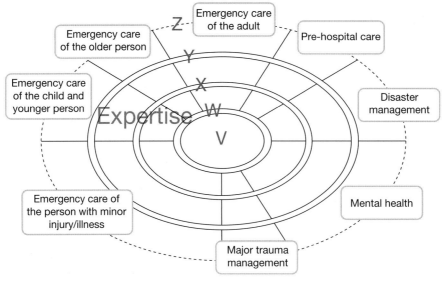

Figure I.2 Faculty of Emergency Nursing Concentric Model

CONCLUSION

From the development of the casualty service in the 19th century to today's modern emergency care services, the nurse has always been an essential and influential member of the multidisciplinary team. It was emergency nurses who developed the RCN A&E forum, who developed the emergency nursing course, and who pioneered the developments of nurse triage, the emergency nurse practitioner, bereavement care, trauma nursing and nurse-run minor injury units. It is emergency nurses who continue to develop the service despite many of the current challenges and the ongoing debate about how, when and where emergency care should be provided.

With increased patient attendance and the extra demands placed on the nurse from the patient, statutory bodies and government departments, stress is inevitable. Stress invokes tension and anxiety (Walsh & Dolan 1999), and there is a need for more awareness and openness regarding stress within emergency nursing. Many things contribute to stress and the result of unrelieved stress and emotional burn-out is often multifactorial (Wilson 1991).

So what of the future for emergency nurses? Well, there are numerous developments to be taken forward: the faculty of emergency nursing, trauma care, primary health care, e-health, health promotion and accident prevention, to name but a few. Emergency nurses need strong leadership at all levels. All emergency care areas should have clinical nurse managers who will take the speciality forward. The Nurse Consultant role brings research and clinical practice together. Care must be properly evaluated and practice changed where necessary.

In an 'activity scoping exercise' undertaken for the Department of Health, Jones (1997) reported a range of initiatives to improve emergency care. Many are now reality. Emergency nurses are not a doctor substitute but a new type of practitioner who legitimately is providing a service that is new.

Emergency nurses have a great future ahead, but must never forget that however much we strive to develop the role of the emergency nurse, however much we push to move the boundaries of our practice forward, it must never be at the expense of patient care. Any change must always be for the good of the patient and his/her relatives and friends. Wilson (1991) stated, that:

'When we take away all the high-tech equipment, human beings are still there with all their needs, some fulfilled, some not. Nursing, in essence, requires human to human contact and if we cannot provide such contact, then nursing is a myth, a game and a drain on the financial and moral structure of society'.

References

Alcock K et al (2002) Physiological observations of patients admitted from A & E. *Nursing Standard*, **16**(34), 33–37.

Afilalo J, Marinovich A, Afilalo M, Colacone A, Léger R, Unger B, Giguère C (2004) Nonurgent emergency department patient characteristics and barriers to primary care. *Academic Emergency Medicine*, **11**, 1302–1310.

Ali L (1990) Models in accident and emergency. *Nursing Standard*, **5**(3), 33–35.

Audit Commission (1996) *By Accident or Design: Improving A&E Services in England and Wales*. London: HMSO.

Audit Commission (2001) *Accident & Emergency Review of National Findings*. London: HMSO.

Baly M (1973) *Nursing and Social Change*. Heinemann: London.

British Association of Accident & Emergency Medicine and Royal College of Nursing (1994) *Bereavement Care in A&E Departments. Report to Chief Medical and Nursing Officers*. London: RCN.

British Medical Association (2007) *Emergency Medicine: Report of National Survey of Emergency Medicine*. London: BMA.

Calnan M (1984) The junctions of the hospital emergency departments: a study of patient demand. *Journal of Emergency Medicine*, **2**, 57–63.

Campling EA, Devlin HB, Hoile RW, Lunn JN (1989) *The Report of the National Confidential Enquiry into Perioperative Deaths*. London: Royal College of Surgeons of England.

Chalmers H (1990) Nursing models: enhancing or inhibiting practice? *Nursing Standard*, **5**(11), 34–35.

Chambers J, Johnson K (1986) Predicting demand for A&E services. *Community Medicine*, **8**(2), 93–103.

Clinical Standards Advisory Group (1995) *Urgent and Emergency Admissions to Hospital*. London: HMSO.

Crinson I (1995) Impact of The Patient's Charter on A&E departments. *British Journal of Nursing*, **4**(21), 1280–1287.

Crouch R, Jones G (1997) Towards a faculty of A&E nursing: planning for the future. *Emergency Nurse*, **5**(6), 12–15.

Crouch R, Williams S, Jones J (2000) *Patient Dependency in A&E: Validation of the Jones Dependency Tool (JDT) Final Report to the Department of Health*. Southampton: University of Southampton School of Nursing and Midwifery.

Department of General Practice and Primary Care/ Department of Accident & Emergency Medicine (1991) *Providing for Primary Care: Progress in A&E*. London: King's College School of Medicine and Dentistry.

Department of Health (1989) *The Children Act*. London: HMSO.

Department of Health (1991a) *The Patient's Charter*. London: HMSO.

Department of Health (1991b) *Welfare of Children and Young People in Hospital*. London: HMSO.

Department of Health (1992) *The Health of the Nation. A Strategy for Health in England*. London: HMSO.

Department of Health (1993) *A Vision for the Future*. London: HMSO.

Department of Health (1996) *The Patient's Charter*. London: HMSO.

Department of Health (1997) *Developing Emergency Services in the Community*. London: The Stationery Office.

Department of Health (2000) *The NHS Plan*. London: The Stationery Office.

Department of Health (2001) *Reforming Emergency Care*. London: The Stationery Office.

Department of Health (2006a) *Direction of Travel for Urgent Care: a Discussion Document*. London: Department of Health.

Department of Health (2006b) *A&E Attendances: Hospital Activity Statistics*. London: Department of Health.

Department of Health (2006c) *A Report for Patients, Clinicians and Healthcare Managers*. London: Department of Health.

Derlet R, Young G (1997) Managed care and emergency medicine: conflicts, federal law and California legislation. *Annals of Emergency Medicine*, **30**, 292–300.

Dolan B (1998) Waiting times (Editorial). *Emergency Nurse*, **6**(4), 1.

Health Services Accreditation (1997) *Standards for Accident & Emergency Services*. Battle: Health Services Accreditation.

Endacott R, Edwards B, Crouch R, Castile K, Dolan B, Hamilton C, Jones G, Macphee D, Manley K, Windle J (1999) Towards a Faculty of Emergency Nursing. *Emergency Nurse*, **7**(5), 10–16.

Farmer J, Hinds K, Richards H, Godden D (2004) *Access, Satisfaction and Expectations: A Comparison of Attitudes to Health Care in Rural and Urban Scotland*. University of Aberdeen: Centre for Rural Health, Research and Policy.

Fone DL, Christie S, Lester N (2006) Comparison of perceived and modelled geographical access to accident and emergency departments: a cross-sectional analysis from the Caerphilly Health and Social Needs Study. *International Journal of Health Geographics*, **5**(25), 16–25.

Gribben B (2003) General Practitioners' assessments of the primary care caseload in Middlemore Hospital Emergency Department. *The New Zealand Medical Journal*, **116**(1169), p 329.

Iankova A (2006) The accountability of emergency nurse practitioners. *Emergency Nurse*, **4**(6), 20–25.

Jones G (1990) *Accident & Emergency Nursing: A Structured Approach*. London: Faber & Faber.

Jones G (1993a) The patient's charter in the accident & emergency department. *Accident & Emergency Nursing*, **1**, 211–218.

Jones G (1993b) A&E nursing: all change ahead. *Emergency Nurse*, **1**(1), 7–8.

Jones G (1997) *Accident & Emergency: A Scoping Report*. London: Department of Health.

Jones G (2002) Care of the emergency patient – frameworks for nursing assessment and management. In Jones G, Endacott R, Crouch R (eds), *Emergency Nursing Care: Principles and Practice*. London: Greenwich Medical Media Ltd.

Kenny T (1993) Nursing models fail in practice. *British Journal of Nursing*, **1**(22), 133–135.

Kent H, McDowell J (2004) Sudden bereavement in acute care settings. *Nursing Standard*, **19**(6), 38–42.

McClelland H (2002) *Patient location linked to dependency*. Unpublished work, Leeds General Infirmary.

Mason S, Fletcher A, McCormick S, Perrin J, Rigby A (2005) Developing assessment of emergency nurse practitioner competence: a pilot study. *Journal of Advanced Nursing*, **50**(4), 425–432.

Melia K (1990) Nursing models: enhancing or inhibiting practice? *Nursing Standard*, **5**(11), 36–39.

National Audit Office (1992a) *NHS Accident & Emergency Departments in England*. London: HMSO.

National Audit Office (1992b) *NHS Accident & Emergency Departments in Scotland*. London: HMSO.

National Audit Office (2004) *Improving Emergency Care in England*. London: HMSO.

O'Mahoney C (2005) Widening the dimensions of care. *Emergency Nurse*, **13**(4), 18–24.

Orem D (1980) *Nursing: Concepts of Practice*, 2nd edn. New York: McGraw-Hill.

Paynter M (1993) Trauma support: revolution in care. *Emergency Nurse*, **1**(2), 7–9.

Playfor S (2001) Accident and emergency services for children within Trent region. *Emergency Medicine Journal*, **18**, 164–166.

Purves Y, Edwards S (2005) Initial needs of bereaved relatives following sudden and unexpected death. *Emergency Nurse*, **13**(7), 28–34.

Richards J, White G, Bigg-Wither G, Clearwater C, Hardy I (1979) Emergency services in South Auckland. *New Zealand Medical Journal*, **90**, 217–220.

Roper N, Logan W, Tierney A, (eds) (1983). *Using a Model for Nursing*. Edinburgh: Churchill Livingstone.

RCN Emergency Care Association (2007) *Skill Mix Guidance*. London: RCN.

Royal College of Nursing A&E Association (1994) *Challenging the Boundaries*. London: RCN.

Royal College of Surgeons of England (1988) *Report of the Working Party on the Management of Patients with Major Injuries*. London: Royal College of Surgeons of England.

Royal College of Paediatrics and Child Health (1999) *Accident and Emergency Services for Children. Report of a Multidisciplinary Working Party*. London: Royal College of Paediatrics and Child Health.

Royal College of Paediatrics and Child Health (2007) Services for Children in Emergency Departments: Report of the Intercollegiate Committee for Services for Children in Emergency Departments. London: RCPCH.

Scott S (1990) Nurses in the front line. *Nursing Standard*, **4**(27), 50.

Standing Medical Advisory Committee (1962) *Accident & Emergency Services (Platt Report)*. London: HMSO.

Stockbridge J (1993) Parasuicide: does discussing it help? *Emergency Nurse*, **1**(2), 19–21.

Walsh M, Kent A (2001) *Accident & Emergency Nursing: A New Approach*, 4th edn. London: Butterworth Heinemann Ltd.

Walsh M (1990a) Why do people go to the A&E? *Nursing Standard*, **5**(7), 24–28.

Walsh M (1990b) Patient's choice: GP or A&E department? *Nursing Standard*, **5**(10), 28–31.

Walsh M (1993) Pain and anxiety in A&E attenders. *Nursing Standard*, **7**(26), 40–42.

Walsh M, Dolan B (1999) Emergency nurses and their perceptions of caring. *Emergency Nurse*, **7**(4), 24–31.

Wilkins R (1991) No care, no excuses. Nursing standrard **5**(9) p 44.

Wilson G (1991) Technology and stress. *Nursing*, **4**(32), 31–34.

Windle J, Downing P, Gray A, Morgan J, Neades B (2004) The faculty of emergency nursing: where next? *Emergency Nurse*, **12**(5), 10–13.

Wright B (1986) *Caring in Crisis*. Edinburgh: Churchill Livingstone.

Wright B (1991) *Sudden Death*. Edinburgh: Churchill Livingstone.

PART 1

Trauma management

PART CONTENTS

Chapter 1

Pre-hospital care

Tim Kilner

INTRODUCTION

There has been considerable debate regarding the role for nurses in the provision of pre-hospital care as part of hospital-based mobile teams (Barnes 2006, Moakes & Kilner 2001). In practice the number of hospital-based teams continues to decline although a small number of established teams still function on a regular basis. Two key factors have largely been responsible for this trend: first, the skills and scope of practice of ambulance staff have increased over the years, allowing them to manage increasingly complex clinical situations; and second, the increasing workload of Emergency Departments (EDs) combined with limited staffing makes it impossible for most departments to resource a mobile team on a regular basis. However, there are circumstances, although infrequent, when an ED may be requested to provide medical and nursing support at the scene of an incident to support their ambulance-service colleagues. Given that such incidents are likely to be complex and high profile there is a risk that staff agree to respond without carefully considering if they and their fellow health-care providers can bring additional expertise which will be of clear benefit to patient care and, in addition, to those services already provided.

To achieve this, guidelines for call-out must be established and the role of the team and its members must be clearly defined. Additionally, activity must be supported through education, training, rehearsal and operational experience. Failure to do so will result in ill-equipped, poorly trained, undisciplined team working in an environment in which there is no place for them. With appropriate preparation, it is possible for the emergency nurse to contribute to and improve the quality of care patients receive from the scene of the incident to their transfer to the ED. This chapter will address these issues in relation to the role of the nurse as part of a medical and nursing team providing pre-hospital care at both major incidents and single or small multiple casualty incidents.

Care of the ill and injured is often perceived as beginning when the patient passes over the threshold of the ED. This is far from the reality of the situation, as care provided by the ambulance service at the scene of the accident and en route to hospital has become increasingly sophisticated. Although much of the hands-on care is provided by ambulance service personnel, there are occasions where the team needs to be broadened to include other health-care professionals, in order to provide optimum care for the patient. The concept of pre-hospital care is based upon the team approach, with the involvement of a range of health-care providers and members of the statutory emergency services. This chapter will examine the role of the emergency nurse in the provision of pre-hospital care in the context of the multidisciplinary team.

In exploring this role, it is important to define the philosophy of pre-hospital care from a medical and nursing perspective. Pre-hospital care, in this context, may be viewed as the provision of specific, skilled, medical and nursing intervention for the ill or injured individual at the scene of the incident. However, these interventions should encompass more than just physical care; as Eaton (1993) suggests, 'it [pre-hospital care] extends beyond the preservation of life to the prevention of complications and the relief of suffering'. Definitive care for both the injured and the acutely ill, realistically, can only be carried out in hospital. Therefore, pre-hospital care must not be an attempt to take the ED to the patient, but to provide interventions to stabilize the patient's condition prior to and during evacuation to hospital.

The contemporary problems in pre-hospital care often emerge when the ambulance service requests the attendance of a medical and nursing team from the local ED at the scene of an accident or major incident. As a consequence of this type of request being such a rarity, the team members frequently have no clearly defined role or function, they are poorly trained and inadequately equipped for work outside the ED. Most importantly they will have little or no operational experience in the pre-hospital setting.

Such requests made by the ambulance service are usually in response to difficult situations, for example in the event of a prolonged entrapment of a multiply injured individual where access to the patient is problematic. Thus the least experienced are requested to deal with the most complex situations. This is a reflection of a common phenomenon seen in hospital.

Consider, for example, the experienced nurse who encounters difficulty in placing a nasogastric tube and calls the junior doctor – the doctor may in fact have considerably less experience in this procedure.

MAJOR INCIDENTS

Not all Acute and Foundation Trusts are required to be able to provide a mobile team in the event of a major incident. It is now the responsibility of the Strategic Health Authorities (SHA) to identify those Trusts who will be responsible for deploying a Medical Emergency Response Incident Team (MERIT) to the scene of the incident, if requested to do so (DH Emergency Preparedness Division 2005). However, the SHAs do not have to use Acute and Foundation Trusts to provide MERITs, they may seek to resource MERITs from other organizations such as local Immediate Care Schemes operating under the auspices of the British Association of Immediate Care (BASICS).

It therefore makes it much clearer for those Trusts who are identified as being able to provide a MERIT when necessary and for the staff working in those Trusts to plan, train and rehearse their roles prior to an event taking place. Staff should be familiar with their local plan, to be aware of any requirements for them to provide a MERIT and their role in the team if requested to participate. When previous guidance was in operation there is evidence that nurses were not aware of their role if asked to deploy as part of a mobile medical and nursing team (Moakes & Kilner 2001). It may be the clarity of current guidance that this position is no longer true.

Current guidance states that in planning for a major incident staff should:

- understand the role they are to fulfil in the event of an incident
- have the necessary competencies to fulfil that role
- have received training to fulfil those competencies (DH Emergency Preparedness Division 2005, 2007).

Plans should provide outline guidance on the role of the MERIT; however, it is incumbent upon the Ambulance Incident Commander (AIC) and the Medical Incident Commander (MIC) to clearly define the role and purpose of deploying a MERIT and giving advice on the best way of executing their role (DH Emergency Preparedness Division 2005). This guidance provides examples of the specific skills the team may bring to the scene such as provision of analgesia or the specialist support of children. There is, however, a clear expectation that the team has received appropriate training for this role.

Resourcing the team often results in the hospital being depleted of key, experienced personnel at a time when their expertise is in greatest demand. Plans must take this into account, ensuring that those required by the SHA to provide a MERIT are able to take action to ensure that a team can be assembled with appropriately skilled staff, when required to do so. The plan should not require action which would knowingly deplete essential services and expose the organization and patients to unacceptable risk.

The plan should also identify the equipment that is available to the MERIT, ensuring that it is appropriately packaged for both clinical needs, operation and manual handling. The team must also have access to appropriate personal protective equipment, primarily for their safety but with due consideration to the identification of team members and key roles. Staff must therefore be familiar with clinical and safety equipment they require and the safe and appropriate use of that equipment in the pre-hospital environment.

Deployment of the team is often delayed, principally for logistical reasons, such as assembly of the team, collection of the equipment and availability of transport for the team. Transport is a particular problem as most ambulances and their staff will be committed to patient care and transport and it may be some time before a vehicle is made available to transport the team. Lee et al. (2002) found the length of time taken to form teams and for them to reach incident sites means that they do not provide care for *any* patients, or are left caring only for those with minor injuries.

Key roles at the scene

The Ambulance Incident Commander (AIC) is responsible for coordinating ambulance resources at the scene of the incident and, in conjunction with the Medical Incident Commander (MIC) coordinating the activity of other NHS resources at the scene of the incident. On arrival at the scene the MERIT must report to the MIC, or the AIC if the MIC has not yet arrived on scene. Under no circumstances should the MERIT self-task at the scene.

The function of the mobile team

Close to the incident site, but outside the inner cordon surrounding the actual incident site, a casualty clearing point will be established. This is the interface between the incident site and the chain of evacuation. It is at this point that the MERIT may be of most use.

Casualties will initially be treated by ambulance personnel prior to evacuation to the casualty clearing point. At the casualty clearing station the mobile team will triage the casualties for transport, identifying those patients who should be dispatched to hospital immediately and those who may wait a short time. The team may also become involved in stabilizing patients awaiting transportation to hospital. A further role the team may play is in the confirmation of death or recognition of life extinct, thus preventing resources being deployed where they will be of no practical benefit. While ambulance staff are authorized to undertake the recognition of life extinct (ROLE) they may be more usefully engaged in the extrication, initial treatment and transportation of the living. It is important that, if life has been declared extinct, the body should be clearly labelled to that effect, as it is not uncommon for a doctor to be requested to see the same casualty several times by different rescuers.

Triage at a major incident

In a mass casualty situation, there is a serious risk of prioritizing casualties without regard for need. Thus triage for transport is essential so that the greatest benefit is achieved for the greatest number. It is important to stress that triage at the scene of a major incident is philosophically different from triage occurring on a day-to-day basis in the ED. As numbers of casualties will outstrip resources, triage includes a category not used routinely in hospital – dead/expectant. 'Dead' is self-explanatory; 'expectant' refers to those casualties whose injuries are so severe that they are expected to die in the absence of involved care. These patients are those who would receive the care of the hospital trauma team at the ED under normal circumstances. If the team become involved in treating these people, however, a greater number of others may die because of being denied simple life-saving interventions. This form of triage is often difficult for nurses and doctors to accept, but the aim is to do the greatest good for the greatest number (Barnes 2006).

Triage for initial treatment must be rapid, using a simple method of assessment (Box 1.1).

Triage for transport

After initial treatment in situ and in the casualty clearing station, patients must be prioritized for transport to hospital. Some patients who receive a high priority for treatment may receive a lower priority for transportation. For example, an unconscious person with a simple airway obstruction would receive 'immediate priority' for treatment; however, once the airway problem is resolved they would become a lower priority than a patient with time-critical hypovolaemia.

Triage for transport employs the triage sort system, which is somewhat less crude than the triage sieve. The triage sort requires the measurement of the Glasgow Coma Score, respiratory rate and systolic blood pressure (Box 1.2).

NON-MAJOR INCIDENTS

At the request of the ambulance service, the hospital may provide a medical and nursing team to attend an incident where there is either one or a small number of casualties. These incidents usually involve entrapment of the casualty or casualties, where removal to hospital is delayed and where interventions may be required which fall outside the scope of practice of the paramedics.

The teams provided by the hospital fall into two distinct groups: the team arranged on an ad hoc basis, as described in the section on major incidents; and the established team who attend incidents on a regular basis.

There are potential difficulties in the operation of these teams, which differ slightly from the teams deployed at a major incident. It is essential that, prior to deployment of a team, there is a clear indication that the team's intervention will be of benefit to the patient. One may well argue that additional resources at the scene of the accident will naturally enhance patient care. However, this is not strictly true as there is a risk that the team may attempt to provide definitive care at the roadside, delaying transfer to hospital. Once release of the casualty has been effected and immediate management of early life-threatening conditions has been initiated, the patient should be transported to hospital. This is essential if mortality and morbidity are to be reduced in those patients with time-critical injuries.

One of the major contributory factors to this potential delay in transfer to hospital is the lack of understanding of the concept of pre-hospital care. Pre-hospital is the provision of skilled care at the roadside and en route to hospital. It is not an attempt to take the ED to the patient. Definitive care can only be carried out in the hospital setting, and pre-hospital care should aim to facilitate the removal of the stabilized patient to hospital at the earliest and most appropriate opportunity.

Expeditious removal to hospital of the polytraumatized patient is based upon the notion of the 'golden hour', the maximum time it should take from injury to definitive care. The golden hour does not belong to the pre-hospital providers, nor does it belong to the ED; it belongs to the patient. Ideally, on-scene treatment of the patient should last no longer than 10 minutes, the 'platinum 10 minutes'. This may be somewhat compromised if the patient is trapped, and in such circumstances the delay should be reduced to an absolute minimum.

Difficulties may be experienced by medical and nursing staff, when working in the pre-hospital environment, in adapting to the subtle changes in their respective roles. This is illustrated in the situation where the hospital team focuses upon the medical and nursing care of the individual to the exclusion of everything else, rather than considering the scene in its broadest context. For example, the patient may have had her airway secured, been provided with high-flow oxygen, had intravenous volume replacement, be connected to monitoring equipment, and had her fractures immobilized and her wounds dressed. During this time, however, the fire service may have been prevented from continuing the rescue and the ambulance service may have been deployed fetching and carrying equipment. The result is that the patient will have received medical and nursing care but is still trapped and no nearer to being transported to hospital.

This lack of understanding of teamwork in its broadest sense is largely explained by a lack of operational experience of the team and is therefore less likely to be a problem where the team is used frequently, as opposed to those teams that are rarely mobilized. Many of these problems may be addressed through multidisciplinary training in both theory and practice, the practical element being reinforced through supervised operational experience. This means that a less experienced, not necessarily junior, member of staff is mentored by an experienced colleague, during 'live' call-outs.

FORMAL TRAINING

Historically, formal training in pre-hospital care for both doctors and nurses, if it existed at all, was based upon in-house training schemes and informal discussion with colleagues. However, this situation has changed with the advent of now well-established courses such as the Pre-hospital Trauma Life Support Course (PHTLS), the Pre-hospital Emergency Care Course (PHEC) and the Pre-hospital Paediatric Advanced Life Support Course. All courses are open to doctors, nurses and ambulance service paramedics, thus promoting multidisciplinary dialogue.

DELIVERY OF CARE

Safety

The delivery of care in the pre-hospital environment is fraught with hazards, some of which are common to many areas of practice and others of which are unique to the pre-hospital environment. Those hazards to which the nurse is exposed on a day-to-day basis in the ED are likely to be recognized and appropriate precautions taken. In the pre-hospital environment, these precautions may not always be taken. For example, when caring for a multiply injured person in the ED, few nurses would consider not wearing gloves, yet at the scene of the accident gloves may not be worn because they become torn on the wreckage or when carrying equipment, or may not be easily accessible. Similarly, gloves are not always replaced when they do become torn.

As with major incidents the team must liaise with the senior officers from the emergency services on arrival at the scene of the incident and take expert advice regarding specific hazards (Barnes 2006). Accident scenes are intrinsically hazardous; the rescuer is at risk from a whole range of potential or actual hazards, such as wreckage, chemicals, electricity, moving vehicles and the weather. In addition, when moving about accident sites, the nurse should beware of jagged metal edges, glass, extrication equipment, rubble and blood. In a highly stressed situation, it is easy to lose sight of hazards in an eagerness to be of assistance. For instance, when arriving at the scene of an accident on the motorway it is easy to step out of an ambulance or police car into a 'live' traffic lane. High-visibility fluorescent jackets offer the nurse no protection in such circumstances, and in fact may lull nurses into a false sense of security. Those who work in the pre-hospital environment need to develop a sixth sense, having a heightened awareness of the environment which surrounds them. As the nurse becomes 'streetwise', he may react to these hazards in an intuitive way.

The personal safety of the rescuers is paramount, and this question of safety extends beyond the duration of the incident, particularly in respect of psychological safety. By the very nature of the work, the nurse who attends the serious incident is exposed to sights which would be psychologically disturbing to anyone who witnessed them. Consideration should be given to arranging multidisciplinary post-incident debriefings which may assist some individuals in dealing with the after-effects. These debriefings need to be carefully planned, timed and managed sensitively, taking professional advice where appropriate. It is also important that these sessions are made available to staff rather than being mandatory, as individuals deal with stress in different ways and some may not find the sessions helpful.

PATIENT ASSESSMENT

Assessment of the patient at the scene of an incident relies heavily on basic clinical assessment skills, rather than the more sophisticated methods employed in hospital. It is a pointless exercise to attempt to auscultate the chest at the side of a motorway as the fire service are cutting the car apart, as is attempting to listen to a blood pressure in the same circumstances. It is almost impossible to see central cyanosis at 4 a.m. in the rain at the side of railway track. A high index of suspicion based upon the mechanism of injury is an invaluable assessment tool.

Technological aids are not always helpful; for example, a pulse oximeter is of little use if the patient is cold and peripherally shut down. If the patient is attached to a number of monitors, as well as the oxygen and bags of intravenous fluid, it becomes quite difficult to remove them without one or more of the appendages snagging. The assessment must be based on identifying the problems the patient is likely to have (reading the wreckage) and then identifying or excluding them. Assessment at the scene should be based upon the primary survey, with the secondary survey being carried out, if possible, en route to hospital. Transport to hospital should not be delayed in order to carry out the secondary survey.

Airway with cervical spine control

The rationale and techniques for airway management and cervical spine control in the trauma patient are well-documented (National Association of Emergency Medical Technicians 2003). It is essential that the emergency nurse considers these interventions in the pre-hospital context rather than relying entirely on the skills acquired in the hospital setting.

When managing the airway, as with much of the practice of pre-hospital care, the nurse needs to have thought two or three steps ahead. It is extremely frustrating to have gained access to a small space to treat the patient, armed with a size three oropharyngeal airway, only to find that the patient needs a size four. This lack of preplanning could be disastrous to patient outcome, e.g. if the patient vomits during an airway intervention and the suction equipment has not been requested as routine.

Similarly, it is frustrating for clinical staff to have successfully intubated the patient but still be unable to inflate the cuff as no syringe is available, with the patient aspirating in the interim. These problems are less likely to occur in the ED, where equipment is readily available and staff are familiar with its whereabouts. Members of the team should be skilled in a range of airway-management techniques, and it is important that these skills have been practised in a range of scenarios. The team member is likely to experience difficulty if faced with an unconscious person with a compromised airway who is trapped upside down, when he has learned the jaw thrust manoeuvre on supine patients.

In the ED, the cervical spine is immobilized with a semi-rigid collar, sandbags and tape, whereas in the pre-hospital environment immobilization is often provided by the rescuer's hands. It may not be possible to apply a collar because of space restrictions and while the patient is trapped it will not be possible to use sandbags and tape.

With the advent of extrication devices, used in conjunction with a cervical collar, protection may be offered to the cervical, thoracic and lumbar spine. The extrication devices (such as the Russel Extrication Device, RED™, or the Kendrick Extrication Device, KED™) are short, moulded, rigid boards which are placed along the spine and strapped to the patient. The device may be inserted from above or from the side, depending on the space available. The use of this equipment requires some skill, which the hospital team needs to acquire. Failing this, the ambulance staff who are trained in its use and who work with the equipment on a daily basis are well placed to carry out this procedure. Ambulance services are now routinely using long spinal boards as a means of extrication as well as providing spinal immobilization during transport. Again, the team should be familiar with the equipment and skilled in its use. This is best achieved through training with staff from the ambulance service.

If an extrication device or long spinal board is not used, it is important that the patient's head is not taped to a conventional ambulance trolley. It is extremely difficult to turn the patient quickly and in a controlled manner, should they vomit en route to hospital, while they are taped to the trolley.

It is also not uncommon to have several people who are mobile post-incident but who have been exposed to similar forces to those who appear to be more severely injured. The fail-safe position may be to provide full spinal immobilization for all these patients. This would rapidly exhaust the available ambulance resources on scene and ultimately create unnecessary pressures on the ED. Emergency nurses deployed to the scene should be familiar with guidance on the clearance of the cervical spine at the scene based on history and clinical examination (Joint Royal Colleges Ambulance Liaison Committee and Ambulance Service Association 2004).

Breathing and ventilation

The use of high concentration of inspired oxygen in the management of the seriously injured patient is well established in practice. However, its use in the pre-hospital environment may raise important, but manageable, safety issues. First, high-flow oxygen used in a confined space may result in an oxygen-rich atmosphere which presents a potential fire hazard. Fire service personnel should be made aware of this as it may have implications for the techniques they use to extricate the patient. Second, there is a potential explosion and fire risk if oxygen therapy equipment comes into contact with grease. This hazard is limited in the hospital setting, but is significantly increased at the scene of an accident.

The environment may present the team with difficulties in performing certain procedures. For instance, it may be difficult to identify the surface anatomy required to site a needle for a needle thorocentesis, because of the position of the patient. This may change priorities in terms of the speed of extrication. Should the extrication be slow with greater control, or should it be rapid with less control, in order to undertake a life-saving procedure?

Circulation

In recent years the National Institute for Health and Clinical Excellence (NICE) has brought some clarity to the debate of pre-hospital fluid replacement in trauma. The guidance recommends intravenous fluid replacement in trauma of 250-ml aliquots titrated to the presence of the radial pulse (National Institute for Health and Clinical Excellence 2004). However, in prolonged entrapments the management of volume replacement may become complex and as such may require the intervention of an experienced critical-care clinician and thus the MERIT.

There are some additional factors which must be considered in the provision of pre-hospital fluid replacement. The environment may complicate volume replacement in the pre-hospital setting. Intravenous fluids rapidly cool when working outside in the winter months. The temperature of the fluid falls prior to and during administration to the patient, with much of the heat being lost as the fluid flows along the giving set tubing. Fluids may be cold before dispatch to the scene if they are stored in cupboards in draughty corridors or in store huts. Rapid infusion of cold fluid may have a catastrophic effect on the physiology of a traumatized patient, yet currently available equipment designed for warming fluid and maintaining its temperature in the pre-hospital setting is suboptimal.

Disability

Neurological assessment may be conducted in the form of the mini-neurological assessment (ATLS), based upon the AVPU acronym:

- A – alert
- V – responds to verbal stimuli
- P – responds to painful stimuli
- U – unresponsive.

The National Institute for Health and Clinical Excellence have provided useful guidance regarding the assessment and management of those patients with head injury (National Institute for Health and Clinical Excellence 2003). This guidance suggests that in the presence of any of the following the patient requires transport by emergency ambulance for further assessment in the ED:

- unconsciousness, or lack of full consciousness
- any focal neurological deficit since the injury
- any suspicion of skull fracture or penetrating head injury
- any seizure
- high energy head injury.

Exposure and environmental control

Exposure of the patient should be sufficient to conduct the primary survey, while being conscious of the patient's dignity in such a vulnerable position. It is also essential to be aware of the effects the environment is having on the patient. The carer may have warm, waterproof clothing, but the patient will not be so well prepared. Protection of the patient from the elements is vital, yet it is often forgotten, partly because it assumes a relative low priority. Hypothermia has both physiological and psychological implications for the patient and should be avoided if at all possible.

Transport

Most of the patients to whom the hospital team are called out will have time-critical injuries. They should therefore be transported by the most appropriate means, to the most appropriate hospital, being that which has the facilities on site to provide the patient with definitive care. This is not necessarily the closest hospital with an ED or the hospital which is the team's base. There is no place to 'stay and play' in the pre-hospital environment. Once extricated, there is little, if any, reason to delay transport to hospital.

UNIQUE ROLE PLAYED BY NURSES IN PROVIDING PRE-HOSPITAL CARE

Some of the skills which nurses refine in the ED are transferable into the pre-hospital arena and of these skills many form the uniqueness of the nurse's role in this environment. The nurse may be a skilled communicator who is able to establish a rapport with the patient early into the incident and follow this through into the hospital phase of care. This may have a significant impact on the psychological well-being of the patient, especially as the nurse has already established a degree of credibility, through having been there at the scene and therefore knowing what it was like. This continuity is more than a familiar face, although this is important; rather, it is reassurance for the patient through a relationship based upon security and trust.

The psychological support is not undertaken in isolation, as the nurse is able to assimilate information from the scene in order to support the patient and gain her or his cooperation. The nurse may become the interface between the patient and the rescue team, interpreting events for the patient and protecting him or her from a barrage of repetitive questions. The nurse is able to provide the rescue team with vital information that the patient is unable to verbalize, e.g. if the patient winces in pain when a particular activity is undertaken.

A nurse is well placed to act as the patient's advocate, which is an acknowledged skill of nurses and is less likely to be taken on by other team members. The nurse may also be skilled in caring for distressed relatives who may be at the scene and who may accompany the patient to the hospital. Again, establishing and sustaining a rapport with the relatives will enhance the quality of care those relatives receive.

CONCLUSION

Nurses can make a valuable contribution to the delivery of pre-hospital care as part of a multidisciplinary team. Yet, with a few exceptions, the service which is currently provided is suboptimal. Optimal care may be achieved through effective planning, multi-agency training and education, research, operational experience and adequate funding, with standards developed and agreed at a national level.

Failure to address these issues will result in the continuation of a fragmented service of dubious quality, which ultimately may result in the demise of nursing input in the provision of pre-hospital care.

References

Barnes J (2006) Mobile medical teams: do A&E nurses have the appropriate experience? *Emergency Nurse*, **13**(9), 18–23.

Department of Health Emergency Preparedness Division (2005) *The NHS Emergency Planning Guidance 2005.* London: Department of Health.

Department of Health Emergency Preparedness Division (2007) *Mass Casual Incident: A Framework for Planning.* London: Department of Health.

Eaton CJ (1997) *Essentials of Immediate Medical Care.* Edinburgh: Churchill Livingstone.

Hodgetts T, McNeill I, Cooke M (2000) *The Pre-Hospital Emergency Management Master.* London: BMJ Publishing Group.

Joint Royal Colleges Ambulance Liaison Committee and Ambulance Service Association (2004) *Clinical Practice Guidelines for use in UK Ambulance Services.* London: JRCALC/ASA.

Lee W, Chie T, Ng C, Chen J (2002) Emergency medical preparedness and response to a Singapore airliner crash. *Academic Emergency Medicine*, **9**(3), 194–199.

Moakes S, Kilner T (2001) Nurses' understanding of their role as part of a mobile medical and nursing team during a major incident. *Pre-hospital Immediate Care*, **5**(1), 34–37.

National Association of Emergency Medical Technicians (2003) *PHTLS Basic and Advanced Prehospital Trauma Life Support.* St Louis: Mosby.

National Institute for Health and Clinical Excellence (2003) *Head Injury: Triage, Assessment, Investigation and Early Management of Head Injury in Infants, Children and Adults.* London: NICE.

National Institute for Health and Clinical Excellence (2004) *Technological Appraisal (No 74) The Clinical and Cost Effectiveness of Prehospital Intravenous Fluid Therapy in Trauma.* London: NICE.

Chapter 2

Trauma life support

Lynda Holt

INTRODUCTION

The multiply injured patient presents a challenge to the ED and trauma team. Trauma remains the leading cause of death among those under 40 years of age and it is suggested that after cardiovascular disease and cancer, traumatic injury is the leading cause of death across all ages in the developed world (Span et al. 2007, Greaves et al. 2001, O'Reilly 2003) and injury is also the main cause of hospital bed day usage (Rainier & de Villiers Smit 2003). As Cole (2004) notes, the human cost of trauma on society is incalculable.

Failure to recognize and correctly treat traumatic injuries promptly will have a detrimental effect on early and delayed mortality and morbidity (Royal College of Surgeons 1988), so careful and thorough assessment must be made as quickly as possible, supported by life-saving interventions. A trauma team may comprise an informal group of individuals who care for the multiply injured patient, or a more formal resuscitation team identified as the 'trauma team'. Activation of a prepared trauma team results in better patient care and improved patient survival (Petrie et al. 1996). Whatever the formation, all team members, including nurses, should be appropriately prepared to care for the trauma patient in a systematic manner, with appropriate leadership. Nurses have a number of roles to fulfil. These include:

- Assessment
- Intervention
- Monitoring
- Communication
- Leadership
- Team building (Hadfield-Law 1993).

The Advanced Trauma Life Support (ATLS®) programme (American College of Surgeons 2004), which follows a sequence of priorities of care, with the objective of minimizing mortality and morbidity, has been widely adopted for trauma patients throughout the world. The initial assessment component of the system comprises:

- Preparation
- Primary survey
- Resuscitation
- Secondary survey
- Continuous monitoring and evaluation
- Definitive care.

This chapter will follow through the sequence of events; in reality, however, many activities occur in parallel or simultaneously and involve a number of team members. For the multiply injured patient, resuscitation of physical condition takes immediate priority, but psychological needs must not be overlooked. In practice, if considered, this often falls to one member of the team. However, all health professionals involved should be careful not to cause further emotional or spiritual distress to patients (Edwards 1995).

PREPARATION

In the pre-hospital phase, emphasis should be placed on airway management, control of bleeding and shock, immobilization of the patient and immediate transport to the closest, appropriate facility. Time spent on scene with the patient should be kept to the minimum (PHTLS Committee 2002). In many instances, the ambulance service alerts the ED to the impending arrival of a multiply injured patient. This allows time for appropriate preparation of personnel and environment. The size and mix of the team will depend on the level of resources available and will vary widely. Some will comprise a junior ED nurse and doctor, while others will have specialist nursing and medical support available 24 hours a day. Irrespective of the level of staffing, a systematic approach to care should apply on every occasion and it should be constantly monitored to maintain optimum effectiveness and efficiency (Sexton 1997). Each team member should have a clear role and pre-designated responsibilities.

A safe and suitable environment is essential, which requires careful preparation. All team members who have direct patient contact must be immunized against hepatitis B and wear protective clothing. This should include goggles, gloves and aprons to protect against contamination from the patient's body fluids. Universal precautions should be taken with all trauma patients. Such patients also need protection from nosocomial infection and death due to sepsis. The use of lead aprons for all those involved means that care can continue while X-rays are taken, without undue risk

to staff. The treatment area should be kept warm to reduce the risk of hypothermia. It should also be spacious enough for team members to work safely and simultaneously.

Adequate numbers of personnel will be required to transfer the patient safely from the ambulance trolley onto the ED trolley.

PRIMARY SURVEY

Each patient should have an initial examination to set priorities for treatment of potentially life-threatening injuries, which should take place immediately and systematically using an ABCDE approach:

- Airway maintenance with cervical spine protection
- Breathing and ventilation
- Circulation with haemorrhage control
- Disability: neurological status
- Exposure/environmental control: completely undress the patient, but prevent hypothermia.

The primary survey and resuscitation aspects of initial assessment are completed together.

Airway with cervical spine control

To prevent secondary cervical spine injury, the patient should be approached from an angle at which he can see the assessor without moving his head. A simple statement which requires a response can then be made, e.g. 'How are you Mr Smith?' or 'Hello, what's your name?' If the patient is able to speak, two important assumptions can be made. First, the airway is clear, and second the patient's brain is being adequately perfused. Even if a patient's airway sounds clear, the assessor should not move onto the next stage without physically checking the airway for potential problems: looking for foreign bodies or damage to the mouth and neck.

Simultaneous cervical spine precautions must be taken from the outset. Any trauma patient, particularly with injuries above the clavicle or those with an altered conscious level, should be considered to have a cervical spine injury until proven otherwise. Manual immobilization of the head and neck should be followed as soon as possible by the application of a semi-rigid collar and specifically designed immobilizers. This is the minimum intervention in terms of acceptable precautions. Specifically designed boards for complete spinal immobilization are most effective. For those patients who are unable to remain still and might be thrashing around on the trolley, a semi-rigid collar can be applied until the patient is calm enough to tolerate more confining measures. Neurological examination alone does not exclude a cervical spine injury. Remember also that a patient who is agitated should be considered hypoxic until proven otherwise.

If the patient does not respond to a simple question, airway obstruction should be assumed and measures should be taken to relieve this immediately. The most common reason for obstruction in the unconscious patient is partial or complete occlusion of the oropharynx by the tongue. Saliva, vomit and blood may exacerbate the problem. Interventions should begin with the simplest, progressing to the more complex if necessary. A chin lift or jaw thrust should pull collapsed soft tissues out of the airway. Any debris or foreign bodies must be physically removed. Suction can be very effective, using a tonsil tip/rigid (Yankeur) suction catheter. Cole (2004) recommends the tip of the Yankeur suction catheter be kept in sight to ensure it is not inserted too deeply causing the patient's gag reflex to be stimulated. Equally, blind finger sweeps should not be used as this may further push foreign objects into the airway.

For those patients who vomit profusely and unexpectedly, airway and cervical spine control can be difficult. Mechanical suction apparatus, including a Yankeur sucker, must always be available for use immediately, so that the patient can be tipped, head downwards, on the trolley and his airway cleared, minimizing the risk of aspiration of gastric contents.

More active measures may be required for those who are unable to maintain their own airway. A nasopharyngeal airway will ensure patency in the conscious patient, without causing a gag reflex. This may be particularly useful for those with a fluctuating conscious level. For the unconscious patient, an oropharyngeal (guedal) airway may be helpful; however, its use increases the risk of vomiting.

Many multiply injured patients need emergency endotracheal (ET) intubation early on in their management. This procedure carries with it certain risks, particularly in the trauma patient. Cervical spine immobilization must be maintained throughout intubation, making the procedure more complex. The patient is often shocked, can have a damaged airway, and frequently has a full stomach. ET intubation in inexperienced hands can be fraught with danger. Ideally, it should be performed by someone with appropriate trauma and anaesthetic skills.

If oral or nasal intubation fails to secure an airway in the patient with obstruction, within 60 seconds, and the patient cannot be ventilated with a bag-valve-mask system for reasons such as facial fractures, the nurse should prepare for an emergency cricothyroidotomy. Several periods of apnoea caused by repeated attempts at intubation can result in dangerous levels of hypoxia. A needle cricothyroidotomy can establish a temporary airway swiftly, but will need to be followed by a surgical cricothyroidotomy or a tracheostomy within 30–45 minutes.

A cuffed tube placed in the trachea is the gold standard for securing and protecting the airway. However, the oesophageal-tracheal combitube and the intubating laryngeal mask airway (ILMA) are recent advances in airway management that can facilitate intubation in the patient with a difficult airway (Stoneham et al. 2001).

A definitive airway should be established if there is any doubt about the patient's ability to maintain airway integrity (American College of Surgeons 2004). After any intervention, though, the patency of the airway should be rechecked.

Breathing

A patent airway does not automatically mean that the patient is able to breathe properly. The patient's chest should be watched carefully, for the rise and fall of the chest wall, on both sides. The assessor should listen for breath sounds and feel for exhaled breath. If the patient is not breathing or is breathing inadequately, mechanical ventilation using a bag-valve-mask system (Ambu bag) with high-flow oxygen should be instituted. This is usually more effective when performed by two people, one to seal the airway and one to squeeze the Ambu bag.

Efficiency of breathing should be established by observing for rate and depth, cyanosis, use of accessory muscles, tracheal shift from the midline, engorged neck veins, any sucking chest wounds, and, of great importance, any change in conscious level. Breathing that is unequal or asymmetrical may indicate bony injury or an underlying pneumothorax. Pulse oximetry is a valuable monitor, as peripheral oxygen saturation is a good measure of breathing efficiency; however, it must be remembered that the reading may not be accurate in a shocked, hypothermic or burned trauma patient (Casey 2001). All trauma patients should receive high-flow oxygen (American College of Surgeons 2004), to reduce further strain on the heart. A concentration of approximately 95% arterial saturation can be achieved by administering oxygen at 15 l/min through a clear mask with a reservoir bag attached.

Any life-threatening condition encountered during the assessment of breathing should be corrected immediately. These include:

- airway obstruction
- tension pneumothorax
- open pneumothorax (sucking chest wound)
- massive haemothorax

- flail chest
- cardiac tamponade

Sucking chest wounds should be covered. Chest decompression will be required immediately in the event of a tension pneumothorax, as this dramatically compromises ventilation and circulation. Equipment for inserting a chest drain should be prepared following a needle thoracentesis. A large flail segment with pulmonary contusion or a massive haemothorax should be treated straight away. If the patient is unable to maintain adequate ventilation unassisted, endotracheal intubation may be required, with mechanical ventilation. After any manoeuvre is used to correct inadequate ventilation, breathing should always be rechecked.

Circulation with haemorrhage control

Despite improvements in trauma care, uncontrolled bleeding contributes to 30–40% of trauma-related deaths and is the leading cause of potentially preventable early in-hospital deaths (Span et al. 2007, Kauver & Wade 2005). Haemorrhage is the predominant cause of post-injury deaths. Assessment of the patient's circulatory status should be made by measuring the level of consciousness, skin colour and pulse. Ashen face and white extremities are ominous signs of hypovolaemia, as is an altered level of consciousness. If the patient does not have a pulse, external cardiac massage should be commenced. It may be appropriate to prepare for open thoracentesis, pericardiocentesis or needle thoracentesis if cardiac tamponade or tension pneumothorax is suspected. Full, slow and regular pulses are *usually* signs of normal circulating volume in those who are not taking beta-blockers.

Any external bleeding should be controlled by direct pressure or by elevation, as there is little point in trying to replace fluid if no attempt is being made to conserve it. Tourniquets should not be used, as the tissue damage incurred can be irreversible. By checking the skin of the patient, other indicators of circulatory status may be available, e.g. colour, warmth, sweating and capillary refill. Every trauma patient should be presumed hypovolaemic until proved otherwise. Erring on the side of caution may prevent some of the unnecessary deaths and disability which occur.

A critical pitfall in the assessment of the trauma patient's circulatory status is the failure to recognize the presence or severity of potentially unstable pelvic ring fractures, which can be life-threatening. Bleeding can be minimized in this event, by tying the patient's legs together.

At least two short, wide-bore cannulae must be inserted (14–16 gauge) with an initial fluid bolus of two litres of warmed Hartmann's solution, given through a blood-giving set. It is important to remember that the rate of intravenous (I.V.) infusion is not determined by the size of the vein, but by the internal diameter of the cannula, and is inversely affected by its length. At this time a blood sample can be taken for grouping and cross-matching of at least six units. Full blood count, urea and electrolyte baselines should also be taken. Women of child-bearing years should have a pregnancy test.

The two peripheral I.V. lines should be started in upper extremities if not contraindicated. Lines should not be placed in injured extremities if they can be avoided. If difficulties arise with insertion, or more lines are required, venous cut-downs should be performed.

Restoration of adequate circulating blood volume and oxygen-carrying capacity is essential. Fluid best suited to the trauma patient remains controversial (Nolan 1999). However, as crystalloids are cheaper than colloids, and are more effective in restoring intravascular volume (Schierhout & Roberts 1998), Hartmann's solution is a good option. It is important to remember that for every millilitre of estimated blood volume lost, three millilitres of crystalloid should replace it. Crystalloids cannot enhance oxygen-carrying capacity, and therefore the best fluid replacement is blood, which should be transfused as soon as possible, if the patient does not respond to a rapid infusion of three litres of crystalloid solution.

Ideally, blood should be typed and cross-matched, but this can mean an unacceptable delay. If so, type-specific blood can be used, as risk of reaction is relatively low. In dire emergencies, O-negative blood can be used and should be stored in small quantities in the ED for such cases. Patient blood samples should be taken early, as infusion of large quantities of O-negative blood can cause difficulties with grouping and cross-matching later.

Aggressive and continued volume resuscitation is not a substitute for manual or surgical control of haemorrhage (Knoferl et al. 1999). The rate of fluid resuscitation will need to take into account mechanism of injury (Soucy et al. 1999). Some studies have shown an increase in survival by limiting fluid resuscitation, until surgery, in cases of unrepaired vascular injury following penetrating trauma (Bickell et al. 1994). In contrast, infusing fluids to achieve a normal blood pressure will increase blood loss, although the reasons for this are not known (Greaves et al. 2001).

Monitoring the patient's fluid intake and output is a vital part of the ED nurse's role. Knowing precisely how much and what kind of fluid the patient has received is essential in determining subsequent fluid management.

Cardiac monitoring provides circulatory information from the heart rate and rhythm. It also provides an indicator of hypoxia, hypoperfusion and hypothermia in the form of ectopic beats, aberrant conduction and bradycardia. Electromechanical dissociation (EMD) is suggestive of profound hypovolaemia, cardiac tamponade or tension pneumothorax and has a poor prognosis unless the underlying cause can be determined and treated immediately.

Urinary catheters and nasogastric tubes should be considered part of the resuscitation of the patient. Urine output is a sensitive measure of renal perfusion and an invaluable way to assess success of the resuscitation. A urinary catheter attached to a urometer should be inserted, providing no contraindications exist, such as blood at the urinary meatus, scrotal haematoma or a high riding prostate, which would indicate urethral damage. A urometer will ensure that accurate hourly measurements of urine output can be taken. If urethral catheterization is contraindicated, due to urethral damage, a suprapubic catheter should be inserted by a suitably skilled team member. A urinary output of more than 50 ml/h in an adult is a good indicator of satisfactory tissue perfusion. The urine which is voided initially should be tested for blood and saved for microscopy and subsequent possible drug analysis.

A nasogastric tube should be inserted to decompress the stomach, thereby helping to avoid regurgitation. This can be caused by a paralytic ileus or air in the stomach as the result of assisted manual ventilation. A gastric tube may also identify blood in the gastric contents. A nasogastric tube should not be inserted if a cribriform plate fracture is suspected, in case it is inadvertently passed into the cranial cavity. In this event, the tube can be inserted orally.

Disability: neurological status

A simple and rapid assessment of neurological status should take place during the primary survey. The evaluation should establish level of consciousness, pupil size and reaction. The Glasgow Coma Score (GCS) is the commonest method used for the assessment of level of consciousness and a sequence of readings will tend to show fairly subtle changes quickly. So, continuity in measurement is important and measurements should be made by the same person.

As part of the GCS, painful stimulus is sometimes required. Safe methods include supraorbital pressure (not in facial fractures), trapezius pinch, and sternal rub. In order to differentiate the motor response to pain, the stimulus should be applied centrally. Be aware of patients with spinal cord injury and upper limb fractures as they may feel painful stimulus but

be unable to respond with limb movement. In all cases painful stimuli should be kept to a minimum.

Normal pupil size ranges from 2 to 5 mm, with a difference of 1 mm being acceptable. As the light is shone in each eye, both eyes should be tested for responsiveness.

A decreased level of consciousness should alert the assessor to four possibilities (Pre-Hospital Trauma Life Support Committee 2002):

- Decreased cerebral oxygenation (hypoxia and hypoperfusion)
- Central nervous system injury
- Drug or alcohol overdose
- Metabolic derangement (diabetes, seizure, cardiac arrest).

Exposure/environmental control

At the end of the primary survey, every item of clothing must be removed, without risking any further damage to the patient (American College of Surgeons 2004). It is prudent at this point to log-roll the patient so that the back, which comprises 50% of the body, can be fully examined and the rescue board can be removed, along with any debris or retained clothing. Failure to assess the back of the patient can mean that the assessor misses a life-threatening injury. However, rolling a patient with an unstable pelvic fracture can result in further pelvic haemorrhage, so minimal movement and gentle handling is crucial (Little et al. 2001).

Trauma patients are at risk from hypothermia (Cochrane 2001). Many have been exposed to low temperatures outside. Wet conditions, wind and blood loss contribute further to a drop in core temperature. Hypothermia increases morbidity and mortality and must be prevented or reversed. Secondary hypothermia should be prevented from occurring in the resuscitation room. Various measures can be used, including:

- warm blankets over the patient from a warming cabinet, radiator or microwave
- I.V., blood and lavage fluids warmed to 39°C
- adequate environmental temperature in resuscitation area
- specifically designed warming plate suspended over patient trolley
- controlled exposure of the patient
- external warming device, e.g. Behr Hugger.

Full history

A comprehensive history surrounding the patient and event will ensure a quicker idea of the status of the patient. Ambulance crews, paramedics, witnesses and relatives are an invaluable source of information. If the patient is conscious, they may possibly hold the most relevant information.

An AMPLE history helps plan patient care:

A Allergies
M Medication currently used
P Past illness/Pregnancy
L Last ate or drank
E Events/environment related to the injury.

Details regarding the mechanism of injury can indicate the site and seriousness of many potential injuries. This can save a great deal of time, which may be a lifesaver for the patient (Halpern 1989). Any pre-existing disease in a trauma patient increases their chances of dying, so clinicians need as much information as possible about medical history. X-rays should be used carefully and should not delay resuscitation. Chest and pelvic X-rays may provide guidance for the resuscitation of patients with blunt trauma. A clear cervical spine X-ray may provide valuable information about serious injury. However, when appropriate, these and any other X-rays required can be deferred to the secondary survey. A major pitfall in the immediate assessment of cervical spine integrity is a failure to recognize that early imaging on its own is inadequate to safely clear the spine (Little et al. 2001).

Pain relief can be overlooked during the activity of resuscitation, but it is an essential part of good patient care. Intravenous opiates work well, but intramuscular routes are not appropriate in acute situations. Entonox can provide useful pain relief during the early stages, but should be avoided if there is the possibility of a pneumothorax. Any drug administered should be carefully recorded in the appropriate place. It is easy to lose track of what drugs have been given during a busy resuscitation.

Good communication, explanation and gentle handling are important preliminaries to analgesia. Correct immobilization of fractures will also relieve a great deal of pain. Other sources of discomfort should be excluded, e.g. full bladder. Analgesia should not be avoided just because the patient has a head injury. But it should be carefully administered and the patient must be monitored afterwards.

SECONDARY SURVEY

The primary survey and resuscitation must be completed before the secondary survey begins. If, at the end of the primary survey, the patient's condition remains unstable, each step should be repeated until stability is achieved. During the secondary, head to toe, survey less obvious injuries, which may pose a latent threat to life, should be detected.

At this stage assessment of vital signs every five minutes should be initiated:

- temperature – rectal or tympanic membrane
- pulse – radial, femoral or carotid
- respirations
- blood pressure
- Glasgow Coma Score.

Vital signs should be monitored by the same person, to avoid assessor variability.

Trauma patients are vulnerable to the effects of pressure on their skin, and every effort should be made to prevent any unnecessary risk (Swartz 2000). Patients who arrive in ED on a spine board should be transferred from it as soon as is safe (Cooke 1998). Wet and soiled linen must be removed as soon as possible.

Head and face

The patient should be asked about any pain he may be experiencing and examined for evidence of injury to the bones or soft tissue, mouth or eyes. Otorrhoea or rhinorrhoea should be noted.

Swelling may prevent adequate examination of the eyes, later, so assess:

- visual acuity
- pupil size
- bleeding into the eye
- penetrating injury
- contact lenses (remove before swelling occurs)
- dislocation of the lens
- ocular nerve entrapment.

Neck

Patients with facial or head trauma must be presumed to have cervical spine injury until this has been excluded by an expert. Cervical spine immobilization should be maintained at all times. If immobilizing devices must be removed, manual in-line immobilization should be substituted. While maintaining careful cervical spine immobilization, the neck should be examined for any obvious injury to the bones or soft tissues. Any evidence of damage should lead the assessor to be concerned about potential airway obstruction. The assessor should check for tracheal deviation or distended neck veins, which may indicate a missed tension pneumothorax or cardiac tamponade.

Chest

The patient should be asked about pain or dyspnoea. Any sign of obvious injury should be noted, e.g. sucking chest wounds, surface/penetrating trauma, paradoxical movements, subcutaneous emphysema, bruising or crepitus over the ribs. Life-saving interventions should already have been performed for open chest wounds or tension pneumothorax.

It is important to remember that every patient has a posterior chest, which should already have been examined during the log-roll at the end of the primary survey. A 12-lead ECG will determine dysrhythmias and may indicate cardiac contusion. This is demonstrated by elevation of the ST-segment of the affected area, atrial fibrillation or an unexplained tachycardia. Elderly patients may not cope with even relatively minor chest injuries. Potential acute respiratory insufficiency should be anticipated and appropriate preventative measures taken. Children can sustain significant injury to the intrathoracic structures without evidence of any skeletal trauma.

Abdomen

An assessment of pain should be made, providing the patient is conscious. The abdomen should be examined for any obvious injury, distension, rigidity, guarding, contusions, scars and bowel sounds. Such an examination should be careful and thorough, as bleeding into the abdomen from damaged organs is frequently the cause of life-threatening hypovolaemia. The most important aspect of the abdominal assessment is to determine whether the patient requires surgery or not.

A naso- or orogastric tube and a urinary catheter should have been inserted during the primary survey and is always inserted before diagnostic peritoneal lavage (DPL) is performed. Such measures will ensure that abdominal and pelvic organs are less likely to be damaged during the procedure. DPL and focused abdominal ultrasonography (FAST) are quick diagnostic procedures to determine intra-abdominal bleeding. They are indicated when results of physical examination are equivocal or the patient is unable to participate in the assessment. They should always be performed by, or in the presence of, the surgeon who will be acting upon any positive findings. Remember that DPL in an unstable patient is looking only for frank blood. If the DPL does not reveal gross blood, then the search must be continued for another site of blood loss (D'Amours et al. 2002).

Pelvis and genitalia

Patients should be asked about pain and whether they have an urge to pass urine. Male patients should be examined for bruising, blood at the urinary meatus, priapism and oedema. The presence of femoral pulses should be ascertained. If a rectal examination was not performed when the patient was log-rolled at the end of the primary survey, it should be carried out now.

The assessor should look for blood in the rectum, which may indicate damage to the gut or pelvis. A high-riding prostate may be indicative of urethral injury, and loss of sphincter tone is often associated with spinal injury. Bony fragments may also be felt, indicating pelvic damage.

A vaginal examination should be performed in women, to look for blood and lacerations resulting from either direct damage or pelvic fractures. The pelvic ring should not be 'rocked' by applying heavy manual pressure to the iliac crests, but should be carefully examined to investigate for lack of continuity. 'Rocking' can be extremely painful and causes further damage and bleeding.

Extremities

Both arms and legs should be examined for contusion or deformity. Each should be assessed for:

- pain
- pallor
- pulse
- paraesthesia
- paralysis
- cold
- perspiration
- instability
- crepitus.

Any injuries should be realigned and splinted. Every time this is done, the limb must be reassessed. Any open wounds should be covered with a sterile dressing. If at any time during the secondary survey a patient's condition deteriorates, returning to the primary survey with institution or reinstitution of resuscitative measures is essential. The primary and secondary surveys should be repeated to ascertain any deterioration in the patient's condition.

Special care should be taken to examine body regions where injuries are easily missed or underestimated:

- back of head and scalp
- neck beneath semi-rigid collar
- back, buttocks and flanks
- groin creases, perineum and genitalia (D'Amours et al. 2002).

TRAUMA IN CHILDREN

Trauma is a major cause of death in children. Many of the principles for managing children are exactly the same as for adults, but it is essential that team members with paediatric experience are available. The priorities for assessment and management are identical. The only differences lie in certain aspects of children's anatomy, physiology and emotional development. It can be difficult for the inexperienced to recognize early problems.

The small size and shape of the child tends to mean that from the mechanism of injury, different patterns of injury result, and there is an increased chance of multiple injuries with the same force. Bones are flexible, which mean they tend to bend, and the structures underneath can be damaged. The high ratio between body surface area and volume puts children at higher risk of hypothermia, due to loss of heat through the skin. Children have not had the experience to develop the emotional coping strategies of adults. Particular attention should be paid to psychological considerations. If at all possible, someone known to the child is almost always a helpful support in the trauma room and should be given the opportunity to stay throughout the resuscitation.

TRAUMA IN THE ELDERLY

There are an increasing number of elderly trauma patients, not least because of demographic changes in the population. The elderly trauma patient has special needs when they are shocked as they often have:

- slower blood circulation
- decreased lung volume and compliance
- decreased cardiac function
- structural and functional changes in the skin
- decreased ability to produce heat
- delayed and decreased shivering response
- slower metabolic rate
- more sedate life-style
- decreased vasoconstrictor response
- diminished or absent sweating
- poor nutrition
- decreased perception of heat or cold.

The elderly are more at risk of developing irreversible shock than younger people. They are more likely to be chronically dehydrated, which, in addition to shock, can move the process very quickly to irreversibility.

DEFINITIVE CARE

Once the trauma patient has been assessed using the ABCDE approach, has been successfully resuscitated and has undergone a head-to-toe assessment to find all injuries, they can be moved on to the next stage of care. Definitive care may be provided in the operating theatre, intensive care unit, trauma ward or another hospital. Serious injuries are treated and definitive plans for the comprehensive care of the patient are made. It is essential the patient is in the best condition possible to undergo transfer either within the hospital

or to another care facility. Many of the areas and routes are limited, in terms of facilities, should the patient's condition deteriorate, and therefore the team should be as confident as possible about the stability of the situation. Nevertheless, appropriate items of resuscitation equipment should accompany the patient, along with suitably skilled staff.

Copies of the comprehensive records and reports, which must be kept up to date, should accompany patients wherever they are transferred. While a resuscitation is in progress, it is tempting to leave documentation until afterwards. Unless there are very few members of the team present, someone should be made responsible for recording all assessments, interventions, evaluations and plans. Pre-printed trauma sheets can be useful, both to save time and to act as an aide memoire. Fully comprehensive notes, regarding all details of the patient, contribute significantly to high standards of communication supporting the patient, and are vital to good care, not to mention medico-legal and audit purposes.

Family members and loved ones should be kept fully informed of the proceedings. The distress experienced by this group of people during resuscitation can be far longer lasting than that experienced by the patient. If possible, someone should be allocated to liaise between the resuscitation room and relatives. Although the nurse may be the ideal person, chaplains, social workers or staff from other areas of the hospital can often assume this role. Relatives can provide important information, and they should be included in patient care planning. Inviting relatives into the trauma room appears to be appropriate in some instances (Kidby 2003, Barratt & Wallis 1998, RCN & BAEM 1995).

PSYCHOLOGICAL ASPECTS

Over recent years trauma management has continued to develop alongside technical advances and evidence-based practices. As this has grown, so has the deeper understanding of the effects of trauma at a psychological level. Where trauma care has expanded from the ED setting to definitive and specialist care, so the psychological needs and the long-term social effects of events must be considered.

Most of the resources associated with trauma management in terms of funding, education and research are directed towards physiological and life-threatening aspects. However, some of the more lasting effects are from the emotional damage trauma has inflicted on patients and their relatives (Larner 2005).

Psychological aspects of care must be addressed early if long-term damage is to be avoided. There is strong belief that immediate intervention assists with the healing of any psychological trauma. Basic interventions, including clear explanations, addressing patient's fears and considering physical comfort, will make a difference during the acute phase of resuscitation. As members of the trauma team everyone takes a role assisting with the psychological support of the patient, although practically this role is often considered to be the remit of the nurse, who can make a significant contribution by combining nursing skills with the increasingly sophisticated methods of managing trauma.

CONCLUSION

Good trauma care relies heavily on a multidisciplinary approach. Not all trauma team members give 'hands-on' care, but each department and speciality has a valuable part to play. Successful initial assessment using a systematic approach every time, by every team member, will ensure that injuries are not missed. This gives the trauma patient the best possible chance of a complete and speedy recovery.

A great deal of progress has been made over the last two decades, but there still remains a great deal to do. In the past, trauma patients have died as the result of relatively simple problems such as hypovolaemia and hypoxia. Many of us are now aware of ways to prevent such deaths. However, it is essential that all those who come into contact with trauma patients have the necessary skills and knowledge. Investment in training of this nature is a small price to pay for a reduction in trauma deaths.

References

American College of Surgeons (2004) *Advanced Trauma Life Support*, 7th edn. Chicago: American College of Surgeons.

Barratt F, Wallis DN (1998) Relatives in the resuscitation room: their point of view. *Journal of Accident and Emergency Medicine*, **15**, 109.

Bickell W, Wail M, Pepe P et al. (1994) A comparison of immediate versus delayed fluid resuscitation for hypotensive patients with penetrating torso injury. *New England Journal of Medicine*, **331**, 1105–1109.

Casey G (2001) Oxygen transport and the use of pulse oximetry. *Nursing Standard*, **15**(47), 46–53.

Cochrane DA (2001) Hypothermia: a cold influence on trauma. *International Journal of Trauma Nursing*, **7**, 8–13.

Cole E (2004) Assessment and management of the trauma patient. *Nursing Standard*, **18**(41), 45–51.

Cooke MW (1998) Use of the spinal board within the accident and emergency department. *Journal of Accident and Emergency Medicine*, **15**, 108–109.

D'Amours SK, Sugrue M, Deane SA (2002) Initial management of the polytrauma patient: a practical approach to an Australian major trauma service. *Scandinavian Journal of Surgery*, **91**, 23–33.

Edwards B (1995) Management of spiritual distress. *Emergency Nurse*, **3**(2), 23–25.

Greaves I, Porter K, Ryan J (2001) *Trauma Care Manual*. London: Arnold.

Hadfield L (1993) Preparation for the nurse as part of the trauma team. *Accident & Emergency Nursing*, **1**(3), 154–160.

Halpern JS (1989) Mechanisms and patterns of trauma. *Journal of Emergency Nursing*, **15**(5), 380–388.

Kauvar DS, Wade CE (2005) The epidemiology and modern management of traumatic hemorrhage: US and international perspectives. *Critical Care*, **9**(Suppl. 5), S1–9.

Kidby J (2003) Family-witnessed cardiopulmonary resuscitation. *Nursing Standard*, **17**(51), 33–36.

Knoferl MW, Angele MK, Ayala A, Cioffi WG, Bland KI, Chaudry IH (1999) Do different rates of fluid resuscitation adversely or beneficially influence immune responses after trauma-hemorrhage? *Journal of Trauma: Injury, Infection and Critical Care*, **46**(1), 23–33.

Larner S (2005) Common psychological challenges for patients with newly acquired disability. *Nursing Standard*, **19**(28), 33–39.

Little G, Kelly M, Glucksman E (2001) Critical pitfalls in the immediate assessment of the trauma patient. *Trauma*, **3**, 43–51.

Nolan JP (1999) Fluid replacement. *British Medical Bulletin*, **55**, 821–843.

O'Reilly M (2003) Majory trauma management. In: Jones G, Crouch R, eds. *Emergency Nursing Care: Principles and Practice*. London: Greenwich Medical Media.

Petrie D, Lane P, Stewart TC (1996) An evaluation of patient outcomes comparing trauma team activated versus trauma team not activated using TRISS analysis Trauma and Injury Severity Score. *Journal of Trauma*, **41**, 870–873.

Pre-Hospital Trauma Life Support Committee (PHTLS) (2002) *Basic and Advanced Pre-hospital Trauma Life Support*. St Louis: Mosby Lifeline.

Rainier T, de Villiers Smit P (2003) Trauma and emergency medicine. *Emergency Medicine*, **15**(1), 11–17.

Royal College of Nursing (RCN) and British Association for Accident and Emergency Medicine (BAEM) (1995) *Bereavement Care in Accident and Emergency*. London: RCN.

Royal College of Surgeons of England (1988) *Report of the Working Party on the Management of Patients with Major Injuries*. London: Royal College of Surgeons of England.

Schierhout G, Roberts I (1998) Fluid resuscitation with colloid or crystalloid solutions in critically ill patients. *British Medical Journal*, **316**(7136), 961–964.

Sexton J (1997) Trauma epidemiology and team management. *Emergency Nurse*, **5**(1), 14–16.

Soucy DM, Rudner M, Hsia WC, Hagedorn FN, Illner H, Shires GT (1999) The effects of varying fluid volume and rate of resuscitation during uncontrolled hemorrhage. *The Journal of Trauma: Injury, Infection and Critical Care*, **46**(2), 209–215.

Span DR, Cerny V, Coats TJ et al. (2007) Management of trauma following major trauma: a European guideline. *Critical Care*, **11**, R17.

Stoneham J, Riley B, Brooks A, Matthews S (2001) Recent advances in trauma management. *Trauma*, **3**, 143–150.

Swartz C (2000) Resuscitation considerations to prevent pressure ulcers in trauma patients. *International Journal of Trauma Nursing*, **6**, 16–18.

Chapter 3

Major incidents

Tim Kilner

INTRODUCTION

Incidents involving large numbers of injured individuals are not as uncommon as people may like to believe, although over the years the profiles of these incidents have changed. Incidents are often associated with industry, transportation, mass gatherings and terrorism. The following are a few examples of incidents occurring over the last 20 years in the UK (Box 3.1).

At a local level the threat of a major incident occurring in the UK has often been viewed as remote; however, the terrorist events in New York and Washington on September 11th 2001 and more recently on the London Underground on 7th July 2005 have certainly heightened awareness. Consequently, major incident planning has assumed a greater priority than previously although there may still be an element of denial, assuming that such events will happen elsewhere.

By their very nature, major incidents are unpredictable, the only certainty being that at some time, somewhere, the unexpected will happen. But when it does, the health services must be able to respond rapidly, mobilizing additional human and material resources. Procedures must also be in place to make the most efficient use of those resources in the given circumstances. Achieving this requires the health services to be proactive in the planning of emergency management measures, thus reducing the need for reactive management in an extremely stressful situation. The Emergency Department (ED) provides the focus for the hospital's patient-care activity during the response to an incident.

This chapter discusses the role of the health services in contingency planning and service provision for major incidents. Consideration will be given to hospital-based activity, both in general terms and

Box 3.1   Examples of major incidents in the UK since 1996

Year	Incident	Dead	Injured
1996	Terrorist bomb Canary Wharf	2 dead	100 injured
1996	Shooting Dunblane	17 dead	13 injured
1996	Rail collision Watford South Junction	1 dead	69 injured
1997	100-vehicle collision A12 Essex		50 injured
1997	26-vehicle collision A19 north Yorkshire	1 dead	4 injured
1997	110-vehicle collision M42 Worcestershire	3 dead	62 injured
1997	Rail collision Southall	7 dead	160+ injured
1997	Hot-air balloon crash into cables Yorkshire	1 dead	13 injured
1997	Gas explosion south London		8 injured
1998	Gas leak in factory York		31 injured
1998	Terrorist bomb Omagh	29 dead	200+ injured
1999	Rail collision Cheshire		27 injured
2000	Rail collision Hatfield	4 dead	35 injured
2001	Explosion in steelworks Port Talbot	2 dead	13 injured
2001	Rail/road vehicle collision Selby	10 dead	76+ injured
2002	Coach collision Cumbria		43 injured
2002	Coach collision Berkshire	7 dead	35 injured
2002	100-vehicle collision Oxford	2 dead	20+ injured
2002	30–50-vehicle collision north Yorkshire		24 injured
2002	Coach collision Heathrow	5 dead	40 injured
2003	Rail collision Chancery Lane		32 injured
2003	Minibus collision Manchester	7 dead	7 injured
2004	Fire at care home Glasgow	10 dead	6 injured
2004	Factory explosion Glasgow	9 dead	40+ injured
2004	Rail collision Upton Nevet	7 dead	150 injured
2005	Multiple terrorist explosion London	52 dead	700+ injured

specifically in relation to in-hospital emergency services. The on-scene response to a major incident is considered in Chapter 1.

In England the primary source of guidance to assist the NHS in planning a response to a major incident is contained in DoH Mass Casualties Incidents – a Framework for Planning (2007), which is influenced by the requirements of the Civil Contingencies Act 2004 (Cabinet Office 2004). Guidance for Scotland, Wales and Northern Ireland is issued by the Health Departments of each of the Administrations.

DEFINITION

Guidance from the Department of Health (1996a,b) defines a major incident as: 'Any occurrence that presents serious threat to the health of the community, disruption to service or causes (or is likely to cause) such numbers or types of casualties as to require special arrangements to be implemented by hospitals, ambulance trusts or primary care organizations'.

This definition reflects the departure from the view that major incidents only result from the 'big bang' scenario such as a rail collision or a building collapse. Guidance now recognizes that major incidents can also occur in a variety of different ways (NHS Management Executive 1998, National Audit Office 2002), such as

- rising tide – such as a developing infectious disease epidemic or an outbreak of legionnaires' disease (Smith et al., 2005)
- cloud on the horizon – a serious incident elsewhere which may develop and need preparatory action such as a cloud of toxic gas from a fire at an industrial plant
- headline news – public alarm about a personal threat
- internal incident – such as a fire in the hospital or power failure
- deliberate release of chemical, biological, radiation or nuclear material
- pre-planned major events – such as sporting or entertainment mass gatherings.

PLANNING

Each NHS organization must have a major incident plan based upon risk assessment, cooperation with partners, communicating with the public and information sharing. It is the Chief Executive's responsibility to ensure such a plan is in place and to keep the Trust Board up to date with the plan.

The plan should outline actions for the acute trust to discharge its responsibilities, namely:

- provide a safe and secure environment for the assessment and treatment of patients
- provide a safe and secure environment for staff that will ensure the health, safety and welfare of staff including appropriate arrangements for the professional and personal indemnification of staff
- provide a clinical response including provision of general support and specific/specialist healthcare to all casualties, victims and responders
- liaise with the ambulance service, SHA, local Primary Care Organizations (including GPs, out-of-hours services, Minor Injuries Units (MIUs) and other primary care providers), other hospitals, independent sector providers, and other agencies in order to manage the impact of the incident
- ensure there is an operational response to provide at-scene medical cover using, for example, BASICS and other immediate-care teams where they exist; members of these teams will be trained to an appropriate standard; the Medical Incident Commander should not routinely be taken from the receiving hospital so as not to deplete resources
- ensure that the hospital reviews all its essential functions throughout the incident
- provide appropriate support to any designated receiving hospital or other neighbouring service that is substantially affected
- provide limited decontamination facilities and personal protective equipment to manage contaminated self presenting casualties
- acute Trusts will be expected to establish a Memorandum of Understanding (MOU) with their local Fire and Rescue Service on decontamination
- acute Trusts will need to make arrangements to reflect national guidance from the Home Office for dealing with the bodies of contaminated patients who die at the hospital
- liaise with activated health emergency control centres and/or on call SHA/PCO Officers as appropriate
- maintain communications with relatives and friends of existing patients and those from the incident, the Casualty Bureau, the local community, the media and VIPs.

The very nature of major incidents brings together diverse groups of professionals in large numbers, each group having distinct roles and responsibilities. When faced with the complexities of a major incident, it is unrealistic to expect such a large multidisciplinary team to function in an effective and coordinated manner without detailed prior planning. It is therefore essential that planning assumes an appropriately high priority.

TRAINING

There is an expectation that staff understand the role they would adopt in a major incident, have the competencies to fulfil that role and have received training to fulfil those competencies. There is some evidence to suggest that staff are not entirely familiar with the action they should take in a major incident (Carr et al. 2006). It is suggested that acute trusts should consider providing annual training and development for staff to enable them to meet these expectations. There is also a requirement for all NHS organizations to undertake a live exercise every 3 years, a table-top exercise each year and a test of communication cascades every 6 months (DH Emergency Preparedness Division 2005).

Large-scale exercises serve a number of purposes: enabling major incident plans to be tested; allowing the rehearsal of practical skills in realistic environments; and working alongside other services, establishing working relationships with individuals and organizations likely to be involved in a true response. However, large exercises do not allow detailed scrutiny of any one aspect of the plan; rather, there is a superficial overview of the plan as a whole. Large-scale exercises should be as realistic as possible in all respects and be based upon the more likely incidents that may occur locally, to gain full benefit from testing the emergency response and making the experience as meaningful as possible.

The timing of an exercise is also of importance. If possible, it is preferable not to advise personnel exactly when the exercise will take place, as forewarning will inevitably create a false state of preparation and readiness which will not truly reflect the response to a 'real' incident. However, there is a need to ensure that exercises do not unduly disrupt the normal functioning of the service, so an acceptable compromise must be reached when planning and informing staff of exercises. The organization and enactment of full or 'live' exercises are expensive in terms of time, personnel and resources, and these factors make exercises of considerable financial cost. Combining exercises with other services and agencies, many of which also have statutory requirements to exercise, can keep costs to a minimum. It may be that in some circumstances other forms of exercise, which may be more cost-effective and appropriate in meeting response and training needs, should also be considered.

Small-scale exercises allow part of the plan to be examined in detail, utilizing skill and task-specific activities, but do not always highlight problems which may occur when influenced by the activity of other departments or organizations. Table-top exercises allow a greater range of activities to be scrutinized in detail, but are largely theoretical and may not highlight logistical problems or poor skill levels resulting from inadequate training.

Given that each method has limitations, there is a case for exercise and training to make use of a combination of these techniques and not to be reliant upon one method.

The hospital should carry out an internal communications/call-in exercise at least every 6 months and exercise communications systems between themselves and the ambulance service at regular intervals. Exercising of plans also provides an opportunity to review procedures and make amendments in the light of lessons learned from testing implementation. Lack of practice in implementing the plan allows deficits, inconsistencies and errors to go undetected until a major incident occurs.

MAJOR INCIDENT ALERTING PROCEDURES

In the event of a 'big bang' major incident it is likely the ambulance service will be the first to become aware of the incident. In this case they will be responsible, on confirmation of the incident, for alerting all appropriate partners within the health community.

The acute trust should be alerted by one of two messages: either 'major incident standby' indicating a major incident may need to be declared, or 'major incident declared – activate plan', indicating that the major incident plan should be implemented and all appropriate action should commence.

The alert will be terminated with either 'major incident – cancelled', indicating a stand down from the alert and a halt to the implementation of the plan, or 'major incident stand down', indicating that all live casualties have left scene, but some may still be en route to hospital.

In the event of a 'rising tide' incident the alert is most likely to come from either the Strategic Health Authority or from one of the Primary Care Organizations. Acute trusts may declare a major incident, initiated by the most senior person available in the trust at that time, and this may result from an incident where casualties self-present prior to the ambulance service being aware. In such cases it is essential that the ambulance service are immediately alerted and updated as a matter of urgency.

THE HOSPITAL'S RESPONSE TO A MAJOR INCIDENT ALERT

The emergency department

The primary responsibility of the ED is the reception and treatment of patients. This will include the establishment of reception areas and treatment areas with appropriate access and egress to control patient flow, and decontamination facilities where necessary. Systems should be implemented to provide clinical records for each patient and for the management of patients' possessions.

During this stage of the incident, relevant nursing and medical staff will be contacted and deployed to activity pre-determined by individual action cards. If additional nursing staff are required by the ED, then an appropriately designated person should initiate a 'call-in' procedure. Other involved areas in the hospital will also activate similar procedures, which may also involve the use of personnel from voluntary organizations. It is often advisable to call in staff rostered for the next shift but one in the department, as this allows for an already rostered fresh shift to come in to relieve those involved in the initial response and allows the present and called-in shifts an opportunity to rest. This is not always possible as the bulk of the current shift may be rostered for the shift after next, e.g. today's late shift staff are tomorrow's early shift staff.

It may also be advisable to distinguish ED nurses and doctors from other staff deployed to the department from elsewhere by the use of identifying tabards. If possible, additional staff deployed into ED should have ED or critical-care experience and should not be utilized in treatment teams without the presence of at least one experienced ED nurse. Nurses from other areas can play useful roles in dealing with minor injuries and in transferring casualties from the treatment areas to admission wards.

Receipt of casualties

Within ED, all of the patients in the department at the time of the major incident alert should have the situation explained to them and their conditions reassessed. Those awaiting treatment or with minor injuries should be given any appropriate first-aid treatment and advised to go home, attend their local community hospital or see their GP. More seriously injured or ill patients should be rapidly stabilized and transferred to a ward.

It should be borne in mind that during a major incident the ED may still receive casualties who have not been involved in the incident, especially if they make their own way to the department. It may be prudent to make facilities available to treat such casualties and to ensure their details and documentation do not become included with those of the major-incident casualties. The department should prepare facilities for the reception and treatment of casualties according to their priority for treatment. This commonly involves the utilization of appropriately identified areas, adjacent to the ED if possible, for the collection and treatment of those with a lower clinical priority. Within the ED and other areas identified for casualty reception and treatment, appropriate types and amounts of equipment should be prepared. To enable this essential equipment to be rapidly available for use, stocks should be held in an easily accessible place within the department, and planning with the central sterile supply department, pharmacy and other departments should enable additional supplies to be quickly procured to replenish the stocks held in ED, such as chest drain packs and controlled analgesic drugs.

Each patient should receive a uniquely numbered identification bracelet and set of records. As immediate identification of the casualty may be difficult and time-consuming, this unique number will accompany the patient throughout the hospital system. The triage labels used at the incident scene should also be uniquely numbered and, if it is practical to use this number within the hospital as well, tracking of the casualty will be assisted.

In the ED, arrangements should be made to receive and treat casualties with appropriate priority. On arrival at the hospital all patients should be re-triaged, documented and directed to an appropriate treatment area. Triage should be carried out by a triage team consisting of an experienced ED doctor and nurse. If separate entrances have been designated for minor and other categories, due to the geography of the hospital, two triage teams may be needed. Each patient will be assigned a triage category and a unique identification number – preferably the same as on the triage label from the scene. Further identification and documentation of patients will take place as their condition allows and will be carried out by members of the police documentation team and hospital administrative staff. Information regarding the numbers and identities of patients will be compiled by the police documentation team and relayed at regular intervals to the police's casualty bureau, where it will be combined with information from the scene, rest centres, mortuary and other sources, such as transport companies' passenger lists.

Patient care

Treatment may be facilitated by organizing available staff into 'treatment teams'. A treatment team can consist of two doctors and two nurses. At least one of the nurses should be an ED nurse. Each 'immediate priority' patient will require one treatment team for their care in the department. However, one team should be able to manage the care of two or three urgent priority patients, and the area designated for delayed priority ('minor') patients should be manageable using two teams. The medical and nursing staff in ED should aim to treat, stabilize and transfer immediate and urgent casualties out of the initial treatment areas as rapidly as possible, to allow treatment of the maximum number of casualties. However, in reality, the number of immediate and urgent patients that a hospital will be able to accept will be limited by the number of intensive care, high-dependency care and operating theatre spaces available.

While casualties in the minor area may be initially regarded as having a low priority, their conditions may change. It is therefore important that at least some of the nurses allocated to this area are suitably experienced and are able to re-triage casualties into higher categories when required and arrange for their transfer to a more appropriate treatment area as necessary, especially as areas designated for the treatment of minor injuries may be geographically separated from the main ED treatment areas, such as an outpatients department.

Transfer teams will also be required to transfer critically ill patients from the treatment area to critical care areas or to the operating theatres. These teams may consist of a doctor and a nurse, preferably both with critical care experience, and preferably two porters, as medical and nursing staff are needed for patient care and should not be pushing trolleys. The transfer of non-critical casualties to their admission destination can be facilitated by a nurse and a porter. In order that there is continuity of care for casualties and of record-keeping and handover, it may prove useful for one nurse to remain with the patients in immediate and urgent categories during their stay in the ED. However, the practicality of this arrangement will depend upon the number of casualties involved and the number of nurses available. It may be that this role should be fulfilled by a nurse drafted into the department from elsewhere in the hospital. During a major incident the knowledge and skills of the emergency nurse are at a premium and if their numbers are limited then they are probably best utilized in the care of critical casualties and in a resource and organization of care role, making use of other hospital nurses drafted into the department.

Hospital response

The hospital will establish a Hospital Coordinating Team (HCT) typically made up of a senior clinician, a senior nurse and a senior manager. The primary function of the HCT is to manage the hospitals response and ensure effective deployment of staff.

If the hospital is to receive patients, it is also likely that routine operating lists will be suspended and as many intensive care and high-dependency spaces as possible made free. In addition, it may be thought necessary to clear as many beds as possible in other wards by means of early discharges and by transferring patients to other, unaffected hospitals – the use of the voluntary aid societies and their vehicles may be indicated for this task as the ambulance service is unlikely to be able to support this activity. The Civil Contingencies Home Office Act (2004) now places statutory responsibilities on primary care organizations to cooperate with other responders to an incident and to have a plan in place. It should be possible, in theory at least, for beds to be made available in a major incident but there is a reliance on primary care organizations having plans for some surge capacity in the event of such an emergency.

Restriction of access

Maintaining security, controlling access to the hospital and the containment of casualties, relatives and the media in specified areas of the hospital are vital tasks essential to the effectiveness of the hospital's response. Full security and containment arrangements must be in place as soon as possible after the hospital has received notification to activate its plan.

If possible, access to all involved areas should be limited to one entrance and egress to one exit. All other entrances should be locked or closed by security personnel. Only those staff with appropriate identification should be allowed into the hospital, the ED and associated treatment and collection points. Major incidents cause a convergence of individuals and groups on the hospital, focusing upon the ED. Well-meaning and interested hospital and non-hospital nursing and medical staff, various volunteers and voluntary groups will cause a disrupted and confused response and their access must be prevented.

It is advisable that hospital staff do not leave their own departments or come to the hospital until they are requested to do so via the recognized communication channels. A decision will also have to be made whether or not to use non-requested, non-hospital medical, nursing and other volunteers who offer their services. The potential legal ramifications of using possibly unqualified impostors and/or the possibility of negligence claims resulting from their practices may well outweigh any useful function that they may be able to perform.

The media

The media, who will no doubt have gathered at the hospital, should be provided with regular and accurate press releases. The media are under pressure during a major incident to meet deadlines and if they do not receive adequate and appropriate information they may set about seeking it out for themselves. The needs of the media should be addressed in ways which will not compromise the emergency response of the hospital and its staff or the confidentiality of casualties and relatives. Only designated members of staff, who preferably have been prepared for this role, should address the media and only statements prepared in consultation with the appropriate emergency services and approved by the hospital's major incident coordination team should be released. Any access to casualties and staff should be very carefully controlled, with ground rules being agreed and consent obtained before any interviews take place.

MEDICOLEGAL ISSUES

During the response to a major incident in the hospital or at the scene, nurses must consider a number of legal and professional issues. Major incident scenes are considered to be 'scenes of crime' until proven otherwise and consideration must be given to the preservation of forensic evidence. Such evidence, e.g. clothing, debris, etc., may leave the scene with casualties and, as a result, be present in the emergency department and other areas of the hospital. Every effort should be made to collect and preserve this evidence in collaboration with the police. Of course, in all circumstances, preservation of life takes priority over the preservation of evidence.

Criminal investigations and prosecutions, civil actions, official inquiries and inquests are all possible following a major incident. Some of the staff involved in the management of the incident are likely to be required to provide statements and/or give evidence. It should also be remembered that all documentation completed during the incident can be used not only as a source of evidence to explain what happened, but possibly also to suggest negligence.

Although staff are working under considerable pressure at the time of an incident, all documentation should be adequate, clear and accurate. Nurses should consider that the pressures of a major incident do not remove their professional accountability for practice, and they may well be asked to justify the actions that they took, both inside and outside the ED, at a later date. Staff should also be aware that the plan, including any action cards, is a written document and, as such, essentially becomes an approved policy document of the organization and provides standards and descriptions of expected activities against which the actions of staff may be judged by any investigation, whether internal or external.

AFTERMATH

During and in the aftermath of a major incident, it is important to recognize that both casualties and staff may be psychologically and/or spiritually affected by events that are outside the normal range of experience. As a consequence they may be at risk of developing post-trauma stress reactions and doubting long-held beliefs.

Hospital major incident plans must include arrangements to provide patients, relatives and staff with appropriate psychological and spiritual support during and after the event. Psychological support may be provided by appropriately trained personnel from the mental health professions or other statutory or voluntary bodies. Religious representatives from the major groupings should also be available, as well as a contact list of representatives from a broad range of spiritual beliefs so that individual needs may be met as far as is possible. Both psychological and spiritual support should be available from the outset and throughout the incident. Follow-up services such as psychological debriefing should also be made available to all of those involved as part of the plan.

CONCLUSION

Major incidents are rare, but they do happen. It is essential that the acute trust plan is based on risk assessment and takes into account other major incident plans within the health community and the work of Local Resilience Fora. For the plan to be successful individuals need to be familiar with their role within the plan and the actions they need to take and to be appropriately skilled, trained and rehearsed for that role.

References

Carr ERM, Chatrath P, Palan P (2006) Audit of doctors' knowledge of major incident policies. *Annals of the Royal College of Surgeons of England,* **88**(3), 313–315.

Department of Health Emergency Preparedness Division (2007) *Mass Casualty Incidents – a Framework for Planning.* London: Department of Health.

Home Office (2004) *Civil Contingencies Act.* London: Home Office.

HSE (1996a) *Emergency Planning in the NHS: Health Services Arrangements for Dealing with Major Incidents,* vol. 1. London: Department of Health.

HSE (1996b) *Emergency Planning in the NHS: Health Services Arrangements for Dealing with Major Incidents,* vol. 2. London: Department of Health.

National Audit Office (2002) *Facing the Challenge: NHS Emergency Planning in England.* London: National Audit Office.

NHS Management Executive (1998) *Planning for Major Incidents: The NHS Guidance.* London: Department of Health.

Smith AF, Wild C, Law J (2005) The Barrow-in-Furness legionnaires' outbreak: qualitative study of the hospital response and the role of the major incident plan. *Emergency Medicine Journal,* **22**(4), 251–255.

PART 2

Trauma care

PART CONTENTS

Chapter 4

Head injuries

Karen Lesley Sanders

INTRODUCTION

One million patients attend emergency departments in the UK each year with head injuries. For most their head injury is minor. Nine out of ten people seen in hospital have a minor head injury and are not admitted to hospital. Of those admitted to hospital, most will be able to go home after 48 hours (NICE 2003).

There are many causes of head injuries, with road traffic accidents (RTAs) being the single largest cause. Other common causes include falls, assaults and sports injuries. There is an increased incidence of head injuries in young males and children (NICE 2003). Eighty per cent of head injuries in the UK are minor (Glasgow Coma Scale (GCS) 13–15), 10% are moderate (GCS 9–12) and 10% are severe (GCS less than 8). Severe head injuries account for 50% of trauma-related deaths in the UK. Five to ten per cent of patients who suffer a severe head injury also suffer a cervical spine injury.

Severe head injuries, i.e. brain injuries, are uncommon because the skull and scalp absorb most of the impact of the assault. The amount of damage suffered is relative to the power of the assault. A high-energy head injury results from the following circumstances: when a pedestrian is struck by a motor vehicle, an occupant is ejected from a motor vehicle, a person falls from a height of greater than 1 metre or more than five stairs (a lower threshold for the height of falls should be used when dealing with infants and young children under 5 years old), following a diving accident, following a high-speed motor vehicle collision, following a rollover motor accident or a bicycle collision (NICE 2003).

It is vital that the emergency nurse caring for patients with head injuries has a good knowledge and understanding of the anatomy and physiology of the skull, the brain and its related structures along with the physiological processes that maintain homeostasis. Such knowledge and understanding allows the nurse to relate the mechanisms of injury to the brain injuries suffered and thus assess, plan, evaluate and implement the care and management needed by the patient at any particular stage following the injury.

A structured approach to the care of head-injured patients should be initiated. The system advocated by the Advanced Trauma Life Support (ATLS) system (American College of Surgeons 2004) provides a mechanism for assessment and immediate management and minimizes the risk of secondary brain injury in adults. For children the advanced paediatric life support (APLS) system should be employed (NICE 2003).

ANATOMY AND PHYSIOLOGY

The skull

The skull is a rigid bony cavity composed of 29 individual bones: the 8 bones of the cranium, 14 facial bones, the 6 ossicles of the ear and the hyoid bone. To ensure maximum protection, strength and support, bony capsules surround the brain, the eyes, the nasal passages and the inner ear; and bony buttresses extend upwards from the teeth through the facial bones. To relieve the potential weight, the skull is made lighter by the paranasal sinuses, which also give resonance to the voice.

The cranium is one of the strongest structures in the body and provides the bony protection for the brain. It is composed of the parietal (2), occipital, frontal, temporal (2), sphenoid and ethmoid bones. Figure 4.1 shows an exploded view of the cranial skull; however, the bones are fused along main sutures, the saggital, coronal, lambdoidal and squamosal. The facial bones form the framework for the nasal and oral cavities and include the zygomatic bones (2), palatine bones (2), mandible, maxilla (2), lacrimal bones (2), nasal bones (2), vomer and the inferior nasal concha (2) (see Fig. 4.2).

Figure 4.3 shows the irregular internal surfaces of the skull. These irregular surfaces/bony protrusions account for injury to the brain as it moves within the skull under acceleration/deceleration forces.

The meninges

The brain and the spinal cord are encased by three layers of membrane – the dura mater, the arachnoid mater and the pia mater known collectively as the meninges (see Fig. 4.4).

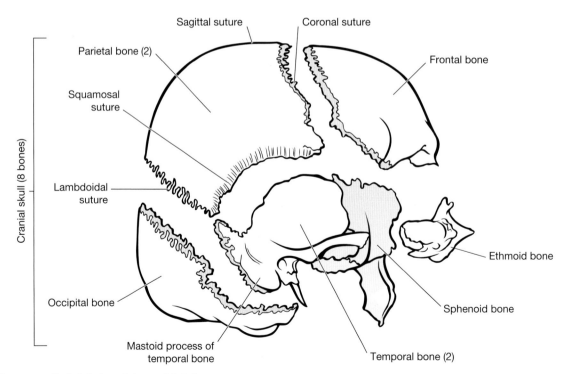

Figure 4.1 Exploded view of the cranial skull.

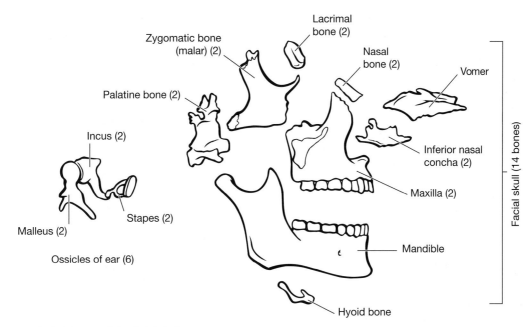

Figure 4.2 Exploded view of the facial skull.

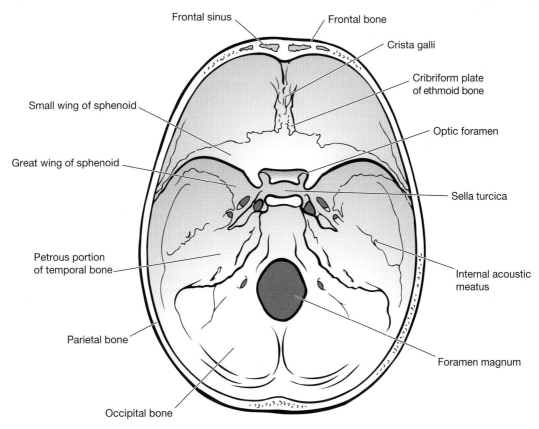

Figure 4.3 View of the base of the skull from above.

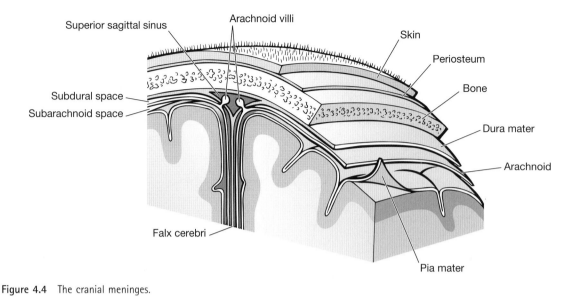

Figure 4.4 The cranial meninges.

The dura mater

The dura mater consists of two layers: the outer layer is the periosteal layer of the skull, which terminates at the foramen magnum, and the inner layer is a strong, thick membrane that is continuous with the spinal dura mater. There is a potential space between the two dura, except at the falx cerebri, which divides the left and right hemispheres of the cerebrum; the tentorium cerebelli, which divides the cerebrum and cerebellum; the falx cerebelli, which divides the lateral lobes of the cerebellum; and the diaphragm sellae. The dura creates a roof for the sella turcica (which houses the pituitary gland). These compartments provide support and protection for the brain and form the sinuses, which drain venous blood from the brain (Lindsey et al. 2004, Crossman & Neary 2000).

The arachnoid mater

The arachnoid mater is fine serous membrane that loosely covers the brain. There is a potential space between this and the inner dura mater, known as the subdural space. Between the arachnoid mater and the pia mater is an actual space, known as the subarachnoid space, which contains the arachnoid villi, cerebrospinal fluid (CSF) and small blood vessels.

The pia mater

The pia mater follows the convolutions and is attached to the surface of the brain. It consists of fine connective tissue, housing the majority of the blood supply to the brain.

The ventricles and cerebrospinal fluid

Within the brain there are four connected cavities called ventricles, which contain cerebrospinal fluid (CSF). These are the left and right lateral ventricles, the third ventricle and the fourth ventricle. The lateral ventricles lie in the cerebral hemispheres, the third in the diencephalon and the fourth in the brain stem. The lateral ventricles are connected to the third ventricle by the interventricular foramen, sometimes known as the foramen of Munro, and the third ventricle is connected to the fourth by the cerebral aqueduct, sometimes known as the aqueduct of Sylvius (see Fig. 4.5).

CSF is a clear, colourless fluid composed of water, some protein, oxygen, carbon dioxide, sodium, potassium, chloride and glucose. Its purpose is to protect the brain from injury by providing a cushioning effect. The major source of CSF is from the secretions of the choroid plexus, found in the ventricles. The choroid plexus produce approximately 500 ml of CSF daily; however, the average adult brain only holds between 125 and 150 ml. CSF is renewed and replaced approximately three times daily, being reabsorbed through the arachnoid villi, which drain into the superior saggital sinus, when the CSF pressure exceeds the venous pressure. Normal CSF pressure is 60–180 mmH$_2$O in the lumbar puncture position (lateral recumbent) and 200–350 mmH$_2$O in the sitting position.

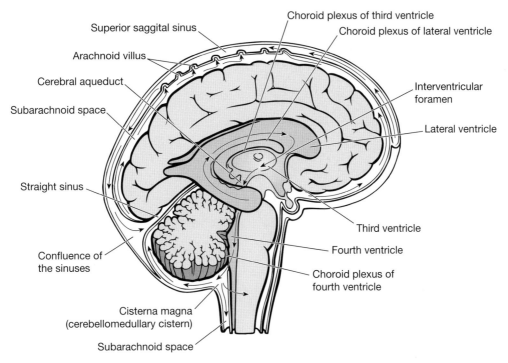

Figure 4.5   Ventricles of the brain and circulatory path of cerebrospinal fluid through the cranial pathways.

The brain

The brain consists of three main areas:

- cerebrum
- cerebellum
- brain stem.

The major structures within the brain are summarized in Box 4.1.

Cerebrum

The cerebrum consists of two cerebral hemispheres, which are partially separated by the longitudinal fissure and connected at the bottom by the corpus callosum. It is generally accepted that one hemisphere (usually the left) is more highly developed than the other. The left side of the brain has been shown to control the right side of the body, spoken and written language, scientific reasoning and numerical skills, whereas the right side is more concerned with emotion and artistic and creative skills. However, at birth, the hemispheres are of equal ability and very early injury to one side or another usually results in skills being acquired by the opposite side of the brain. Each cerebral hemisphere has an area of grey matter called the basal ganglia, which assists in the motor control of fine body movements.

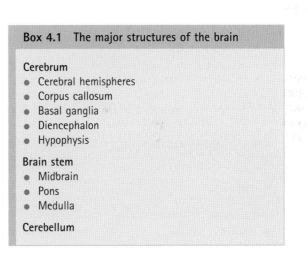

Box 4.1   The major structures of the brain

Cerebrum
- Cerebral hemispheres
- Corpus callosum
- Basal ganglia
- Diencephalon
- Hypophysis

Brain stem
- Midbrain
- Pons
- Medulla

Cerebellum

The surface area of the cerebral cortex (grey matter), on the surface of the brain is much increased by the presence of gyri and sulci (see Fig. 4.6), resulting in a 3:1 proportion of grey to white matter. Below the cortex lies the white matter. The cerebral hemispheres are composed of four lobes, the frontal, parietal, temporal and occipital lobes. Box 4.2 summarizes the main functions of these lobes.

The diencephalon is located deep into the cerebrum and consists of the thalamus, hypothalamus,

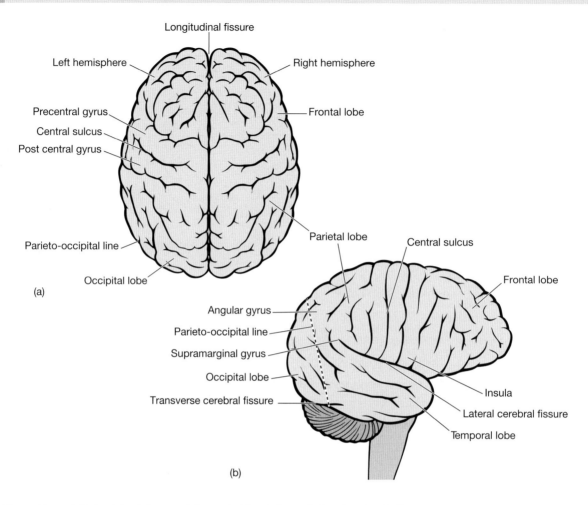

Figure 4.6 a, b Gyri, sulci and fissures of the cerebral hemispheres. A: Superior view. B: Right lateral view.

Box 4.2 The functions of the cerebral cortex by lobe

Frontal
- Motor
- Expression
- Moral

Parietal
- Sensation
- Spatial

Temporal
- Auditory
- Equilibrium
- Interpretive
- Intellectual

Occipital
- Visual

---

sub-thalamus and epithalamus. It connects the mid-brain to the cerebral hemispheres. The hypothalamus includes several important structures, such as the optic chiasma, the point at which the two optic tracts cross and the stalk of the pituitary gland (hypophysis).

Cerebellum
The cerebellum is situated behind the pons and attached to the midbrain, pons and medulla by three-paired cerebellar peduncles. It consists of three main parts:

- the cortex
- the white matter, which forms the connecting pathways for impulses joining the cerebellum with other parts of the central nervous system
- four pairs of deep cerebellar nuclei.

The cerebellum is the processing centre for co-ordination of muscular movements, balance, precision, timing and body positions. It does not initiate any movements and is not involved with the conscious perception of sensations.

Brain stem

The brain stem is the connection between the brain and the spinal cord and is continuous with the diencephalon above and the spinal cord below. Within the brain stem are ascending and descending pathways between the spinal cord and parts of the brain. All cranial nerves except the olfactory (1) and the optic (2) nerves emerge from the brain stem (see Fig. 4.7). The brain stem is formed from three main structures:

- Midbrain connects the pons and the cerebellum to the cerebrum. It is involved with visual reflexes, the movement of the eyes, focusing and the dilatation of the pupils. Contained within the midbrain and upper pons is the reticular activating system, which is responsible for the 'awake' state.
- Pons is located between the midbrain and the medulla and serves as a relay station from the medulla to higher structures in the brain. It is involved with the control of respiratory function.
- Medulla connects the pons and the spinal cord. The point of decussation of the pyramidal tract occurs within the medulla. The vital centres

associated with autonomic reflex activity are present in its deeper structure. These are the cardiac, respiratory and vasomotor centres and the reflex centres of coughing, swallowing, vomiting and sneezing.

Cerebral circulation

The brain is supplied with blood by four major arteries: two internal carotid arteries, which supply most of the cerebrum and both eyes; and two vertebral arteries, which supply the cerebellum, brain stem and the posterior part of the cerebrum. Before the blood enters the cerebrum it passes through the circle of Willis, which is a circular shunt at the base of the brain consisting of the posterior cerebral, the posterior communicating, the internal carotids, the anterior cerebral and the anterior communicating arteries (see Fig. 4.8 and Fig. 4.9). These vessels are frequently anomalous; however, they allow for an adequate blood supply to all the brain, even if one or more is ineffective.

The venous drainage from the brain does not follow a similar pathway (Fig. 4.10). Cerebral veins empty into large venous sinuses located in the folds of the dura mater. Bridging veins connect the brain and the dural sinuses and are often the cause of

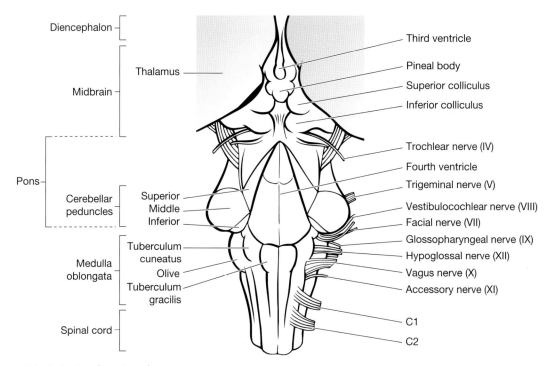

Figure 4.7 Brain stem (dorsal view).

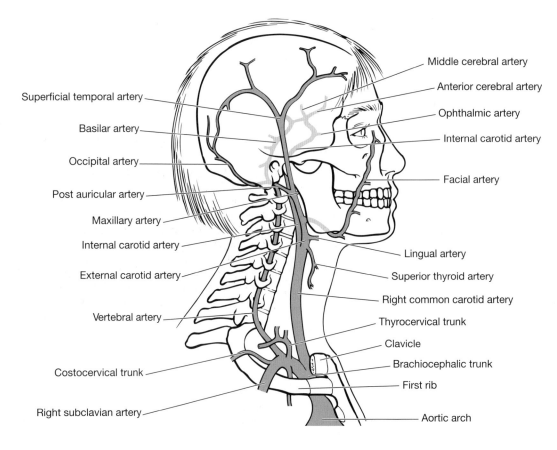

Figure 4.8 Major arteries of the head and neck.

subdural haematomas. These sinuses empty into the internal jugular veins, which sit on either side of the neck and return the blood to the heart via the brachiocephalic veins.

The brain, especially the grey matter, has an extensive capillary bed, requiring approximately 15–20% of the total resting cardiac output, about 750 ml/min. Glucose, required for metabolism in the brain, requires about 20% of the total oxygen consumed in the body for its oxidation. Blood flow to specific areas of the brain correlates directly with the metabolism of the cerebral tissue.

PHYSIOLOGY OF RAISED INTRACRANIAL PRESSURE

Intracranial pressure (ICP) represents the pressure exerted by the cerebrospinal fluid (CSF) within the ventricles of the brain (Hickey 1997). The exact pressure varies in different areas of the brain. Its normal range is 0–15 mmHg in adults, 3–7 mmHg in children and 1.5–6 mmHg in term babies when measured from the Foramen of Munro.

ICP is fundamental in maintaining adequate brain function. The brain lies in the skull, a rigid compartment. The contents of the skull are non-compressible, i.e. brain tissue (80%), intravascular blood (10%) and cerebrospinal fluid (10%). Normally these components maintain a fairly constant volume, therefore creating dynamic equilibrium therein. Should one or more component increase for whatever reason the Monro-Kellie hypothesis states that another component must decrease in quantity in order to maintain the dynamic equilibrium and thus maintain adequate cerebral blood flow (CBF). If this does not occur, ICP rises, leading to brain injury (Hickey 1997). Dynamic equilibrium is maintained by a number of compensatory mechanisms: these include

● increasing CSF absorption
● decreasing CSF production
● shunting of CSF to the spinal subarachnoid space
● vasoconstriction – reducing cerebral blood flow.

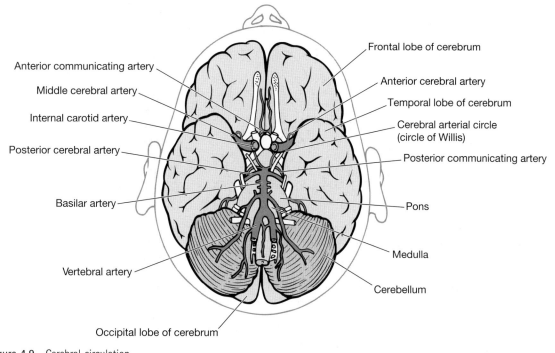

Figure 4.9 Cerebral circulation.

Maintenance of the dynamic equilibrium in the brain is further aided by autoregulation. Autoregulation is the ability of the brain to maintain a relatively constant CBF over a wide range of perfusion pressures (60–160 mmHg). Autoregulation is initiated by cerebral perfusion pressure (CPP), which is defined as the blood pressure gradient across the brain and is calculated by subtracting ICP from the systemic mean arterial pressure (MAP)

$$CPP = MAP - ICP$$

In healthy adults CPP is 60–70 mmHg. Should the patient's MAP fall and/or the patient's ICP increase, there is a risk that the cerebral perfusion pressure will fall to too low a value to maintain adequate cerebral blood flow. This will result in hypoxia and cerebral ischaemia, causing secondary brain injury. CPP should be maintained between 70 and 100 mmHg. Autoregulation fails should the CPP fall below 60 mmHg or rise above 160 mmHg. It is raised ICP, decreased MAP or reduced CPP, which is responsible for most secondary brain injury.

Chemoregulation is triggered by changes in extracellular pH and metabolic by-products. Changes in PCO_2 or a dramatic reduction in PO_2 (see Fig. 4.11) may also trigger it. In the head-injured patient, maintaining adequate oxygenation is vital, because allowing the PCO_2 to rise initiates chemoregulation, which in turn increases ICP, because it increases overall brain mass due to the resulting vasodilatation. Cerebral vasoconstriction reduces brain mass, and it is for this reason that ventilated head-injured patients are hyperventilated, as this reduces PCO_2 and activates chemoregulation, thus inducing vasoconstriction which helps to reduce ICP.

The mechanisms which compensate for rises in ICP in the healthy adult brain fail as ICP reaches 20 mmHg. From then on, small increases in brain mass, blood volume or CSF have a profound effect on ICP. Chestnut (1993) demonstrated a clear correlation between the length of time the patient's ICP remains greater than 20 mmHg and an increased mortality and morbidity rate.

CLASSIFICATION OF HEAD INJURIES

Head injuries can be classified under three anatomical sites:

- the scalp
- the skull
- the brain.

Patients often present with a combination of injuries.

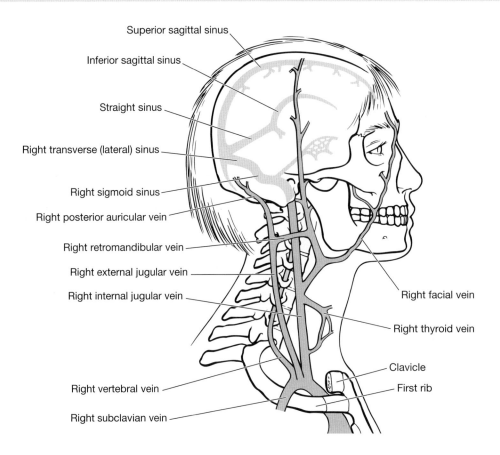

Figure 4.10 Major veins of the head and neck.

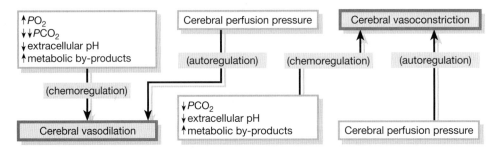

Figure 4.11 Chemoregulation of the brain.

Scalp injuries

There are four types of injury to the scalp:

- Abrasion – minor injury that may cause a small amount of bleeding. Treatment may not be required, but ice applied to the area may reduce any haematoma formation.

- Contusion – no break in the skin, but bruising to the scalp may cause blood to leak into the subcutaneous layer.
- Laceration – a cut or tear of the skin and subcutaneous fascia that tends to bleed profusely. Bleeding from the scalp alone is unlikely to cause shock in the adult. In small children, a scalp

laceration may be sufficient to cause hypovolaemia. Scalp lesions should be explored under local anaesthetic for foreign bodies and/or skull fracture with a skull X-ray if there is any doubt about the diagnosis. Lesion(s) should be sutured or glued according to their depth and position.

- Subgaleal haematoma – a haematoma below the galea, a tough layer of tissue under the subcutaneous fascia and before the skull. The veins here empty into the venous sinus, and thus any infection can spread easily to the brain, despite the skull remaining intact. There is controversy surrounding the treatment of subgaleal haematomas, due to the risks of infection; therefore some doctors argue that it is best to evacuate the haematoma, while others suggest that it is best to let it reabsorb.

If the scalp injuries are only part of other injuries, it is important they are documented to allow further investigation at a more appropriate time. They may need to be cleaned and dressed or temporarily sutured. Abrasions may not require any treatment, but ice applied to the area may reduce any haematoma formation (Hickey 1997). Lacerations can bleed extensively; however, bleeding from the scalp alone is unlikely to cause shock in the adult patient.

The skull

Skull fractures indicate that the head has suffered a major impact. Patients who suffer skull fractures have a high incidence of intracranial haematoma.

Skull fractures are classified into five groups:

- *Linear.* These are the most common types of injury. They usually result from low-velocity direct force. They are usually diagnosed from skull X-ray and need no specific treatment.
- *Depressed.* Usually evident clinically, but a skull X-ray to discover the full extent of the potential brain damage is usually necessary. Management is dependent on the severity of the fracture and whether there are any accompanying injuries. If there are no other injuries requiring surgical management, they may not be surgically elevated, due to the risks of infection. However, surgical intervention will normally be necessary if there are bone fragments imbedded in the brain so as to elevate the bone fragments and manage the brain trauma.
- *Open.* Usually evident clinically. Usually managed according to the severity of the injury. If debris is dispersed in the brain tissue then surgery will be required and there is a heightened risk of infection.

- *Comminuted.* These are detected on skull X-ray. These patients should be closely observed and any neurological deficits managed appropriately. Surgical intervention is usually required. If there are bone fragments imbedded in the brain tissue then surgery will be required to elevate the bone fragments and manage the brain trauma.
- *Basal.* Are diagnosed clinically as they are difficult to detect on X-ray. Signs include CSF leakage from the nose (rhinorrhoea) or the ear(s) (otorrhoea). Rhinorrhoea or otorrhoea indicates that a skull base fracture has breached the dura and formed a communication between the intracranial contents and an air sinus. This places the patient at risk of meningitis while the CSF leak continues. If CSF leakage is suspected, the fluid should be tested for glucose and the 'halo test' performed, where a small amount of fluid is placed on blotting paper; if CSF is present it will separate from blood and form a yellow ring around the outside of the blood. Patients with a base of skull fracture may also have retroauricular bruising (Battle's signs) and peri-orbital bruising ('panda eyes' or 'raccoon eyes'): 80–90% of cases seal within 2 weeks and usually neurosurgical intervention is not considered until this time has elapsed. An exception is a fracture of the posterior wall of the frontal sinus, visualized on CT scan, where anterior fossa repair may be undertaken early.

Patients with CSF leakage are usually prescribed prophylactic antibiotics, because of the high risk of bacterial meningitis. The available evidence, however, does not support the use of prophylactic antibiotics (Watkins 2000). If gastric decompression is indicated, the orogastric route should be used, as the nasogastric route carries the risks of trauma to the brain and the introduction of infection.

The brain

Damage to the brain as a result of trauma includes both the immediate (primary) injury which is the damage caused at the moment of the impact and the secondary injury that develops during the first few hours or days after the impact (Box 4.3). These secondary injuries may have extracranial or intracranial causes.

There are no interventions that can prevent the primary brain injury. Secondary brain insults, which further exacerbate neuronal injury and lead to a worsening outcome depending on their duration and severity, are largely preventable. The two main causes of secondary injury are delayed diagnosis and treatment of intracranial haematomas and failure to correct

---

Box 4.3   Types of brain injury

Primary brain injury

- Disruption of brain vessels
- Haemorrhagic contusion
- Diffuse axonal injury

Secondary brain injury
Extracranial insults

- Systemic hypotension
- Hypoxaemia
- Hypercarbia
- Disturbances of blood coagulation

Intracranial insults

- Haematoma (extradural, subdural, intracerebral)
- Cerebral oedema (see Fig. 4.12)
- Infection

---

systemic hypoxaemia and hypotension. Over one third of all patients who suffer a severe head injury appear to experience either hypoxia or hypotension or both during the acute post-injury period and these secondary insults correlate with a doubling of mortality and an increase in morbidity (Chesnut 1995) (see Fig. 4.12).

Brain injuries are usually categorized as either focal or diffuse injuries.

Focal injuries

Focal injuries occur in a specific area of the brain. The mechanism of injury is usually blunt injury and acceleration/deceleration injury.

Cerebral contusion – bruising of the surface of the brain is sustained as the brain hits the bony protuberances of the skull at the site of the impact (coup injury) and at the opposite side of the brain during deceleration (contrecoup injury). Cerebral contusion is a common type of brain injury, which is diagnosed by computed tomography (CT) scan, and is most commonly seen at the frontal and temporal lobes as a result of the irregular surfaces/bony protrusions of the skull. The term contusion is used when the pia mater has not been breached. The brain swells around the site(s) of the contusion(s). Bleeding may occur into the contusion(s). If the contusion(s) is (are) large and/or widespread, the swelling may cause the ICP to rise. Nausea, vomiting and visual disturbances are common clinical signs.

Cerebral lacerations – of the cortical surface commonly occur in similar locations to contusions and are most commonly seen at the frontal and temporal lobes as a result of irregular surfaces/bony protrusions of the skull. The term laceration is used when the pia mater is torn.

Haematoma

Extradural haematoma (EDH) is an accumulation of blood in the extradural space between the periosteum on the inner side of the skull and the dura mater (see Fig. 4.13). Most are associated with skull fracture and are commonly caused by a laceration to the middle meningeal artery or vein, or less commonly to the dural venous sinus, following an insult to the

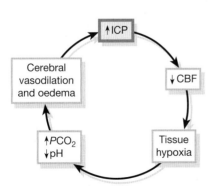

Figure 4.12   Cycle of progressive brain swelling.

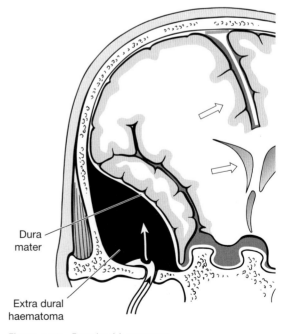

Figure 4.13   Extradural haematoma.

temporal-parietal region. Consequentially the parietal and parieto-temporal areas of the brain are affected. In 85% of patients the EDH will be accompanied by a skull fracture (Hudak & Gallo 1994).

Patients with skull fractures may be neurologically intact on admission and later deteriorate as the EDH develops. Most often the primary brain injury causes some disturbance of consciousness and the developing haematoma results in rapid neurological deterioration (Kwiatkowski 1996). Patients with EDHs most commonly present with a history of transient loss of consciousness, followed by lucidity for a period (hours to days) dependent on the rate of the bleed, irritation and headache. Patients then rapidly lose consciousness and deteriorate very quickly. Late signs are seizures, ipsilateral pupil dilatation, unconsciousness and contralateral hemiplegia. Surgical treatment is required to evacuate the haematoma and ligate the damaged blood vessel.

Relatives, friends and/or carers often require a great deal of reassurance, as they often feel responsible for not bringing the patient to hospital earlier.

Subdural haematoma (SDH) is an accumulation of blood between the dura mater and arachnoid mater. SDHs are caused by the rupture of bridging veins from the cortical surfaces to the venous sinuses (cortical veins) (see Fig. 4.14).

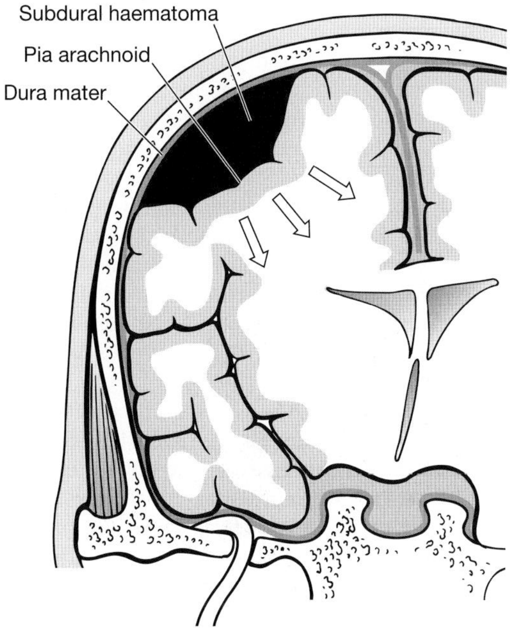

Subdural haematoma

Pia arachnoid

Dura mater

Figure 4.14   Subdural haematoma

SDHs can be seen in isolation, but more commonly are associated with accompanying brain injury, i.e. cerebral contusions and/or intracerebral haematomas. They are the most common intracranial mass result from head trauma (Maartens & Lethbridge 2005). In most cases a large contusion is found at the frontal or temporal surface of the brain. SDHs are predisposed with increasing age and alcoholism. Both groups can suffer regular falls and have a degree of cerebral atrophy, which puts strain on the bridging veins and coagulopathy. Subdural haematomas are classified as acute, subacute and chronic:

– *Acute* (ASDH) refers to symptoms which manifest before 72 hours post-injury. Most patients harbouring an acute SAH are unconscious immediately following major cerebral trauma. The expanding haematoma then causes additional deterioration (Duffy 2001).

– *Subacute* refers to symptoms which manifest between 72 hours and 3 weeks post-injury.

– *Chronic* refers to symptoms which manifest after 3 weeks post-injury. The injury may have been considered as minor and the patient often does not remember a particular predisposing injury.

The most common symptom of a SDH is a headache, which progressively intensifies and is eventually accompanied by vomiting, cognitive impairment(s), a depressed level of consciousness and a focal deficit, which will vary depending on severity of the injury. Even in the absence of focal deficit, increasing ICP may lead to cognitive impairment and eventually a depressed level of consciousness (Watkins 2000). SDHs are often associated with other injuries, and therefore the symptoms can become confused within a general head injury picture. Small SDHs may be treated conservatively, as they will reabsorb over time. Larger SDHs will require evacuation, due to the secondary damage they cause.

A poor outcome is likely if the SDH is bilateral, it accumulates rapidly or there is a greater than 4 hour delay in the surgical management of an acute subdural haematoma. Increased patient age and underlying accompanying brain injury also lead to a poor outcome.

Intracerebral haematoma (ICH) **is** caused by bleeding within the substance of the brain (see Fig. 4.15). ICH usually affects the white matter and the basal ganglia found deep within the brain parenchyma. ICHs are related to contusions as a result of a major impact, which are usually found in the frontal, temporal and parietal lobes. Other causes include penetrating and missile injuries and shearing of blood vessels deep within the brain following an acceleration/deceleration injury. Symptoms include headache,

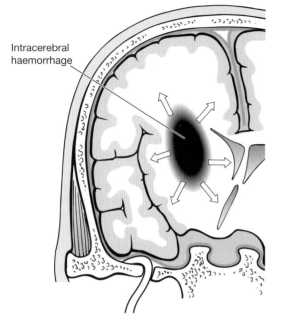

Intracerebral
haemorrhage

Figure 4.15   Intracerebral haematoma.

contralateral hemiplegia, ipsilateral dilated/fixed pupil and deteriorating level of consciousness, progressing to deep coma (Glasgow coma scale < 8). Treatment tends to be conservative, due to the difficulties of evacuating haematomas situated so deeply within the brain. Mortality is high within this group of patients.

Subarachnoid haemorrhage (SAH) is seen in 30–40% of patients following severe traumatic brain injury. Mortality and morbidity is double in these patients compared to those with similar injury without the SAH component (Dearden 1998). The patient either suffered the SAH prior to the insult and thus the SAH is possibly the cause of the incident (Sakas et al. 1995), or the vessels in the subarachnoid space are damaged by the shearing forces at the time of the insult.

Diffuse injuries

Diffuse injuries occur throughout the brain rather than in a specific area of the brain. They result in generalized dysfunction. Diffuse injuries range from concussion, with no residual damage, to diffuse axonal injury and persistent vegetative state. Diffuse injury occurs in 50–60% of patients with severe head trauma and is the commonest cause of unconsciousness, the vegetative state and subsequent disability (Graham 1995).

Concussion – This is a transient form of diffuse injury, which occurs following blunt trauma. It causes a temporary neuronal dysfunction because of transient ischaemia or neuronal depolarization. This manifests as a headache, dizziness, inability to concentrate, disorientation, irritability and nausea. Concussion can occur with or without memory loss. Concussion is graded in line with the severity of symptoms (see Box 4.4).

Recovery is usually rapid, but if neurological symptoms persist, a CT scan should be performed to rule out more severe injuries. Skull X-ray should only be performed if the mechanisms of injury or existing clinical findings are suggestive of a skull fracture. Most patients with concussion can be discharged with an accompanying adult. If there has been a loss of consciousness greater than 10 minutes, the patient should be admitted for observation even if he appears fully recovered.

Approximately one-third of patients with head injuries who are discharged from emergency departments have persistent post-concussion-type symptoms, such as headache, fatigue, inability to concentrate, irritability and anxiety, persisting for several months due to mild diffuse axonal injury (Jackson 1995). The majority of these patients will have been knocked out for a short time and may have other mild neurological signs. As there is no treatment for mild diffuse axonal injury, and recovery is usually spontaneous, reassurance and psychological support are vital to the patient's recovery (see Box 4.5).

Acute axonal injury – This is usually the result of an acute rotation/deceleration injury, typically following a road traffic accident (Fig. 4.16). The patient usually becomes unconscious rapidly after injury, due to the shearing injury to the brain. Mortality is high in this patient group, and those who do survive usually suffer severe neurological dysfunction.

Initially a CT scan may show little abnormality, but gradually with repeated scans, many small diffuse haemorrhagic areas will begin to appear, commonly in the corpus callosum, often associated with traumatic intraventricular haemorrhage and the brain stem. As a result of these injuries the patient may also develop autonomic dysfunction and exhibit symptoms such as excessive sweating, hyperpyrexia and hypertension. Severe generalized cerebral oedema usually accompanies such injuries. Management and treatment involves maximizing cerebral perfusion and the prevention of secondary brain injury.

Cerebral oedema – This is a consistent reaction of the brain to an insult and it usually develops during the first 3–5 days following the insult causing an increase in ICP. Cerebral oedema following severe traumatic brain injury affects almost all patients to a greater or lesser degree. The opening of the blood brain barrier is a central prerequisite to the development of cerebral oedema (Fernandex & Landolt 1996). Four pathophysiological mechanisms of cerebral oedema have been proposed (Box 4.6).

Cerebral ischaemia – This occurs whenever the delivery of oxygen and substrates to the brain falls below its metabolic needs, as a result of hypoxia (cardiac arrest, obstructive airway, cervical spinal injury and prolonged epileptic-type seizures), hypotension and/ or intracranial hypertension (raised ICP).

Blood flow in and around areas of brain tissue damaged by trauma may be abnormal. Vasomotor paralysis also occurs in and around areas of brain tissue damaged by trauma. Blood vessels lose the ability

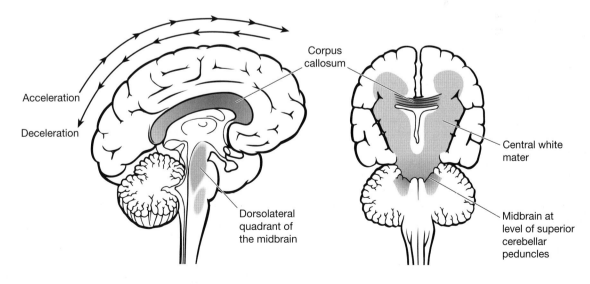

Figure 4.16 Diffuse axonal injury.

to control their own resistance actively with subsequent loss of blood pressure autoregulation and reactivity to CO_2. Cerebral blood flow thus becomes pressure dependent, rendering these areas of brain more susceptible to ischaemia at lower blood pressures and more likely to sustain injury at higher pressures.

Cerebral ischaemia may be global or focal, complete or incomplete. Incomplete ischaemia differs from complete ischaemia in that there is a continuing supply of glucose to the brain tissue despite tissue hypoxia. The glucose sustains anaerobic metabolism, which increases the brain lactic acid level. Neuronal damage occurs above a certain threshold. This effect is the basis for concern that increased peri-ischaemia glucose levels may increase and/or hasten the ischaemia tissue damage. Ischaemia leads instantly to cerebral oedema, which in turn worsens ischaemia (Farnsworth & Sperry 1996).

As the $PaCO_2$ increases, unaffected normal blood vessels dilate, however blood is shunted away from the abnormal areas of the brain that do not respond to CO_2 and is known as the 'steal phenomenon'. An inverse steal (Robin Hood Phenomenon) occurs when the $PaCO_2$ is reduced and the unaffected, normal blood vessels vasoconstrict, shunting blood to the abnormal areas of the brain that do not constrict (Darby et al. 1988).

The concept of *ischaemia penumbra* states that the area of the brain around an ischaemic brain, where blood flow is providing sufficient oxygenation for the cells to survive, but insufficient oxygenation for the cells to maintain normal neuronal function, can re-establish normal function if blood flow and oxygenation to this area is rapidly improved. Cerebral ischaemia is the single most important factor in determining outcome in severe traumatic brain injury: ischaemia lesions are found in 90% of patients at post-mortem (Dearden 1998).

MANAGEMENT

Patients who have sustained a head injury should initially be assessed and managed according to clear principles and standard practice as embodied in the advanced trauma life support (ATLS) system (American College of Surgeons 2004) and for children the advanced paediatric life support (APLS) system (Bavetta & Benjamin 2002, NICE 2003). The main focus of the assessment should be the risk of clinically important brain and cervical spine injuries. Due attention should also be paid to co-existing injuries and other concerns the healthcare team may have, e.g. non-accidental injury.

External referrals

Community health services, e.g. general practice, paramedics, NHS walk-in centres, dental practitioners and NHS minor injury clinics and telephone advice services, e.g. NHS Direct, should refer people who have sustained a head injury to the ambulance services for emergency transport to ED if they have experienced any of the following:

- GCS less than 15 at any time since the injury
- any loss of consciousness as a result of the injury
- any focal neurological deficit since the injury, e.g. problems understanding, speaking, reading or writing, loss of sensation in a part of the body, problems balancing, general weakness, problems walking and any changes in eyesight
- any seizure since the injury
- any suspicion of a skull fracture or penetrating head injury, e.g. CSF leakage from the nose (rhinorrhoea) or the ear(s) (otorrhoea), black eye(s) with no associated damage around the eye(s), bleeding from one or both ears, new deafness in one or both ears, bruising behind one or both ears, penetrating injury signs or visible trauma to the scalp or skull
- a high-energy head injury
- or the injured person or their carer is incapable of transporting the injured person safely to the hospital emergency department without the use of ambulance services, providing any other risk factors indicating emergency department referral are present (NICE 2003).

Telephone advice services, e.g. NHS Direct, should refer people who have sustained a head injury to an hospital emergency department if the related history indicates any of the following risk factors:

- amnesia for events before or after the injury: the assessment of amnesia will not be possible in pre-verbal children and is unlikely to be possible in any child under 5 years old
- persistent headache since the injury
- any loss of consciousness as a result of the injury from which the injured person has now recovered
- any vomiting episode since the injury: clinical judgement should be used regarding the cause of vomiting in those aged less than or equal to 12 years and whether referral is necessary
- any previous cranial neurosurgical intervention
- history of bleeding or clotting disorders
- current anticoagulant therapy such as warfarin
- current drug or alcohol intoxication
- age greater than or equal to 65 years

- suspicion of non-accidental injury
- irritability or altered behaviour particularly in infants and young children
- continuing concern by the Helpline's personnel about the diagnosis (NICE 2003).

In the absence of the factors listed above the telephone advice services should advise the injured person to seek medical advice from community health services, e.g. general practice and NHS walk-in centres if any of the following factors are present:

- adverse social factors, e.g. no one able to supervise the injured person at home
- continuing concern by the injured person or their carer about the diagnosis (NICE 2003).

History

Accurate history-taking gives vital clues to the type and potential severity of the head injury (Shah 1999) (see Box 4.7). This may have to be obtained from a witness or paramedic. If the history is obtained from the patient, it should be corroborated by a witness/relative if possible.

Assessment

Management of head injury in the emergency department revolves largely around the assessment of the risks of, and the prevention or limiting of secondary brain injury (the causation of secondary brain injury is shown in Box 4.8) and of injury to the cervical spine, whilst the patient awaits definitive treatment such as surgery to evacuate haematoma. Due attention should also be paid to co-existing injuries.

Patients presenting to the emergency department with a GCS less than or equal to 8 should be assessed early by an anaesthetist or critical-care physician to provide appropriate airway management and to assist with resuscitation (NICE 2003). The recommended primary investigation of choice for the detection of acute clinically important brain injuries is CT imaging (NICE

> **Box 4.8   Causes of secondary brain injury**
>
> - Hyperpyrexia
> - Cerebral ischaemia
> - Cerebral oedema
> - Raised intracranial pressure
> - Infection
> - Metabolic disorder
> - Evolving intracranial bleed
> - Hypotension

2003). MRI for safety, logistic and resource reasons is not currently indicated as the primary investigation, although additional information of importance to the patient's prognosis can sometimes be detected using MRI. MRI is contraindicated unless there is certainty that the patient does not harbour an incompatible device, implant or foreign body. Skull X-ray(s) are the recommended primary investigation of choice for skull fractures (see Box 4.9). If CT scanning is not available then skull X-rays along with high quality patient observations have a vital role. Early imaging, rather than admission and observation for neurological deterioration, reduces the time needed to detect life-threatening complications and is associated with a better outcome (NICE 2003). Indications for CT scanning are listed in Box 4.10.

Neurological assessment

Full neurological assessment forms part of the secondary survey, as should thorough examination of the scalp for lacerations, haematomas or evidence of a depressed skull fracture. The assessment and classification of patients who have suffered a head injury should be guided primarily by the adult (16 years or older) and paediatric versions of the Glasgow Coma

---

> **Box 4.7   History-taking in head injury**
>
> - Mechanism of injury
> - Time elapsed
> - Period of loss of consciousness
> - Any pre/post-traumatic amnesia
> - Condition since injury, such as nausea, vomiting, confusion, visual disturbance, lethargy or dizziness

---

> **Box 4.9   Indications for skull X-ray**
>
> - Suspected penetrating injury
> - Decreased consciousness (if GCS below 8/15, CT is indicated)
> - Altered neurology
> - CSF from nose or ear
> - Significant scalp bruising or swelling
> - Difficulty in clinical examination, where mechanism of injury is suggestive of fracture

---

Box 4.10   Indications for urgent CT scanning following a head injury

- GCS less than 13 at any point since the injury
- GCS 13–14, two hours after the injury
- Suspected open or depressed skull fracture
- Clinical symptoms of basal skull fracture
- Post-traumatic seizure
- Focal neurological deficit(s)
- More than one episode of vomiting (clinical judgement should be used regarding the cause of vomiting in those children 12 years or younger, and whether imaging is necessary)
- Amnesia for greater than 30 minutes of events prior to the assault. This assessment is not possible in children 5 years or younger.

CT should be immediately requested in patients with any of the following risk factors, providing they have experienced some loss of consciousness or amnesia since the assault.

- Age 65 years or older
- Coagulopathy (clotting disorder or current treatment with warfarin)
- A high-energy head injury

CT Scanning and the results should be analysed within one hour of the request having been received by the radiology department in patients with the following risk factors

- GCS less than 13 at any point since the injury
- GCS 13–14, 2 hours after the injury
- Suspected open or depressed skull fracture
- Any signs of basal skull fracture
- Post-traumatic seizure
- Focal neurological deficit(s)
- More than 1 episode of vomiting (clinical judgement should be used regarding the cause of vomiting in those children 12 years or younger, and whether imaging is necessary)
- Amnesia for greater than 30 minutes of events prior to the assault. This assessment is not possible in children 5 years or younger.
- Age 65 years or older providing that loss of consciousness or amnesia has been experienced.
- Coagulopathy (history of bleeding, clotting disorder or current treatment with warfarin) providing that loss of consciousness or amnesia has been experienced.
- A high-energy head injury (NICE 2003).

Scale (GCS) and its derivative the Glasgow Coma Score (NICE 2003). The paediatric version should include a 'grimace' alternative to the verbal score to facilitate assessment in the pre-verbal or intubated patients (NICE 2003).

The Glasgow Coma Scale (GCS), developed by Teasdale & Jennett (1974), provides an objective, standardized and easily interpreted tool for neurological assessment without relying on subjective terminology such as 'stupor', 'semi-coma' and 'deep coma' (see Box 4.11 and Fig. 4.17). The GCS records what you see, measuring arousal, awareness and activity, by assessing eye opening, verbal response and motor ability. Each activity is allocated a score, therefore enabling objectivity, ease of recording and comparison between recordings. It also provides useful information for patient outcome prediction. The score should be based on the sum of 15 and to avoid confusion this denominator should be specified, e.g. 13/15 (NICE 2003). When recording the GCS it is important to record the three separate response scores as well as the total GCS score, i.e. E2, V3, M4. GCS = 9 (NICE 2003)

When applying verbal stimulus, it is good practice to commence with normal voice and then increase volume to elicit a response. It is important to ascertain

whether the patient is deaf, wears a hearing aid and whether English is the patient's spoken language. When applying a painful stimulus, it is good practice to commence with light pressure and then increase to elicit a response. When assessing motor function, always record the response from the best arm. There is no need to record left and right differences, as the GCS does not aim to measure focal deficit. It is not appropriate to measure leg response unless unavoidable, i.e. injury to both arms, as a spinal reflex rather than a brain-initiated response might be initiated (Teasdale & Jennett 1974).

The GCS may be misleading in patients who have a high cervical injury, or brain stem lesion, and in those who are hypoxic, haemodynamically shocked fitting or post-ictal. These patients may be unable to move their limbs or may show no responses at all. It is important to attempt to assess the spinal patient using facial movements, being aware of the possibility of a combined head and neck injury. Patients who show no response should be re-evaluated following correction of any shock or hypoxia (NICE 2003).

The GCS assessment should be accompanied by an assessment of pupil size and reactivity, limb movement and vital signs observations:

Box 4.11   Adult and Paediatric Glasgow Coma Scale

Adult (16 years and older)

Eye opening		Motor response		Verbal response	
Spontaneous	4	Obeys	6	Orientated	5
To speech	3	Localizes	5	Confused	4
To pain	2	Normal flexion	4	Inappropriate	3
None	1	Abnormal flexion	3	Incomprehensible	2
		Extensor response	2	None	1
		None	1		

Child

Eye opening		Motor response		Verbal response	
Spontaneous	4	Obeys commands or performs normal spontaneous movements	6	Alert, babbles, coos, words or sentences to usual ability	5
To speech	3	Localizes to painful stimuli or withdraws to touch	5	Less than usual ability and/or spontaneous irritable cry	4
To pain	2	Withdrawal to painful stimuli	4	Cries inappropriately	3
None	1	Abnormal flexion	3	Occasionally whimpers and/or moans	2
		Abnormal extension	2	None	1
		None	1		

Pre-verbal child or intubated patient

Eye opening		Motor response		Grimace response	
Spontaneous	4	Obeys commands or performs normal spontaneous movements	6	Spontaneous normal facial/oro-motor activity	5
To speech	3	Localizes to painful stimuli or withdraws to touch	5	Less than usual Spontaneous ability or only response to touch stimuli	4
To pain	2	Withdrawal to painful stimuli	4	Vigorous grimace to pain	3
None	1	Abnormal flexion	3	Mild grimace to pain	2
		Abnormal extension	2	None	1
		None	1		

- blood pressure
- respiration rate
- heart rate
- temperature
- blood oxygen saturation.
  (NICE 2003).

As well as providing a baseline for assessing the patient's progress, vital signs give important information about potential secondary brain injury, e.g. respiration rate and cerebral hypoxia. When assessing vital signs in conjunction with GCS, it is important to remember the following:

- Hypotension is only of neurological origin in end-stage brain injury or spinal shock. Other causes of hypotension, such as hypovolaemia, should be investigated.

- Cushing's triad (hypertension, bradycardia and bradypnoea) indicates a life-threatening rise in ICP.
- Pyrexia with hypertension may indicate autonomic dysfunction.

Limb movement is useful to assess for focal damage. However, although it is usual for a hemiparesis or hemiplegia to occur on the contralateral side to the lesion, it may occur on the ipsilateral side. This is due to indentation of the contralateral cerebral peduncle and is known as a false localizing. Spontaneous movements are observed for equality. If there is little or no spontaneous movement, then painful stimuli must be applied to each limb in turn, comparing the result. It is most appropriate to complete this while assessing the motor component of the GCS.

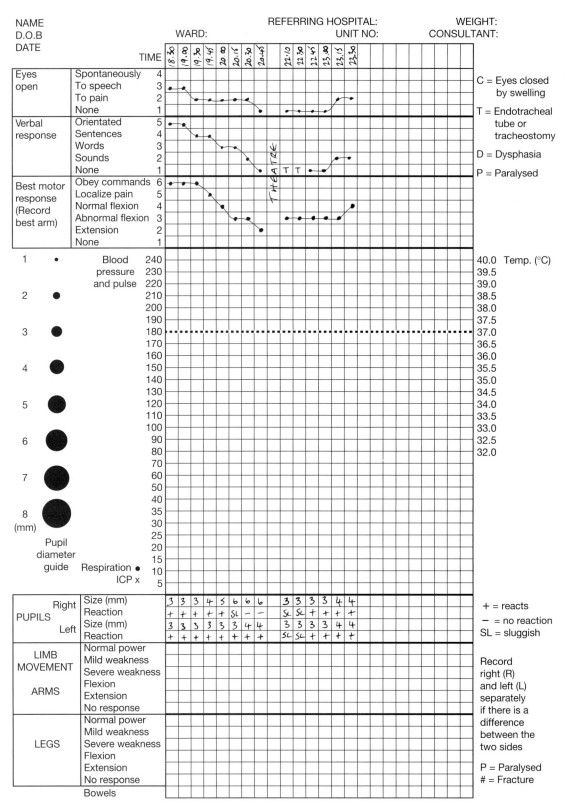

Figure 4.17 Glasgow Coma Scale.

Pupils are assessed for their reaction to light, size and shape, i.e. cranial nerves II (optic) and III (oculomotor) activity. Each pupil needs to be assessed and recorded individually. Pupils are measured in millimetres, the normal range being 2–6 mm in diameter. They are normally round in shape and abnormalities are described as ovoid, keyhole or irregular (Hickey 1997). A bright light is shone into the side of each eye to assess the pupils' reaction to light. This should produce a brisk constriction in both pupils, the consensual light reaction. Herniation of the medial temporal lobe through the tentorium directly damages the oculomotor (IIIrd) nerve, resulting in dilation of the pupil and an impaired reaction to light. The pupil dilates on the side of the lesion.

Patients with head injuries can be classified into three groups depending on their GCS:

- A score of 13–15 is indicative of a minor head injury. In some patients, a one-point drop in their GCS can be alcohol- or drug-induced. This necessitates extra vigilance from nursing staff as alcohol and/or drugs may mask subtle changes in the patient's cognition or conscious level.
- A GCS of 9–12 suggests a moderate head injury, or a more serious injury evolving. Any changes in the patient's condition should be closely monitored.
- A severe head injury is classed by a GCS of 8 or less. These patients are potentially at risk of secondary brain injury, and their GCS and vital signs should be monitored at frequent intervals.

ADMISSION TO HOSPITAL

Patients should be admitted if

- they have suffered a new surgically significant abnormality on imaging
- the patient has not returned to a GCS equal to 15 after imaging, regardless of the imaging results
- they fulfil the criteria for CT scanning but this cannot be done within the appropriate period, either because CT is not available or because the patient is not sufficiently co-operative to allow scanning
- the patient has continuing worrying signs of concern to the clinicians, e.g. persistent vomiting and severe headache
- the patient has received sedation or general anaesthetic during CT imaging
- the patient has other sources of concern to the clinicians, e.g. drug or alcohol intoxication, other injuries, shock, suspected non-accidental injury, meningism and cerebrospinal fluid leak (NICE 2003).

Urgent re-assessment by the clinician in charge of the case

Any of the following should prompt an urgent response:

- development of agitation or abnormal behaviour.
- a sustained (at least 30 minutes) drop of one point in GCS level (greater weight should be given to a drop of one point in the motor score of the GCS).
- any drop of greater than two points in GCS level regardless of duration or GCS sub-scale.
- development of severe or increasing headache or persisting vomiting.
- new or evolving neurological symptoms or signs such as pupil inequality or asymmetry of limb or facial movement (NICE 2003).

MANAGEMENT OF MINOR HEAD INJURY

The majority of patients treated in emergency departments with head injury will have a 'minor' head injury. Some 92% of these patients will have normal neurology (Klauber 1993) and the majority will be discharged home. A thorough assessment of the patient's condition should be performed, which should include pulse, respiration, blood pressure, pupil size and reaction, and the patient's GCS. Although only 1% of head-injured patients have skull fractures (Ramrakha & Moore 1997), there are certain circumstances where a skull X-ray is appropriate (see Box 4.9).

The key to managing minor head injury is giving adequate information and advice to the patient and his carer. The patient should be advised to rest quietly, avoid stressful situations, should be discouraged from taking part in strenuous activities and from undertaking long periods of VDU work or watching TV which will exacerbate any headache. The patient should not stay at home alone for the first 48 hours after leaving hospital. Simple analgesia should be suggested, such as paracetamol, which should be sufficient to alleviate headaches without masking other signs of deterioration. The patient should be discouraged from taking alcohol or drugs until symptoms have subsided. The patient should not play any contact sport for at least 3 weeks after the injury without talking to their doctor or other appropriately qualified clinician first. Written advice should always be given to the patient/carer to reinforce any verbal information (Box 4.12). (See also Chapter 33 – Health Promotion.)

When discussing the outcomes of a minor head injury, it is important that the emergency nurse explains post-concussion-type symptoms to the patient. Head-injured patients should be discharged into the care of a responsible adult. Not all patients with minor head injury are appropriate for discharge (see Box 4.13).

Box 4.12   Typical head injury advice sheet

- General advice about observing a patient every 2 hours; ensure he wakes easily and is orientated when awake. Ensure the patient is able to move all limbs
- You should return to hospital if any of the following occur:
  - persistent vomiting
  - confusion
  - excessive sleeping; difficulty in rousing patient
  - severe headache
  - double vision
  - limb weakness
  - convulsions or 'passing out'
  - discharge of blood/fluid from nose/ears
- You should not drink alcohol until all symptoms have subsided
- The name and telephone of the hospital should be included

Box 4.13   Indications for hospital admission

- Decreased consciousness
- Neurological deficit
- Severe headache and persistent vomiting
- Confusion
- Intoxification rendering clinical assessment unreliable
- Coexisting conditions such as clotting disorders
- Social circumstances making discharge unwise

Particular care is needed with patients who are intoxicated and/or have taken drugs where neurological assessment is unreliable.

MANAGEMENT OF SERIOUS HEAD INJURY

Despite the fact that patients who have suffered severe injury to the brain may recover completely if they are treated quickly and appropriately, it is also possible that the patient may suffer serious disability or even death (NICE 2003). Age is a significant factor in determining outcome, especially in patients who become deeply unconscious. Mortality is 19% in patients aged 20, but 71% in those aged 60 and over (Hickey 1997).

The aim of management of the head-injured patient is to prevent and treat secondary physiological insults. There is a developing base of evidence to guide the management of patients with traumatic brain injury (TBI) but a study carried out by Matta & Menon (1996) suggests that there is considerable room for improvement, with many centres not following basic recommendations for monitoring and principles of treatment. A study by Patel et al. (2002) looked at the effect of neurocritical care, delivered by specialist staff and based on protocol driven therapy. They found improved outcomes, supporting, though not proving, the notion that treatment directed at ICP and CPP improves outcome.

It is universally accepted that initial management of severe TBI requires urgent cardiopulmonary resuscitation, emergency CT scan, transfer to a neurosurgical centre and appropriate surgical intervention, and guidelines covering this initial care are generally well established (McNaughton & Harwood 2002, Intensive Care Society 1997). Monitoring of ECG, direct arterial blood pressure, central venous pressure and pulse oximetry is mandatory in all patients. Regular arterial blood gas analysis, measurement of blood glucose and sodium and core temperature monitoring are also required to optimize treatment strategies.

In an attempt to address variability in practice, the European Brain Injury Consortium (EBIC) set out to define general standards of severe TBI management (Maas et al. 1997). The resulting guidelines were published in 1997 and were based on consensus and expert opinion (see Box 4.14). In 1996 the American Brain Injury Consortium (ABIC) had produced evidence-based guidelines for the management of severe TBI (Brain Trauma Foundation 1996). Despite the different approaches used in formulating the guidelines, the conclusions and recommendations of both the ABIC and EBIC guidelines are similar, reflecting the consensus that exists in many countries on the management of severe TBI.

Extracranial complications of severe TBI and treatment

Extracranial complications occur frequently in severe TBI and studies suggest that some complications are highly influential in determining patient outcome.

Respiratory

In patients with isolated head injury, acute lung injury (ALI) is common. Studies show ALI occurrence in 20% of patients with a post-resuscitative GCS of 8 or less. ALI is an additional marker of the severity of brain

---

Box 4.14   EBIC guidelines for management of severe head injury in adults (Maas et al. 1997)

Monitoring and general care

- Minimal monitoring requirements include ECG, SpO_2 invasive arterial BP, temperature and end tidal CO_2
- Maintain $SpO_2 > 95\%$, MABP > 90 mmHg
- Central venous pressure monitoring to ensure normovolaemia
- If ICP monitored – continuous monitoring of arterial blood pressure (ABP) and calculation of cerebral perfusion pressure (CPP)

Ventilatory parameters

- Adjust ventilation to maintain $PaO_2 > 13$ kPa (100 mmHg) and $PaCO_2$ 4.0–4.5 kPa (30–35 mmHg)

Management of ICP and CPP

- Treat ICP elevations above 20–25 mmHg.
- Maintain CPP 60–70 mmHg
- There is no consensus whether patients should be nursed flat or with the head up to a maximum of 30° elevation

Accepted methods of management of ICP and CPP

- Sedation
- Analgesia
- Mild to moderate hyperventilation ($PaCO_2$ 4.0–4.5 kPa, 30–35 mmHg)
- Volume expansion and inotropes or vasopressor when ABP insufficient to maintain CPP in a normovolaemia patient
- Osmotic therapy – preferably mannitol, repeated in bolus infusions, maintaining serum osmolarity >315

- If osmotherapy has insufficient effect, frusemide can be given additionally
- CSF drainage
- If these methods fail, more intensive hyperventilation ($PaCO_2 < 4.0$ kPa or 30 mmHg), preferably with monitoring by jugular oxymetry of cerebral oxygenation to detect ischaemia
- Alternatively, the use of barbiturates, inducing increased sedation, may be considered
- There is no established indication for steroids in the management of acute head injury

Timing and indications for operative therapy

- A surgically significant EDH or ASDH should be evacuated immediately upon detection.
- For small haemorrhagic contusions or other small intracerebral lesion, a conservative approach is generally adopted, but operation should be considered urgent for large intracerebral lesions with high or mixed density on CT scan
- Depressed skull fracture: operation is definitely indicated only if it is a compound (open) fracture (not over sagittal sinus) or if the fracture is so extensive that is causes mass effect
- Closed depressed skull fractures are usually treated conservatively, but operation may be appropriate in selected cases to reduce mass effect or correct disfigurement
- Decompressive craniotomy may be considered in exceptional situations.

---

injury and is associated with an increased risk of morbidity and mortality (Bratton & Davis 1997). Neurogenic pulmonary oedema (NPE) represents the most severe form of ALI and is typically reported in cases of fatal or near fatal head injuries (Bratton & Davis 1997). The exact mechanism responsible for this acute condition seen after severe TBI and after abrupt elevations in ICP is unclear. It is generally accepted that there is a neurological pathway following central nervous system injury and that it is the result of massive sympathetic outflow, possibly mediated by the hypothalamus.

The pathophysiological changes result in the rapid development of interstitial oedema and subsequent increased pulmonary shunt, decreased compliance and loss of lung volume. Signs and symptoms include dyspnoea, cyanosis, pallor, sweating, a weak rapid pulse and the production of pink frothy sputum. The development of neurogenic pulmonary oedema can be remarkably rapid and is usually associated with an acute and significant rise in ICP. The classic form appears early, within minutes to a few hours, after injury while the delayed form progresses slowly over a period of 12 to 72 hours (Durieux 1996). Primary treatment consists of employing therapeutic interventions aimed at reducing ICP and providing appropriate ventilation support and management, increasing inspired oxygen concentration, controlling carbon dioxide levels and increasing positive tracheal end pressure (PEEP) to maximize oxygenation with minimal effect on ICP and cardiac output.

The development of non-cardiogenic pulmonary oedema complicates the management of severe TBI because many of the therapies used to protect the lungs causes a rise in ICP or decreased CPP. The ventilatory strategies used to protect the lungs, e.g. reduced tidal volume, permissive hypoxia and hypercarbia, increased levels of PEEP, and prone lying, pose management problems during the management of the acute head injury when intracranial hypertension may be high and delay the early rehabilitation therapy which is essential to maximize recovery (Robertson et al. 1999).

Some studies have shown a link between CPP management and acute respiratory distress syndrome (ARDS) (Contant et al. 2001, Robertson 2001). Induced hypertension to raise CPP can cause increased pulmonary hydrostatic pressures and thereby increase the amount of water accumulating within the lungs. The results of a randomized trial comparing two head injury management strategies, one ICP targeted and the other CPP targeted, showed a fivefold increase in the incidence of ARDS in the CPP targeted group where CPP was maintained > 70 mmHg (Robertson 2001). Approximately 60% of patients with severe TBI become hypoxaemic without ventilatory support or added oxygen and require advanced ventilatory support within a short period of time.

Management should follow the sequence laid down by ATLS (American College of Surgeons 2004). Airway management is paramount in preventing hypoxia and therefore secondary brain injury. Oedema and/or debris following injury, loss of the gag reflex and/or vomiting may threaten airway patency. If a clear airway cannot be maintained with simple aids, such as a guedal or oro-pharyngeal airway then intubation should be performed. Cervical spine immobilization should be maintained until a full risk assessment (and imaging if deemed necessary) has been undertaken and the possibility of a neck injury has been excluded. Suctioning should be kept to a minimum as it raises ICP.

The neurophysiology of breathing is complex and involves several areas of the brain. Following head injury the normal pattern of breathing is easily disrupted, leading to hypoxia. It is important to maintain adequate oxygenation, as a rise in PCO_2 levels initiates autoregulation, causing cerebral vasodilatation and a rise in ICP. If unchecked, this can lead to secondary brain injury. As good oxygenation is imperative, head-injured patients should be given oxygen via a facemask and reservoir bag: if bradypnoeic, this should be assisted by mechanical ventilation as soon as possible following the severe TBI. Induced

hyperventilation should be used to reduce PCO_2 levels, but this should be discussed with a neurosurgeon first (Bullock & Teasdale 1996).

If urgent intubation is indicated, it should be assumed that the patient has a full stomach, and cricoid pressure should be applied to prevent vomiting or gastric regurgitation. In adults, this should be maintained until the cuff of the ET tube is inflated, creating a secure airway. Short-acting sedatives and muscle relaxants should always be used for intubation, to minimize the impact on the brain. Hypoxia is a major cause of cerebral ischaemia and care should always be taken to maintain adequate oxygenation levels by monitoring respiratory effort closely with arterial blood gases (ABGs) and O_2 saturation measurement and intervening with supportive therapy at an early stage.

Intubation and ventilation should be implemented immediately in the following circumstances:

- GCS less than or equal to 8
- loss of protective laryngeal reflexes
- ventilatory insufficiency as judged by arterial blood gases:
  - hypoxaemia (PaO_2 less than 9 kPa on air or less than 13 kPa on oxygen) or
  - hypercarbia ($PaCO_2$ greater than 6 kPa)
- spontaneous hyperventilation (causing $PaCO_2$ less than 3.5 kPa)
- respiratory arrhythmia (NICE 2003).

Intubation and ventilation should be implemented before the start of a transfer in the following circumstances in addition to the above:

- significantly deteriorating conscious level
- bilateral fractured mandible
- copious bleeding into the mouth, e.g. base of skull fracture
- seizures (NICE 2003).

Cardiovascular complications

High levels of sympathetic activity and of circulating catecholamines after severe TBI can have an adverse effect on cardiac function, basal metabolic rate and vascular and neuronal function in the central nervous system (Clifton et al. 1983). The magnitude of this hyperdynamic cardiovascular state occurring after severe head injury does not necessarily correlate with ICP, GCS or CT findings (Clifton et al. 1981). There is both clinical and experimental evidence that cerebral neurogenic factors cause arrhythmias in normal hearts, with fatal arrhythmias being reported in otherwise healthy brain-injured patients (McLeod 1982,

Oppenheimer et al. 1990). A wide variety of atrial and ventricular arrhythmias, abnormalities of the QRS complex, T-wave and ST segment and QT prolongation have been documented and occur most commonly in patients with diffuse injury, oedema and contusions. In two seminal studies, 31% of patients admitted with head injury exhibited some form of cardiac arrhythmia (Hersch 1961) and cardiac arrhythmias were observed in 41 of 100 patients admitted with acute subdural haematoma, with more than half of these showing ventricular arrhythmias ranging in severity from premature ventricular contractions to ventricular tachycardia and ventricular fibrillation (Van der Ark 1975). Elevations of pulse greater than 120 beats per minute have been found in one third of patients with severe TBI.

It is generally accepted that hypotension related to trauma is not caused by head injury, although it can be related to head injury per se in children. However, there is some evidence that episodes of hypotension following severe TBI may be of neurogenic origin in a small proportion of patients, and that this is not simply attributable to devastating, unsurvivable brain injury (Chesnut 1998).

Hypotension is usually a result of systemic hypovolaemia following multiple traumas. Causes of hypotension should be identified and fluid resuscitation is imperative to prevent a drop in cerebral ischaemia and secondary brain injury. In the late stages of head injury, hypertension occurs with bradycardia and bradypnoea. Hypertension is a late sign of pending brain injury. Arterial blood pressure increases in an attempt to maintain the cerebral perfusion pressure in the brain. The decreases in respiration and heart rate are due to pressure on the medulla. These signs often precede death. This is referred to as Cushing's triad.

Coagulopathy

Severe TBI can be complicated by the development of a coagulopathy that can worsen blood loss and delay invasive neurosurgical treatment. Studies have reported a positive correlation between the presence and severity of disseminated intravascular coagulation (DIC) and the degree of brain injury, assessed by plasma fibrinogen degradation product levels. Although most of the acute coagulopathies associated with brain injury are not preventable, prompt treatment can be effective in reducing morbidity. Clotting studies at the time of admission to ED can be valuable in predicting the occurrence of delayed injury and early follow-up CT scanning is advocated in the patient with coagulopathy (Piek et al. 1992, May et al. 1997).

MANAGEMENT OF INTRACRANIAL COMPLICATIONS

Raised intracranial pressure

Uncontrolled elevation in ICP is the most common cause of mortality, morbidity and secondary brain injury after severe TBI. More than one third of patients' ICP exceeds 20 mmHg at some stage (Chan et al. 1995). This is because it alters tissue perfusion, causing cerebral ischaemia. It is therefore important to ensure that signs of raised ICP are noted and treated early. Disorientation, irritation, headache, seizures, nausea and vomiting are all possible indicators of raised ICP, and later signs include deterioration in the GCS, limb and pupil changes and finally alteration in the vital signs (Cushing's triad).

Hypercapnia can cause secondary brain injury, which results from either inadequate ventilation or a response to hypermetabolism following trauma. High PCO_2 levels result in cerebral vasodilation in an attempt to increase oxygenation. This increases cerebral blood flow and, therefore, intracranial pressure. Hyperventilation is controversial (Harrahill 1997), but is the most common treatment for inducing vasoconstriction, and reduces PCO_2 and thus intracranial pressure. Arterial blood gas analysis should be frequently recorded in-patients being artificially hyperventilated/ventilated.

While it has never been shown definitively that lowering ICP in patients with raised ICP improves outcome, an ICP >20 mmHg has been shown to be the fourth most powerful predictor of outcome after age, admission GCS and pupillary signs (Marmarou et al. 1991) and there is evidence to suggest that treatment should be initiated if the ICP is 20–25 mmHg (Lang & Chesnut 1995). Both ICP and CPP correlate strongly with outcome after TBI with the worse outcomes occurring in patients with an ICP >20 mmHg and/or a CPP <60 mmHg (Chesnut 1995). One study, which examined early versus late treatment of raised ICP, reported that early aggressive management based on ICP monitoring significantly reduced the overall mortality rate from 84% to 69% without causing a disproportionate number of severely disabled or vegetative patients (Rosner et al. 1995).

Focal increases of ICP lead to distortion of brain parenchyma and secondary ischaemic damage, while diffusely raised ICP leads to tentorial hemiation and brain stem death. Early intracranial hypertension is confirmed as a sign of poor prognosis. The ABIC and EBIC guidelines recommend that ICP be maintained ICP < 20–25 mmHg during the acute course of head injury. They also advise that treatment for raised

ICP should only be continued if it is effective in decreasing ICP and/or increasing CPP (Maas et al. 1997, Brain Trauma Foundation 1996).

Maintenance of cerebral perfusion pressure

One of the most controversial areas in the management of severe TBI is the level of CPP required to adequately perfuse the brain, and to date no study has shown that any one approach with a particular CPP threshold improves clinical outcome more than any other. Substantial clinical and experimental evidence shows that hypotension following TBI has an adverse effect on outcome, and particularly so if it occurs in the first few hours after injury. Hypotension (defined as a systolic BP <90 mmHg) has been uniformly identified as the most predominant factor in secondary brain injury and has the highest correlation with morbidity and mortality (Chesnut et al. 1993).

There is general agreement on the need to maintain CPP between 60 and 70 mmHg, either by reducing ICP or by elevating MAP. Aggressive fluid replacement and cardiovascular support with vasopressors and inotropes to increase MAP and maintain CPP >70 mmHg has been associated with a reduction in the incidence of secondary ischaemic events by approximately 50% (Rosner et al. 1995). However, this treatment has been shown to lead to a fivefold increase in the incidence of acute ARDS. Robertson (2001) advocates a target CPP of 60 mmHg, with higher CPP levels being reserved for patients who demonstrate a specific indication for induced raised ICP such as regional or global ischaemic.

The ABIC and EBIC guidelines recommend that episodes of hypotension be avoided whenever possible, or if they do occur, corrected immediately to maintain a mean arterial blood pressure (MABP) >90 mmHg or a systolic BP >120 mmHg (Maas et al. 1997, Brain Trauma Foundation 1996).

Blood haemoglobin concentration

CBF can be influenced by blood viscosity, of which haematocrit is the single most important determinant. Blood viscosity increases logarithmically with increasing haematocrit and the optimal level is probably about 35%. Cerebral blood flow is reduced by haematocrit levels over 50% and increased with haematocrit levels below 30%. This compensatory mechanism allows sufficient oxygen delivery in healthy individuals even with haematocrit levels of 20%.

Studies suggest that a haematocrit of 30–34% may result in optimal oxygen delivery to brain tissue. However, if maximum vasodilatation already exists, haemodilution may decrease oxygen delivery and

lead to increases in cerebral blood volume (CBV) and therefore ICP (Cesarini 1996).

Control of ICP

Mannitol is an effective agent to reduce cerebral oedema and ICP (Bullock 1995). In addition to its osmotic effects, mannitol may also reduce ICP by improving cerebral microcirculatory flow and oxygen delivery. However, repetitive administration can potentially increase ICP since mannitol accumulates within brain tissue, reversing osmotic shift and increasing cerebral oedema. The peak effect of mannitol on ICP occurs within 15 minutes of administration, but its effects on serum osmolarity last 2 to 6 hours, depending on the dose and clinical condition of the patient. Adverse effects of mannitol include:

- opening of blood-brain barrier – this effect may become harmful after multiple doses and actually exacerbate ICP by increasing brain swelling
- accumulation of mannitol in the brain is most marked when mannitol is in the circulation for long periods as occurs with continuous infusion administration, therefore mannitol should be administered in repeat boluses
- mannitol is excreted entirely by the urine, therefore there is increased risk of acute renal failure (acute tubular necrosis) if administered in large doses, particularly if serum osmolarity is > 320 mosmol/l)
- increased serum sodium levels
- mannitol raises urine osmolarity and specific gravity, therefore these variables cannot be used to diagnose diabetes insipidus.

The ICP-lowering effect of bolus administration of mannitol appears to be equal over the range 0.25 to 1.0 g/kg, although the duration of activity may be somewhat shorter with the lower dose. Under most circumstances, the lower dose should be used in order to minimize the risk of hyperosmolality and avoid a negative fluid balance. The ABIC and EBIC guidelines recommend mannitol 20% be given as an intravenous infusion over 15 to 20 minutes, and repeated as necessary. Blood osmotic pressure must be monitored and serum osmolarity kept below 315 mosmol/l. They also recommend that if mannitol has insufficient effect then frusemide can be given additionally (Maas et al. 1997, Brain Trauma Foundation 1996).

Drugs

It is common practice for severe TBI patients to be empirically managed with a protocol that includes the routine use of sedatives, analgesics and neuromuscular blocking agents to facilitate mechanical ventilation and to treat intracranial hypertension.

Intravenous anaesthetic agents cause a dose-dependent reduction in cerebral metabolism, CBF and ICP while maintaining pressure autoregulation and CO_2 reactivity. The use of barbiturates in TBI is controversial and has largely been replaced by propofol, which has similar cerebrovascular effects but a more favourable pharmacological profile. Propofol has become the sedative of choice but care must be taken to avoid hypotension (Kelly 2000, Kelly et al. 1999).

Fentanyl and morphine are frequently administered to limit pain, facilitate mechanical ventilation and potentiate the effect of sedation. Neuromuscular blocking drugs have no direct effect on ICP but may prevent rises produced by coughing and straining on the endotracheal tube. However, such agents are not associated with improved outcome and their use is the subject of much debate (Prielipp & Coursin 1995).

The ABIC and EBIC guidelines suggest that sedation and neuromuscular blocking drugs can be useful in optimizing transport of the head-injured patient. In the absence of outcome-based studies the choice of sedative is left to the physician, and neuromuscular blocking agents should only be employed when sedation alone proves inadequate (Maas et al. 1997, Brain Trauma Foundation 1996).

Hyperventilation

The aim is to reduce PCO_2, cerebral blood volume and thus ICP; it also causes a significant reduction in CBF. Hyperventilation only has a short-lived effect on ICP. The ABIC and EBIC guidelines advocate that, in the absence of increased ICP, prolonged prophylactic hyperventilation should be avoided. Prophylactic hyperventilation should be reserved for only brief periods in the event of acute neurological deterioration, or for longer periods when intracranial hypertension is unresponsive to sedation, paralysis, CSF drainage and osmotic diuretics (Maas et al. 1997, Brain Trauma Foundation 1996).

Temperature control

Following TBI, temperature regulation may be disrupted as a result of damage to the hypothalamus. Injury to the CNS is temperature dependent. Fever can make an existing neurological dysfunction more apparent and may worsen an ongoing insult. The brain's metabolic rate for oxygen increases by 6–9% for every degree Celsius rise in temperature. In the acute phase of head injury, therefore, hyperthermia should be treated since it will exacerbate cerebral ischaemic and adversely affect outcome.

Hypothermia as a treatment in severe TBI has been a major area of research during the last decade. The interim results of a large multicentre study showed that cooling to 32–33°C within 10 hours of injury improved neurological recovery in patients presenting with head injury and a GCS of 5–7 but not those with a lower GCS. However, this study was terminated early with no clear benefit established (Marion et al. 1997).

Some studies suggest that while hypothermia may not attenuate damage from the primary injury, it provides protection against secondary injury, specifically hypotension and hypoxia, and that there may be a therapeutic window for neuroprotection in the early stages following injury (Yamamoto et al. 1999). Whether this protection can be sustained over longer periods remains to be determined.

A randomized trial evaluating the use of mild hypothermia during intracranial aneurysm surgery found that, compared with normothermic patients, more patients in the hypothermic group had good outcomes and fewer of these patients had neurological deficits at the time of discharge (Hindman 1999). In a further study on CBF and oxygen metabolism during mild hypothermia (33–34°C) in elective aneurysmal surgery, positron emission tomography (PET) showed luxury perfusion in almost all cases, providing the first PET evidence of decreased CBF and metabolic rate of O_2 during hypothermia in humans (Kawamura 2000).

There is some evidence of increased mortality in the general trauma population for patients admitted with hypothermia and at least one early study demonstrated an increased incidence of infection in head injured patients subjected to hypothermia (Sutcliffe 2001). Both the ABIC and EBIC guidelines, while recognizing the need to treat pyrexia after severe TBI, consider therapeutic hypothermia as experimental at present (Maas et al. 1997, Brain Trauma Foundation 1996).

Seizure activity

This reflects disordered electrical discharges in the damaged brain and results in local loss of autoregulation, increased metabolic activity in the brain with concomitant increases in cerebral blood flow and tissue lactacidosis, which may aggravate ICP. Seizures are common after TBI in 5–15% of patients, especially in those who have suffered a haematoma, penetrating injury, including depressed skull fracture with dural penetration, and focal neurological signs or intracranial sepsis (Watkins 2000, Dunn 1996).

If seizure activity is continuous, i.e. status epilepticus or serial fitting, severe cerebral oedema may occur. Patients having seizures should be protected from harm, but if they are not in any danger then they should not be handled. The seizure should be observed for origin, sequence of events and time of start/finish. This information should be clearly recorded in the patient's notes. In the conscious patient a single seizure requires only supportive treatment, but in the comatose patient every seizure can threaten life or neurological function and should be treated appropriately. Anticonvulsants should be used if two or more seizures occur (Watkins 2000). Both the post-ictal state and medication may alter the neurological observations, so extra vigilance is required. Regular GCS observations should be completed until the pre-seizure state is regained.

No generally accepted classification of seizures exists, but it is useful to distinguish between non-focal seizures, where loss of consciousness is the primary event, followed by convulsions affecting all four limbs, and focal or partial seizures, where activity is confined to one area of the cerebral cortex. The continuous neuronal firing, which occurs during non-focal seizure activity, causes a massive increase in the brain's requirement for oxygen. As these demands can rarely be met by a corresponding increase in the supply of oxygen, ischaemia and neuronal death may occur.

Neuroprotective drugs

Corticosteroids have been used in the treatment of certain neurological conditions since the 1950s. There is no doubt about their value in producing rapid improvement in patients with brain tumours associated with oedema and there is evidence of benefit in the early administration of high-dose methylprednisolone in spinal cord injury.

CRASH Trial collaborators (2004, 2005) state, after a major study involving over 10 000 adults, that patients with head injuries should *not* be given corticosteroids, as they increase the risk of death or severe disability. The ABIC and EBIC guidelines also do not recommend steroids in the treatment of severe TBI.

Fluid management

Fluid management is crucial to ensuring adequate maintenance of ICP. As previously stated, patients should have adequate fluid resuscitation to ensure they are normotensive. Several factors need to be considered in the fluid management of patients following severe TBI:

- clinical and laboratory assessment of volume status
- the effects of different fluids on CPP and cerebral oedema

- osmotic therapy
- water and electrolyte disturbances.

Following TBI the blood-brain barrier (BBB) is likely to be disrupted, and different solutions can have an effect on cerebral oedema. If the serum osmolarity falls, water moves across the BBB along the altered osmotic gradient, causing cerebral oedema, increased ICP and decreased CPP. The use of hypotonic fluids should, therefore, be avoided.

Since 0.9% saline is isotonic, with an osmolarity of 308 mosm/l, it has a negligible effect on brain water and has become the crystalloid of choice in the management of TBI. Resuscitation with 0.9% saline requires 4 times the volume of blood lost to restore haemodynamic parameters; therefore, blood loss from other injuries should be replaced with blood products (Spiekermann & Thompson 1996).

The use of hypertonic saline solutions (7.5%) has recently been studied in the context of fluid resuscitation in TBI. Theoretically, hypertonic saline, like mannitol, through its osmotic effect on the brain should decrease brain oedema and potentially decrease ICP when used for volume resuscitation. This assumption is supported by several laboratory studies and one clinical study that reported improved survival when hypertonic saline was compared to isotonic crystalloid for initial fluid replacement in patients with severe TBI. A decrease in CSF production with the use of hypertonic saline has also been reported. Hypertonic saline solutions may improve outcome in patients with multiple trauma because of a favourable effect on ICP; however, further studies are needed before they can be used routinely in clinical practice (Spiekermann & Thompson 1996)

Based on data from various studies, it is widely accepted that glucose-containing solutions should not be used in the fluid management of patients following severe TBI unless specifically indicated to correct hypoglycaemia. The mechanism by which glucose worsens neurological injury is not fully understood; however, it is believed that, in the presence of ischaemia, glucose is metabolized anaerobically leading to an accumulation of lactic acid. Increased lactic acid is thought to decrease intracellular pH, compromise cellular function and ultimately cause cell death. An alternative explanation proposes that hyperglycaemia worsens ischaemia by decreasing CBF. Other studies suggest that hyperglycaemia decreases cerebral adenosine levels, and adenosine is an inhibitor of the release of excitatory amino acids that are thought to play a major role in ischaemic cell death (Spiekermann & Thompson 1996). Accurate fluid input and output observations are essential. For this reason, because of diuretic therapy (mannitol) and to reduce discomfort, patients should have a urinary catheter.

Positioning

Many studies have been undertaken to determine the influence of body position on ICP and CPP and establish the best practices for positioning of severe TBI patients (Sullivan 2000). It has been demonstrated that head elevation decreases ICP and that head rotation and neck flexion are associated with increased ICP, decreased jugular venous return and localized changes in cerebral blood flow. In the light of these findings, it is common practice to position head-injured patients in bed with the head elevated above the heart to varying degrees (0–30°) provided they have an adequate blood pressure and there are no contraindications, in neutral alignment with the trunk, in order to reduce ICP.

Referral to a neurosurgeon

Patients should be referred where

- a new surgically significant abnormality on imaging is seen
- a persisting coma (GCS less than or equal to 8) after initial resuscitation
- unexplained confusion, which persists for more than 4 hours
- deterioration in GCS score after admission. Greater attention should be paid to motor response deterioration
- progressive focal neurological signs
- a seizure without full recovery
- definite or suspected penetrating injury
- a cerebrospinal fluid leak (NICE 2003).

Transfer to a specialist neurosurgical unit

The most common reason for interhospital transfer in the head-injured patient is the need for surgical intervention, such as evacuation of haematoma or treatment of a depressed skull fracture. Once the decision to transfer has been made, it is imperative that the patient is thoroughly resuscitated and stabilized prior to transfer to avoid complications during the journey.

The neck should be fully examined to identify or exclude cervical injury (see also Chapter 6). Chest or abdominal injuries (Chapters 7 and 8) should be treated if potentially life-threatening and fractures splinted where appropriate (see Chapter 5). Airway management is a major cause for concern during transfer. Unconscious patients, those who are vomiting or those whose condition appears to be deteriorating (GCS less than 8) should be intubated and ventilated prior to transfer (NICE 2003).

Any patient being transferred should be accompanied by a clinician with at least 2 years experience in an appropriate specialism, e.g. anaesthesia, or a paediatrician and one who has received supervised training in the transfer of patients with a severe head injury, along with a competent nurse escort (NICE 2003). During transfer, the patient should be carefully observed and ECG, oxygen saturation levels and blood pressure should be monitored continuously (Parkins 1998). All patients with a GCS less than or equal to 8 requiring transfer should be intubated and ventilated. If the patient is not sedated, pupil size and reaction and GCS should be recorded. All documentation and results of clinical investigations, such as CT, should accompany the patient (Jones 1993).

Surgical treatment

Delay in surgical treatment of TBI has been shown to be a major preventable cause of morbidity and mortality. In a typical series of patients who had surgery for acute sub-dural haematoma (ASDH), more than 70% had a functional recovery, that is, good recovery or moderate disability, if the delay from injury to operation was less than 2 hours. Where the delay was 2–4 hours, just over 60% made a functional recovery. Where the delay was more than 4 hours after the injury, fewer than 10% made a functional recovery (Watkins 2000). The Royal College of Surgeons of England recommends that, in all circumstances, life-saving decompressive surgery must be available, to all patients who require it, within 4 hours of the injury (Royal College of Surgeons 1999, Flannery & Buxton 2001).

Some lesions may be inaccessible to the neurosurgeon or be in such sensitive areas of the brain that the risks of surgery are too great. Alternatively, brain injury may be diffuse and surgical intervention inappropriate. Whether all haematomas must be removed remains controversial and this is particularly so in the management of intracerebral haematomas and haemorrhagic contusions. While some surgeons advocate early surgery in such cases, experience has shown that despite surgical treatment, post-operative intracranial hypertension continues to occur in virtually all patients. The ABIC and EBIC guidelines outline specific indications for surgery based on biological and pathophysiological principles, published evidence and practical experience (Maas et al. 1997, Brain Trauma Foundation 1996).

Indications for decompressive surgery:
- intracranial mass lesions with > 5 mm midline shift or basal cistern compression on CT scan
- a surgically significant (1 cm thick) EDH or ASDH needs evacuation within 2–4 hours of injury to achieve optimal chance of recovery
- for small haemorrhagic contusions or other small intracerebral lesions a conservative approach is generally adopted but operation should be considered urgent for a large ICH (> 20–30 ml) based on position, clinical condition and ICP
- skull fracture depressed greater than the thickness of the skull or compound fractures with a torn dura require surgery (Maas et al. 1997, Brain Trauma Foundation 1996).

Decompressive craniectomy/craniotomy

The practice of wide bone removal for the treatment of intracranial hypertension due to cerebral oedema, refractory to medical management, has a long history and remains controversial. Polin et al. (1997) concluded that provided surgery was performed before ICP exceeded 40 mmHg for a sustained period and within 48 hours of injury, decompressive craniectomy showed a statistical advantage over medical treatment.

Surgical excision of a contused lobe to give the swelling brain more space is also a controversial issue. It has been shown to produce a worthwhile outcome in some cases and seems to be indicated especially in young patients with deteriorating coma scores and CT evidence of widespread bilateral swelling. Contraindications are primary brainstem injury or established signs of herniation, that is, bilateral dilated and unreactive pupils. Decompressive craniectomy, which can also increase oedema formation, is usually reserved as a last resort (Maas et al. 1997).

BRAIN STEM DEATH TESTING

The diagnosis of brainstem death is usually made in the intensive care unit.

Preconditions
- Diagnosis compatible with brainstem death
- Presence of irreversible structural brain damage
- Presence of apnoeic coma preconditions

Exclusions
- Therapeutic drug effects (sedatives, hypnotics, muscle relaxants)
- hypothermia (temp >35°C)

- metabolic abnormalities
- endocrine abnormalities
- intoxication

Clinical tests
1. Confirmation of absent brain stem reflexes

- no pupillary response to light
- absent corneal reflex
- no motor response within cranial nerve distribution
- absent gag reflex
- absent cough reflex
- absent vestibulo-ocular reflex

2. Confirmation of persistent apnoea

- pre-oxygenation with 100% oxygen for 10 minutes
- allow $PaCO_2$ to rise above 5.0 kPa before test
- disconnect from ventilator
- maintain adequate oxygenation during test
- allow $PaCO_2$ to climb above 6.65 kPa
- confirm no spontaneous respiration
- reconnect ventilator

3. Two experienced practitioners should perform clinical tests

- at least one should be a consultant: both must be competent to perform the tests, i.e. intensivists/neurologists/neurosurgeons
- neither should be part of the transplant team
- the tests should be performed on two separate occasions
- there is no necessary prescribed time interval between the tests.

These conditions limit the probability of the full testing occurring in the emergency department; however, some or all of the tests may be performed, either to complete a clinical picture or to reach an endpoint in an inevitable situation. This is a very difficult situation to manage, even in the intensive care unit, when the nurse may be familiar with the patient's family and friends.

CONCLUSION

Head trauma can have a devastating effect on a person's life and some mortality and morbidity are inevitable. The emergency nurse is fundamental to keeping morbidity to a minimum by being vigilant and preventing secondary brain injury

References

American College of Surgeons (2004) *Advanced Trauma Life Support*, 7th edn. Chicago: American College of Surgeons.

Bavetta S, Benjamin JC (2002) Assessment and management of the head-injured patient. *Hospital Medicine*, **63**, 289–293.

Brain Trauma Foundation (1996) American Association of Neurological Surgeons' Joint section on neurotrauma and critical care guidelines for the management of severe head injury. *Journal of Neurotrauma* **13**, 641–734

Bratton Sl, Davis RL (1997) Acute lung injury in isolated traumatic brain injury. *Neurosurgery* **40**(4), 707–712

Bullock R (1995) Mannitol and other diuretics in severe neurotrauma. *New Horizons* **3**(3), 443–452.

Bullock R, Teasdale G (1996) Head injuries. In: Skinner D, Driscoll R, Earlam R (eds), *ABC of Trauma*. London: BMJ Publishing Group.

Cesarini KG (1996) Pathophysiology of cerebral ischaemia. In: Palmer JD (ed.), *Manual of Neurosurgery*. London: Churchill Livingstone

Chan K, Dearden NM, Miller JD, Andrews PJD, Midgley S (1995) Multimodality monitoring as a guide to treatment of intracranial hypertension after severe brain injury. *Neurosurgery* **32**(4), 547–553.

Chesnut RM, Marshall LF, Klauber MR (1993) The role of secondary brain injury in determining outcome from severe head injury. *Journal of Trauma* **34**, 216–222.

Chesnut RM (1995) Secondary brain insults after injury: clinical perspectives. *New Horizons* **3**, 366–375.

Chesnut RM, Gautille T, Blunt BA, Kaluber MR, Marshall LF (1998) Neurogenic hypotension in patients with severe head injuries. *Journal of Trauma* **44**(6), 958–963.

Clifton GL, Ziegler MG, Grossman A (1981) Circulating catecholamines and sympathetic activity after head injury. *Neurosurgery* **8**, 10–14.

Clifton GL, Robertson CS, Kyper K et al. (1983) Cardiovascular response to severe head injury. *Journal of Neurosurgery* **3**, 447–454.

Contant CF, Valadka AB, Shankar MD et al. (2001) Adult respiratory distress syndrome: a complication of induced hypertension after severe head injury. *Journal of Neurosurgery*, **95**, 560–568.

CRASH Trial collaborators (2005) Final results of MRC CRASH, a randomized placebo-controlled trial of intravenous corticosteroid in adults with head injury – outcomes at 6 months. *The Lancet* **365** (9475), 1957–1959.

CRASH Trial collaborators (2004) Effects of intravenous corticosteroids on death within 14 days in 10 008 adults with clinically significant head injury (MRC CRASH Trial): randomized placebo-controlled trial. *Lancet* **364** (9442), 1321–1328.

Crossman AR, Neary D (2000) *Neuroanatomy – An Illustrated Colour Text*, 2nd edn. Edinburgh: Churchill Livingstone.

Darby J, Yonas H., Marion DW et al. (1998) Local 'inverse steal' induced by hyperventilation in head injury. *Neurosurgery*, **23**, 84.

Dearden NM (1998) Mechanism and prevention of secondary brain damage during intensive care. *Clinical Neuropathology* **17**(47), 221–228.

Duffy C (2001) Anaesthesia for head injury. In: Gupta AK and Summors A (eds), *Notes in Neuroanaesthesia and Critical Care*. London: Greenwich Medical Media.

Dunn LT (1996) Post-traumatic epilepsy. In: Palmer JD (ed), *Manual of Neurosurgery*. London: Churchill Livingstone.

Durieux ME (1996) Anaesthesia for head trauma. In: *The Neuroanaesthesia Handbook* (eds. Stone DJ et al.). St. Louis: Mosby

Farnsworth ST, Sperry RJ (1996) Neurophysiology. In: Stone JD, Sperry RJ et al. (eds), *The Neuroanaesthesia Handbook*, St Louis: Mosby.

Fernandes C, Landolt H (1996) Blood brain barrier and cerebral oedema. In: Palmer JD (ed.), *Manual of Neurosurgery*. London: Churchill Livingstone.

Flannery T, Buxton N (2001) Modern management of head injuries. *Journal of the Royal College of Surgeons (Edinburgh)* **46**, 150–153.

Graham DI, Hume Adams J, Nicoll JAR, Maxwell WL, Gennarelli TA (1995) The nature, distribution and causes of traumatic brain injury. *Brain Pathology* **5**, 397–406.

Harrahill M (1997) Management of severe head injury: new document provides guidelines. *Journal of Emergency Nursing* **23**(3), 282–283.

Hersch C (1961) Electrocardiographic changes in head injuries. *Circulation* **23**, 853–860.

Hickey JV (1997) *The Clinical Practice of Neurological and Neurosurgical Nursing*, 4th edn. Philadelphia: JB Lippincott.

Hindman BJ, Todd MM, Gelb AW et al. (1999) Mild hypothermia as a protective therapy during intracranial aneurysm surgery: a randomized prospective pilot trial. *Neurosurgery* **44**, 23–33.

Hudak CM, Gallo BM (1994) *Critical Care Nursing*, 6th edn. Philadelphia: JB Lippincott.

Intensive Care Society (1997) *Guidelines for the transport of the critically ill adult*. London: Intensive Care Society.

Jackson S (1995) Not so minor head injuries? *Emergency Nurse* **3**(1), 19–22.

Jones H (1993) Safe transfer. *Nursing Times* **89**(41), 31–33.

Kawamura S, Suzuki A, Hadeishi H et al. (2000) Cerebral blood flow and oxygen metabolism during mild hypothermia in patients with subarachnoid haemorrhage. *Acta Neurochir* (Wein) **142**(10), 1117–1121.

Kelly DF, Goodale DB, Williams J, Herr DL et al. (1999) Propofol in the treatment of moderate and severe head injury: a randomized prospective double-blind trial. *Journal of Neurosurgery* **90**(6), 1042–1052.

Kelly DF (2000) Sedation after severe head injury: beneficial to final outcome? *European Journal of Anaesthesiology* **17** Suppl. 18, 43–54.

Klauber K (1993) Rehabilitation of the trauma patient. In: Neff JA, Kidd PS, eds. *Trauma Nursing: the Art and Science*. St Louis: Mosby Year Book.

Kwiatkowski S (1996) Traumatic acute intracranial haematoma. In: Palmer JD, ed. *Manual of Neurosurgery.* London: Churchill Livingstone.

Lang EW, Chesnut RM (1995) Intracranial pressure and cerebral perfusion pressure in severe head injury. *New Horizons* 3, 400–409

Lindsey KW, Bone I, Callander R (2004) *Neurology and Neurosurgery Illustrated*, 4th edn. Edinburgh: Churchill Livingstone.

Maartens N, Lethbridge G (2005) Head and neck trauma. In: RA O'Shea, ed. *Principles and Practice of Trauma Nursing.* Edinburgh: Elsevier Churchill Livingstone.

Maas AIR, Dearden M, Teasdale GM, Braakman R, Cohadon F, Lannotti F et al. (1997) European Brain Injury Consortium Guidelines for management of severe head injury in adults. *Acta Neurochir* (Wien), **139**, 286–294.

Marion DW, Penrod, LE, Kelsey SF et al. (1997) Treatment of traumatic brain injury with moderate hypothermia. *New England Journal of Medicine* **336**(8), 560–566.

Marmarou A, Anderson RL, Ward JD et al. (1991) Impact of ICP instability and hypotension on outcome in patients with severe head trauma. *Journal of Neurosurgery* **75**, 559–566.

Matta BF, Menon DK (1996) Severe head injury in the United Kingdom and Ireland: a survey of practice and implications for management. *Critical Care Medicine* **24**, 1743–1748

May AK, Young JS, Butler K et al. (1997) Coagulopathy in severe closed head injury: is empiric therapy warranted? *American Journal of Surgery* **63**(3), 233–236.

McLeod AA, Neil-Dwyer G, Meyer CHA et al. (1982) Cardiac sequelae of acute head injury. *British Heart Journal* **47**, 221–226

McNaughton H, Harwood M (2002) Traumatic brain injury: assessment and management. *Hospital Medicine* **63**, 8–12.

National Institute for Clinical Excellence [NICE] (2003) *Head Injury Triage, Assessment, Investigation and Early Management of Head Injury in Infants, Children and Adults.* London: NICE.

Oppenheimer SM, Cochetto DF, Hachinski VC (1990) Cerebrogenic cardiac arrhythmias. *Acta Neurology* **47**, 513-519

Parkins DR (1998) Transportation of the injured: head injuries. *Pre-hospital Immediate Care* **2**, 25–26.

Patel HC, Menon DK, Tebbs S et al. (2002) Specialist neurocritical care and outcome from head injury. *Intensive Care Medicine* **28**, 547–553

Piek J, Chesnut RM, Marshall LF et al. (1992) Extracranial complications of severe head injury. *Journal of Neurosurgery* **77**, 901–907.

Polin S, Shaffrey ME, Bogaev CA et al. (1997) Decompressive craniectomy in the treatment of severe refractory post-traumatic cerebral oedema. *Neurosurgery* **41**, 84–94.

Prielipp RC, Coursin DB (1995) Sedative and neuromuscular blocking drug use in critically ill patients with head injuries. *New Horizons* **3**(3), 456–468.

Ramrakha P, Moore K (1997) *Oxford Handbook of Acute Medicine.* Oxford: Oxford University Press.

Robertson CS, Valadka AB, Hannay HJ et al. (1999) Prevention of secondary insults after severe head injury. *Critical Care Medicine* **27**, 2086–2095.

Robertson CS (2001) Management of cerebral perfusion pressure after traumatic brain injury. *Anaesthesiology* **95**(6), 15, 13–17.

Rosner MJ, Rosner SD, Johnson AH (1995) Cerebral perfusion pressure – management protocol and clinical results. *Journal of Neurosurgery* **83**, 949–962.

Royal College of Surgeons (1999) *Report of the Working Party on the Management of Patients with Head Injury.* London: Royal College of Surgeons.

Sakas DE, Dias LS, Beale D (1995) Subarachnoid haemorrhage presenting as a head injury. *British Medical Journal* **310**, 1186–1187.

Shah S (1999) Neurological assessment. *Nursing Standard* **13** (22), 49–56.

Spiekermann BF, Thompson SA (1996) Fluid management. In: Stone D and Sperry RJ et al. (eds) *The Handbook of Neuroanaesthesia.* St Louis: Mosby.

Sullivan J (2000) Positioning of patients with severe traumatic brain injury: research based practice. *Journal of Neuroscientific Nursing* **32**(4), 204–209.

Sutcliffe A (2001) Hypothermia (or not) for the management of head injury. *Care of the Critically Ill* **17**(5), 162–165.

Teasdale G, Jennett B (1974) Assessment of coma and impaired consciousness: a practical scale. *The Lancet,* **2** (7872), 81–84.

Van der Ark GD (1975) Cardiovascular changes with acute subdural haematoma. *Surgical Neurology,* **5**(3), 305–308.

Watkins LD (2000) Head *injuries*: general principles and management. *Surgery* **18**(7), 219–224.

Yamamoto M, Marmarou CR, Stiefel MF et al. (1999) Neuroprotective effect of hypothermia on neuronal injury in diffuse traumatic brain injury coupled with hypoxia and hypotension. *Journal of Neurotrauma,* **16**(6), 487–499.

Chapter 5

Skeletal injuries

Mary Dawood & Lynda Holt

CHAPTER CONTENTS

INTRODUCTION

Skeletal and soft tissue injuries range in severity from life- or limb-threatening to self-limiting minor injuries. International research has demonstrated that patients with musculoskeletal injuries represent approximately 25% of the emergency department workload. It is imperative for emergency nurses to be able to assess musculoskeletal injury and identify life- or limb-threatening trauma, some of which may not seem devastating at first glance.

This chapter will provide the underpinning anatomy and physiology of the musculoskeletal system, before looking at areas such as pelvis, neck of femur and limb injuries. Each of these will be examined in detail, principles of assessment and management will be discussed, and particular problems related to specific injuries will be identified.

ANATOMY AND PHYSIOLOGY

In order to appreciate the impact of injury, it is necessary for the emergency nurse to have a thorough understanding of the make-up and purpose of the human skeleton (Fig. 5.1) and skeletal muscle. The skeleton comprises two parts with specific functions:

- *the axial skeleton*, consisting of the skull, vertebral column, ribs and sternum – supports and protects vital organs
- *the appendicular skeleton*, consisting of the shoulder girdle, pelvic girdle and limbs – provides shape and facilitates movement.

Bone is a form of connective tissue comprising three major components:

- organic matrix of collagen – creates tensile strength
- mineral matrix of calcium and phosphate – creates rigidity and strength

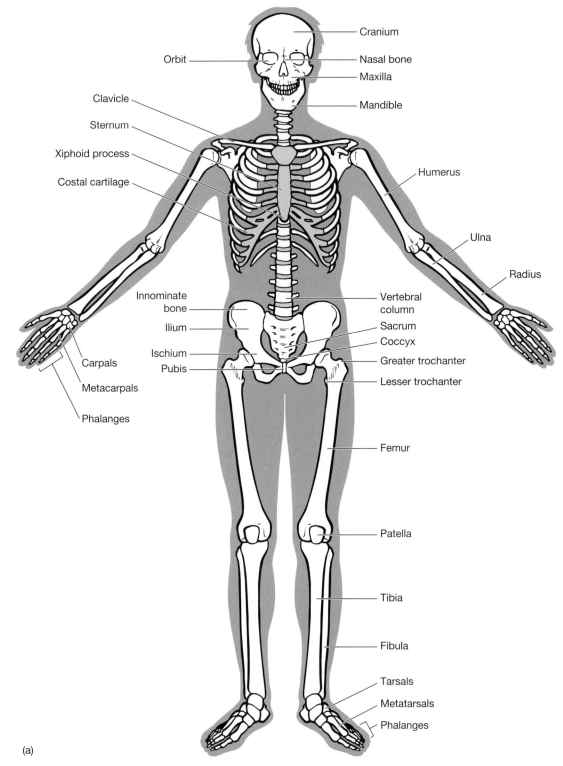

(a)

Figure 5.1 The skeleton. (a) Anterior view and

(Continued)

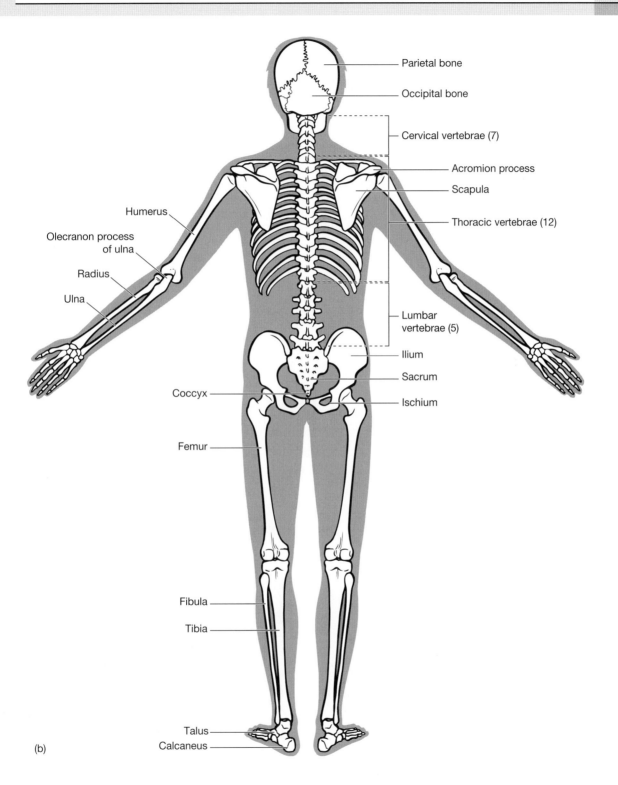

Parietal bone

Occipital bone

Cervical vertebrae (7)

Acromion process

Scapula

Thoracic vertebrae (12)

Humerus

Olecranon process
of ulna

Radius

Ulna

Lumbar
vertebrae (5)

Ilium

Sacrum

Coccyx

Ischium

Femur

Fibula

Tibia

Talus

Calcaneus

(b)

Figure 5.1 Cont'd   (b) Posterior view.

- bone cells, including osteoblasts, osteoclasts, osteocytes and fibroblasts.

Compact cortical bone, which is found on outer parts of all bone, forms the shaft of long bones and encloses marrow cavities (see Fig. 5.2). Compact bone contains Haversian canals with osteocytes which facilitate the exchange of nutrients and waste. Cancellous bone (trabeculae) is organized in a lattice system and contains fewer Haversian canals. Red and fatty bone marrow fills the cavities in the lattice. Cancellous bone is found at the ends of the long bone and in the vertebrae and flat bones.

The periosteum is a fibrous tissue layer covering bone, but not cartilage or synovial joints. It transmits blood vessels and nerve fibres. The periosteum also provides attachments for ligaments and muscles. Beneath this layer are osteoblasts which aid bone growth, as a result, the periosteum does not attach to the bone surface until adulthood when growth is complete. Because of the abundant nerve supply, the periosteum is responsible for bone pain. Damage to periosteum or pressure on it from tumours or trauma can cause severe pain.

Bone cells

Osteoblasts These are present on all bone surfaces and form a uniform layer. Their purpose is the synthesis and secretion of collagen and protein, and they promote calcification during rapid phases of this process.

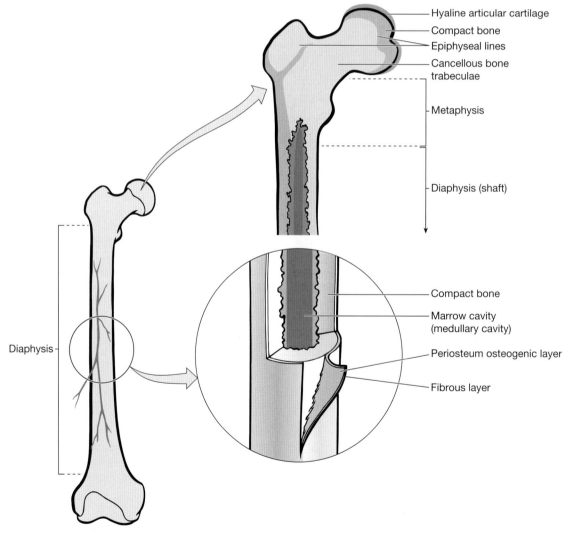

Hyaline articular cartilage
Compact bone
Epiphyseal lines
Cancellous bone trabeculae
Metaphysis
Diaphysis (shaft)
Diaphysis
Compact bone
Marrow cavity (medullary cavity)
Periosteum osteogenic layer
Fibrous layer

Figure 5.2   Cross-section of bone.

Osteocytes These form from osteoblasts trapped in matrix. The exact function of these cells is not known, but they appear to act as a pump, controlling calcium release in response to hormones.

Osteoclasts These are found near bone surfaces and are responsible for reabsorption of bone. They are very mobile and are found in great numbers where bone is undergoing erosion. Their activity is controlled by a number of hormones including parathyroid and thyroxin.

Joints

Joints are the area of contact between bone and bone, or bone and cartilage. They are classified by the type of movement they permit.

Fibrous joints permit no movement at all, e.g. skull joints. Fibrous connective tissue merges into the periosteum of each bone.

Cartilaginous joints permit limited movement because of flexible cartilage between bones. The symphyses have cartilage pads, or discs, between bones, e.g. symphysis pubis or intervertebral joints. Complex ligament arrangements stabilize these cartilage pads to limit movement and facilitate recoil. Synchondroses are cartilage joints which ossify in adulthood and prevent movement, e.g. epiphysis of long bone.

Synovial joints form most of the body's joints. They are further classified by the type and range of movement they allow (see Table 5.1). All synovial joints have a number of similar structured features. They are enclosed in a capsule which is lined with synovial membrane, which secretes synovial fluid. Bone ends are not in direct contact and are covered by hyaline cartilage. The fibrous capsule is held in place by a number of ligaments.

Muscular system

Muscle tissue is formed to convert chemical energy into mechanical contraction, creating movement. Movements are generated both at joints and in soft tissue. Muscles also assist in maintaining body posture and muscular activity is associated with maintaining body heat.

Muscles are made up of bundles of fibres (fasciculi). The length of these fibres relates to the range of movement the muscle performs; that is, the longer the fibre, the greater is the range of movement. The number of fibres relates to the strength of the muscle. Muscles are attached to the periosteum by tendons. There are two points of attachment, the origin of which remains fixed during contraction while the insertion moves. Skeletal muscles have a rich blood supply which increases dramatically during exercise.

Table 5.1 Classification of synovial joints

Type of joint	Site	Range of movement
Hinge	Elbow Fingers Ankle Toes	Flexion Extension
Pivot	Vertebral column	Rotation
Gliding	Shoulder girdle Vertebral column	Limited motion in several directions
Ball and socket	Hip Shoulder	Extensive range of movement: Flexion Extension Rotation
Saddle	Hand Base of thumb	Flexion Extension Abduction Adduction Opposition
Ellipson	Wrist Hand Foot	Flexion Extension Abduction Adduction Opposition

Tendons

Tendons are made up of fibrous connective tissue carrying parallel bundles of collagen fibres. This gives greater flexibility but prevents stretching when under pressure, such as in muscle contraction. They act like a spring, allowing the transition of movement from muscle to bone. Tendons have a sparse blood supply which inhibits healing if damaged.

Ligaments

Ligaments are made up of bundles of collagen that are not designed to stretch. They are attached to bone and are responsible for maintaining joint stability. Undueforce may tear some fibres, resulting in them being painful, swollen and in severe cases can result in unstable joints.

PELVIC INJURY

Anatomy and physiology

The pelvis is designed to provide structure, strength for weight-bearing, and protection of internal organs. It houses the rectum, bladder and, in women, the reproductive organs. The pelvis forms a ring, comprising

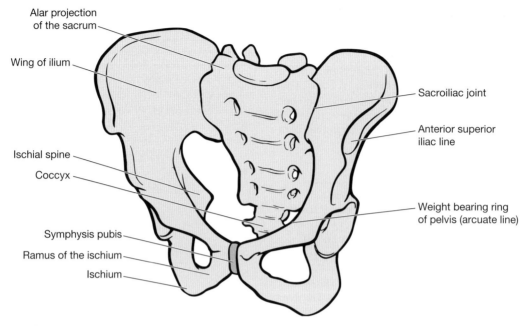

Alar projection
of the sacrum

Wing of ilium

Sacroiliac joint

Anterior superior
iliac line

Ischial spine

Coccyx

Symphysis pubis

Ramus of the ischium

Ischium

Weight bearing ring
of pelvis (arcuate line)

Figure 5.3   The pelvis.

the sacrum and two innominate bones, each made up of an ilium, pubic bone and ischium (see Fig. 5.3).

The bones are supported by strong ligaments at the sacroiliac joint, and cartilaginous joint at the symphysis pubis. The innominate bones do not fuse until around 16–18 years of age, and in children are supported by cartilage. The pelvis has a rich blood supply from the internal and external iliac arteries. The stability of the pelvic ring is dependent on the strong posterior sacroiliac, sacrotuberous and sacrospinous ligaments. Disruption of the pelvic ring can result in significant trauma to the neurovascular and soft tissue structures it protects.

Mechanism of injury

Major trauma to the pelvic girdle is relatively uncommon and accounts for approximately 3–6% of all skeletal injuries and 20% of polytrauma cases (Smith 2005); however, the mortality associated with major pelvic fractures ranges from 4 to 50% (Monsell & Ross 1998, Muir et al. 1996). Most pelvic fractures are caused by motorcycle accidents, accidents involving pedestrians, direct crush injuries or falls from a height (American College of Surgeons 2004).

Fracture patterns

In adults, isolated pelvic fractures rarely occur. This is because of the strength and ligamentous stretch of the pelvic ring. If significant force is applied, two or more breaks in the pelvic ring are likely to occur. The pelvis

has predictable areas of strength and weakness, and therefore, in adults, potential patterns of fractures are easy to predict. In children, the increased elasticity of the pelvis prior to fusion of the innominate bones makes isolated fractures far more likely.

Lateral compression fractures (graded I, II, III) are caused by a side impact, usually to motorcyclists or pedestrians in collision with vehicles. A compression fracture of the pubic bone or rami is combined with compression fracture on the side of impact (see Fig. 5.4a). With greater force of impact, the iliac wing on the side of the impact will also break; this is a grade II injury (Fig. 5.4b). A grade III injury also involves the opposite side to the impact (Fig. 5.4c).

Anteroposterior compression fractures (graded I, II, III) are caused by direct pressure or crushing and result in the pelvis opening outwards from wings rather like a book. The result is fracturing of the pubis or rami together with sacroiliac distribution. In grade I injuries, the symphysis is separated by less than 2 cm (see Fig. 5.5a); in grade II injuries the sacrospinous and sacrotuberous ligaments rupture (Fig. 5.5b); and in grade III injuries the iliolumbar ligament can rupture (Fig. 5.5c). This type of pelvic fracture has double the mortality rate of the lateral compression injuries.

Vertical shearing force fractures result from falls or from knees hitting a car dashboard with great speed. The pattern of injury is similar to anteroposterior compression, but with vertical displacement (see Fig. 5.6). With combined mechanical forces, such as being run

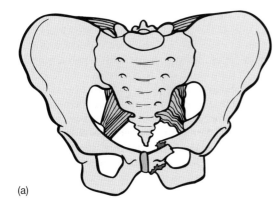

(a)

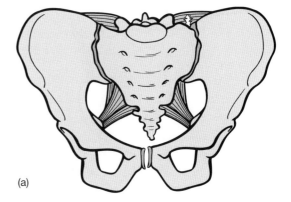

(a)

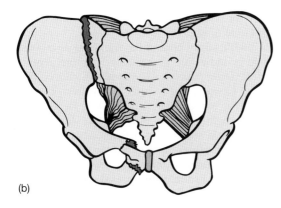

(b)

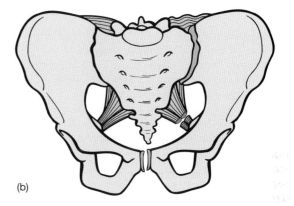

(b)

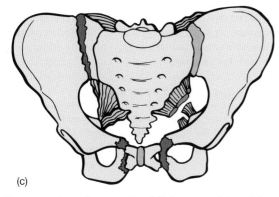

(c)

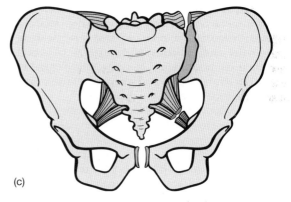

(c)

Figure 5.4   Lateral compression (LC) fractures of the pelvis. (a) Grade I, (b) Grade II, (c) Grade III.

Figure 5.5   Anteroposterior compression (APC) fractures of the pelvis. (a) Grade I, (b) Grade II, (c) Grade III.

over by a motor vehicle, a combination of the above fracture patterns may occur simultaneously.

Patterns of single fracture injury to the pelvis include:

- a*cetabulum* – these are not common in isolation, but can occur with direct force to the leg, driving the head of the femur into the acetabulum

- *sacrum* – again these are uncommon in isolation, but can result from a backward fall or falls from a height
- *coccyx* – this is often fractured by falls onto the buttocks, particularly in women where the coccyx is more prominent
- *single pubic ramus* – these appear to be common in elderly patients following falls; however, evidence

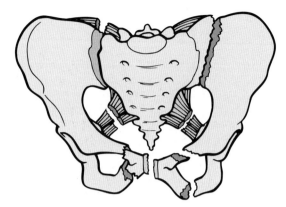

Figure 5.6 Pelvic ring fracture.

suggests that they usually occur with other pelvic injuries that are not initially detected

- *avulsion fractures* – these occur in young athletes, where excessive muscle strain can avulse growth cartilage on the apophyseal plates
- *iliac wing fractures* – these injuries commonly result from direct trauma and should always be considered in conjunction with intra-abdominal injury.

Assessment of pelvic ring injury

Fractures involving the pelvic ring carry potentially life-threatening complications if not rapidly identified and treated. Because of the force exerted to cause such fractures, attendant injury to underlying organs and haemorrhage is common and associated with high morbidity and mortality rates. Injuries can include rectal, urethral or vaginal bleeding; neurological deficit; haematuria; and haemodynamic instability due to hypovolaemic shock (Routt et al. 2002).

Mechanisms of injury should give some clues as to a potential pelvic fracture. The assessing nurse should carry out a primary assessment following the ABCDE approach laid out in ATLS guidelines (American College of Surgeons 2004). A patient with a pelvic ring fracture will have severe pelvic pain and progressive flank, perianal or scrotal swelling and bruising. Disruption of the pelvic ring can also be identified by differences in leg length and external rotation of a leg without an associated limb fracture.

Mechanical instability of the pelvis can be tested by manual manipulation or compression of the pelvis. This should be carried out once by an experienced clinician and only when X-rays have excluded unstable pelvic fractures. It is a very painful procedure for the patient and undue force carries the risk of exacerbating haemorrhage. When the clinician manipulates

the pelvis, pressure should be applied gently to the iliac crest. If the pelvis has rotated, the clinician will be able to close the ring by gently pushing the iliac crests together. Most patients with a pelvic ring fracture will have moderate to severe hypotension.

Assessment should also include examination of groins, perineal area and genitalia. Femoral pulses should be checked on both sides. Absent pulses are indicative of damage to the external iliac artery and surgery is required to preserve the limb of the affected side. Decreased pulse pressure should be closely monitored, as it may be indicative of a worsening systemic condition or damage to the iliac artery. The perineum should be inspected for laceration and bleeding. Prophylactic antibiotics should be prescribed for wounds because of the high infection risk from faecal flora (Ruiz 1995).

In men testicles should be examined as a swollen testicle is indicative of testicular rupture requiring surgical decompression. The penis should be examined for blood at the meatus, suggestive of urethral damage. In women the vulva should be examined, and the vagina and urethral meatus inspected for blood. In male and female patients where there is no evidence of urethral injury, a urinary catheter should be inserted. If urethral injury is likely then suprapubic catheterization should be considered for bladder decompression. A rectal examination should be performed to test sphincter tone; a reduction in tone is suggestive of a sacral fracture. Frank blood is usually indicative of a rectal tear and surgical intervention is necessary. In men, the position of the prostate should be established as a high, boggy prostate indicates a urethral transection.

Management of pelvic ring fractures

Pelvic fracture can be a life-threatening injury often accompanied by significant haemorrhage and injury to the genitourinary system (Kellman & Browner 1998). Arterial injuries occur in 20% of patients and posterior fractures are more likely than anterior fractures to cause bleeding Initial management focuses on volume replacement, stabilization of fractures and, therefore, the rate of haemorrhage and pain control. Fluid replacement should follow ATLS guidelines with a rapid infusion of warmed crystalloid fluid, ideally Ringer's lactate or Hartman's Solution (American College of Surgeons 2004). Ringer's solution closely resembles the electrolyte content of plasma and therefore provides transient intravascular expansion followed by interstitial and intracellular replacement. Normal saline can be used, but large amounts are not recommended because it can induce hypercholaemic acidosis. After an initial 2 L, or 20 ml/kg in children, blood or colloid solutions should be commenced. The patient's haemodynamic condition should be continuously monitored during this period.

Haemorrhage control relies on fracture stabilization. This can be achieved in a number of ways. The use of a pneumatic anti-shock garment (PASG) serves a dual purpose of haemorrhage and pain control. It provides mechanical stabilization of the fractures and external counter-pressure. Circulation to extremities should be regularly checked. Decompression of the PASG should take place in a controlled environment, at a pace which does not exacerbate haemodynamic instability. Usually this takes place in the operating theatre. If a PASG is not available, longitudinal skin traction can be used (American College of Surgeons 2004). Early external fixation provides definitive haemorrhage control. Pain control is initiated by fracture immobilization, but inhaled analgesia, such as Entonox in the conscious patient, and i.v. opiates are also necessary.

Uncomplicated, isolated pelvic fractures not involving the pelvic ring should be assessed in a similar manner. The management of these injuries is usually conservative. Patients usually require hospital admission for initial bed rest, pain control and rehabilitation support. Most of these fracture injuries have an uncomplicated recovery pattern. Acetabular fractures, however, have a high morbidity. They are caused by extreme force, commonly road traffic accidents (RTAs), where the knees hit the dashboard at speed. Long-term prognosis is improved by surgical intervention (Snyder 1998).

HIP INJURY

Anatomy and physiology

The femoral head and neck lie within the joint capsule of the hip joint. The head of the femur moves within the acetabulum. This is supported by three ligaments: iliofemoral, ischiofemoral and pubofemoral. Blood supply to the head of the femur is largely from the profunda femoris artery, which has circumflex branches around the neck of femur, off which smaller branches supply the head. This pattern of blood supply is particularly vulnerable to disruption from impacted fractures – hence the high risk of vascular necrosis with neck of femur fractures. The periosteum is very thin or non-existent around the neck of femur, therefore making it very susceptible to fractures. This susceptibility increases with age, particularly for women where osteoporosis has further weakened bone strength.

Classification of fractures

Neck of femur

Garden's classification of neck of femur (NOF) fractures has been used for over 40 years (Garden 1964). He highlighted four stages of fracture (Fig. 5.7):

Stage I represents impacted fractures. The trabeculae and cortex are pushed into the femoral head. This is considered a stable fracture as the inferior cortex usually remains intact. This type of fracture is not very susceptible to avascular necrosis and therefore operative treatment usually entails pinning rather than prosthetic replacement of the femoral head. Union rates are good and morbidity is low following this treatment (Ruiz 1995).

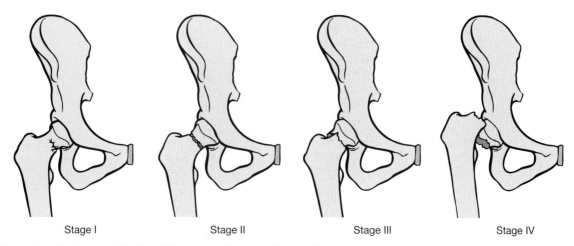

| Stage I | Stage II | Stage III | Stage IV |

Figure 5.7   Garden's classification of femoral neck fractures: Stages I–IV.

Stage II   These are non-displaced fractures across the entire femoral neck. Because there is no impaction, the fracture is unstable, but as there is no displacement the risk of avascular necrosis is low. These injuries are therefore fixed with screws.

Stage III   These are displaced fractures, with the femoral head abducted in relation to the pelvis. Fragments of the fracture are in contact with each other. Disruption of the blood supply is common and for this reason operative repair usually involves the insertion of a prosthesis to replace the femoral head.

Stage IV   Similar to stage III fractures, these are displaced, but the femoral head is adducted in relation to the pelvis, fracture fragments are completely separated and avascular necrosis is likely. In most cases, prosthetic replacement of the femoral head is the treatment of choice in younger patients; however, attempts may be made to reduce and internally fixate the fracture. This prevents degeneration of the acetabulum caused over time by a prosthesis.

Intertrochanteric fractures

Although these have specific differences from NOF fractures, the assessment of injury and initial emergency management is similar. In terms of anatomy, the main difference is in bone density, as periosteum is present over the trochanters, although osteoporosis has a detrimental effect in women. In younger people and older men these fractures are far less common than NOF fractures. These injuries are not affected by avascular necrosis as the circumflex arterial branches of the NOF are not damaged. Because of the periosteum, the risk of non-union is also lower.

Several fracture classifications are used and all have slight variations from each other. To provide a general idea of fracture classification, Kyle et al. (1979) described four types of injury (see Fig. 5.8):

- Type I – stable, undisplaced intertrochanteric fracture, requiring simple internal fixation.
- Type II – stable but displaced with fragmentation of the lesser trochanter; these are internally fixed.
- Type III – unstable fractures of the greater trochanter with postero-medial comminuted bone and deformity. These are fixed, but if a stable reduction cannot be achieved because of the amount of comminuted bone, osteotomy to the base of greater trochanter may be performed.
- Type IV – these have the components of type III fractures, but also have subtrochanteric fractures. Internal fixation is attempted using screws and sliding plates.

In children, NOF or intertrochanteric fractures are uncommon and are caused by severe force. Internal

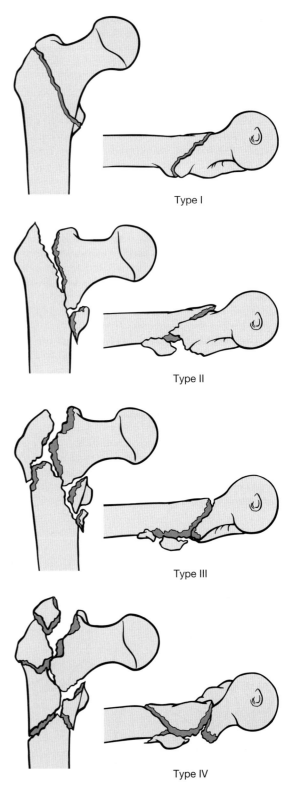

Type I

Type II

Type III

Type IV

Figure 5.8   Kyle's classification of intertrochanteric fractures.

fixation is not the treatment of choice because of growth patterns. Children are treated with bed rest and traction.

Assessment of patients with hip injury

These patients are usually elderly, predominantly women and commonly attend the emergency department following a fall (Audit Commission 2000). Although these injuries are rarely immediately life-threatening, attributed mortality is as high as 20% (Ruiz 1995). The patient usually complains of groin pain, and pain through the thigh to the knee. Pain is worsened by any movement and the majority of patients will have been unable to weight-bear since injury. In most NOF and intertrochanteric fractures, the injured limb will be externally rotated, and is shortened if displacement exists at the fracture site. Neurovascular integrity should be checked distally to the fracture, although damage of this type is extremely uncommon. The patient's haemodynamic status should be regularly observed, particularly with intertrochanteric fractures where blood loss from surrounding tissues is higher than NOF fractures. The patient's general health should be discussed and pre-existing medical conditions and medication established. It is also necessary to establish the cause of the fall to rule out medical reasons. The patient's hydration and nutritional status should be assessed, as should skin integrity and risk level for pressure sores (Wickham 1997a).

Initial management

In most instances, these fractures can be broadly diagnosed clinically. X-rays provide supplementary information which is necessary for ongoing management. As a result, patients with clinically diagnosed fractures should receive appropriate analgesia, such as morphine sulphate, prior to X-ray. Hydration at an early stage reduces mortality, and therefore intravenous fluids should be commenced, particularly for patients with intertrochanteric fractures where blood loss is greater. Regular observations should be undertaken to ensure haemodynamic stability is maintained, and to ensure the patient is neither dehydrated nor becomes overloaded by fluid replacements. Most hospitals now have fast-track policies to get patients into a ward bed and off hard emergency trolleys (Audit Commission 2000). If tissue viability is to be maintained, this together with regular pressure area care is vital (Wickham 1997b). If the patient's general condition prohibits internal repair of the fracture, skin traction is advised at the earliest opportunity.

Hip dislocation

The majority of hip dislocations occur in people with total hip replacements or femoral head replacements. Hip dislocations in patients who have not had previous hip surgery are uncommon and demand a great deal of force. Posterior dislocation is commonly caused by high-impact road traffic accidents where the patient's knee hits the dashboard. Posterior dislocation accounts for about 90% of non-prosthetic dislocations. The patient will present in severe pain, with an internally rotated, flexed leg. Neurological examination is important as those particularly with marked internal rotation may compress the sciatic nerve and its branches, resulting in deficits especially in the peroneal nerve region. Anterior dislocation is much less frequent and results from a fall from a height where the patient lands on an extended leg. This type of injury can be confused with a fractured NOF in elderly patients, and therefore careful history-taking and limb assessment are vital.

In both anterior and posterior dislocations, early limb relocation is essential. Closed reduction should be performed, provided associated fractures of the femoral head have been excluded. Management priorities in ED involve pain relief, X-ray and relocation of the hip joint under sedation. Once the hip is relocated, the patient should be admitted for traction. If relocation attempts are unsuccessful with conscious sedation in the emergency department, then urgent transfer to theatre for closed or open reduction under general anaesthetic is appropriate.

LIMB INJURY

Anatomy and physiology

Limbs form part of the appendicular skeleton and are vital for movement. Both arms and legs comprise long bones, with complex joints and bone systems in the hands and feet. Limb injuries treated in the emergency department fall into two categories: fractures and soft tissue injury.

Classification of fractures

A break or fracture of the bone occurs when it is no longer able to absorb the mechanical energy placed on it. This usually results from trauma (Bickley & Szilagyi 2003). Fractures are classified into the following groups (see Fig. 5.9):

- *simple* – this is a closed fracture; therefore the skin is intact and the fracture is undisplaced. These can be further categorized by the direction in which the fracture travels:

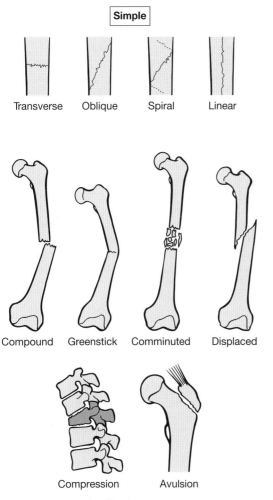

Figure 5.9 Fracture classification.

- transverse: across the bone
- oblique: at an angle to the length of the bone
- spiral: encircle the bone in a spiral around its diameter
- linear: runs parallel to the axis of the bone
- *compound* – an open fracture where bone has punctured skin. These can exist with any of the above types of fracture. It is also possible for fracture fragments to puncture blood vessels, nerves and organs
- *greenstick* – these occur in children and are incomplete fractures, like a bend which disrupts the bone cortex but does not pass right through
- *comminuted* – fragmented fracture with two or more pieces
- *displaced* – bone ends are completely separated at the fracture site
- *compression* – adjacent bones are compacted

- *avulsion* – bone ends or condyles pulled off when the ligaments remain intact under extreme force.

Fracture healing follows a specific pattern. It has three main phases: inflammatory, reparative and remodelling.

The inflammatory phase lasts approximately 72 hours. Initially a homeostatic response to the physiological damage to bone, tissue and blood vessels occurs. A dot is formed in which the fibrin networks collect debris, blood and marrow cells. Capillary network increases over 24 hours and neutrophils invade the area. In the following 48 hours, phagocytosis takes place. In the reparative stage, chondroblasts and osteoblasts proliferate. The chondroblasts unite fracture ends in a fibrous tissue called callus which begins to calcify after 14 days. Osteoblasts create the trabeculae of cancellous bone and osteoclasts destroy dead bone. Remodelling takes several months; osteoblasts and osteoclasts restore bone shape, replacing cancellous with compact bone (see Fig. 5.10).

Assessment of limb injury

Following ATLS principles, assessment of extremity injury should take place after only the primary survey is completed and more serious injuries are dealt with. The assessment has three stages:

- *identification* and intervention in life-threatening haemorrhage (primary survey)
- *identification* and intervention in limb-threatening haemorrhage (secondary survey)
- *identification* and management of other limb injuries.

Assessment should follow a set pattern regardless of how severe or trivial an injury may appear. The assessing nurse should establish the history, perform an examination and, if appropriate, refer the patient for X-ray. When assessing the history, the nurse should establish a number of factors (see Box 5.1). Mechanism of injury should include what happened, the direction and magnitude of force, and how long the patient was exposed to the force. When determining symptoms, the nurse should establish pain, loss of function and perceived swelling. The nurse should also enquire about the duration of symptoms and whether they are worsening or improving. Past history should include pre-existing injuries to that limb, medical conditions which affect the musculoskeletal system or bone density and factors which would influence recovery.

Examination

Examination should follow a specific pattern, starting from the joint above, moving through the site of

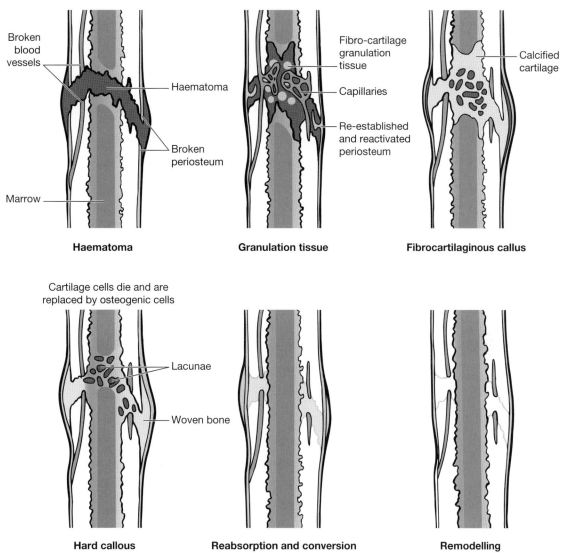

Haematoma
- Broken blood vessels
- Haematoma
- Broken periosteum
- Marrow

Granulation tissue
- Fibro-cartilage granulation tissue
- Capillaries
- Re-established and reactivated periosteum

Fibrocartilaginous callus
- Calcified cartilage

Hard callous
- Cartilage cells die and are replaced by osteogenic cells
- Lacunae
- Woven bone

Reabsorption and conversion to lamellar bone

Remodelling

Figure 5.10   Bone healing process.

Box 5.1   Establishing history of musculoskeletal injury

- Mechanism of injury
- Symptoms
- Duration
- Pain
- Previous relevant injury, iliness, medication

the injury, and finally checking neurovascular function distal to the injury. Principles of examination are shown in Box 5.2. Examination starts from the joint above the injury site both to assess function and limits of injury and to gain the patient's cooperation and confidence. The examination should also include assessment of pain, and factors influencing it, such as movement, pressure and guarding (Mooney 1991).

carefully assessed for signs of hypovolaemic shock as blood loss from a closed shaft of femur fracture averages 1200 ml (Cadogan 2004). Although isolated femoral fractures rarely cause significant shock, fractures occurring with other traumatic injury do contribute to significant hypovolaemia. Observation should therefore be vigilant and X-ray will confirm diagnosis. Severe muscle spasms cause significant pain following femoral fracture and also cause the limb to shorten. Crepitus occurs over the fracture site as bone pieces move (O'Steen 2003).

Management priorities

Management priorities in the emergency department are twofold: preventing secondary damage and pain control. Preventing secondary damage includes managing blood loss by initiating intravenous fluid replacement. Reduction in blood loss and significant pain reduction can be achieved by correct application of an appropriate traction splint, such as a Donway traction splint. Alternatively a traditional Thomas splint may be used. These stabilize the fracture until definitive repair can take place. In doing this, the extent of the trauma to surrounding soft tissue is minimized. Pain is reduced because bone ends are immobilized. Distal and proximal pulses, capillary refill and sensation should be rechecked after splint application. If the fracture is open, broad-spectrum antibiotics should be given and the patient's tetanus status checked. The wound should be covered with a wet dressing. Povidone-iodine soaks are commonly used because of the devastating effects of infection (see also Chapter 23). Intravenous analgesia should also be given. Fractured femurs take about 8–16 weeks to heal in an adult and 6–12 weeks in a child. Definitive treatment is usually internal fixation for an adult, which means they can usually be walking within 2 weeks post-surgery. Surgery is not recommended for children because of growth and speed of repair;

If a patient presents with a mechanism of injury or the clinical examination is suggestive of a fracture then X-ray should be requested. X-rays should not, however, be performed for purely medico-legal reasons (Ward 1999).

FEMORAL FRACTURES

The femur is the longest, strongest human bone. It is surrounded by muscles and is fed by the profunda femoris artery. The shaft of femur also has a good collateral blood supply in the periosteum. Most of the bleeding associated with femoral fracture is due to rupture of small branches of the profunda femoris artery. The femur only fractures under great force and the most common cause of injury is road traffic accidents, particularly motorcycle accidents (Crimmins & Ruiz 1995).

Assessment

Fractures of the femur fall into three anatomical categories: proximal, mid-shaft and distal. Examination findings are shown in Box 5.3. The patient should be therefore traction is recommended for older children, and plastering with hip spica for toddlers and small children.

Supra-condylar fractures of the femur are assessed in the same way as shaft fractures. The mechanisms of injury are similar, with pain usually localized to the knee. Fractures involving the femoral condyles usually involve the knee joint and there may be associated knee joint injuries particularly osteochondral fractures of the patella (Rowley & Dent 1997). These fractures do not cause the same extent of blood loss as shaft fractures and are repaired by either long leg casting or surgery.

LOWER LEG INJURY

The principles of assessment are common to all limb injuries and have been highlighted earlier in the chapter. This section describes specific advice, identifying common mechanisms of injury, assessment findings and initial management.

Fractures and dislocations

Patellar fractures occur following a direct blow or fall onto the knee. Indirect twisting injury can also result in a fracture as the patella is ripped apart by the quadriceps muscles. The patient presents with pain, swelling and a knee effusion. As a result, range of movement is restricted, particularly full extension. Usually, patellar fractures can be repaired by long leg cylindrical casting for 4–6 weeks. Surgical intervention is necessary for open fractures; those fractures where fragmentation of the patella leaves gaps greater than 4 mm; and longitudinal fractures.

Patellar dislocation results from a direct blow to the medial aspect of the knee, common in football or similar contact sports. The knee locks and remains in a flexed position. On examination, obvious lateral deformity is present with medial tenderness and pain on attempted movement. Acute swelling between 2 and 12 hours of injury is likely to indicate haemarthrosis (Adams 2004, Rourke 2003). Treatment seeks to relocate the patella. This is usually straightforward and achieved by extension of the knee. It is painful because of muscle spasm and therefore analgesia and muscle relaxants should be used. A supportive long leg bandage should then be applied, or a long leg cast.

Tibial plateau fractures

Tibial plateau injury commonly occurs from pedestrian/car accidents, usually at lower speeds where the car bumper hits the standing pedestrian. Fractures also occur as a result of a fall from a height, causing compression of the plateau, or they may occur in elderly patients with osteoporotic bones. Patients usually present with pain and swelling over the fracture site and inability to weight-bear. Swelling varies considerably, with haemathrosis sometimes present. Conservative treatment with long leg casting is less common than internal fixation because of the morbidity risk of long immobilization, particularly in older patients (Harris & Haller 1995).

Tibial shaft fractures

Mechanisms of injury are varied. The tibia has little muscular protection, so fractures from direct blows are the commonest long bone fracture. They are also the most common open fracture. Torsional or indirect forces are also common causes of fracture, particularly in children. Similar mechanisms cause tibial and fibular fracture, although much more force is needed to break both bones. Direct trauma tends to cause transverse or comminuted fractures, and indirect trauma causes oblique and spiral fractures. The patient presents with localized pain and is usually unable to weight-bear. Surrounding soft tissue damage varies from a haematoma, causing swelling, to an open wound caused by fracture ends. Treatment for tibial fractures varies: children with greenstick fractures need casting for 6 weeks; in adults, displaced fractures may need internal fixation. Open fractures warrant prophylactic antibiotics and tetanus prophylaxis if not covered (Beales 1997). ED documentation of the neurovascular status is vital as the risk of compartment syndrome is high. Therefore admission for 24 hours observation and limb elevation should be considered in very swollen proximal tibial fractures. Pain is managed with i.v. opiates and the lower leg should be plastered as soon as possible. Circumferential casts must *never* be applied in the acute phase because of the inherent risk of compartment syndrome.

Fibula fractures

Isolated fibular fractures are not common and usually occur in conjunction with tibial fractures. Isolated fibular fractures usually occur as a result of direct trauma to the lateral aspect of the calf. Distal fibular/malleolar fractures occur with excessive rotational forces. They are discussed in more detail under ankle injury below. As the tibia is vulnerable to torsional injuries, for example in sporting injuries, and force transmitted through the feet is high, the incidence of injury is high (Smith 2005). The patient will complain of pain over the fracture site, with radiation along the length of the fibula on palpation. Because the fibula is not a weight-bearing bone, the patient may be walking with discomfort. Swelling is usually minimal. Depending on the degree of pain, isolated fractures are treated by either plaster cast or compression bandage.

Tibial and fibular fractures

Combined tibial and fibular fractures are fairly common in contact sports, such as football. In injuries where indirect force causes the fracture, the tibia and fibula may be fractured in different places. Commonly, the tibial shaft fractures at the distal third, and because of a twisting mechanism the fibula fractures at the proximal end. This reinforces the need to assess from the joint above to the joint below the injury. If injury is caused by direct force and both bones are fractured at the same level, the leg will appear unstable and flexible at the fracture site. It is important that temporary immobilization occurs as soon as possible, both to reduce pain and to prevent further soft tissue damage. These fractures will need surgical fixation.

Ankle fractures

Most ankle injuries seen in the emergency department are soft-tissue injuries (Wilkerson 1992). Patients with fractures risk significant morbidity if these are not identified and treated early. The ankle is a complex hinge joint made up of three bones – the tibia, fibula and talus – and three collateral ligaments – the lateral, medial and interosseous. These ligaments stabilize the ankle joint; the lateral ligament allows for some inversion of the joint, whereas the medial and interosseous have less stretch (see Fig. 5.11). Injury patterns can be classified by the mechanism of injury (see Box 5.4 and Fig. 5.12).

Box 5.4 Lange–Honsen classification of ankle injury (After Mayeda 1992.)

Supination – adduction (inversion injury)

Stage I	Fracture of lateral malleolus at joint level or below, or tear of lateral collateral ligament
Stage II	As above with fracture of medial malleolus

Supination – lateral rotation

Stage I	Rupture of anterior tibiofibular ligament
Stage II	As above with spiral fracture of distal fibula
Stage III	As above with posterior tibiofibular ligament disruption with/without avulsion fracture of posterior malleolus
Stage IV	As above with medial malleolar fracture

Pronation – abduction

Stage I	Transverse fracture of medial malleolus or deltoid ligament tear
Stage II	As above with posterior and anterior tibiofibular ligament disruption with/without avulsion fracture of posterior malleolus
Stage III	As above with fracture of distal fibula at ankle joint level

Pronation – lateral rotation

Stage I	Transverse fracture of medial malleolus or tear or deltoid ligament
Stage II	As above with disruption of anterior tibiofibular ligament and interosseous membrane
Stage III	As above with fracture of distal bone 6 cm or greater above joint
Stage IV	As above with posterior tibiofibular ligament disruption with/without avulsion fracture of posterior malleolus

---

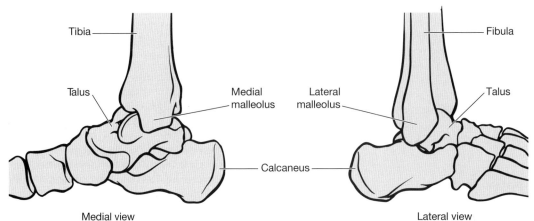

Figure 5.11 Bony anatomy of the ankle.

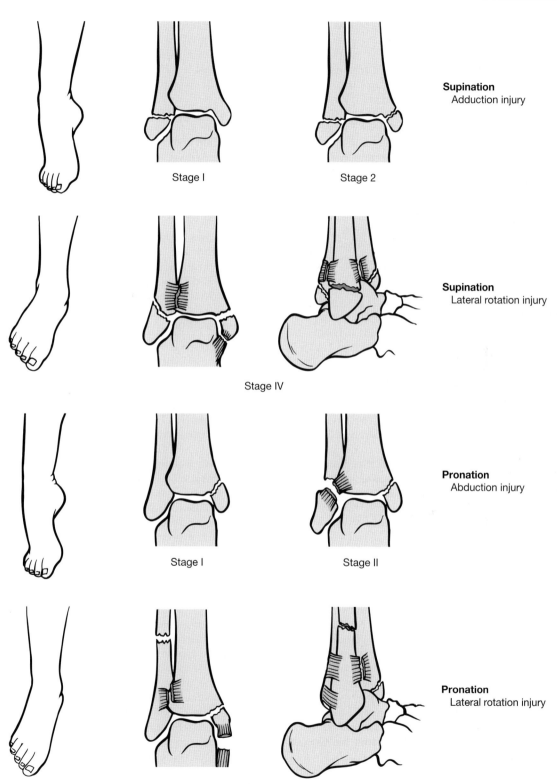

Stage I   Stage 2   **Supination** Adduction injury

Stage IV   **Supination** Lateral rotation injury

Stage I   Stage II   **Pronation** Abduction injury

Stage IV   **Pronation** Lateral rotation injury

Figure 5.12   Ankle fracture (based on Lange–Hansen classification). (After Mayeda 1992.)

Isolated lateral malleolar fractures can occur following inversion injury. Patients present with swelling and bony tenderness on the lateral aspect of the ankle and are usually unable to weight-bear (Whelan 1997). Most isolated fractures are either a chip or avulsion fracture with ligament injury. These can be treated by a below-knee weight-bearing cast. Some fractures above the joint line or comminuted fractures may warrant surgical intervention. Isolated medial malleolar fractures are less common and usually result from a direct blow or eversion and, occasionally, inversion injury. The patient presents with pain over the medial aspect, swelling and limited range of movement. Usually, the patient will be non-weight-bearing (Wyatt et al. 1999). Simple avulsion fractures can be managed by below-knee casting. Fractures into the joint space should be referred for specialist opinion as internal fixation may be necessary.

Bi-malleolar fractures involve two of the lateral, medial and posterior malleoli, usually the lateral and medial. The patient presents with a history of inversion or eversion injury and will have bilateral bony tenderness and swelling, with or without deformity, and will be non-weight-bearing. These are unstable fractures with a significant risk of ankle dislocation. The ankle should be temporarily immobilized, adequate pain relief should be given and hospital admission facilitated. Restoration of function requires accurate medial malleolus reduction and joint space alignment (Mayeda 1992). Good outcomes are also dependent on skilled plastering and surveillance for weeks. Increasingly surgeons prefer to avoid these uncertainties by routine accurate internal fixation (McRae 1999). Lateral malleolar reduction is desirable but less crucial. This is usually achieved by open reduction and fixation in theatre, but can be achieved by closed methods if surgery is contraindicated.

Tri-malleolar fractures involve the posterior malleolus as well and are usually combined with ankle dislocation. They are caused by falls or, most commonly, tripping, e.g. off a kerb. Management priorities are limb realignment (see discussion of dislocations below) and subsequent internal fixation, using the same principles as for bi-malleolar fractures.

The standard X-ray evaluation for the acutely injured ankle includes lateral, anteroposterior and mortice views. The requirement for X-ray of the adult ankle or foot may be determined using the Ottowa Ankle Rules (Steill et al. 1992). These have shown that X-rays are only required for the ankle if there is any pain in the malleolar region and:

- bone tenderness over the posterior aspect of the distal 6 cm of the lateral malleolus or
- bone tenderness over the posterior aspect of the distal 6 cm of the medial malleolus or
- inability to weight-bear for at least 4 steps both immediately after the injury and at the time of assessment in ED
- foot X-ray is required if there is pain in the mid-foot region and:
- bone tenderness at the navicular or
- bone tenderness at the base of the fifth metatarsal or
- inability to weight-bear for at least 4 steps both immediately after the injury and at the time of assessment in ED.

The Ottowa Ankle Rules (see Fig. 5.13) apply to adults (>18 years) and have a >98% sensitivity for detecting clinically significant malleolar ankle injuries. They also reduce the number of ankle X-rays by up to 40% (Bachmann et al. 2003).

Ankle dislocation

Ankle dislocation occurs when significant force applied to the joint results in loss of opposition of the articular surfaces.

Dislocation occurs in one of four directions: anterior, lateral, superior and posterior. Posterior is the most common (see Fig. 5.14). Stability of the ankle is normally maintained by tight articulation of the talus with the tibia and fibula. Because of the amount of force needed, isolated ankle dislocation is extremely rare (Greenbaum & Papp 1992). It is usually associated with malleolar fractures and ligament rupture. Common causes of dislocation are sports injuries, direct force or road traffic accidents (Harris 1995). Complicated dislocations associated with multiple ankle fractures are most common in osteo-porotic women.

On examination the ankle will be oedematous, the joint locked, with the distal tibia prominent under stretched skin. Management priorities in the emergency department are to preserve neurovascular integrity. Early reduction is crucial, since delay may increase risk of neurovascular compromise or damage to articular cartilage. If there appears to be neurovascular compromise, the ankle dislocation should be reduced urgently, without waiting for X-rays. If neurovascular integrity appears intact, X-rays can be obtained, but the foot should remain supported to prevent further injury. Reduction should be carried out swiftly after X-ray. Nitrous oxide is a useful initial pain relief, for its therapeutic effects of analgesia, increasing oxygen intake and for its distraction potential, i.e. by getting

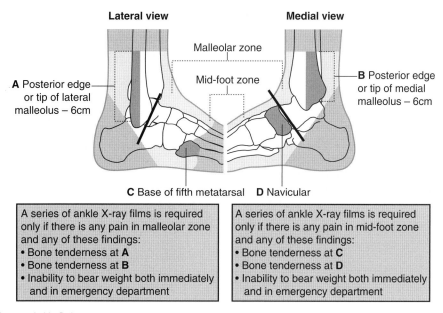

Figure 5.13   Ottowa Ankle Rules assessment.

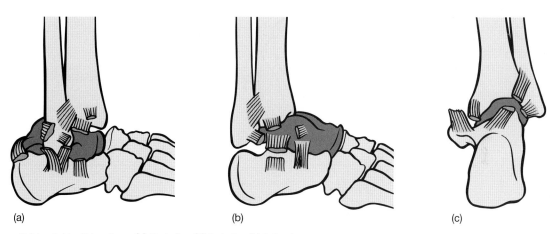

Figure 5.14   Ankle dislocations. (a) Posterior, (b) Anterior, (c) Lateral.

the patient to concentrate on breathing. While dislocation is being reduced, the patient should have adequate intravenous analgesia and muscle relaxant. The patient's cardiac and respiratory function should be monitored during this procedure.

Ankle reduction is a two person job. It is achieved by flexing the patient's knee to reduce tension on the Achilles tendon. One carer supports the lower leg while the other applies downward traction to the foot and force is applied in the opposite direction to that of the original injury. When reduction is completed, neurovascular integrity should be rechecked, by checking for pedal pulse, capillary refill and sensation. The ankle should then be immobilized in an above-knee plaster which is either bivalved or guttered, because of the degree of swelling associated with fracture manipulation. Most patients need internal fixation of associated fractures.

FOOT FRACTURES

The foot has 28 bones and 57 articulating surfaces and is divided into three anatomical areas (see Fig. 5.15). It is considered vital for balance, movement and as a shock absorber for movement.

The hindfoot

The talus supports the body weight and forces above by allowing movement at the ankle joint and between the calcaneus and midfoot. It is well secured by ligaments surrounding the ankle joint and therefore

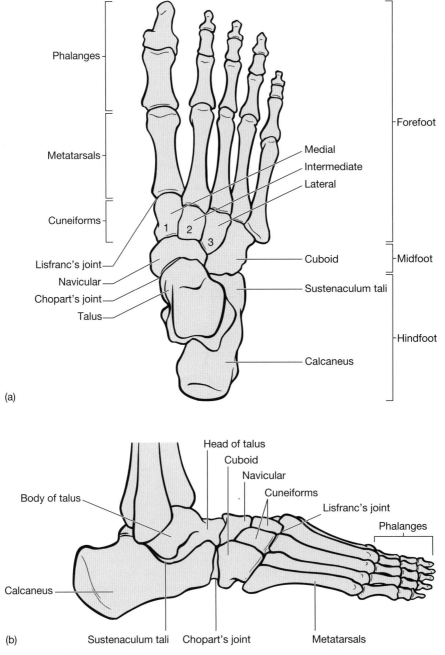

Figure 5.15   The right foot (a) Dorsal view, (b) Lateral view.

fracture is uncommon (Harris 1995). In the event of injury to the talus, the risk of complication is high because 60% of the surface is covered by articular cartilage and vascular supply is low, creating a significant threat of avascular necrosis. It is usually injured as a result of falls, landing on the heel or forefoot, causing fractures through the body or neck of the talus. Fractures to the neck of the talus also result from head-on road traffic accidents, where the driver's foot is pressed against compressed floors or pedals, causing extreme dorsiflexion.

The patient will present with ankle pain, there may be visible disruption to normal ankle anatomy and swelling is common. Fractures to the talar neck are usually treated by below-knee casting, but if any displacement cannot be reduced, open reduction is necessary. Fractures to the talar body frequently require internal fixation. Fractures of the talar head are extremely uncommon and management varies with the extent of the injury and associated injuries. Specialist orthopaedic advice should be sought for specific management.

The calcaneus

This is the largest bone of the foot and it absorbs the body's weight when standing or moving. The calcaneus is a relatively hollow bone consisting of an outer thin cortical shell filled with cancellous bone. As a result, it fractures when subjected to vertical forces such as falling from a height. There is an associated crush fracture of the lumbar spine in about 10% of cases resulting from a fall. The Achilles tendon attaches to the tuberosity and can cause an avulsion fracture when damaged. Fractures resulting from a fall are most common in men between 30 and 50 years old (Clisham & Berlin 1981), whereas avulsion fractures are more common in women showing signs of osteoporosis.

The patient presents with pain over the rear of the foot and both sides of the heel. Swelling is usually present and patients are usually unable to weight-bear on their heel. If the presentation to ED is a few hours post-injury, a horseshoe-shaped bruise may be present. Calcaneal fractures are categorized into two groups: those involving the subtalar joint and those which do not, i.e. extra-articular fractures. The outcome for patients with extra-articular fractures is considerably better than those involving the subtalar joint. Extra-articular fractures are managed conservatively with compression and elevation in the first instance. After swelling has subsided, the injury is immobilized in a cast. The majority of fractures do involve the subtalar joint and the prognosis for these patients is poor. About 50% have some long-term problems from the injury (Mayeda 1992), including restricted movement, pain and subtalar arthritis. Most are treated with internal fixation. Fractures to other bones of the foot are not uncommon, and patients with suspected calcaneum fractures, or those who have fallen over six feet, must have a full examination of the spine and lower leg (Larsen 2002).

The midfoot

This region includes the navicular, cuboid, cuneiform and metatarsal bones. The midfoot provides foot flexibility. Fractures to this area are uncommon and result from direct force, such as crush injuries. Transverse dislocation of the forefoot results from direct force. Patients present with localized tenderness and swelling. These injuries heal well and can usually be treated with below-knee non-weight-bearing casts. There are two exceptions to this: the first relates to avulsion fractures of the navicular, which occur as a result of eversion injury. If 20% or more of the articular surface is avulsed, the fracture should be internally fixed. If less than 20% is avulsed, a below-knee cast should be adequate. The second exception is the Lisfranc dislocation, which occurs when the forefoot is dislocated across the metatarsal joints. This is an extremely rare condition, occurring in one in 55 000 cases (Mayeda 1992). Neurovascular compromise is common, partly because the force necessary to cause dislocation also causes extensive soft tissue damage, resulting in oedema and vascular compromise. The patient presents with moderate to severe midfoot pain and large amounts of swelling which can hinder diagnosis. There is usually a shortening of the foot length, compared with the uninjured foot, and the injured foot will have transverse broadening.

Patients with Lisfranc dislocation will not be able to stand on their toes. Treatment of this injury revolves around rapid reduction of the dislocation and cast immobilization, because the risk of circulation compromise and subsequent necrosis is so high. If a base of second metatarsal fracture coexists, an accurate reduction may not be possible, or will prove unstable. In such cases, internal fixation should be considered. Hospital admission is usually necessary during the initial days post-injury, whatever the method of reduction.

The forefoot

The forefoot consists of the five metatarsal bones and the phalanges.

Metatarsal fractures

The metatarsals are susceptible to fractures because of their length. The mechanisms of fracture vary; the second and third metatarsals are relatively fixed and therefore susceptible to stress fractures. The first, fourth and fifth metatarsals are more mobile. Fractures are caused by direct blows to the foot, e.g. a heavy object falling across the foot.

Twisting injury can also result in fractures, particularly of the second to fourth metatarsals. The patient presents with swelling over the foot, localized pain and inability to weight-bear. Reduction of swelling is imperative as skin necrosis and neurovascular compromise can occur. Elevation of the foot is essential. Most fractures can be managed by immobilization in a short leg cast.

Fifth metatarsal fracture is one of the most common foot injuries (Larsen 2002). It usually results from an inversion injury causing sudden contraction of the peroneus brevis muscle. The tendons joining this muscle with the base of the fifth metatarsal can cause an avulsion fracture. The management of fifth metatarsal fractures is either neighbour (or buddy) strapping and crutches or a below-knee cast, depending on the patient's pain. Occasionally, displaced fractures require internal fixation.

First metatarsal fractures warrant special consideration because of the weight-bearing capacity of the first metatarsal and its contribution to balance and stability. If the metatarsal head has been displaced in plantar rotation, the patient will have trouble with weight-bearing and with the 'push-off' mechanism in walking. Many of these fractures can be reduced in ED with adequate analgesia, and then immobilized in a cast. If reduction cannot be achieved in this manner, internal fixation should be considered.

Phalangeal fractures

These result from stubbing injury or from dropping heavy objects on toes. The patient presents with pain, swelling and often bruising or a subungal haematoma. The clinical symptoms can make fracture diagnosis difficult and often X-rays do not offer much assistance (Mayeda 1992). If angulation or deformity of the toe exists, then X-rays are more helpful. Most fractures can be managed by neighbour strapping and elevation. Obviously angulated fractures should be reduced using a digital block, then the toe neighbour strapped. Big toe fractures needing reduction may warrant immobilization in a cast with toe support.

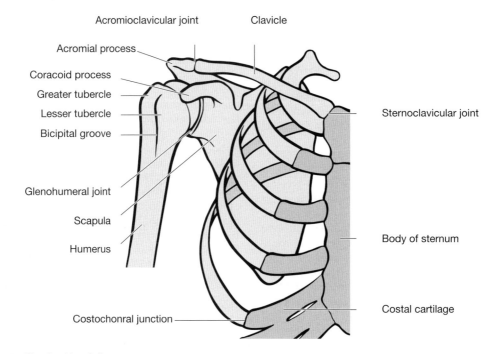

Figure 5.16 The shoulder girdle.

INJURY TO THE SHOULDER

The shoulder girdle consists of three bones: the scapula, the clavicle and the humerus (see Fig. 5.16). The shoulder attaches the arms to the axial skeleton. These are interconnected at the acromioclavicular, glenohumeral, coracoclavicular and sternoclavicular articulations (ACJ) and muscles from the rib cage and cervical spine. The SCJ, deltoid, pectorals and trapezius muscles maintain the normal position of the shoulder. The clavicle is attached to the scapula by acromioclavicular and coracoclavicular ligaments, the latter incorporating both the conoid and trapezoid ligaments and is the stronger of the two. The ACJ permits a 'gliding' motion of the articular end of the clavicle on the acromion and rotation of the scapula on the clavicle during abduction of the arm (Knapton 1999). If the ligaments weaken or tear, the shoulder has a greater tendency to dislocate.

Scapular fractures

The scapula is situated above and lateral to the posterior thorax. It is well protected from injury by thick muscle and extreme force is necessary to fracture it. Injury commonly results from high-speed road traffic accidents, crush injury or falls. Occasionally, a scapular fracture occurs as a result of electric shock, when both scapulae are fractured (Dumas & Walker 1992). Fractured scapulae most frequently occur in young men (O'Steen 2003) because of the force needed to cause fractures and associated injuries such as pneumothorax, chest wall injury or related shoulder girdle injuries.

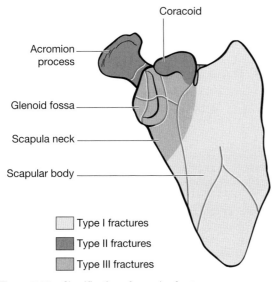

Figure 5.17   Classification of scapular fractures.

Anatomically, scapular fractures fall into three categories (Fig. 5.17):

Type I fractures   They are difficult to palpate because of thick muscle and pain. An adducted shoulder and the mechanism of injury should suggest possible fracture, which can be confirmed on X-ray (Knapton 1999). Treatment is usually conservative and involves pain relief and simple immobilization using a broad arm sling on the injured side. Controversy exists over the benefits versus risks of plating scapular body fractures. It has been suggested that fractures in young patients where extensive displacement exists are best treated by plating (Nordqvist & Petersson 1992). However, a high complication rate has been identified following surgical management of fractures (Schmidt et al. 1992).

Type II fractures   acromion and coracoid process. They occur from direct trauma and are similar in that patients have pain over the site of injury and adduction of the shoulder. They differ in that acromion fractures cause pain on elbow flexing, while in coracoid fractures the patient actively flexes the elbow as a form of pain relief. Both types are usually managed conservatively unless concurrent shoulder girdle injury exists, such as dislocation or clavicular fracture.

Type III fractures   involve the scapul neck or glenoid fossa. A result from lateral to medial rotation of the humeral head. The patient presents with pain around the humeral head and on shoulder adduction, and is usually supporting an injured arm. Treatment involves immobilization of the arm on the injured side; however, difficulty in regaining full range of movement following this injury is high.

Clavicular fractures

The clavicle provides anterior support for the shoulder. It is a slightly S-shaped bone which articulates laterally with the acromion process and medially with the sternum. The clavicle gives definition to body shape as well as providing protection for the subclavian neurovascular bundle. Clavicle fractures make up 5% of all fractures, so are not uncommon and in children and adolescents it is a particularly common fracture (O'Steen 2003). Fracture of the clavicle is most commonly due to a violent upwards and backwards force such as a fall on the outstretched hand. Less commonly the clavicle may be fractured by blows or falls on the point of the shoulder.

Clavicular fractures are divided into three groups: proximal third fracture, mid-clavicular fracture and distal fractures (see Table 5.2).

Table 5.2   Classification of clavicular fractures

Type	Mechanism of injury	Frequency (% of all clavicular fractures)
Proximal third	Direct blow to anterior chest	5%
Mid-third	Indirect force to lateral aspect of shoulder	80%
Distal third	Direct blow to top of shoulder	15%

Common presenting symptoms include pain over the fracture site, crepitus and sometimes a palpable deformity. The patient is usually supporting the arm of the injured side. In mid-clavicular fractures, deformity is common. The patient presents with a downward shoulder stump, sometimes rotated inward and forward. This is due to gravitational forces and contraction of the pectoralis major. The proximal fragment is displaced upward. Because of the location of the neurovascular bundles and the great blood vessels, a careful assessment of neurovascular function of the arm on the injured side must be carried out. Management of clavicular fracture is usually conservative. Immobilization with a simple sling is as effective as other less comfortable methods and is therefore the treatment of choice. Displaced fractures of the distal third often require surgical repair because of the risk of non-union. Complications frequently include malunion, regardless of the support mechanism used. While Newman (1988) suggests that this malunion is of little functional or cosmetic consequence, others believe that a persistent sharp clavicular spike may cause discomfort against clothes and require excision (Kelly 2004, McRae 1999). Patients should be advised that a residual palpable or visible deformity may be present after healing has occurred (Smith 2005).

Shoulder dislocation

The glenohumeral joint of the shoulder girdle is a shallow synovial ball and socket joint that comprises five joints and three bones. The wide range of movement carried out at the shoulder, and its lack of bony stability, predisposes the joint to dislocation. Two main patient groups can be identified: men between the ages of 20 and 30, and women over 60 (Kroner at al. 1989), and approximately 55–60% of shoulder dislocations are recurrent (Proehl 1999). Glenohumeral joint dislocation can be categorized into four groups:

anterior (>90% of dislocations), posterior (<5%), inferior (<1%) and superior (<1%).

Anterior dislocation

Anterior dislocations occur following a fall onto an outstretched hand where the arm is extended and externally rotated. They can also be caused by direct trauma to the postero-lateral aspect of the shoulder.

The patient presents in extreme pain, usually holding the injured arm in abduction and external rotation (Genge Jagmin 1995). On examination, the shoulder will be obviously deformed when compared with the uninjured side. It will have a square appearance and the acromial process will be prominent (see Fig. 5.18). Assessment should include a detailed examination of neurovascular function (Box 5.5).

Before shoulder dislocation is treated, humeral fracture should be excluded on X-ray. Fractures of the humeral head or neck prohibit early reduction of dislocation in the emergency department and orthopaedic opinion should always be sought. If no fracture exists, reduction of shoulder dislocation should be carried out as soon as possible. Prompt reduction

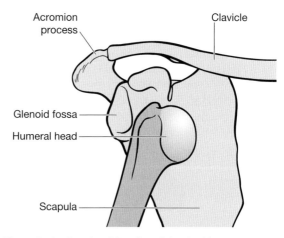

Figure 5.18   Anterior dislocation of the shoulder.

Box 5.5   Assessment of neurovascular function following shoulder injury

Posterior cord of brachial plexus – test for wrist extension
Axillary nerve damage – test for sensation over lateral aspect of upper arm
Axillary artery damage – test for brachial pulse

is always necessary as the procedure becomes more difficult as time passes and the dislocation may prove irreducible (Mills et al. 1995), partly because muscle spasm increases with the length of time the joint is dislocated. Early relocation is also vital in maintaining the integrity of the humeral head. Because the scapular neck is harder than the humeral head, a compression fracture occurs, causing long-term deformity to the humeral head (Hill-Sachs deformity), which leads to recurrent dislocation. This is thought to occur in between 11 and 50% of patients with anterior dislocation (Tullos et al. 1984).

Four types of anterior dislocation exist, classified by the exact position of the humeral head. Management is broadly the same. Successful reduction of shoulder dislocation depends on overcoming muscle spasm. This is achieved by intravenous administration of muscle relaxant, such as midazolam, together with appropriate analgesia, usually opiates. The mechanics of shoulder reduction are achieved by traction or leverage, or a combination of both.

Traction methods include laying the patient on her front with the injured arm over the side of the trolley and hanging a 5–7 kg weight, depending on the patient's muscularity, on the affected arm. Over 20–30 minutes this reduces muscle spasm by gently elongating muscles, pulling the humeral head off the scapular and allowing the rotator cuff muscles to relocate it in the glenoid fossa. This method is thought to be less painful than some more aggressive relocations and the risk of complication is low (Quaday 1995). The most commonly used and safest method of reduction is a two-person traction/counter-traction approach. One person applies longitudinal traction to the injured arm, reducing muscle spasm, while the other person applies counter-traction by wrapping a sheet around the patient's chest and under the axilla of the injured side and then pulling towards the patient's ear on the unaffected side. This helps to disengage the humeral head from the scapula. The arm should then be adducted and immobilized.

Traditional traction/counter-traction methods of putting a foot in the patient's armpit and then pulling on the arm is not recommended because of its high association with neurovascular injury and lower success rate than other methods (Quaday 1995). Leverage techniques involve some traction to lift the humeral head off the scapula, but then lever it back into place. These methods are fast, but increase the risk of injury to the glenoid rim or humeral shaft. The external rotation method of reduction is the least traumatic. It works by slowly adducting the injured arm and then flexing the elbow to 90°. The elbow is then held in place while the forearm is externally rotated by its own weight and gravity, not by force. This allows the smallest profile of the humeral head to be relocated into the glenoid fossa. The traditional method of leverage is Kocher's technique. This involves a three-step external/internal rotation manoeuvre which is both painful for the patient and dangerous because of the high risk of vascular tearing, rotator cuff injury and humeral fracture (Riebel & McCabe 1991). If reduction cannot be achieved, orthopaedic referral should be made for manipulation under general anaesthetic.

Whatever method of reduction is used, it is important that neurovascular integrity is rechecked, and an X-ray taken to check position. The affected arm should be immobilized to prevent re-dislocation. The arm should be adducted and internally rotated. To prevent shoulder stiffness, the patient should be advised to extend the elbow and rotate the arm to a neutral position several times a day. In older patients, the risk of joint stiffness is greater, and therefore it is usual to remobilize the arm sooner than in younger people. Patients over 40 should not be immobilized for longer than 3 weeks. The rate of re-dislocation is higher in younger people, and therefore those patients under 40 years of age are immobilized for up to 6 weeks

Posterior dislocation

The anatomy of the shoulder girdle makes posterior dislocation difficult because the glenoid fossa is positioned posteriorly to the humeral head. The angle of the scapula helps to buttress this structure. When dislocation occurs, the humeral head sits behind the glenoid and usually below the acromion (see Fig. 5.19).

Posterior dislocation is caused by a fall onto an outstretched hand where the arm is flexed and internally rotated. Posterior dislocation also occurs

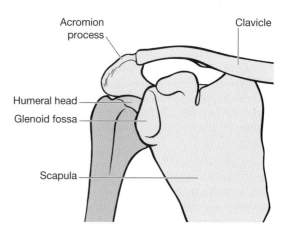

Figure 5.19   Posterior dislocation of the shoulder.

following significant electric shock, epileptic seizures and, occasionally, from direct force to the anterior aspect of the shoulder. The patient will have severe pain and will present holding the arm in internal rotation, supported in a sling type position. There is usually a loss of definition of the anterior shoulder and a prominent acromial and coracoid process, with the humeral head sometimes palpable posteriorly. The patient is unable to lift the arm above 90° and cannot externally rotate.

Diagnosis should be made from the mechanism of injury and patient presentation as anteroposterior X-rays are inconclusive and up to 50% of posterior dislocations are missed initially (Quadray 1995). Lateral and axillary X-ray views will confirm diagnosis. Neurovascular injury is less common with posterior dislocation because the major structures lie anterior to the joint and are thus protected. Although closed reduction with muscle relaxant and analgesia may be attempted, orthopaedic consultation should determine this.

Because of the strong anterior muscle mass, reduction in ED is usually only recommended for elderly or frail patients and reduction under general anaesthetic is generally required. If attempts at reduction are made in ED, the process involves slow in-line traction, while maintaining internal rotation, with gentle pressure on the humeral head to lift it off the glenoid. If reduction is attempted, neurovascular integrity should be checked afterwards and X-rays performed. The affected arm should be immobilized but not internally rotated. For this reason, shoulder spicas are often used to create slight external rotation (Brown 1992). Immobilization should not exceed four weeks.

UPPER ARM INJURY

The humerus is surrounded by strong muscle compartments – anteriorly the biceps and posteriorly the triceps. The neurovascular bundle lies on the medial border of the biceps and contains the brachial artery, the brachial vein and the medial and ulnar nerves. The radial nerve runs posteriorly until it reaches the distal humerus, where it travels laterally until it is anterior to the humerus. The muscle design of the upper arm is appropriate for pulling or hanging activities.

Humeral fractures are common in two main patient groups:

- women aged between 56 and 65 years, usually with osteoporosis – fractures occur as a result of a fall and occasionally direct force; injury is usually to the proximal humerus, neck or shaft
- young men aged between 16 and 24 years – mechanisms of injury include road traffic accidents

(transverse humeral fractures), falls from a significant height (oblique or spiral fractures) and stress fractures from throwing actions.

The patient will present holding their arm close to their chest, with localized pain, extensive bruising or shoulder pain in fractures of the humeral neck. The upper arm is usually swollen and may have obvious shortening with normal movement at the point of fracture. Very careful neurovascular assessment is necessary, especially with distal third fractures as both the brachial plexus and axillary nerve may be damaged. Circulation should be assessed at the brachial pulse, radial pulse and along the ulnar and brachial arteries. The axillary artery is the most common to sustain vessel injury and may be present with any combination of limb pain, paraesthesia, pallor, pulselessness, a cool limb and paralysis. Capillary refill of the fingertips and hand should also be assessed. Sensory and motor function should be checked in line with radial, ulnar and median nerve activity.

The muscle masses help to splint humeral fractures, and gravity helps with lengthening and aligning the bone. However, this is a very painful option for the patient, and non-union is common. Although exact alignment is not vital because the shoulder's mobility can compensate, four basic steps to fracture management should be followed:

- traction to restore length and align fragment
- any angulation should be reduced
- initial immobilization for pain control and healing
- encourage mobilization of shoulder and elbow to prevent loss of function.

A number of immobilization methods exist. Open reduction with internal fixation is one option, usually performed for open or severely comminuted fractures and in patients with multiple fractures where conservative management would delay overall recovery and mobility. Hanging casts and U-slabs have been used for many years as a method of immobilizing the upper arm. As well as being extremely uncomfortable and restrictive for patients, these casts can cause posterior angulation of the fracture (Ciernick et al. 1991). Slings are commonly used, but these offer little immobilization or pain control. The treatment of choice appears to be an interlocking upper arm brace with forearm support. These have 95% excellent functional rotation and 85% minimal shortening of the limb (Zagorski et al. 1988).

ELBOW INJURY

The elbow joint is a hinge-like articulation and consists of the distal humerus, radius, ulna and olecranon (see Fig. 5.20). The distal humerus forms two

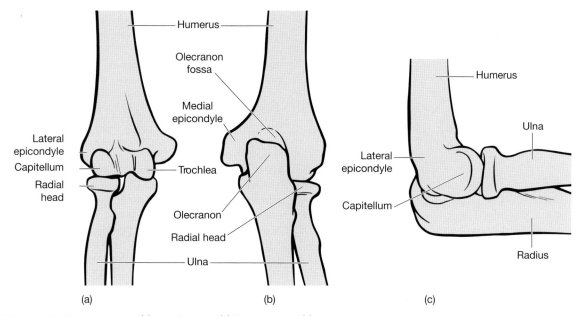

Figure 5.20   The elbow joint. (a) Anterior view, (b) Posterior view, (c) Lateral view.

columns; the lateral and medial epicondyles form the proximal part of these columns and are significant for their muscle attachment facilitating wrist movement. The wrist extensors originate from the lateral epicondyle, and flexors from the medial epicondyle. The trochlea articulates with the olecranon to allow flexion/extension at the elbow, and the capitellum allows pronation and supination of the forearm by articulation with the radial head. The radial nerve travels around the humerus to the anterior of the lateral epicondyle, and supplies the wrist and finger extensors. Because of its proximity to the distal humerus, it is very susceptible to injury. The medial nerve travels anterior to the humerus with the brachial artery. It provides sensation to the thumb and index finger and coarse hand movement, such as grip. If the nerve is damaged above the elbow, the index finger cannot be flexed (Ochsner's test). If damaged in the forearm, the interphalangeal thumb joint cannot be flexed if the base of the thumb is held to immobilize it.

The ulnar nerve crosses behind the medial epicondyle and is therefore susceptible to damage when elbow injury occurs. It supplies the flexor muscles and intrinsic hand nerves. Sensation to the ulnar side of the hand is also provided by the ulnar nerve. The brachial artery travels down the anterior aspect of the humerus and crosses the elbow with the median nerve. This is the major blood supply to the hand and forearm and compromise of this supply following injury can result in Volkmann's ischaemia. This is muscle wasting of the hand and forearm which leads to contracture.

Supracondylar fractures

These are distal humerus fractures, proximal to the epicondyles. They are the most common fracture in children, accounting for 60% of childhood fractures (Nicholson & Driscoll 1995). Supracondylar fractures are categorized into two groups depending on mechanism of injury: extension and flexion fractures.

Extension fractures

This type of fracture is caused by a fall onto an outstretched hand with the elbow locked in extension (see Fig. 5.21). This results in posterior displacement of the distal fragment of the humerus, and puts neurovascular structures at risk because of the jagged proximal humerus which becomes anteriorly angulated. This injury is most common in those under 15 years of age, because the tensile strength of the ligaments and joint capsule is greater than that of bone, and therefore fracture occurs. In adults, the reverse is true and dislocation of the elbow joint is more common (Magnusson 1992).

The patient will present holding the arm partially flexed. There is usually severe pain and swelling above the elbow. A thorough assessment should be made of neurovascular and motor function, as injury to the radial nerve occurs in about 8% of patients (Tsai & Ruiz 1995) (see Table 5.3).

Management depends on clinical findings. If circulatory compromise exists then immediate reduction should be considered in the emergency department.

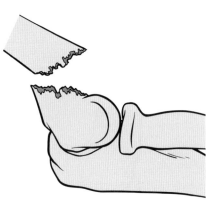

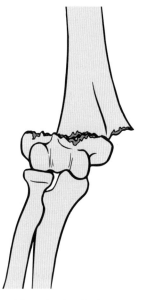

Figure 5.21 Supracondylar extension fracture.

This carries significant risk of neurovascular damage and should only be carried out in limb-threatening situations (St Claire-Strange 1982). In most cases prompt reduction of the fracture should be carried out in theatre. In undisplaced fractures, a plaster backslab can be applied, and provided neurovascular integrity is maintained the patient can be discharged with limb care advice and fracture clinic follow-up.

Flexion fractures

These are less common than extension fractures and comprise approximately 2–4% of the total number of supracondylar fractures (Tsai & Ruiz 1995). They are caused by direct force to a flexed elbow, from a fall or a blow (see Fig. 5.22). The patient will have significant pain around the site and will be supporting the injured arm in a flexed position, but the olecranon prominence will be decreased. There may be a prominent proximal fragment of the humerus anteriorly, and these injuries are commonly seen in open fractures. Although nerve damage is less likely with flexion fractures, the ulnar nerve is at risk because of fracture displacement. Vascular injury is uncommon. If only minimal displacement exists, the fracture can be treated by closed reduction and an above-elbow back-slab in flexion. Fractures with significant displacement or open injuries should have open reduction and internal fixation of the fracture.

Elbow dislocation

Although elbow dislocation is not uncommon in adults, considerable force is needed to cause dislocation. As a result, a 1 in 3 likelihood of an associated fracture exists. The most common type of dislocation is posterior, where the coronoid process slips back

Table 5.3 Assessing neurological function following elbow injury

Nerve	Position	Motor function	Sensory function
Radial	Spirals humerus to anterior of lateral epicondyle	Wrist and finger extensor muscles – test for wrist drop on elbow flexion and forearm pronation	Snuff box area and dorsal aspect of thumb – test for sensation
Median	Anterior to humerus	Coarse hand movement, e.g. grip Test location of injury – above elbow there will be inability to flex index finger: below elbow there will be inability to flex thumb	Thumb and index finger – test for sensation
Ulna	Posterior to medial epicondyle	Flexor muscles of wrist and fingers and intrinsic muscles of the hand – damage can present as claw-like hand	Palmar and dorsal aspects of ulnar half of hand

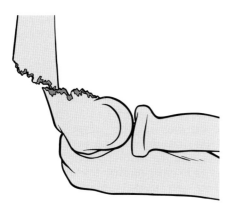

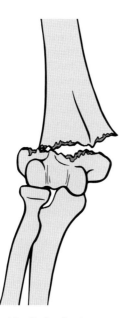

Figure 5.22 Supracondylar flexion fracture.

and lies in the olecranon fossa, or impacts into the distal humerus. The joint capsule is damaged and collateral ligaments are torn.

The patient will have pain, the arm will be supported in mid-flexion and the limb will appear shortened. The olecranon is prominent. Careful neurovascular examination is essential especially of the nerve and brachial artery. The median nerve may be assessed by feeling the muscle while the patient attempts to resist the thumb being pressed from a vertical position against the plane of the hand (Smith 2005). The brachial artery can be assessed by checking the radial pulse.

Management involves urgent relocation for both pain control and neurovascular integrity. This is achieved with muscle relaxants and adequate analgesia followed by a traction/counter-traction approach

where one carer applies sustained traction distally from the wrist followed by flexion with posterior pressure. When the reduction is completed, range of movement should be checked to rule out a mechanical blockage, neurovascular integrity should be rechecked, and then the arm should be immobilized in at least 90% flexion. Medial, lateral and anterior dislocations can also occur, but these are less common and should be managed by the orthopaedic team.

Radial head fractures

In this type of fracture the radial head becomes compressed upwards against the capitilum following a fall onto an outstretched hand. It is an important feature in elbow flexion/extension and forearm rotation. The patient will present with localized pain, which is worse with passive rotation of the forearm and an inability to fully extend the forearm. The presence of an anterior fat pad alone on X-ray is associated with an underlying radial head fracture in up to 50% of patients (Irshad et al. 1997). For management purposes, fractures are classified into three types (see Table 5.4).

FOREARM INJURY

The forearm consists of two long bones: the radius and ulna. They run essentially parallel, although the ulna is straight and the radius bows laterally to allow supination and pronation. The radius and ulna articulate with each other at both ends and are held together by the elbow and wrist joints and their ligaments. The radiocarpal joint connects the radius and the articular disc of the ulna with the carpal bones. This allows palmar and dorsiflexion of the wrist and abduction of the ulna. The union and alignment of the radius and ulna are vital to the function of the forearm and wrist.

Table 5.4 Classification and management of radial head fractures

Type	Description	Management
I	Undisplaced	Sling with early mobilization
II	Marginal fracture with displacement	Joint aspiration if necessary Sling and early mobilization
III	Comminuted fracture	Treatment options vary from internal fixation to partial or total extension of the radial head

Fracture of both radius and ulna

This occurs following a direct blow, fall or road traffic accident involving significant force or longitudinal compression. These fractures are commonly open and nearly always displaced because of the force needed to break both bones. Injury commonly occurs where the mid- and distal thirds merge because there is less muscle protection. These fractures are easy to diagnose as the patient presents with severe pain and marked deformity, sometimes with abnormal movement of the forearm, which mainly depends on the degree of deformity. If there is no angulation or displacement, a long arm Plaster of Paris (POP) slab with 90° flexion of the elbow is applied. Usually open reduction with internal fixation is required because displacement is common. If good reduction is not achieved and maintained, non-union of the bones or union with loss of function will occur.

Ulnar fractures

Ulnar shaft fractures are caused by direct force to the arm, commonly when it is raised to protect the face from injury. The patient presents with pain over the area, and swelling and deformity if the fracture is displaced. Management depends on the degree of displacement. Fractures with more than 50% displacement or 10% of angulation should be internally fixed as they carry a significant risk of non-union (Dymond 1984). Fractures with less displacement/angulation can be treated in a long arm POP cast with the elbow in 90° flexion and the forearm in a neutral position. Non-displaced fractures initially treated by immobilization respond well to early remobilization at about 10 days post-injury.

Proximal ulnar fractures rarely occur independently and are associated with radial head dislocation. This is called a Monteggia fracture. Several classifications of these fractures exist, usually defined by the position of the radial head (Carr 1995). The patient presents with localized pain and, depending on the position of the radial head, it may be palpable and shortening of the forearm may also be noted. The patient will resist any movement of the elbow. Management involves open reduction and internal fixation in adults, as non-union and persistent dislocation of the radial head is common. Greenstick fractures of the ulna are often difficult to detect, which in part accounts for the reason that Monteggia fractures are frequently overlooked in children. A closed reduction under general anaesthetic can usually be achieved in children, as slight radial angulation of the ulna will not restrict movement. In adults, about 95% have some morbidity following this injury (Oveson et al. 1990), i.e. non-union, loss of reduction and infection. Radial nerve paralysis can also occur as a result of compression from the displaced radial head. This causes weak wrist and hand extensors.

Fractures of the radius

Proximal third fractures are rare because of the muscular support attached to the forearm. When they do occur, these fractures are usually caused by direct force to the forearm. The patient usually has pain around the fracture site and pain on longitudinal compression of the radius. Deformity is not as easy to detect as in other forearm fractures because of the amount of soft tissue surrounding the proximal radius. Associated ulnar injury is common because of the force needed to fracture the radius at this level.

The shape of the radius must be maintained to restore function. In proximal third fractures this is complicated by the force exerted by the supinator and biceps brachii muscles, creating supination and displacement of the proximal fragment. The pronator teres muscle causes pronation of the distal fragment which compounds deformity. This deforming process can occur within a POP cast, and therefore if fractures occur proximal to the point of pronator teres insertion in the mid-third of the radius, internal fixation of the fracture is recommended. Fractures in the proximal fifth of the radius are unsuitable for internal fixation because orthopaedic metalwork/hardware cannot be accommodated. These fractures should be treated in a long arm cast with 90° elbow flexion and forearm supination to minimize muscle forces and maintain reduction. The outcome of closed reduction is better in children than in adults.

Distal third shaft fractures also occur because of direct force, but are more common because of the lack of soft tissue protection. Isolated fractures are less common than more complicated injury (Goldberg et al. 1992). Dislocation of the radio-ulnar joint is usually concomitant with fractures around the mid-shaft and distal shaft junction. This is called a Galeazzi fracture. Pain is the primary diagnostic feature. Tissue swelling may obscure deformity, but shortening is sometimes apparent. The deforming forces, shown in Table 5.5, make closed reduction less successful than open reduction with internal fixation.

WRIST INJURY

Anatomically, the wrist is an area which contains multiple joints connected by ligaments. It extends from the distal radius and ulna to the distal carpal bones (see Fig. 5.23). Injury to the wrist usually results from a fall onto an outstretched hand, which causes hyperextension of the hand and force to be exerted on the volar aspect of the radius causing fracture.

Table 5.5	Deforming forces in Galeazzi fractures
Mechanism	Deformity
Gravity	Subluxation or dislocation of radioulnar joint
	Angulation of radial fracture
Pronator quadratus	Rotation of distal fragment in a proximal and volar direction
Brachioradialis	Shortening because of distal fragment rotation
Thumb abductors and extensors	Compounds shortening

Injury pattern varies with age, gender and the amount of force involved.

Distal radius fractures

The distal radius is a common site of injury in adults. Fractures of this area are broadly grouped into three categories depending on the displacement of the distal radius and ulna. The most common of these is the Colles' fracture (see Fig. 5.24). This describes a distal radius fracture with dorsal displacement of the distal fragment. This causes a loss of the usual volar tilt and pronation of the distal fragment over the proximal fragment. An associated ulnar styloid fracture is present in 60% of cases (Cooney et al. 1991). The injury is most prevalent in women over 50, particularly those with signs of osteoporosis. Colles' fractures are easy to identify at initial assessment as the patient presents with classic dinner-fork

deformity of the wrist because of dorsal displacement and loss of volar angulation.

The patient usually has significant swelling around the fracture site and localized pain. Nerve involvement is not uncommon and paraesthesia may be present in areas served by the median or ulnar nerve. Severe swelling can cause vascular compromise and compartment syndrome. Neurovascular function should therefore be carefully checked on assessment. All the digits should be touched to ensure there is feeling and therefore neurological deficit is present and capillary refill should be checked. Patients need adequate analgesia and a full explanation of what is going to happen before any examination of the wrist is undertaken (Summers 2005). Management priorities involve restoration of anatomical alignment, in particular the degree of volar tilt, and the exact

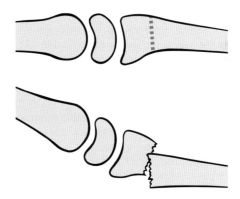

Figure 5.24   Colles' fracture.

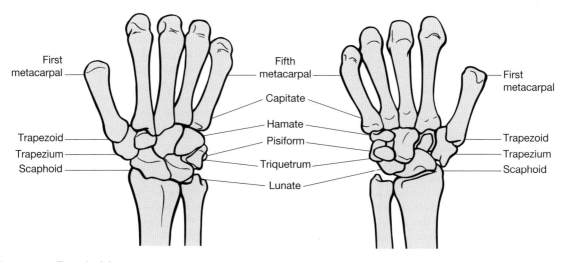

Figure 5.23   The wrist injury.

restoration of a neutral radio-ulnar joint if good function of the wrist is to be restored. Fractures with minimal displacement with no shortening and maintenance of volar tilt are managed in a forearm POP back-slab or split cast with the hand pronated and ulnar deviation, and flexion at the wrist (Brown 1996).

Most displaced fractures can be managed by closed reduction in the emergency department. To facilitate this, adequate analgesia is required. Debate persists as to which method of anaesthesia is most appropriate, and various methods are discussed in Chapter 25. Bier's block is often favoured by orthopaedic staff, but demands skilled operators. Haematoma block carries the risk of subsequent tissue toxicity from the lidocaine used, and has been criticized for providing inadequate anaesthesia to complete the reduction (Cooney et al. 1991). Despite this, haematoma block is commonly used and is successful in the treatment of elderly women. As a general rule, haematoma block is not suitable for Colles' fracture reduction in younger patients, particularly men with greater muscle spasm creating resistance to reduction. An accurate reduction is vital for restoration of full function in younger patients, and therefore multiple attempts at manipulation are sometimes needed. This is more easily facilitated under Bier's block.

The reduction involves a traction/counter-traction approach, with the first person applying longitudinal traction through the hand to lengthen the radius, while the other applies counter-traction through the forearm until disimpaction of the distal fragment can be felt. Then the first person applies pressure to the top of the distal fragment to reduce it. Again, volar movement will be felt and visible deformity should be resolved. The wrist should be immediately immobilized in a POP slab with ulnar deviation and wrist flexion. Post-reduction X-rays should be obtained to establish the degree of volar tilt, length and neutral radio-ulnar joint position (Greaves & Jones 2002). If this cannot be achieved by closed manipulation, open reduction and internal fixation should be considered. In complicated or severely comminuted injuries, open reduction and internal fixation should be considered and closed manipulation not attempted in ED.

Compartment syndrome, which is the compression of nerves and blood vessels in an enclosed space, can lead to permanent damage of these structures. Summers (2005) recommends the following symptoms of compartment syndrome – the 'five Ps' – should be discussed with patients, stressing that, if any of these symptoms manifest themselves, patients should contact their ED for advice.

The five Ps are:

- persistent pain
- pallor, when fingers lose their healthy colour
- pulselessness: instruction needs to have been given on how to perform capillary refill testing and interpret results
- paraesthesia
- paralysis.

As patients with Colles' type fracture are often older, their social circumstances should be established before discharge to make sure they can cope at home.

Smith's fractures

In both anatomical presentation and mechanism of injury, a Smith's fracture represents the opposite of a Colles' fracture. The distal radius is displaced proximally and the distal fragment is volar to the radial shaft. There are three classifications depending on the direction of the fracture (see Fig. 5.25).

The mechanism of injury is an impact on the distal aspect of the hand. Because significant force is needed to cause this fracture, the cause is usually a road traffic accident or cyclist going over the handlebars. Smith's fractures are most common in young men. The patient presents with severe pain, obvious volar deformity of the wrist, making the hand appear anteriorly displaced, and often swelling to the dorsal aspect of the wrist. Neurological compromise to median and ulnar nerves is possible with significant deformity, as is vascular compromise. Careful triage will highlight these complications.

Type I fractures can usually be treated in the emergency department. Closed manipulation involves restoring length and dorsal alignment of the radius. This can be achieved using Bier's block anaesthesia and manual traction. Once deformity is corrected, the arm should be immobilized in an above-arm split POP cast with the forearm in a supinated position.

Type II and type III fractures are unstable injuries and, to ensure maximum functional recovery, orthopaedic advice should also be sought. Open reduction with internal fixation is usually required.

Carpal fractures

The carpal bones form two rows (see Fig. 5.23). The proximal row consists of the scaphoid, lunate, triquetrum and pisiform bones. The scaphoid has a bridging position with the distal row which consists of the trapezium, capitate and hamate bones. These bones are supported by three strands of ligaments stemming from the radial styloid. The radial and ulnar arteries

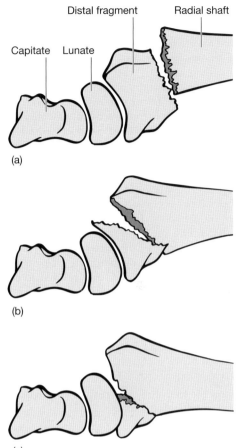

(a)

(b)

(c)

Figure 5.25 Smith's fracture: Classification of anterior displacement. (a) Type I–transverse fracture, (b) Type II–oblique fracture from proximal volar surface through dorsal particular surface, (c) Type III–oblique fracture with joint space involvement (same as Barton fracture-dislocation).

& Gillespie 2004). It occurs in both adults and children, most often between early teens and mid-life. The oblong-shaped scaphoid bone derives its name from the Greek word 'skaphos' meaning 'boat' and is divided into four anatomical areas (see Fig. 5.26).

The scaphoid has a good vascular supply to the middle and distal areas, but the proximal pole has no dedicated blood supply. This results in a high incidence of vascular necrosis if fracture union is not rapidly achieved (Gumucio 1989). Scaphoid fractures are usually classified as stable or unstable according to Herbert & Fisher (1984), and time taken to union differs with the fracture location (Box 5.6). Stable fractures that are incomplete or completely undisplaced, heal rapidly and are treated with immobilization. An unstable fracture has been defined as displacement of the fracture by 1 mm or more on X-ray.

The most common mechanism of injury is a fall onto an outstretched hand. Externally, there is little visible evidence of a fracture, although swelling can sometimes be present. The patient will have generalized pain,

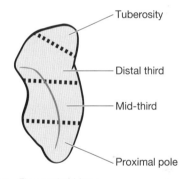

Figure 5.26 The scaphoid bone.

provide vascular supply, and the radial, ulnar and median nerves provide neurological function.

Fractures of the carpal bones are less common than other wrist injuries (Collier 1995), but are often associated with ligament injury, creating an unstable wrist joint. Long-term disability is not uncommon in missed fractures. Assessment of wrist injury should focus on the mechanism of injury, force involved and exact site of impact as well as the age of the patient, as wrist anatomy and relative strengths change with age.

Scaphoid fracture

Because of its unique position in relation to the radius and both rows of carpal bones, the scaphoid is the most commonly fractured carpal bone and accounts for between 2 and 7% of all orthopaedic fractures (McNally

---

Box 5.6   Herbert's classification of scaphoid fractures

Type A (stable)
A1	Crack fractures
A2	Tubercle fractures

Type B (unstable)
B1	Distal third
B2	Waist
B3	Proximal pole
B4	Carpal dislocation
B5	Comminuted

which is worse on wrist movement, particularly gripping actions. On examination, patients will have specific tenderness in the anatomical snuff box. They may also have pain when longitudinal pressure is applied to on the thumb and index finger, and pain on dorsiflexion of the wrist. Because of the location of pain and lack of external signs, patients often delay attending the emergency department as they do not automatically relate symptoms with a broken bone.

X-ray findings can be misleading as up to 20% of patients with scaphoid fracture have normal initial X-rays (McNally & Gillespie 2004). For this reason, diagnosis should be based on clinical findings, specifically, mechanism of injury and localized tenderness in the anatomical snuffbox. Although management of scaphoid fractures can be controversial (Hunter 2005), a general consensus exists that all fractures, whether clinical or radiological, should be immobilized as failure to do this can result in delayed or non-union healing or avascular necrosis. A POP cast or splint which incorporates the forearm and thumb, with the wrist in slight volar flexion, should be used. Complicated fractures should be referred to the orthopaedic team because of the risk of avascular necrosis. Some fractures are internally fixed at an early stage to prevent non-union and to ensure good functional recovery. Fractures not initially visible on X-ray will be apparent between 10–14 days post-injury (Hunter 2005).

Lunate fracture

The lunate is in the middle of the proximal carpal row and rests in the lunate fossa of the radius. Injury of the lunate bone is relatively uncommon because it is protected by the lunate fossa. When fracture does occur it is usually due to a fall onto an outstretched hand, where force is taken through the heel of the hand. The patient presents with mid-dorsal pain and wrist weakness; however, swelling is uncommon. As a result, attendance in the emergency department is sometimes days or weeks after the initial injury.

Radiological evidence of fracture is not always obvious, therefore clinical diagnosis is necessary based on location of pain and mechanism of injury. Non-displaced fractures should be treated in a forearm POP cast, with orthopaedic follow-up. Displaced fractures are prone to avascular necrosis and non-union, with a potential for secondary osteoarthritis. For this reason, patients should be referred to the orthopaedic team for possible internal fixation.

Triquetrum fractures

The triquetrum is the second most commonly fractured carpal bone. Such fractures often occur with other carpal fractures or peri-lunate dislocation. Isolated injury is less common and usually minor. Triquetrum fractures are usually caused by hyperextension injury of significant force. The patient usually complains of pain over the dorso-ulnar area of the wrist. Management involves a short arm POP cast or splint for 3–6 weeks in the case of isolated injury or referral to the orthopaedic team where the fracture is associated with other wrist injuries. Other carpal fractures generally occur as part of a more complicated hand or wrist injury, and demand specialist orthopaedic input after initial diagnosis in the emergency department.

Perilunate and lunate dislocation

These dislocations occur as a result of disruption to the lesser arc of ligaments. They can be graded into four groups depending on the degree of disruption (see Box 5.7). They are caused by extreme hyperextension, which might occur due to a motorcycle accident or fall from a height. Because of the force needed to cause perilunate and/or lunate dislocation, concurrent injury is common. The patient presents with extreme pain and a fork-type deformity, and is usually unable to hold the fingers in a flexed position. Nerve disruption is not uncommon, so paraesthesia may also be present. Fractures and severe ligament disruption are usual with these injuries, which should always be managed by the orthopaedic team and often require open reduction when associated with fractures.

HAND INJURY

The hand is a complex structure whose skeletal outline is shown in Fig. 5.27. The back of the hand is referred to as the dorsal aspect and the palm of the hand the volar aspect. The intricate mechanisms of hand movement are particularly vulnerable to injury because of its environmental exposure and functional

---

Box 5.7   Stages of perilunate disruption and midcarpal dislocation (After, Mayfield 1984.)

- **Stage 1: scapholunate instability** – due to torn radioscaphoid and scapholunate interosseous ligaments with/without scaphoid fracture
- **Stage 2: dorsal perilunate dislocation** – capitate dislocates dorsally from lunate at the midcarpal joint
- **State 3: disruption of lunate and triquetrum** – occurs with avulsion fracture of triquetrum with/without scaphoid or capitate fracture
- **Stage 4: volar dislocation of lunate**

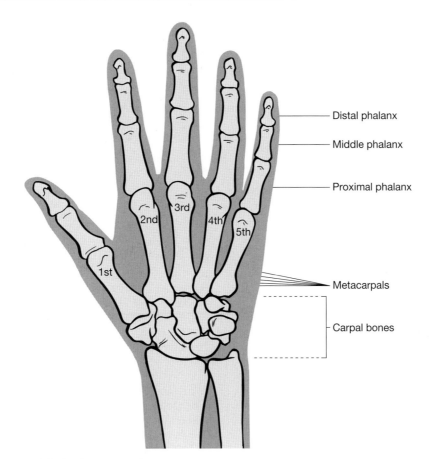

Figure 5.27   Anatomy of the hand.

purpose. Hand function relies on intact muscle and tendon structures and sensory motor connection to the central nervous system, as well as adequate circulation. The treatment of any hand injury revolves firstly around restoring function and secondly around appearance. Anatomy will be considered in greater detail where relevant to specific injuries.

Thumb injury

The flexor surface of the thumb is perpendicular to that of the fingers and has a saddle joint which allows 45° of rotation. The range of thumb movements includes flexion/extension, adduction/abduction and opposition. It provides both strength and grip.

First metacarpal fractures

These are treated differently from other metacarpal fractures because of the degree of functional restoration needed.

Metacarpal shaft fractures

These usually occur in the proximal half of the bone and are often associated with adduction of the distal segment. Management usually involves longitudinal traction and POP cast incorporating the thumb. Early orthopaedic follow-up is advisable.

Base of metacarpal fractures

These are usually more complicated and result from flexion injuries, commonly from clenched fists. They can be classified as intra-articular fractures, such as Bennett's fractures, or extra-articular transverse or oblique fractures. Extra-articular fractures are the most common fracture types. The fracture occurs within the joint capsule but does not involve the articular surface of the joint (see Fig. 5.28). These injuries are usually managed by closed reduction and POP cast incorporating the thumb. In order to retain good function, it is important not to hyperextend the thumb at the metacarpophalangeal joint. Some oblique fractures

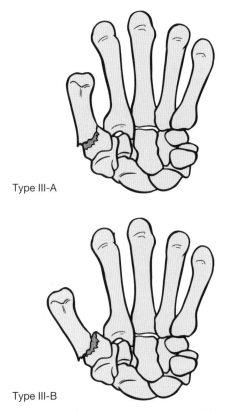

Type III-A

Type III-B

Figure 5.28 Extra-articular fracture to the base of the first metacarpal.

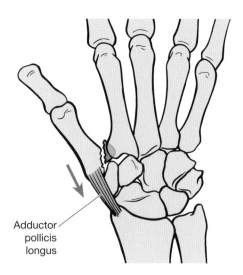

Adductor pollicis longus

Figure 5.29 Intra-articular fracture to the base of the first metacarpal (Bennett's Fracture).

may remain unstable with closed reduction and plaster immobilization alone, and therefore orthopaedic referral for percutaneous pinning is necessary.

Intra-articular fractures can be divided into two groups: the more common Bennett's fracture and Rolando's fracture. The Bennett's fracture is categorized by the displacement of the metacarpal shaft while the palmar articular fragment retains its correct anatomical location as shown in Fig. 5.29. The mechanism of injury is similar to that of an extra-articular fracture, with interpersonal fracas being a common cause of injury. The patient has limited movement of the base of the thumb with pain and swelling around the area. Effective emergency management is essential to prevent degenerative post-traumatic arthritis and to restore adequate range of movement.

The injury is considered unstable because of the adductor pollicis longus tendon, which is attached to the base of the first metacarpal. Its tensile strength prevents union of fracture without the aid of percutaneous pins or orthopaedic reduction and internal fixation.

Rolando's fracture is similar to a Bennett's fracture, but in addition to the palmar articular fragment remaining in place, the dorsal fragment displaces from the base, creating a Y-shaped or more severely comminuted base of metacarpal fracture. Mechanism of injury and patient presentation are similar to those of a Bennett's fracture, but the prognosis is poor as functional integrity is difficult to restore with orthopaedic reduction and internal fixation or closed reduction and immobilization. Persistent pain and degenerative arthritis are common. Phalangeal fractures of the thumb are generally managed in the same manner as fingers.

Second to fifth metacarpal fractures

The metacarpals are anatomically sectioned into base, shaft, neck and head. Unlike other long bones, the base is at the proximal point and the head at the distal end.

Base of metacarpal fractures (II–IV)
The patient presents with a history of a fall onto an outstretched hand or punch injury. The fractures are often associated with carpal fractures and second and third metacarpal base fractures often have intra-articular involvement, but this causes little or no disability because of the relative immobility of the second and third carpo-metacarpal (CMC) joint. As a result, treatment focuses on maintaining patient comfort. A removable splint is the treatment of choice. Fractures of the fourth and fifth metacarpal bases are usually associated with CMC dislocation. Fourth metacarpal base 'fractures can usually be managed in the

emergency department with closed reduction and splinting followed up by the orthopaedic team. Fifth metacarpal base fractures will usually require pinning because of displacement.

Good fracture alignment is necessary to retain normal mobility of the CMC joint. When splinting hand injuries, it is vital that metacarpo-phalangeal joints are immobilized in at least 70° of flexion to prevent shortening of the collateral ligaments. If these ligaments contract during immobilization, the patient is left with considerable disability because of joint stiffness.

Shaft of metacarpal fracture

These are caused by a number of mechanisms of injury (see Table 5.6). Principles of management revolve around correction of any rotation, angulation and shortening of the finger to ensure functional recovery. Even a small degree of rotation can cause problems with flexion of the metacarpo-phalangeal joint. Effective closed reduction and immobilization are usually achievable in A&E unless severe swelling or open fractures exist. If rotation cannot be corrected with manipulation, the patient should be referred for percutaneous pinning or orthopaedic reduction and internal fixation.

Metacarpal neck fractures

Second and third metacarpal neck fractures often need wiring to correct angulation in order to restore functional mobility, and therefore orthopaedic opinion should be sought. The fourth metacarpal is more mobile and neck fractures will heal without functional deficit even if volar angulation at the metacarpal neck exists. Any rotation in these fractures must be corrected to prevent functional deficit.

Fifth metacarpal neck fracture (boxer's fracture)　This is one of the most common hand injuries treated in the emergency department and usually results from a punch injury. Management of these fractures is controversial, but there is a consensus that any rotational injury needs manipulation and either splinting or wiring. Volar angulation can, however, be treated in a number of ways, ranging from orthopaedic

reduction and internal fixation to no treatment and early mobilization (Ford et al. 1989)

Clinical trials (Rusnak 1995) have found that no treatment at all or supportive splinting which facilitates mobilization has quicker functional repair, with minimal cosmetic deformity in the majority of cases. Where closed reduction is carried out, maintaining that reduction is difficult without causing further damage to the function of the hand. This is because 70° of flexion at the metacarpo-phalangeal joint is necessary to prevent contractures, but this position will not provide the three-point fixation needed to stabilize the metacarpal neck.

If the patient is exceptionally concerned about the cosmetic result and the possible loss of knuckle definition, then surgical fixation should be considered; however, recovery is significantly slower with this method. Whatever method is used, the patient should have adequate follow-up from a hand surgeon to ensure the fullest functional potential is achieved. Metacarpal head fractures should be managed conservatively unless they are displaced or comminuted, when an orthopaedic opinion should be sought.

Fracture of phalanges

As with other hand fractures, the key management priority is to maintain good function by correcting rotation. Neighbour strapping is usually the treatment of choice for uncomplicated fractures.

SOFT TISSUE INJURIES

Soft tissue injuries are commonly treated in ED and are usually considered 'minor' in nature by emergency staff. The impact on the patient, however, is far from minor; loss of normal function in the short term is common, usually because of pain. If soft tissue injuries are not detected and treated properly, long-term or recurrent problems can occur. Soft tissue injury (STI) is the all-encompassing term given to injury to muscles, ligaments, tendons and skin. As a result, the diagnosis of a STI has a number of possible causative factors. The common ones are described below.

Sprains

These are injuries to the fibres of ligaments supporting a joint. This results from abnormal movement of the joint which causes stretching and tearing of the ligament. The degree of this varies from some fibrous tearing to total disruption of the ligament complex supporting a joint (see Table 5.7).

The patient will present with mechanisms of injury and symptoms similar to those with fractures. The joint

Table 5.6	Metacarpal shaft fractures
Type	**Cause**
Transverse	Direct blow
Oblique	Torque force
Comminuted	Crush injury/gunshot wound

Table 5.7 Classification of sprains

	Physiology	Clinical signs
First degree	Minor tearing of ligament fibres with mild haemorrhage	Minimal swelling Tenderness over ligaments – worse with motion, stressing the ligaments
Second degree	Partial tear with moderate haemorrhage and reduced active motion	Significant pain – worse with passive movement and swelling Injuries prone to recurrence and can cause joint instability
Third degree	Complete rupture of ligament; moderate haemorrhage with significant loss of function	Less painful with significant swelling and abnormal motion of joint on active/passive movement Usually need surgical repair if joint instability exists.

has often been subjected to forces in opposite or abnormal directions, creating joint stress. The patient will usually describe a sudden onset of acute pain, and often describe hearing a 'snap' at the time of injury. Many patients are convinced this means they have broken their limb and the nurse must therefore be careful to assess the injury thoroughly and provide the appropriate reassurance (Smith 2003, Loveridge 2002). Although specific injury management can vary, common principles of sprain management apply:

Rest Most acute sprains benefit from a 48-hour period of rest, with minimal use.

Ice As well as being a useful first aid measure, ice packs, or wrapped crushed ice, help to decrease both pain and swelling. The patient should be advised to apply the ice for 10–15 minutes every 2–3 hours for the first 12 hours post-injury.

Compression Elastic tubular bandages or strapping provide support for the injury and help to reduce swelling. Tubular bandage should be removed by the patient at night to prevent oedema distal to the injury. In severe sprains, POP casts may be more appropriate for specific injuries.

Elevation Together with ice packs and rest, elevation of the injured part helps to reduce the accumulation of blood and lymph in tissues surrounding the injury, which in turn reduces both pain and healing time (Safran et al. 1999). This is particularly important for distal limb injuries, such as those of the hand, foot or ankle.

Strains

These are injuries to muscles and tendons. They occur after forced stretching or sudden violent contraction. As with sprains, the severity of strain injury is classified by the extent of damage (Table 5.8).

Treatment of strains is similar to that of sprains. Management of first-degree strains involves rest, ice, compression and elevation as described under 'sprains' above. Second-degree injuries may require immobilization, depending on the site affected, and usually take longer to heal. Third-degree injuries should be immobilized and the patient referred for early orthopaedic consultation at the fracture/STI clinic. Some injuries benefit from surgical repair, but many require simple immobilization. Many factors influence this decision: the site of injury, as well as the age, activity level and occupation of the patient (Loveridge 2002).

Table 5.8 Classification of strains

	Physiology	Clinical signs
First degree	Minor tearing of muscle/tendon unit	Spasm, swelling and localized pain
Second degree	More severe pain but incomplete tearing of fibres	Muscle spasm, swelling, localized pain and loss of strength
Third degree	The muscle or tendon is completely disrupted with separation of muscle from tendon, tendon from muscle or tendon from bone	Palpable defect is often present Muscle spasm, pain, swelling and loss of function

Tendinitis

This is an inflammatory condition usually caused by overuse. Less commonly it is caused by direct trauma. The patient complains of pain at the point where the tendon attaches to bone. Pain is worse on movement and function is sometimes restricted. Occasionally, palpable crepitus exists. Common sites include the rotator cuff of the shoulder (supraspinatus tendonitis), the insertion of hand extensors to the humeral lateral epicondyle (tennis elbow), the medial epicondyle (Golfer's elbow), the radial aspect of the wrist (De Quervain's tenosynovitis) and the Achilles tendon. Management involves rest and non-steroidal anti-inflammatories (NSAIDs).

Bursitis

This is inflammation of the bursa. The bursa is a sac of synovial fluid situated between muscle, tendon and bony prominences to facilitate movement. Bursitis can result from friction between the bursa and musculoskeletal tissue, direct trauma or infection. It results in inflammation and oedema, which causes sac engorgement, and the area becomes painful.

This condition is most common in middle age (Genge Jagmin 1995). The patient usually presents to the emergency department with a swelling at 2–3 days post-injury or strain. Pain can increase gradually over this time or may be of sudden onset. It is usually worse on movement and radiates distally from the site of bursitis. The area will appear classically inflamed with erythema and swelling and will be hot to the touch. Areas commonly affected include the knee (Adams 2004), elbow and big toe (gout bursitis).

If infection is suspected, e.g. following a puncture wound, or if the patient has pyrexia, the bursa should be aspirated and the aspirate sent to the laboratory for culture. Otherwise, the injured area should be managed conservatively with rest and NSAIDs.

Haematoma

This is a collection of blood resulting from vascular injury within the soft tissues, bone or muscle. It is a result of direct or blunt trauma. Large haematomas not only threaten homeostasis, due to loss of circulatory volume, but are also a potential host for infection. As a result, surgical drainage and antibiotic therapy may be necessary. Smaller haematomas can be treated with compression bandages, ice as described above, and elevation.

Contusions

These usually result from direct trauma, which results in localized pain, swelling and bruising. Most are self-limiting and symptoms are relieved by ice treatment, analgesia and early mobilization.

Specific soft tissue injuries

There are a number of soft tissue injuries that are so commonly treated in emergency departments that they warrant individual discussion within this chapter.

Knee injury

The knee gives support and flexibility to body movement. Ligaments and musculo-tendinous structures maintain its stability. The knee joint is the most complicated joint in the body (Adams 2004, Snell 2000) and because of its load-bearing task it is very susceptible to injury, particularly during sporting activities such as rugby and football. Medial injuries tend to be the most common; lateral injuries, however, are often more disabling. A history of an audible snap at time of injury is suggestive of anterior cruciate rupture. The mechanism of injury gives a strong indication of the likely structural damage, so accurate history-taking is vital (see Table 5.9).

Examination of the knee should be carried out with the patient undressed and lying on a trolley. The nurse should look at both knees to detect subtle differences. Bruising, swelling or redness are all signs of soft tissue injury. A rapid onset of swelling is indicative of haemarthrosis, which could be the result of

Table 5.9   Mechanisms of knee injury

Force	Cause	Injury
Hyperextension Forced flexion	Running/sudden deceleration, e.g. from rugby tackles	Tearing of anterior cruciate ligament
Twisting or flexed knee injury	Direct or blunt trauma	Meniscal injury
Valgus stress with external rotation	Skiing	Medial collateral ligament injury
Varus stress internal rotation	Skiing in snowplough position	Lateral collateral ligament
Direct force	Fall, hitting dashboard in RTA	Posterior cruciate ligament

ligament/meniscus tear or a fracture of the tibial plateau and is therefore an indication for X-ray. Aspiration may be carried out in strict aseptic conditions, both for symptom relief and for diagnostic purposes. If the aspirate contains fat globules then a fracture is present. All patients with a rapid-onset haemarthrosis have significant knee trauma and should be referred for orthopaedic follow-up. Swelling which has a gradual onset usually represents a reactionary effusion. These may also be aspirated for symptom relief if large or restrictive.

The nurse should carefully assess knee movement, as this will give clues as to what ligamentous damage exists. Most ligament injuries can be healed with the treatment described above for sprains. Because of the load-bearing nature of the knee tendon, ruptures are often associated with fractures and frequently need surgical repair. For this reason, patients with total ruptures should be referred to the orthopaedic team.

Patients may also present to the emergency department with knee pain but no history of trauma. In such presentations other diagnosis such as Baker's Cyst, osteoarthritis or in rare cases septic arthritis should be considered

Achilles tendon rupture

The Achilles tendon is the largest, thickest and strongest tendon in the body and after the quadriceps is the second most ruptured supporting tissue (Kerr 2005). Achilles tendon rupture is a common tennis and badminton injury, associated with sudden jumping movements with a heavy landing. The patient complains of a sudden sharp pain at the back of the ankle, not dissimilar to a direct blow. Swelling is present in some cases, as is bruising, but often it is simply pain and the mechanism of injury which initially indicate Achilles tendon rupture. The calf squeeze test (Simmonds' test) is useful in confirming diagnosis. The patient kneels backwards over a chair or lies face down on a trolley with the ankles over the end. When the calf is squeezed, plantar flexion of the ankle should occur unless the Achilles tendon is ruptured (Bickley & Szilagyi 2003). All of these patients should be referred for orthopaedic follow-up.

Most are initially managed in long leg equinous plaster, with the ankle in plantarflexion. Some patients benefit from surgical repair, particularly young athletic people. Patient outcomes appear similar whether or not open repair is performed (Mayeda 1992). Achilles tendinitis should not be confused with partial rupture. Tendinitis is caused by overuse or sudden change in activity such as dancing or running. The patient will have localized pain, swelling and crepitus over the tendon. The range of movement will be normal but

painful. The patient should be treated with rest and NSAIDs.

Ankle sprain

Large numbers of patients with ankle injuries are treated in ED, and one of the priorities for ED nurses lies with identifying serious or potentially limb-threatening injury (Loveridge 2002). Assessment for all ankle injuries should be systematic and thorough, although the majority will turn out to be straightforward sprains. Assessment should include mechanism of injury, the most common being an inversion injury causing damage to the anterior talofibular ligaments. This results from slipping off kerbs or twisting the ankle in a manner where the sole of the foot turns inwards.

Eversion injury is less common, but is more likely to be associated with an avulsion fracture and causes damage to the deltoid ligament; it is characterized by an injury where the sole of the foot turns outwards. Patients will often have heard a 'snap' or 'crack' at the time of injury which they will probably associate with a broken bone. The nurse needs to provide reassurance as well as a thorough assessment, particularly when an X-ray is not clinically indicated (see Ottowa ankle rules p. 96 Fig 5.13). The patient with an ankle sprain usually has pain at the site of injury, swelling over that area and reduced mobility because of pain. Examination usually identifies the area immediately below the respective malleolus to be the most severe point of pain, as opposed to a fracture where pain is worse over the bony prominence.

Management involves initial rest with compression bandaging, intermittent ice therapy and support. Recovery usually takes 2–4 weeks; however, most long-term problems stem from prolonged immobilization. For this reason, patients should be encouraged to exercise the ankle gently and resume activity after 1–2 weeks as pain and swelling permit.

Rotator cuff injury

The varied mobility of the shoulder joint makes it susceptible to injury (Ryan 2004). Shoulder stability is maintained by the rotator cuff. It comprises a sheath of muscles listed in Table 5.10. Degenerative conditions

Table 5.10	The rotator cuff muscles
Muscle	Action
Infraspinatus	External rotation
Teres minor	External rotation
Subscapularis	Internal rotation
Supraspinatus	Internal rotation

such as rheumatoid arthritis are not uncommon and increase the likelihood of injury. Acute injury includes tearing or tendinitis. The supraspinatus is the most commonly injured area; this results from falls with hyperextension or hyperabduction of the shoulder. Rest and analgesia comprise the management of choice, and most patients benefit from orthopaedic follow-up, as recurrent injury is not uncommon.

Rotator cuff tendinitis is usually a chronic condition, but a patient may present to the emergency department following an acute exacerbation. Unlike a rotator cuff tear, the patient will describe a gradually worsening discomfort, inability to sleep and decreased range of movement. NSAIDs and rest are the treatment of choice.

Thumb sprain

Stability and function of the thumb rely on the ulnar collateral ligament (UCL). Injury to the UCL is caused by hyperextension of the thumb from ball games or a fall, or by hyperabduction, usually from falling while moving, such as during skiing. If the history is suggestive of a UCL injury and the patient has pain in that area, then an X-ray should be performed to exclude a thumb fracture before joint stability is formally tested. If no fracture is present, the joint should be examined with the thumb in flexion and extension to determine stability. If UCL rupture is suspected, the patient should be referred to the orthopaedic team, as open surgical repair is often beneficial. If an uncomplicated sprain exists then elastoplast strapping in the form of a thumb spica will provide the compression and rest the joint to enable the sprain to heal.

Mallet finger

This is caused by a direct blow to the end of the finger or more commonly occurs as a result of forced flexion of the distal interphalangeal (DIP) joint. It is caused by rupture or avulsion of the extensor tendon. If an avulsion fracture of the distal phalanx is present, healing is usually more rapid than a tendon rupture. The patient presents in the emergency department with pain and a deformed finger and is unable to actively extend the fingertip distal to the DIP joint, causing drooping of the distal phalanges which may be slight or severe (Wang & Johnston 2001). Management involves splinting the finger to below the DIP joint in slight hyperextension. Patient education and cooperation are vital to the success of this treatment. The splint is usually plastic and needs to be removed frequently to clean the finger and prevent skin damage. It is important, however, that hyperextension of the DIP joint is maintained during this time. The patient should therefore be taught to apply and remove the splint while supporting fingertip on a firm surface.

Compartment syndrome

Compartment syndrome is a common but potentially life-threatening condition that requires prompt treatment and recognition. Caused by high pressure in a closed fascial space so that capillary perfusion is too low for tissue viability, it is well recognized as a potentially devastating complication of fractures (Edwards 2004). If this pressure is allowed to rise and stay high, it causes permanent damage to the soft tissue structures and nerves within that compartment. The limbs contain compartments, so injuries where swelling occurs have the potential to cause compartment syndrome. The forearm contains dorsal and volar compartments, and the lower leg is divided into four compartments: lateral, anterior, superficial posterior and deep posterior. In addition to internal tissue swelling, constricting dressings or plaster of Paris which is too tight can cause compartment syndrome. This is one reason why casts on new injuries tend to be either split or bivalved or back-slabs are applied.

Tissue pressure rises for a number of reasons, and often the primary injury is not in itself devastating. Any injury with the potential for haemorrhage or tissue swelling can result in compartment syndrome. There is no correlation between fractures and severity and tissue pressure. If pressure rises there is an increased volume in that area. There are two main causes:

- bleeding into the compartment, perhaps following a fracture or rupture of small vessels, will result in clot formation and increased compartmental pressure
- muscle swelling – this usually occurs after a period of ischaemia, e.g. following vascular damage.

During the ischaemic period, fluid leaks into tissues through damaged capillaries and membranes. When blood supply is restored, however, this situation continues because of capillary damage. This results in muscle oedema. This is why compartment syndrome is so common after major burn injury or as a follow-up to major crush injuries. Increased tissue pressure leads to hypo-perfusion of the structure within the affected compartment. Tissue perfusion rises, restricting venous return and causing reduced blood flow in major vessels; therefore the patient will have no tangible change in systemic blood pressure and pulses in the affected compartment will remain palpable. Tissue ischaemia can cause irreversible muscle and nerve damage unless nurses are familiar with the physiology of compartment syndrome and do not rely solely on traditional determinants, such as major pulses, to assume all is well.

The patient will complain of severe pain which is incompatible with the severity of the injury and paraesthesia. Pain may also occur away from the site of the primary injury. Symptoms are usually worse on movement or manual compression of the compartment. The patient often complains of numbness of the extremities distal to the compartment because of neurological compression. Motor function may also be impaired.

If any restrictive splints or dressings are in place these should be removed and the limb elevated in an attempt to reduce swelling. Initial treatment with mannitol can decompress compartment syndrome and avoid the need for surgery (Better 1999, Porter & Greaves 2003); however, if conservative treatment fails to restore sensation and relieve pain, fasciotomy will be necessary to prevent long-term damage. Fasciotomy has a high complication rate, however, as it transforms a closed lesion into an open wound (Fitzgerald et al. 2000). In all patients susceptible to compartment syndrome, early involvement of the orthopaedic and/or vascular team is essential. Specialist tissue-pressure monitoring gives an accurate portrait of how the patient is responding to conservative management and an indication of how quickly to intervene with fasciotomies. If left unchecked, the cycle of oedema and ischaemia results in muscle infarction, nerve injury and permanent loss of function in the extremity (Edwards 2004).

CONCLUSION

Musculoskeletal injury is one of the most common types of presentation to emergency departments. As this chapter has highlighted, it is imperative for emergency nurses to be able to assess musculoskeletal injury and identify life- or limb-threatening trauma, some of which may not seem devastating at first glance. An understanding of the underpinning anatomy and physiology of the musculoskeletal system has been provided in order to inform clinical decision-making and meet the needs of the individual patient and avoid long-term, preventable disability. As most of these patients will be discharged from the emergency department, the nurse has a crucial role as health educator in ensuring the patient looks after their injury, and prevents or minimizes long-term sequelae. In doing so, the emergency nurse may be assured of delivering quality care to this vulnerable group of patients.

References

Adams N (2004) Knee injuries. *Emergency Nurse*, **11**(10), 19–27.

American College of Surgeons (2004) *Advanced Trauma Life Support*, 7th edn. Chicago: American College of Surgeons.

Audit Commission (2000) *United they Stand: Coordinating Care for Elderly People with Hip Fractures*. London: The Stationary Office.

Bachmann LM, Kolb E, Koller MT, Steurer J, Rietter G (2003) Accuracy of Ottawa ankle rules to exclude fractures of the ankle and mid-foot: a systemic review. *British Medical Journal*, **326**, 405–406.

Beales J (1997) Tetanus immunisation: implications in A&E. *Emergency Nurse*, **5**(5), 21–23.

Better O (1999) Rescue and salvage of casualties suffering from crush syndrome after mass disasters. *Military Medicine*, **164**, 366–369.

Bickley LS, Szilagyi PG (2003) *Bates' Guide to Physical Examination and History Taking*, 8th edn. Philadelphia: Lippincott, Williams & Wilkins.

Brown AFT (1996) *Accident & Emergency Diagnosis and Management*. Oxford: Butterworth-Heinemann.

Brown DE (1992) Shoulder injuries. *Primary Care*, **19**, 265–281.

Cadogan M (2004) Femur injuries. In: *Textbook of Emergency Medicine*. (2nd edn) (eds P Cameron, G Jelinek, AM Kelly, L Murray, AFT Brown, J Heyworth) Edinburgh: Churchill Livingstone.

Carr M (1995) Forearm injuries. In: Ruiz E, Cicero JJ, eds. *Emergency Management of Skeletal Fractures*. St Louis: Mosby.

Chin HW, Propp PA, Orban DJ (1992) Forearm and wrist. In: Rosen P, Barkin RM, Braen GR et al., eds. *Emergency Medicine: Concepts and Clinical Practice*, 3rd edn. St Louis: Mosby Year Book.

Ciernick IF, Meier L, Hollinger A (1991) Humeral mobility after treatment with a hanging cast. *Journal of Trauma*, **31**, 230–233.

Clisham MW, Berlin SJ (1981) The diagnosis and conservative treatment of calcaneal fractures – a review. *Journal of Foot Surgery*, **20**(1), 28.

Collier R (1995) The wrist. In: Ruiz E, Cicero JJ, eds. *Emergency Management of Skeletal Fractures*. St Louis: Mosby.

Cooney WP, Linscheid RL, Dobyns JH (1991) Fractures and dislocations of the wrist. In: Rockward CA et al., eds. *Fractures in Adults*, vol. 1. Philadelphia: JB Lippincott.

Crimmins TJ, Ruiz E (1995) Shaft fractures of the femur. In: Ruiz E, Cicero JJ, eds. *Emergency Management of Skeletal Fractures*. St Louis: Mosby.

Dumas JL, Walker N (1992) Bilateral scapular fracture secondary to electric shock. *Archives of Orthopaedic Trauma Surgery*, **111**, 287–288.

Dymond IW (1984) The treatment of isolated fractures of the distal ulna. *Journal of Bone Joint Surgery*, **66**, 408–410.

Dyson S (1997) The diagnosis and treatment of scaphoid fractures in A&E. *Emergency Nurse*, **5**(6), 23–25.

Edwards S (2004) Acute compartment syndrome. *Emergency Nurse*, **12**(3), 32–38.

Fitzgerald AM, Wilson Y, Quaba A, Gaston P, McQueen M (2000) Long-term sequelae of fasciotomy wounds. *British Journal of Plastic Surgery*, **53**, 690–693.

Ford DJ, Ali MS, Steel WM (1989) Fractures of the 5th metacarpal neck – is reduction or immobilisation necessary? *Journal of Hand Surgery*, **14B**(2), 165–167.

Garden RS (1964) Stability and union in subcapital fractures of the femur. *Journal of Bone Joint Surgery*, **46-B**, 630.

Genge Jagmin M (1995) Musculoskeletal injuries. In: Kitt S, Selfridge-Thomas J, Proehl JA, Kaiser J, eds. *Emergency Nursing: A Physiologic and Clinical Perspective*, 2nd edn. Philadelphia: Saunders.

Goldberg HD, Young JWR, Reiner BI (1992) Double injuries of the forearm: a common occurrence. *Radiology*, **185**, 223–227.

Greaves L, Jones J (2002) *Practical Emergency Medicine*. London: Arnold.

Greenbaum MA, Papp GR (1992) Ankle dislocation without fracture – an unusual case. *Journal of Foot Surgery*, **31**, 238–240.

Gumucio CA (1989) Management of scaphoid fractures – a review and update. *South African Medical Journal*, **82**, 1377–1388.

Harris CR (1995) Ankle injuries. In: Ruiz E, Cicero JJ, eds. *Emergency Management of Skeletal Fractures*. St Louis: Mosby.

Harris CR, Haller PR (1995) The tibia and tibula. In: Ruiz E, Cicero JJ, eds. *Emergency Management of Skeletal Fractures*. St Louis: Mosby.

Herbert T, Fisher W (1984) Management of the fractured scaphoid using a new bone score. *Journal of Bone and Joint Surgery*, **71**-A(6), 938, 941.

Hunter D (2005) Diagnosis and management of scaphoid fractures: a literature review. *Emergency Nurse*, **13**(7), 22–26.

Irshad F, Shaw NJ, Gregory RJ (1997) Reliability of fat pad sign in radial head/neck fractures of the elbow. *Injury*, **28**(7), 433–435.

Kellman JF, Browner BD (1998) Fractures of the pelvic ring. In: Browner BD, Jupiter JB, Levine AM, Trafton PG eds. *Skeletal Trauma Fractures, Dislocations, Ligamentous Injuries*. 2nd edn. Philadelphia: WB Saunders.

Kelly AM (2004) Injuries of the shoulder girdle. In: *Textbook of Emergency Medicine*. (2nd edn) (Eds P Cameron, G Jelinek, AM Kelly, L Murray, AFT Brown, J Heyworth) Edinburgh: Churchill Livingstone.

Kerr J (2005) Achilles tendon injury: assessment and management in the emergency department. *Emergency Nurse*, **13**(2), 32–38.

Knapton P (1999) Shoulder injury: a case study. *Emergency Nurse*, **6**(10), 25–28.

Kroner K, Lind T, Jenson J (1989) The epidemiology of shoulder dislocation. *Archives of Orthopaedic Trauma & Surgery*, **108**, 288.

Kyle RF, Gustilo RB, Premer RF (1979) Analysis of 622 intertrochanteric hip fractures: a retrospective and prospective study. *Journal of Bone Joint Surgery*, **61**, 216.

Larsen D (2002) Assessment and management of foot and ankle fractures. *Nursing Standard*, **17**(6), 37–46.

Loveridge N (2002) Lateral ankle sprains. *Emergency Nurse*, **10**(2), 29–33.

Magnusson AR (1992) Humerus and Elbow. In: Rosen P, Barkin RM, Braen GR et al., eds. *Emergency Medicine: Concepts and Clinical Practice*, 3rd edn. St Louis: Mosby Year Book.

Mayeda DV (1992) Ankle and foot. In: Rosen P, Barkin RM, Braen GR et al., eds, *Emergency Medicine: Concepts and Clinical Practice*, 3rd edn. St Louis: Mosby Year Book.

McNally C, Gillespie M (2004) Scaphoid fractures. *Emergency Nurse*, **12**(1), 21–25.

McRae R (1999) *Orthopaedics and Fractures*. Edinburgh: Churchill Livingstone.

Mills K, Morton R, Page G (1995) *Color Atlas and Text of Emergencies*, 2nd edn. London: Mosby-Wolfe.

Monsell FP, Ross ERS (1998) Pelvic injuries. In: Driscoll P, Skinner D eds, *Trauma Care: Beyond the Resuscitation Room*. London: BMJ Books.

Mooney N (1991) Pain management in the orthopaedic patient. *Nursing Circles of North America*, **26**, 73–87.

Muir I, Boot D, Gorman DS, Teanby DN (1996) Epidemiology of pelvic fractures in the Mersey region. *Injury*, **27**, 199–204.

Newman AP (1988) Fractures of the shoulder. *Topics in Emergency Medicine*, **10**(3), 65.

Nicholson DA, Driscoll PA (1995) Elbow. In: Nicholson DA, Driscoll PA eds, *ABC of Emergency Radiology*. London: BMJ Publishing Group.

Nordqvist A, Peterson C (1992) Fracture of the body, neck and spine of the scapula: a long term follow up study. *Clinical Orthopaedics*, **283**, 139–144.

O'Steen D (2003) Orthopaedic and neurovascular trauma. In: Newbery L, ed. *Sheehy's Emergency Nursing: Principles and Practice*, 5th edn. St Louis: Mosby.

Oveson O, Brok KE, Arreskov J et al. (1990) Monteggia lesions in children and adults: an analysis of aetiology and long term results of treatment. *Orthopaedics*, **13**, 529–534.

Porter K, Greaves I (2003) Crush injury and crush syndrome: a consensus statement. *Emergency Nurse*, **11**(6), 26–30.

Proehl J (1999) *Emergency Nursing Procedures*, 2nd edn. Philadelphia: WB Saunders.

Quday K (1995) Shoulder injuries. In: Ruiz E, Cicero, JJ eds, *Emergency Management of Skeletal Fractures*. St Louis: Mosby.

Riebel GD, McCabe JB (1991) Anterior shoulder dislocation: a review of reduction techniques. *American Journal of Emergency Medicine*, **9**(3), 180–188.

Rourke K (2003) An orthopaedic nurse practitioner's practical guide to evaluating knee injuries. *Journal of Emergency Nursing*, **29**(4), 366–372.

Routt ML Jr, Nork SE, Mills WJ (2002) High energy pelvic ring disruptions. *Orthopedic Clinics of North America*, **33**, 59–72.

Rowley DI, Dent JA (1997) *The Musculoskeletal System: Core Topics in the New Curriculum*. London: Arnold.

Ruiz E (1995) Pelvic, sacral and acetabular fractures. In: Ruiz E, Cicero, JJ eds. *Emergency Management of Skeletal Fractures.* St Louis: Mosby.

Rusnak RA (1995) Examination of the hand and management of finger-tip injuries. In: Ruiz E, Cicero JJ, eds. *Emergency Management of Skeletal Fractures.* St Louis: Mosby.

Ryan A (2004) Rotator cuff tears. *Emergency Nurse,* **12**(4), 27–37.

Safran MR, Achazewski JE, Benedetti RS, Bartolozzi AR, Mandelbaum R (1999) Lateral ankle sprains: a comprehensive review. Part 2: treatment and rehabilitation with an emphasis on the athlete. *Medicine and Science in Sports and Exercise,* **31**(7), S438–S447.

Schmidt M, Armbrect A, Havermann D (1992) Results of surgical management of scapula fractures. 78th annual meeting of the Swiss Society of Accident Surgery and Occupational Diseases. *Z-Unfallchir Versicherungsmed,* **85**, 186–188.

Smith M (2003) Ankle sprain: a literature search. *Emergency Nurse,* **11**(3), 12–16.

Smith M (2005) Orthopaedic trauma. In: O'Shea RA ed. *Principles and Practice of Trauma Nursing.* Edinburgh: Elsevier Churchill Livingstone.

Snell RS (2000) *Clinical Anatomy for Medical Students,* 6th edn. Philadelphia: Lippincott Williams, Wilkins.

Snyder PE (1998) Fractures. In: Maher AB, Salmond SW, Pellino TA, eds. *Orthopaedic Nursing,* 2nd edn. Philadelphia: WB Saunders.

St Claire-Strange FG (1982) Entrapment of median nerve after dislocation of elbow. *Journal of Bone and Joint Surgery,* **64B**, 224.

Stiell IG, Greenberg GH, McKnight RD, Nair RC, McDowell I, Worthington JR (1992) A study to develop clinical decision rules for the use of radiography in acute ankle injuries. *Annals of Emergency Medicine,* **21**(4), 384–390.

Summers A (2005) Recognising and treating Colles' type fractures in emergency care settings. *Emergency Nurse,* **13**(6), 26–33.

Tsai AK, Ruiz E (1995) The elbow joint. In: Ruiz E, Cicero, JJ eds. *Emergency Management of Skeletal Fractures.* St Louis: Mosby.

Tullos HG, Bennett JG, Braly WG (1984) Acute shoulder dislocations: factors influencing diagnosis and treatment. In: *The American Academy of Orthopaedic Surgeons Instructors Course Lectures,* vol. 33. St Louis: Mosby.

Wang QC, Johnson BA (2001) Fingertip injuries. *American Family Physician,* **63**, 1961–1966.

Ward W (1999) Key issues in nurse requested X-rays. *Emergency Nurse,* **6**(9), 19–23.

Whelan L (1997) Ankle injury: a case study. *Emergency Nurse,* **5**(7), 24–27.

Wickham N (1997a) Pressure area care in A&E: Part One, *Emergency Nurse,* **5**(3), 23–31.

Wickham N (1997b) Pressure area care in A&E: Part Two, *Emergency Nurse,* **5**(4), 25–29.

Wilkerson CA (1992) Ankle injury in athletes. *Primary Care,* **19**, 377–392.

Wyatt JP, Illingworth RN, Clancy MJ, Munro P Robertson CE (1999) *Oxford Handbook of Accident and Emergency Medicine.* Oxford: Oxford University Press.

Zagorski JB, Latta LI, Zych GA, et al. (1988) Diaphyseal fractures of the humerus treatment with prefabricated braces. *Journal of Bone and Joint Surgery,* **70A**, 607–610.

Chapter 6

Spinal injuries

Mike Paynter

INTRODUCTION

Spinal cord injury is one of the most disabling and catastrophic outcomes of injury in a person's life. The annual incidence of spinal cord injury in the UK is about 10–15 per million of the population, with the majority of patients male, usually below the age of 40, with a quarter of all cord-injured patients being below the age of 20 (Gallagher 2005). Many of these patients are left with permanent disabilities. The overall physical, emotional and financial consequences of disability are devastating for those injured, and for their families and friends.

Although the effect of the initial injury is irreversible, the spine and spinal cord are at further risk from secondary insult either by accidental ill-handling at the accident scene or by subsequent poor management in the emergency department. This chapter explores the identification and management of spinal cord injuries in the ED.

ANATOMY AND PHYSIOLOGY

The vertebral column is a series of stacked bones that support the head and trunk and provide the bony encasement for the spinal cord. It comprises 33 vertebrae – 7 cervical, 12 thoracic, 5 lumbar, 5 fused sacral and usually 4 rudimentary coccygeal vertebrae. With the exception of the atlas (C1) and the axis (C2), all vertebrae are anatomically alike but di\ffer in size and function (see Fig. 6.1).

The human vertebral column enables people to assume an upright position. It provides a base of muscle attachments, protects the spinal cord and vital organs in the thorax, and allows for body movements to occur. A vertebral body consists of the body, a vertebral arch, and a vertebral foramen. The arch of the

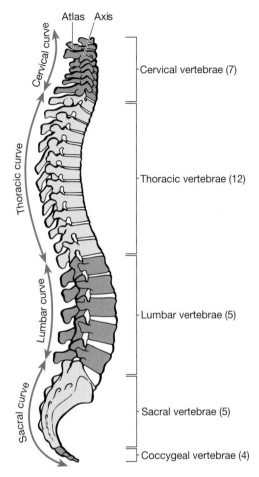

Figure 6.1 Anatomy of spinal vertebrae.

vertebra is composed of two pedicles, two laminae, four facets, two transverse processes and the spinous process, which can be palpated. Intervertebral cartilaginous discs provide cushioning and shock absorption between vertebral segments.

The spinal cord lies protected within the spinal canal, which is a hollow tunnel extending the length of the vertebral column. The spinal cord descends from the medulla oblongata near the atlas to the level of the second lumbar vertebra. The spinal cord is nearly circular in section and about 1 cm in diameter, with two enlargements. On cross-section, the spinal cord has a grey matter, appearing in the form of the letter H. The grey matter consists of nerve cells that act as relay stations for nerve impulses transmitted up and down the spinal cord. White matter surrounds the grey matter and contains longitudinal myelinated fibres organized in tracts or bundles to carry information to and from the brain. Ascending tracts are sensory, and descending tracts are motor (Jaworski & Wirtz 1995).

PATHOPHYSIOLOGY

The cervical vertebrae are the most mobile part of the spine, so this area is the most frequent site of injury. The rib cage keeps the vertebrae from T1 and T10 stable and relatively immobile. The second most common site of injury is the thoracolumbar junction at T11 to L2. This is a transition area between the rigid thoracolumbar region and the more mobile lumbar region (Semonin-Holleran 2003). Force applied to the cervical spine does not always result in localized vertebral damage, however, because the flexibility of the region, and the ability of the neck to move in *anteriorposteriolateral* directions, can help transfer the force downwards to the thoracic spine where there is little or no flexibility (Sheerin 2005).

Vertebral column injury, with or without neurological deficits, must always be sought and excluded in a patient with multiple trauma. Any injury above the clavicle should prompt a search for a cervical spine (c-spine) injury. Approximately 15% of patients sustaining such an injury will have an actual (c-spine) injury. Approximately 55% of spinal injuries occur in the cervical region, 15% in the thoracic region, 15% at the thoracolumbar junction, and 15% in the lumbosacral area. Approximately 5% of patients have an associated spinal injury, while 25% of spinal injury patients have at least a mild head injury (American College of Surgeons 2004).

Approximately 8–10% of patients with a vertebral fracture have a secondary fracture of another vertebra, often at a distant site. These secondary fractures are usually associated with more violent mechanisms of injury, such as ejection or rollover. Owing to the mechanism of injury, many patients with spinal injury often have other associated injuries, including head, intrathoracic or intra-abdominal injuries, which may alter priorities in management (Lowery et al. 2001). Falls account for 46%, road traffic accidents (RTAs) account for 34% and sports-related incidents account for 10% of spinal injuries in the UK (Harrison 2004). The forces involved in RTAs can cause such severe damage to vertebrae C1 and C2 that the cord is affected, so that the person involved cannot self-ventilate. In such circumstances, death is the most common outcome (Schoen 2000).

The majority of spinal cord injuries are closed. Table 6.1 outlines the specific categories of movement that may result in spinal cord injury.

The most common type of injury mechanism is excessive flexion. This usually occurs following road

Table 6.1   Categories of movement that may result in spinal cord injury (Semonin-Holleran 2003)

Category	Mechanism of injury
Hyperextension	The head is forced back and the vertebrae of the cervical region are placed in an overextended position
Hyperflexion	The head is forced forward and the vertebrae are placed in an overflexion position
Axial loading	A severe blow to the top of the head causes a blunt downward force on the vertebral column
Compression	Forces from above and below compress the vertebrae
Lateral bend	The head and neck are bent to one side, beyond the normal range of motion
Overrotation and distraction	The head turns to one side and the cervical vertebrae are forced beyond normal limits

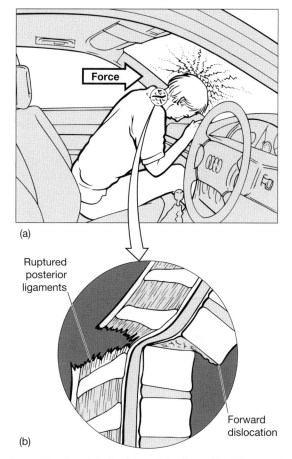

(a)

Ruptured posterior ligaments

(b)

Forward dislocation

Figure 6.2   Spinal flexion injury. (After Jaworski & Wirtz 1995.)

traffic accidents (RTAs) when the patient's head strikes the steering wheel or windscreen and the spine is forced into hyperflexion with the chin thrown forward to the chest. Rupture of the posterior ligaments results in forward dislocation of the spine (see Fig. 6.2).

Axial loading or compression-type injuries can occur when the head strikes an object and the weight of the still-moving body bears against the now stationary head, such as when the head of an unrestrained car passenger is flung into the windscreen or during a dive into shallow water. Vertebral bodies are wedged and compressed, and the burst vertebral fragments enter the spinal canal, piercing the cord (Jaworski & Wirtz 1995) (see Fig. 6.3).

Rotational injuries (e.g. Fig. 6.4) can result from a number of causes. Disruption of the entire ligamentous structure, fracture and fracture-dislocation of spinal facets may occur. Flexion-rotation injuries are highly unstable fractures.

Distraction, or over-elongation of the spine, occurs when one part of the spine is stable and the rest is in longitudinal motion. This 'pulling apart' of the spine can easily cause stretching and tearing of the cord. It is a common mechanism of injury in children's playground accidents and in hangings (Pre-Hospital Trauma Life Support Committee 2006).

PATIENT ASSESSMENT

History–taking

The importance of obtaining the patient's history and establishing the mechanism of injury cannot be overemphasized. Obtaining an accurate history represents 90% of the diagnosis (American College of Surgeons 2004). A fully documented pre-hospital history should be obtained from the ambulance personnel, police officers and others involved in the pre-hospital phase of patient care. If the patient has been injured as the result of an RTA, digital pictures of the accident scene and the damage sustained to vehicles can provide valuable information about the mechanisms involved. If taken, these photographs should be printed off and included in the patient's hospital notes (Greaves & Hodgetts 2005).

A high index of suspicion is needed if patients are to be managed correctly (Caroline 1995).

Spinal cord injury should be suspected with any of the following:

- a history of significant trauma and altered mental status from intoxication
- a history of seizure activity since the accident

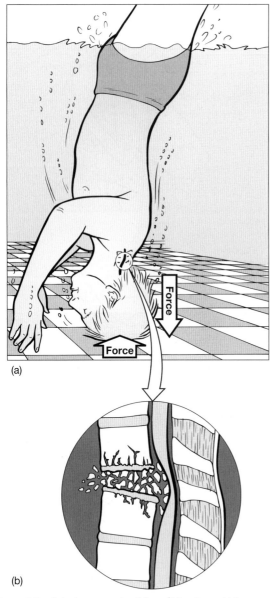

(a)

(b)

Figure 6.3   Spinal compression injury. (After Jaworski & Wirtz 1995.)

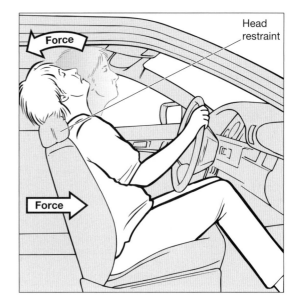

Figure 6.4   Spinal rotation injury.

- any complaint of neck pain or altered sensation in the upper extremities
- a complaint of neck tenderness
- a history of loss of consciousness
- an injury above the clavicle
- a fall greater than three times the patient's height
- a fall that results in a fracture of the heels
- an unrestrained (no seat belt) person with a facial injury

- significant injuries in a RTA that result in chest and intra-abdominal injuries.

The patient may complain of a feeling of 'electric shock' or 'hot water' running down his back. A history of incontinence before arrival in the ED may be reported (Semonin-Holleran 2003). Failure to suspect a spinal injury will lead to failure in its detection, with potentially devastating consequences for the patient.

The patient's ability to walk should not be a factor in determining whether he needs to be treated for spine injury. Not all patients will have a dramatic entrance into the emergency department; in one North American study 17% of patients who required surgical repair of unstable spine injuries were found 'walking around' at the accident scene or walked into the ED in the local hospital (McSwain 1992). A nod of the head or a sneeze in such patients could easily push an unstable fragment of vertebra against the spinal cord. Therefore an unstable spine can only be ruled out by careful physical assessment, X-ray examination or a lack of any potential mechanism.

Spine immobilization

When the patient arrives in the emergency department, extreme care is required in the transfer from the ambulance stretcher to the trauma trolley: total spinal immobilization is the goal. The use of a backboard is ideal for the transfer of such patients.

Once the patient is on the trauma trolley, protection of the cervical spine should be given the same priority as the airway (American College of Surgeons 2004). All emergency personnel involved in caring for the patient must be continuously aware that imprudent movement of the spine has the potential to cause secondary injury. The patient must have the cervical spine immobilized in a semi-rigid well-fitting cervical collar (Aprahamian et al. 1984), have sandbags either side for lateral stabilization and have the forehead taped to the trauma trolley. Semi-rigid cervical collars alone are inadequate. Caution should be exercised with the use of semi-rigid cervical collars in head injury patients, since even correctly fitted collars have been shown to cause a variable rise in intracranial pressure (Kolb 1999, Davies et al. 1996).

It should also be noted that in children the head is large and the posterior musculature is not well developed. If placed on a rigid board or trolley, a child's head is typically moved to severe flexion. When immobilizing children, significant padding under the torso is usually necessary to maintain the immobilization (Pre-Hospital Trauma Life Support Committee 2006).

One member of the ED team must remain at the patient's head and ensure total in-line immobilization of the spine and airway patency. This team member should communicate with the patient, explaining what is happening and why. The patient is in an unnatural environment, probably surrounded by strangers, and is likely to feel out of control of his situation, because of carer interventions. Reassurance and support are therefore vital in gaining the patient's cooperation. If the patient is confused, agitated and restless, it is advisable to leave only the semi-rigid cervical collar on and not to use forcible restraint. Otherwise the patient will be liable to twist and thrash, causing unwanted movement of the neck and trunk and a possible total transection of a partially transected spinal cord. Once the patient has become settled, full immobilization can be initiated.

Airway

Obstruction of the airway is an ever-present threat in managing patients with suspected cervical spine injuries. Normal efforts used for maintaining airway patency are liable to exacerbate the injuries (Aprahamian et al. 1984). If the patient can talk in a normal voice and give appropriate answers to questions, the airway is patent and the brain is being perfused (Driscoll & Skinner 2007). In an unconscious patient, potential problems come from the tongue falling back against the posterior pharyngeal wall and causing an obstruction. Foreign bodies, such as loose teeth and broken denture plates,

and the risk of regurgitation and aspiration all put the airway at risk.

Obstruction caused by the tongue is corrected by the chin lift. The airway can then be maintained by the insertion of an oropharyngeal airway (Safar & Bircher 1988). To perform the chin lift, place the fingers of one hand under the mandible and gently lift the chin upward; the thumb of the same hand lightly depresses the lower lip to open the mouth. The chin lift is the method of choice for the patient with a suspected spinal injury, since it does not risk aggravating a possible fracture.

The jaw thrust is another technique. This is performed by grasping the angles of the lower jaw, one hand on each side; forward displacement of the mandible will open the airway. Again, great care must be taken not to flex or extend the neck. All debris, such as broken teeth or loose denture plates, must be removed in order to prevent potential problems. These can be removed using Magill forceps under direct vision.

Blood and vomit must be removed immediately. A rigid wide-bore suction device, with head-down tilt of the trauma trolley, will help to prevent aspiration. The semi-prone recovery position is contraindicated, since it involves cervical rotation. Endotracheal intubation with a cuffed tube is the definitive method of securing a patent airway, preventing aspiration and aiding ventilation, oxygenation and suctioning. If intubation is required, it must be performed by a suitably skilled and experienced member of the team (Safar & Bircher 1988). During intubation, in-line cervical spinal immobilization must be maintained. Cricoid pressure can be applied through the aperture in the front of the semi-rigid collar. Stimulation of the oropharynx during intubation or suctioning may cause a vagal discharge, resulting in profound bradycardia. The heart rate should be closely monitored during intubation and supported if necessary with intravenous atropine.

Breathing

Ventilation may be affected by the level of the cord injury, aspiration and presence of primary lung injury. In the absence of major airway obstruction and flail chest, the presence of paradoxical breathing is considered highly suggestive of cervical spine injury. Paradoxical breathing occurs because of loss of motor tone and paralysis of thoracic muscle innervated by thoracic spinal segments. Diaphragmatic action results in a negative intra-pleural pressure. As a consequence of chest wall paralysis the tendency is for the soft tissues of the thorax to 'cave in', producing paradoxical chest movement. The diaphragm needs to undertake the full work of breathing, including overcoming added resistance to ventilation caused by paradoxical chest wall movement. In addition to standard respiratory status assessment, continuous pulse oximetry and assessment of vital capacity is necessary. Early intubation should be considered if vital capacity is inadequate or falling (Wassertheil 2004).

Circulation

Complete injuries above T1, and perhaps T4, can be expected to have clinically significant manifestations of neurogenic shock. The clinical signs are bradycardia, peripheral vasodilatation and cessation of sweating. Priapism in a trauma is due to penile vasodilatation from parasympathetic nervous system stimulation and loss of sympathetic nervous system control. It is highly suggestive of spinal cord injury, especially if the patient is unconscious.

Circulatory status is best assessed by conscious state, urine output and venous pressure monitoring. In the early phases of management, close urine output monitoring is of major importance. Early insertion of a urinary catheter not only allows measurement of urinary output but may also assist in identifying occult renal tract injury, and also prevent bladder distension.

Disability

Spinal cord injury has an association with significant head trauma (Wassertheil 2004). In patients with altered conscious state due to head trauma, brief mental assessment and pupillary reflexes are important.

Once the patient has a safe patent airway and full cervical spine precautions are in place, further examination can proceed. All clothing needs to be removed to facilitate examination; this should cause minimum discomfort and not aggravate potential injuries. Under no circumstances must the neck or trunk be flexed, extended or rotated during this process. Extending the arms to the side or elevating them above the head causes angulation of the shoulder girdle and substantial movement of the cervical spine. Therefore, to ensure no disruption to the cervical immobilization, it is often safest to cut away clothing. Clothing that remains under the patient can be removed during the later log roll.

Once the airway and cervical spine are protected, a full set of baseline vital signs must be recorded:

- the patient's neurological status
- respiratory rate
- pulse
- blood pressure
- temperature
- blood glucose levels
- 12-lead electrocardiograph.

In patients who are potentially haemodynamically unstable, cardiac monitoring and measurement of oxygen saturation should be mandatory.

Secondary survey and the log roll

As part of the secondary survey, the patient's back must be fully examined. Obviously this involves turning the injured patient. Without losing control of the in-line cervical spine immobilization, this can be safely accomplished by using the log roll technique (Tippett 1993). Four members of the team are required to safely execute this procedure (see Fig. 6.5). The senior team member assumes manual control of the cervical spine; only then are tapes and sandbags removed. The remaining three members of the team take responsibility for the chest, pelvis and legs (Griffiths & Gallimore 2005). The senior person at the patient's head coordinates the roll. The person holding the leg keeps the lateral malleolus in line with the hip, preventing adduction. The patient is then smoothly rolled in a well-coordinated move, avoiding any rotational movements of individual spinal segments.

The cervical, thoracic and lumbar spines are all examined for areas of deformity, grating crepitus, haematomas and areas of increased pain on palpation. An assessment for paraesthesia is made, noting the location and level. Finally a rectal examination is performed, the aim of which is to assess rectal sphincter tone, and thereby the sacral nerves. If voluntary sphincter contraction occurs, the spinal injury is classified as incomplete (Jaworski & Wirtz 1995). Before the patient is returned to the supine position, all remaining clothing that may have been left under the patient can be removed at this stage. Debris such as windscreen glass fragments can easily be cleared away with the aid of a portable car vacuum, thus minimizing further risk to the patient's skin and pressure areas.

Once full posterior examination of the patient has been performed, the person holding the head gives the command for all members of the team to return the patient to the supine position. Once returned, sandbags and tape are reapplied and manual immobilization can then be discontinued.

CERVICAL SPINE FRACTURES

The cervical spine is the most mobile part of the entire vertebral column and as such is liable to considerable injury. Sudden violent forces can move the spine beyond its normal range of movement, either by impacting on the head and neck or by pushing the trunk out from under the head. Since extreme forces are required to damage the cervical spine, patients will often present with severe head and maxillofacial

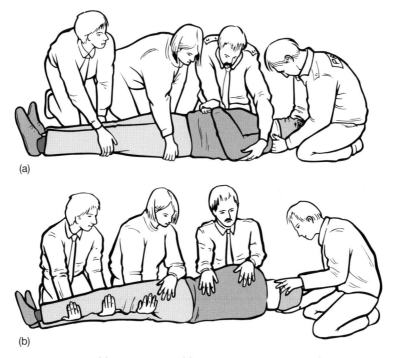

(a)

(b)

Figure 6.5 Log rolling the spinal patient. (a) Initial position, (b) Patient on side during roll. (From Greaves et al. 2005.)

wounds. Despite what may look like horrific injuries, the ATLS principles of patient care should be applied: airway and cervical spine management is first and foremost, followed by breathing and circulatory support as appropriate.

Good-quality X-rays are essential for accurate diagnosis of spinal injury (Raby et al. 2005). There are only three radiographs that are mandatory in the resuscitation room and these can be obtained as soon as life-threatening problems have been identified and controlled. The first is a lateral cervical spine view, and the other two are of the chest and pelvis. The lateral cervical spine views can be obtained without interrupting immobilization (Wyatt et al. 2005).

All seven cervical vertebrae, C1 to the C7/T1 junction, must be identified on the lateral film (Grundy 2002). If problems are encountered viewing C7, the application of downwards traction on the arms will pull the shoulders down and should make viewing easier. Sometimes this proves impossible. If this is the case a 'swimmer's view' of the lower cervical spine and upper thoracic areas can be obtained (McRae 2006). At least 70% of fractures, dislocations or subluxations will be visible on the lateral radiograph with most common injuries around the C1–C2 articulations and between C5 and C7 (Holliman et al. 1991).

The type of vertebral injury most likely to produce neurological damage is a fracture-dislocation. Inadequate or misinterpreted radiographs of the cervical spine are potentially devastating for the patient. It is vital that the ED nurse insists on continued c-spine immobilization until all radiographs have been reviewed and C1 to C7 have been cleared of abnormality. Clinical history and examination must always take precedence over apparently normal radiographs; important neck injuries may still be present despite normal-looking plain films (Jones & Rawlinson 1993). All cervical spine fractures should be treated as unstable in the emergency department and, depending upon neurological examination, be referred to the orthopaedic, neurosurgical or specialist spinal unit teams (McRae 2006).

THORACOLUMBAR SPINE FRACTURES

Fractures of the thoracic spine between T2 and T10 are usually the result of hyperflexion which produces a wedge compression of one or more vertebrae. Wedge compression fractures of the thorax are rarely unstable because the rib cage provides fairly rigid support; however, these fractures can be rendered unstable if there are associated fractures of the ribs and sternum. Fractures of the thoracic vertebrae tend to be slightly more common in elderly patients, where they are often associated with a degree of osteoporosis and can sometimes occur with minimal trauma. In younger patients, severe trauma is required to cause these fractures (McRae 2006). Fractures of the thoracolumbar region are frequently due to the relative immobility of the thoracic spine compared with the lumbar spine. The mechanism of injury is usually acute hyperflexion and rotation, and hence these fractures are commonly unstable.

Falling from a height and landing on the feet can result in compression and axial loading. Typically, falls from a height are from second- or third-storey levels (National Spinal Injuries Unit 2005). The individual falls and the fall is broken by contact with a solid barrier causing a sudden change in the velocity of the body to 0 mph. On impact, an equal and opposite force is created and meets the impacting individual. If the person falls on the feet, the two forces travel longitudinally along the vertebral column, which causes 'axial loading', and meet at a point where the forces are concentrated. This can compress vertebrae and the spinal cord, cause burst fractures, and force bone fragments to enter the spinal canal. There may also be fractures to the lower extremities. If the person falls on the buttocks, a hyperflexion injury to the lumbar area may result, again with compression fractures (Sheerin 2005).

The impact of landing forces the weight of the head and thorax down against the lumbar vertebrae, while the sacral vertebrae remain stationary. Fractures of the lumbar vertebrae are reasonably common, especially at the T12/L1 and L4/S levels (McRae 2006). Twenty per cent of falls greater than 15 feet involve associated fractures of the lumbar vertebrae (McSwain 1992).

Isolated sacral fractures are uncommon and are frequently associated with much more serious fractures of the pelvis. As with cervical spine injuries, the patient must be kept in the neutral position and complete spinal immobilization maintained. The log roll must be employed to facilitate examination of the back.

SPINAL CORD INJURY

The main risk factor associated with spinal fractures is damage to the spinal cord. If the fracture is stable, the cord is safe, but if the fracture is unstable the possibility of cord injury is present. Stable fractures are not likely to displace further than at the time of injury; an unstable fracture or dislocation is, however, liable to further displacement, therefore posing considerable risk to the spinal cord (Crawford-Adams 2001).

The spinal cord is the communication pathway between the brain and the body. A transection of the cord will render all nerves distal to the injury useless. A conscious patient will be able to identify pain at the site of the injury but have no sensation below it; from the moment of injury the patient feels cut in two. Voluntary movement below the level of the cord injury is lost immediately and the muscles become flaccid. The bladder and rectum are paralysed; however the bladder sphincter subsequently recovers and causes acute urinary retention.

The position of the cord injury has a direct effect on the patient's prognosis. Complete transection of the cord at levels C1, 2 or 3 is incompatible with life. Damage to the cord at this level causes both intercostal and diaphragmatic movement to cease, and only intermittent positive pressure ventilation (IPPV) will keep the patient alive. Lower cervical cord damage may leave the phrenic nerve sufficiently intact to maintain diaphragmatic breathing. Diaphragmatic breathing only, provided from C4 to T6, is liable to reduce vital capacity and a subsequent compensatory tachypnoea will develop. If tidal volume and vital capacity are reduced, consideration must be given to intubating and providing IPPV (Robertson & Redmond 1994). See Table 6.2.

Table 6.2 Assessing level of spinal injury (Szilagyi & Bickley 2004)

Muscle group	Nerve supply	Reflex
Diaphragm	C3, C4, C5	
Shoulder abductors	C5	
Elbow flexors	C5, C6	Biceps jerk
Supinators/pronators	C6	Supinator jerk
Wrist extensors	C6	
Wrist flexors	C7	
Elbow extensors	C7	Triceps jerk
Finger extensors	C7	
Finger flexors	C8	
Intrinsic hand muscles	T1	
Hip flexors	L1, L2	
Hip adductors	L2, L3	
Knee extensors	L3, L4	Knee jerk
Ankle dorsiflexors	L4, L5	
Toe extensors	L5	
Knee flexors	L4, L5, S1	
Ankle plantar flexors	S1, S2	Ankle jerk
Toe flexors	S1, S2	
Anal sphincter	S2, S3, S4	Bulbocavernosus reflex Anal reflex

If the patient is unconscious, the following clinical findings will indicate a cervical cord injury:

- diaphragmatic breathing
- weakness or paralysis
- hypotension with bradycardia
- flaccidity
- loss of bulbocavernosus reflex and anal tone
- evidence of painful stimuli above the clavicles
- ability to flex, but not extend, the elbows
- priapism.

Since the urinary bladder is paralysed when the cord is damaged, acute urinary retention will occur. Insertion under strict aseptic technique of an indwelling urinary catheter will be required to decompress the bladder in order to monitor the patient's haemodynamic status. Short periods of local pressure result in pressure sores. It is essential that all clothing and debris are removed from under the patient at the earliest opportunity, ideally during the secondary survey log roll procedure. Loss of gastrointestinal tone will result in the cessation of peristaltic activity with subsequent gastric distension and a paralytic ileus, necessitating the use of a nasogastric tube.

There is considerable debate about the use of high dose methylprednisolone in the management of spinal cord injury. Patients presenting to the ED within 8 hours of acute spinal cord injury should be given methylprednisolone 30 mg/kg as soon as possible, followed 45 minutes later by a continuous infusion of 5.4 mg/kg for 24 hours. Further improvement in motor function recovery has been shown to occur when maintenance therapy is extended for 48 hours (Sauerland et al. 2000, Braken et al. 1997). However, Hugenholtz (2003), citing agreement from the Canadian Neurosurgical and Spine Societies and the Canadian Association of Emergency Physicians, argues this is not a treatment standard or guideline for treatment, but, rather, a treatment *option*.

Early correct management in the emergency department can do much to reduce later complications in the cord-injured patient. Rehabilitation after cord injury requires on-going multidisciplinary commitment to reducing the morbidity from the physical and psychological problems associated with cord injury, long after the patient has left the care of the ED (McDonald and Sadowsky 2002).

NEUROGENIC SHOCK

Neurogenic shock is often confused with spinal shock even though they are different entities. Neurogenic shock is most often associated with acute spinal cord disruption from trauma or spinal anaesthesia. Other causes include brain injury, hypoxia, depressant drug actions and hypoglycaemia associated with insulin shock. It results from impairment of the descending sympathetic pathways in the cord between T1 and L2, resulting in the loss of vasomotor and cardiac sympathetic tone. Loss of vasomotor tone causes vasodilatation and a pooling of blood in the lower extremities, resulting in hypotension. Loss of cardiac tone produces a bradycardia (Driscoll & Skinner 2007). Priapism is seen in male patients and rectal and bladder sphincter control is absent (Chapman 2003)

Patients presenting to the emergency department may have extensive injuries that would normally be associated with a hypovolaemic shock state; bradycardia with hypotension – not tachycardia and hypotension – and this should increase suspicion of spinal cord injury. The peripheral skin is generally warm and dry because of peripheral vasodilatation and may be either flushed or pale (Selfridge-Thomas 1995). Fluid resuscitation is required if circulatory volume is to be restored (Grundy 2002); therefore patients may require a small bolus of crystalloid (up to 500 ml IV) to correct hypotension. No further fluid should be given if spinal cord injury is the sole injury. Overloading the patient who is in purely neurogenic shock can precipitate pulmonary oedema, and therefore all patients must have careful monitoring of their vital signs in order to detect the physiological response to fluid resuscitation (Mitchell 1994). Insertion of an indwelling catheter will drain the dysfunctional bladder and provide information about overall tissue perfusion. Central venous pressure monitoring also provides an accurate method of determining response. Improved cardiac output may be indicated by a heart rate above 50 beats/min and a systolic pressure of greater than 100 mmHg.

SPINAL SHOCK

Spinal shock (or cord shock) is a temporary neurological condition that occurs after injury to the cord above the T6 level. The signs are a loss of all motor, sensory, reflex and autonomic responses below the site of the injury. There will be flaccidity and a positive Babinski sign, i.e. dorsal flexion of the first toe instead of plantarflexion, although all areas below the level of injury will not necessarily be permanently destroyed (Royle & Walsh 1992). Hypotension, bradycardia and hypothermia, because of the loss of sympathetic control and tone, are classic signs of spinal cord shock that occur immediately after injury.

Spinal shock does not resolve abruptly but rather in a series of phases extending over a few hours to several weeks, depending on the segmental level and extent of the cord injury (Ditunno et al. 2004). In areas where no function has returned, flaccid paralysis becomes spastic with increased tone. The diagnosis of spinal shock can only be formally made retrospectively. The immediate management in the emergency department is the same as for any cord-injured patient.

CONCLUSION

Spinal injuries are not a common cause of presentation to emergency departments but their consequences can be devastating. Whatever associated injuries coexist, the priorities – airway with cervical spine control, breathing and circulatory support – remain unchanged, as hypoxia from an upper airway obstruction or transection of the upper cervical cord will kill before hypoperfusion.

The nurse should always listen carefully to the pre-hospital history to find out the mechanism of injury, maintain a high index of suspicion and if in doubt initiate full spinal immobilization (Dickinson 2004). A semi-rigid cervical collar alone will not provide adequate immobilization; sandbags and tape must be used. The initial damage from the injury has already occurred, and ED staff must prevent secondary injury by careful handling of the patient – one false move could result in quadriplegia or paraplegia. Failure to suspect spinal injury can lead to failure in its detection. All vertebral fractures should be treated as unstable in the emergency department until fully examined by senior ED, orthopaedic or neurosurgical staff.

References

American College of Surgeons (2004) *Advanced Trauma Life Support*, 7th edn. Chicago: American College of Surgeons.

Aprahamian C, Thompson BM, Finger WA, Darin JC (1984) Experimental cervical spine injury model: evaluation of airway management and splinting. *Annals of Emergency Medicine*, 13(8), 584–587.

Braken MB, Shepard MJ, Holford TR, Leo-Summers L (1997). Administration of methylprednisolone in the treatment of acute spinal cord injury – National Acute Spinal Cord Injury Study. *Journal of American Medical Association*, 277 (20), 1597–1604.

Caroline N (1995) *Emergency Care in the Streets*, 5th edn. Boston: Little Brown.

Chapman CA (2003) Shock emergencies In: Newberry L, ed. *Sheehy's Emergency Nursing: Principles and Practice*, 5th edn. St Louis: Mosby.

Crawford-Adams J (2001) *Outline of Fractures*, 13th edn. Edinburgh: Churchill Livingstone.

Davies G, Deakin A, Wilson A (1996) The effect of a rigid collar on intracranial pressure. *Injury*, 27(9), 647–649.

Dickinson M (2004) Understanding the mechanism of injury and kinetic forces involved in traumatic injuries. *Nursing Standard*, 12(6), 30–34.

Driscoll P, Skinner D (2007) *ABC of Major Trauma*, 4th edn. London: BMJ.

Ditunno JF, Little JW, Tessler A, Burns AS (2004) Spinal shock revisited: a four-phase model. *Spinal Cord*, 42, 383–395.

Gallagher SM (2005) Spinal trauma. In: *Principles and Practice of Trauma Nursing (Ed. RA O'Shea)*. Edinburgh: Elsevier Churchill Livingstone.

Greaves I, Hodgetts T, Porter T (2005) *Emergency Care: A Textbook for Paramedics*, 2nd edn. London: WB Saunders.

Griffiths H, Gallimore D (2005) Positioning critically ill patients in hospital. *Nursing Standard*, 19(42), 56–64.

Grundy D (2002) *ABC of Spinal Cord Injury*, 4th edn. Bristol: BMJ Publications.

Harrison P (2004) Spinal cord injury incidence update: UK database summary 2001. *Spinal Cord Injury Link*, 3(2), 4.

Holliman CJ, Mayer JS, Cook RT (1991) Is theanteriorposterior cervical spine radiograph necessary in initial trauma screening? *American Journal of Emergency Medicine*, 9, 421–425.

Hugenholtz H (2005) Methylprednisolone for acute spinal cord injury: not a standard of care. *Canadian Medical Association Journal*, 168(9), 1145–1146.

Jaworski MA, Wirtz KM (1995) Spinal trauma. In: Kitt S, Selfridge-Thomas J, Proehl JA, Kaiser J, eds. *Emergency Nursing – a Physiological and Clinical Perspective*. Philadelphia: WB Saunders.

Jones KG and Rawlinson JA (1993) Managing neck injuries. *British Medical Journal*, 307, 868–869.

Kolb JC (1999) Cervical collar induced changes in intracranial pressure. *American Journal of Emergency Medicine*, 17, 135–137.

Lowery D, Marlena M, Browne B, Tiggs S et al. (2001) Epidemiology of spine injury victims. *Annals of Emergency Medicine*, 38, 12–16.

McDonald JW, Sadowsky C (2002) Spinal cord injury. *Lancet*, 359(9304), 417–425.

McRae R (2006) *Pocketbook of Orthopaedic and Fractures*, 2nd edn. Edinburgh: Churchill Livingstone.

McSwain N (1992) *Advanced Emergency Care*. Philadelphia: JB Lippincott.

Mitchell M (1994) Spinal cord injury. In: Hudak C, Gallo BM, eds. *Critical Care Nursing: A Holistic Approach*, 6th edn. Philadelphia: JB Lippincott.

National Spinal Injuries Unit (2005) NSIU Database. Dublin: Mater Misericordiae University Hospital.

Pre-Hospital Trauma Life Support Committee (2006) *PHTLS: Basic and Advanced Pre-Hospital Trauma Life Support.* St Louis: Mosby Lifeline.

Raby N, Berman L, de Lacey G (2005) *Accident and Emergency Radiology.* Philadelphia: Elsevier Saunders.

Robertson C, Redmond AD (1994) *The Management of Major Trauma,* 2nd edn. Oxford: Oxford University Press.

Royle J, Walsh M (eds) (1992) *Watson's Medical-surgical Nursing and Related Physiology,* 4th edn. London: Baillière Tindall.

Safar P, Bircher N (1988) *Cardiopulmonary Cerebral Resuscitation,* 3rd edn. London: WB Saunders.

Sauerland S, Nagelschmit M (2000) Risks and benefits of pre-operative high dose methylprednisolone in surgical patients: a systematic review. *Drug Safety,* **55,** 452–453.

Schoen D (2000) *Adult Orthopaedic Nursing.* Philadelphia, Lippincott Williams.

Segelov P (1986) *Manual of Emergency Orthopaedics.* Edinburgh: Churchill Livingstone.

Selfridge-Thomas J (1995) Shock. In: Kitt S, Selfridge-Thomas J, Proehl JA, Kaiser J, eds. *Emergency Nursing – A Physiological and Clinical Perspective.* Philadelphia: WB Saunders.

Semonin-Holleran R (2003) Spinal trauma. In: Newberry L, ed. *Sheehy's Emergency Nursing: Principles and Practice,* 5th edn. St Louis: Mosby.

Sheerin F (2005) Spinal injury: causation and pathophysiology. *Emergency Nurse,* **12**(9): 29–38.

Swain A (1997) Trauma to the spine and spinal cord. In: Skinner D, Swain A, Peyton R, eds. *Cambridge Textbook of Accident and Emergency Medicine.* Cambridge: Cambridge University Press.

Szilagyi PG, Bickley LS (2004) *Bates' Guide to Physical Examination and History Taking,* 8th edn. Philadelphia, Lippincott Williams & Wilkins.

Wassertheil J (2004). Spinal Trauma. In: *Textbook of Emergency Medicine.* (2nd edn) (eds P Cameron, G Jelinek, AM Kelly, L Murray, AFT Brown, J Heyworth) Edinburgh, Churchill Livingstone.

Chapter 7

Thoracic injuries

Barbara Warncken

INTRODUCTION

Thoracic injury is one of the most serious types of trauma and may result in disruption of the airway, breathing or circulation. It is responsible for approximately 25% of trauma-related deaths and is a major contributory factor to mortality in a further 25% (Greaves et al. 2001, Mansour 1997). Although many of these deaths occur immediately from the combined effects on respiratory and haemodynamic function, namely hypoxia, hypercarbia and acidosis (Rooney et al. 2000), there is a significant group of patients who, having sustained thoracic trauma, may survive with simple prompt effective systematic assessment and management. Westaby & Brayley (1991) found that, in practice, fewer than 15% of patients with chest injuries required surgical intervention. The management of patients with chest injuries can therefore be challenging and rewarding.

MECHANISMS OF INJURY

The ED nurse is likely to be the first contact with the patient on arrival at the hospital. It is therefore imperative that the nurse obtains all available information about the patient and the incident. When recording the history and clinical findings, forensic and medico-legal aspects need to be remembered. It is important to remember that serious intrathoracic injury can occur without obvious external damage to the chest wall. The mechanism of injury is an essential part of the history and can give crucial diagnostic clues to aid patient assessment. The main consideration is whether the chest injury was caused by blunt or penetrating trauma. In addition, an estimate of the velocity (speed) causing the injury may be gleaned from evidence of intrusion or vehicle damage, seat belt usage and steering wheel damage. Known high-velocity trauma, the presence of other seriously injured or dead people, ejection from a vehicle or fall from a great height are indicative of the potential for serious injuries to be present.

In the UK, as ballistic injuries are relatively uncommon, blunt chest trauma is currently more common than penetrating trauma (Driscoll & Skinner 2007). Blunt chest trauma commonly results from rapid deceleration of the chest wall against a solid object. Typically, this is seen following road traffic accidents (RTAs) in which the chest strikes the vehicle steering wheel, causing a high-velocity blunt chest injury. Superficial tissues are mostly affected; however, as the energy transfer increases in direct-force injuries, deeper tissues become involved, producing contusions, haemorrhages, organ ruptures and fractures. Blunt chest trauma can also result from a fall from a height. Shearing forces make organs and tissue planes move relative to each other, resulting in tearing of the communicating structures and blood vessels. This type of chest trauma may be associated with injuries to the great vessels, major airways, lung parenchyma and myocardium, as well as diaphragmatic rupture and fractures to the ribs and/or sternum. Crush injuries may also be caused by RTAs or industrial accidents (Porter & Greaves 2003). Frequently, fractured ribs and cardiac and pulmonary contusion may ensue. Other causes of blunt chest trauma include blast injury and low-velocity impact from direct blows to the chest. Penetrating injuries, such as stabbings or gunshot wounds, cause fewer than 5% of major trauma, in comparison with 20% or more of cases in the United States (Fitzpatrick & Mak 2002, Cole 2004). Penetrating trauma to the chest can be subdivided depending on the energy transfer involved. Stab wounds and impalements are a cause of low-energy chest trauma and cause direct damage along a straight track.

Medium- and high-energy chest wounds are determined by a number of variables, which determine how much energy is transferred to the tissues and how rapidly. These variables depend on the projectiles' physical makeup, the speed, range and characteristics of their flight and the nature of the tissue impacted.

Farming, industrial and road traffic incidents are also less common causes in the UK.

Although this chapter deals predominantly with chest injuries, it is imperative that the chest is not viewed in isolation, as other life-threatening injuries outside the chest may be present. While chest trauma may occur in isolation, it is more common in patients with multiple injuries. Ingestion of alcohol or drugs is particularly noteworthy in patients with chest trauma because the pattern, depth and rate of respiration may be affected.

ANATOMY OF THE CHEST

The chest wall: chest injury occurs when there is damage to the thoracic cage or its contents. The thoracic cage comprises ribs and intercostal muscles. It is divided by the central mediastinum, which acts as a partition between the lungs. The outer surface of each lung is covered by the visceral pleura and this is reflected onto the chest wall as the parietal pleura (see Fig. 7.1). The two pleural layers are effectively sealed together by a film of pleural fluid which exerts a strong surface tension force that prevents separation of the membranes. This seal is essential, since it enables the lungs, which themselves contain no skeletal muscle, to be expanded and relaxed by movements of the chest wall (Tortora & Grabowski 2003). If the pleura is breached, e.g. as a result of penetrating trauma, the integrity of this system is disrupted and the lung will collapse.

The mediastinum forms the central part of the thorax and extends from the sternum to the vertebral column. The mediastinum contains the trachea, oesophagus and major blood vessels, such as the aorta. It also encases the heart. It is important in the assessment of a trauma patient because disruption of its shape, such as widening, is indicative of damage to one of the structures within it, most commonly the aorta.

The heart lies above the diaphragm at the base of the thoracic cavity, with two-thirds of its bulk to the left of the body's midline. The outer surface of the heart is covered by the visceral pericardium. This is reflected onto the surrounding fibrous sac to form the parietal pericardium. A thin film of fluid separates these pericardial surfaces, allowing the heart to move freely, only being anchored by the great vessels (see Fig. 7.2). This potential space can become filled with blood (haemopericardium) following trauma or myocardial infarction. As the fibrous pericardium is unable to distend, any fluid collecting within the potential space (pericardial cavity) will exert pressure on the heart and impair filling.

Below the level of the fourth intercostal space, the thoracic cage surrounds the upper abdominal region, particularly when the diaphragm elevates during expiration. Any injury to the ribs at or below this level should alert the nurse that an intra-abdominal injury, specifically to the liver, spleen or diaphragm, may also be present.

THE PHYSIOLOGY OF RESPIRATION

The key functions of respiration are oxygen uptake and carbon dioxide elimination. To enable this to happen, air is conveyed through the respiratory tract – this is called ventilation (see Fig. 7.3).

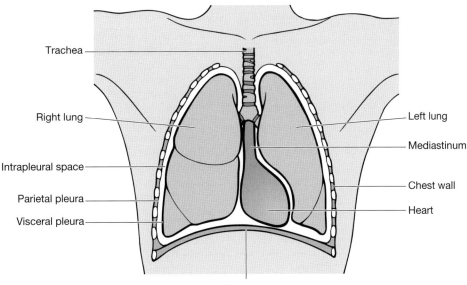

Figure 7.1 Relationship between lungs, thoracic cage and pleurae.

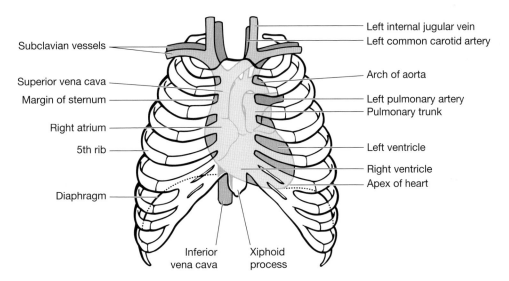

Figure 7.2 Location of the heart and associated blood vessels in the thoracic cavity.

In addition, an adequate blood volume must circulate through the pulmonary capillaries. This is called perfusion. The exchange of oxygen and carbon dioxide between the alveoli and capillaries is called diffusion. Gases move from an area of high partial pressure to one of low partial pressure. When leaving the lungs via the pulmonary veins, blood has its highest partial pressure of oxygen (Po_2) (Dickinson 2000).

Oxygen diffusion requires: a high concentration of oxygen in the alveolus; a low blood concentration of oxygen; solubility of the gas; membrane thickness that the gas has to cross; perfusion pressure; and alveolar ventilation. Damage to either system leads to hypoxia or hypercapnia, which in turn threatens homeostasis. The ratio between ventilation and perfusion is fundamental to the success of respiratory function (see Fig. 7.4).

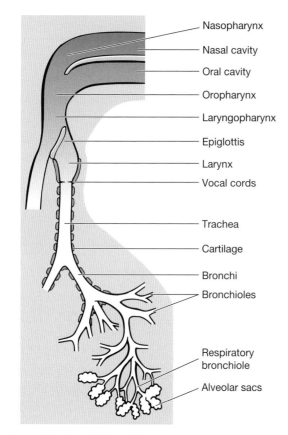

Figure 7.3 Organization of the airways.

results in a high ventilation/perfusion ratio (see Fig. 7.5).

If ventilation decreases, most commonly with an obstructed airway, the amount of oxygen reaching the alveoli is reduced. When perfusion is normal this results in more blood and haemoglobin passing the alveoli than can be saturated with oxygen. As a result, the blood leaving the lungs has a low oxygen content. This is a low ventilation/perfusion ratio (see Fig. 7.6).

Although the ventilation/perfusion ratio varies in different parts of the lung, a high ratio in one area will not offset a low ventilation/perfusion ratio in another. This is because of the reduction in haemoglobin saturation. In the trauma patient, particularly where chest injury has occurred, maintaining adequate ventilation is crucial in preventing hypoxia. A simple and vitally important nursing intervention is the early administration of effective oxygen therapy. This is best achieved by using a reservoir bag attached to a face mask, which allows a high concentration of inspired oxygen. Oxygen therapy helps to prevent respiratory acidosis (Chapman 2003), which results from impaired

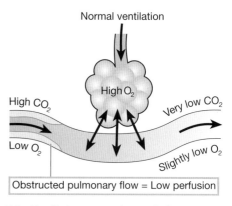

Figure 7.5 Ventilation greater than perfusion.

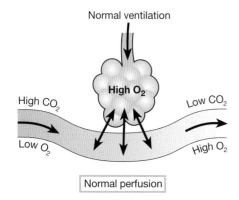

Figure 7.4 Normal ventilation/perfusion ratio.

If a problem occurs with pulmonary flow, most commonly a low circulatory volume in trauma, adequate oxygen cannot be taken up. This is because less blood passes the alveoli and there is subsequently less haemoglobin take-up of oxygen. This results in a decrease in tissue perfusion. Unbound oxygen is expired. This

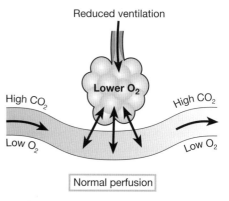

Figure 7.6 Ventilation lower than perfusion.

ventilation associated with chest injury. Metabolic acidosis results from inadequate tissue perfusion secondary to airway, breathing and circulatory problems, further compounding the patient's condition.

PRINCIPLES OF CARE

The trauma team

There may be variation between emergency departments regarding when to activate the trauma team (Khetarpal et al. 1999). Each department or hospital should have an established agreement so that the trauma team knows when and why they need to respond. Many EDs have established a system of care for seriously injured patients based on a team approach which utilizes Advanced Trauma Life Support (ATLS) principles and incorporates well-established objectives of trauma management (American College of Surgeons 2004) (see Chapter 2). The team leader is responsible for the coordination of care and the appropriate delegation of roles whilst maintaining an overview of the situation. The use of a standardized systematic approach not only expedites patient care, but also offers a format enabling less-experienced staff to focus their activities in a predetermined order. Some hospitals have established trauma teams in which each member has a specific role.

Clearly, the ED nurse's role is dynamic and directly related to the patient's needs. The key components of the nursing role when caring for patients with chest trauma are outlined in Box 7.1. The number and experience of other team members may influence the nurse's actual activities, but the needs of the patient and her family/friends must remain paramount. Ideally, a member of the care team will be allocated to care for and liaise with the patient's family and/or friends (see Chapter 13 [Care of the Bereaved] for guidance on this issue).

Box 7.1   The role of the ED nurse

- Prepare the environment for receiving the patient
- Perform a systematic, rapid assessment using the ABC approach
- Prioritize and initiate appropriate interventions and care continually evaluating their effectiveness
- Function as an effective member of a multidisciplinary team
- Act as an advocate for the patient who may be incapacitated
- Ensure patient and staff safety at all times
- Coordinate holistic patient care from receipt to transfer or definitive care

---

Assessment of chest injury

The immediate management of the patient with chest injury should follow the principles laid down in the ATLS guidelines (American College of Surgeons 2004). A primary survey should be carried out to identify and treat any immediately life-threatening conditions (Box 7.2; the management of specific conditions will be discussed later in the chapter). In the stable patient, a secondary survey or head-to-toe examination should then be carried out to identify any other injury.

Greaves et al. (2001) state that actions taken before the patient's arrival to ED need to be established; for example, a tension pneumothorax may have been decompressed. The sequence of questions in the hand-over to the hospital care can be remembered as 'MIST':

> **M**echanism of injury
> **I**njuries found and suspected
> **S**igns (respiratory rate, SpO_2, blood pressure)
> **T**reatment given pre-hospital.

Nursing assessment of the patient's overall condition is part of the overall progress towards definitive care. Nursing observations should include:

- the rate and depth of respiration
- chest wall movement
- blood pressure
- pulse oximetry
- pulse rate and pressure
- pain assessment
- level of consciousness
- urine output

Additional investigations include:

- cardiac monitoring
- chest X-ray/lateral cervical spine and pelvis (trauma series)
- ECG
- blood gas analysis
- blood chemistry (may include CPK and CK-MP, troponin I and troponin T; however, no specific blood test for myocardial injury following trauma exists)

Box 7.2   Immediately life-threatening conditions of the chest

- Airway obstruction
- Tension pneumothorax
- Massive haemothorax
- Open chest wound
- Cardiac tamponade
- Flail chest

- full blood count and cross-match
- ultrasound/echocardiography
- computed tomography/magnetic resonance imaging
- angiography (aortic disruption)
- thorascopy: direct or video assisted if not contraindicated

A specific chest injury assessment is listed in Box 7.3.

Initial management of chest injury

Airway and breathing

Management of chest injury should include high-flow oxygen as described above. The method of delivery depends largely on the patient's condition; in a conscious patient without obvious compromise, use of a tight-fitting mask (NB: be aware of possible parallel facial injuries) and non-rebreathing bag is the method of choice. If the patient is unable to maintain her airway, as is common after chest injury, supportive methods should be found (see Box 7.4).

Airway compromise occurs either because of damage to the airway, resulting in oedema, compression, bleeding, foreign body obstruction, displaced facial bones or suspected cervical spine injuries, or through a deterioration in the patient's consciousness level, resulting in the loss of her gag reflex. If breathing is absent, the airway should be assumed to be blocked. Noisy breathing (stridor) may be indicative of partial upper airway obstruction or laryngospasm. If the patient is able to give a verbal response, then the airway can be assumed to be patent for the present time (see Box 7.5).

The tongue slipping back and occluding the oropharynx causes a significant number of airway obstructions. These can be simply resolved by using a chin lift or jaw thrust manoeuvre. This will pull the tongue forward in the mouth and remove the obstruction. The

---

Box 7.3   Specific assessment of the chest

Visual inspection
- Wounds, bruises, surface trauma
- Symmetry of chest expansion
- Rate, rhythm and depth of respiration
- Use of accessory muscles
- Intercostal recession
- Paradoxical chest movement
- Jugular Venous pressure (JVP)

Palpation
- Tracheal deviation and tracheal tug
- Pain
- Swelling
- Masses
- Pulsation
- Crepitus
- Step defects
- Apex beat
- Subcutaneous emphysema

Percussion
- Resonant (normal)
- Hyper-resonance
- Dullness

Auscultation
- Breath sounds – check rate, quality, type
- Heart sounds

Box 7.4   Assessing and securing the airway in a trauma patient

1. Seek verbal response from patient, by asking, for example, 'Are you all right?', while giving O$_2$ and stabilizing the cervical spine.
   2, 3 & 4 should be simultaneous
2. Look for chest movement – for 10 seconds minimum
3. Listen for breath sounds – for 10 seconds minimum (check simultaneously with chest movement)
4. Feel for expired air – for 10 seconds minimum
5. If the airway is compromised → chin lift or jaw thrust. If airway remains compromised repeat steps 3–5
6. Clear mouth of obvious debris, such as vomit, broken teeth, ill-fitting dentures
7. If airway remains compromised, repeat steps 3–5
8. Intubation with assisted ventilation. If airway remains compromised, repeat steps 3–5

Box 7.5   Indicators of airway obstruction

- Apnoea
- Tachypnoea
- Increased respiratory effort
- Intercostal recession
- Use of accessory muscles
- Tracheal tug
- Stridor/noisy breathing
- Pallor/cyanosis (late sign)

mouth should be inspected with adequate light to identify any debris, which should be removed carefully with suction or angled forceps. It is important not to stimulate the gag reflex during suction because this can induce vomiting.

If the gag reflex is present, or the patient is conscious, a nasopharyngeal airway is best tolerated (Landon et al. 1994). This is inserted via the nostril to the pharynx. This type of adjunct should not be used where a base of skull fracture is suspected or where facial injuries prevent its use. The tube should never be forced. If oedema or potential haemorrhage is likely, alternative airway support should be used.

If the gag reflex is absent, the patient needs endotracheal intubation; however, an oropharyngeal or Guedel airway is the temporary support of choice (Landon et al. 1994). This will prevent the tongue from occluding the pharynx and provide an artificial airway. If simple airway management fails to secure a patent airway, because of either injury or vomiting, endotracheal intubation should be performed (see Box 7.6). It is important to stress the need for in-line immobilization of the cervical spine. This is addressed in detail in Chapter 6.

The effectiveness of all airway management should be assessed by:

- Looking at chest movement
  - Is it symmetrical bilateral?
  - Is there sufficient chest expansion?
- Listening to breath sounds
  - are they present?
  - is there stridor or gurgling from debris?
- Feeling for expired air.

Conditions which compromise breathing will be considered below.

Circulation

The patient's circulatory status should be assessed by:

- pulse rate and volume
- the speed of capillary return
- skin colour or pallor.

Box 7.6 Indications for endotracheal intubation

- Poor airway maintenance with other methods due to injury
- Loss of gag reflex with high risk of aspiration
- Compromised respiratory function due to chest injury
- Need for mechanical ventilation
- Anticipation of airway obstruction, such as increasing oedema
- Raised intracranial pressure

All patients should have i.v. access established with two wide-bore cannulae and a fluid regime appropriate to circulatory status. Blood should also be taken for cross-match, and baseline full blood count and urea and electrolytes during initial management. Conditions posing a specific threat to circulation will be discussed later.

Disability

The hypoxic patient will initially be confused and may become combative. Primary head injury will also cause an altered mental state, and this will be compounded by hypoxia or hypercarbia. It is essential that airway and ventilation are optimized as quickly as possible in the presumed head-injured patient, as the confusion of hypoxia may be reversed and harmful secondary brain injury reversed (Greaves et al. 2001).

IMMEDIATELY LIFE–THREATENING CHEST INJURIES

Pneumothorax

A pneumothorax can be caused by blunt or penetrating trauma. Laceration of lung tissue, often associated with rib fractures and subsequent air leak, is the most common cause of pneumothorax with blunt trauma (Peavey & Newberry 2003). It occurs when the fluid seal between the parietal and visceral pleura is broken. Once the seal is broken, air rushes in, expands the space and the existing negative pressure is lost. The resulting positive pressure in the expanded intrapleural space is exerted onto the adjacent lung. This may result in partial or total collapse of the lung, and serious impairment of gaseous exchange. Because the pleural layers are separated by the mediastinum, the opposite lung continues to move with the chest wall and functions normally, unless it becomes compressed by the volume of air accumulating on the injured side (see Fig. 7.7).

Pneumothoraces are classified in Box 7.7.

Tension pneumothorax

This is an immediately life-threatening chest injury and should be dealt with as soon as it is identified in the primary survey. Tension pneumothorax can result:

- from blunt or penetrating trauma
- from baro-trauma associated with positive pressure ventilation
- where chest injury such as rib fracture exists
- following invasive procedures, such as insertion of a central line
- as a complication of a simple pneumothorax

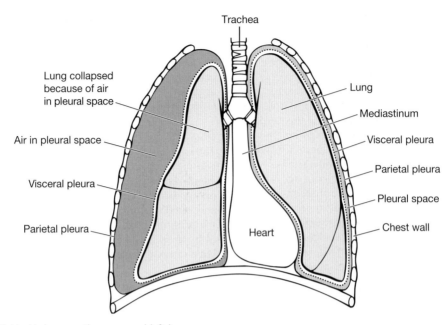

Figure 7.7 Right-sided pneumothorax, normal left lung.

Box 7.7   Classification of pneumothoraces

- **Simple** – Occurs spontaneously or as a result of blunt trauma. It is not initially life-threatening but has the potential to develop into a tension pneumothorax. A simple pneumothorax may compromise respiratory function, particularly on mild exertion

- **Open** – Results from a penetrating injury, where the integrity of the chest wall is breached and air is sucked into the pleural cavity

- **Tension** – Results from blunt or penetrating trauma, mechanical ventilation or from a simple pneumothorax. It occurs when air enters the pleural space and becomes trapped. The volume of air increases and causes compression of other organs

---

It is imperative that the ED nurse remains vigilant as a tension pneumothorax can occur at any stage of the patient's treatment.

A tension pneumothorax is a clinical diagnosis. It occurs when air is sucked into the pleural space, either from the lung or from outside the chest wall. The pleura acts as a one-way valve, trapping air in the pleural space, therefore allowing air in to, but not out of, the cavity. The pressure of this causes a total collapse of the lung on the affected side. As the intrathoracic pressure increases, the mediastinum and trachea shift towards the unaffected side, causing impaired venous return and cardiac compression. This results in reduced cardiac output and severe hypotension. The increasing pressure also causes compression of the unaffected lung, compounding the patient's already compromised ventilation, systemic hypotension, shock and, ultimately, cardiac arrest (Gallon 1998). A tension pneumothorax is a condition of rapid onset and demands immediate decompression of the pleural space to maintain life. Time should not be wasted by attempting to obtain a chest X-ray (see Fig. 7.8).

Assessment

Priorities for care of the patient with a tension pneumothorax lie with correct identification of the condition. A conscious patient will be very distressed because of the rapid worsening of the dyspnoea. Hypoxia may also make the patient confused, agitated and restless. Specific clinical features are highlighted in Box 7.8.

A tension pneumothorax can expand rapidly. This increase in size correlates with a decrease in functional lung space. Therefore, as the condition worsens, the patient's dyspnoea, respiratory function and tissue oxygenation all deteriorate.

Immediate management

Immediate management entails maintaining oxygenation. This is a twofold activity. First, oxygen intake

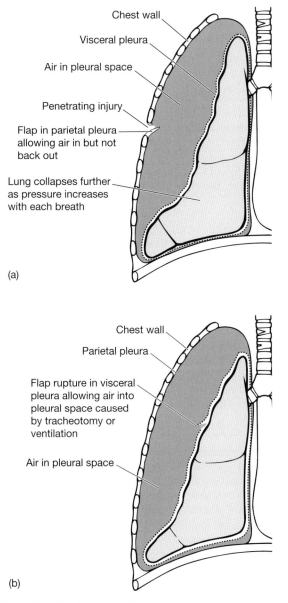

(a)

(b)

Chest wall

Visceral pleura

Air in pleural space

Penetrating injury

Flap in parietal pleura
allowing air in but not
back out

Lung collapses further
as pressure increases
with each breath

Chest wall

Parietal pleura

Flap rupture in visceral
pleura allowing air into
pleural space caused
by tracheotomy or
ventilation

Air in pleural space

Figure 7.8   Tension pneumothorax.

must be maintained either through a high-flow mask with oxygen reservoir or with assisted manual or mechanical ventilation. The second life-saving intervention is to remove the 'tension' from the pneumothorax to reduce further loss of lung capacity. This is achieved by providing an artificial escape route for the trapped air. To facilitate this, a needle thoracentesis is performed. While this is a rapid and simple procedure which buys time for the resuscitation team, it is not definitive treatment.

> **Box 7.8   Clinical signs of tension pneumothorax**
>
> - Tachypnoea
> - Tachycardia
> - Shock
> - Decreased air entry to affected side
> - Hyper-resonance on affected side
> - Distended neck veins – if the patient is not hypovolaemic (late sign)
> - Tracheal deviation away from affected side (late sign)
> - Cyanosis (late sign)

Chest decompression by needle thoracentesis is carried out by inserting a wide-bore (16 g) cannula into the pleural space. The cannula is inserted in the second intercostal space midclavicular line over the superior aspect of the third rib. The cannula is attached to a syringe, and once in situ, the rapid release of air confirms initial diagnosis. This procedure should dramatically reduce the patient's discomfort and clinical symptoms.

At this stage, it is important to obtain intravenous access as bleeding may lead to hypovolaemia. A chest drain will facilitate the removal of remaining air from the pleural cavity. The chest drain is inserted in front of the midaxillary line through the fifth intercostal space. The drainage tube is connected to an underwater sealed system which allows air out of the pleural space, but not back in. Fluid levels in the drainage system should rise and fall with respiration (Landon et al. 1994). While a chest X-ray will verify the presence of collapsed lung and demonstrate a mediastinal shift towards the unaffected lung, if the patient has severe cardiopulmonary instability and a high suspicion of tension pneumothorax exists, immediate treatment should be instituted without obtaining a chest X-ray (Greaves et al. 2001).

Open pneumothorax

Open pneumothorax may occur following penetrating trauma in which the chest wall is pierced. When chest wall integrity is breached, e.g. by a stab wound, air can enter the pleural space creating a pneumothorax. This occurs because of a loss of negative pressure and an equalling of atmospheric and intrathoracic pressures. If the external damage to the chest wall is large enough, i.e. greater than two-thirds of the diameter of the trachea, air will enter the pleural cavity via the wound rather than via the normal respiratory tract, because air tends to follow the path of least resistance.

It is for this reason that an open pneumothorax is often referred to as a 'sucking chest wound', as air can be heard entering the pleural space on inspiration. As air enters the thoracic cavity by this route, respiratory efficiency is rapidly decreased. This is because of alveolar hypoventilation despite increased respiratory effort. This results in a low ventilation/perfusion ratio and tissue hypoxia.

Assessment

The mechanism of injury is the main factor in assessment. The patient will have a history of penetrating trauma and may or may not have an impaled object in situ. On examination, the patient will be tachypnoeic and tachycardic and may be hypotensive. Breath sounds may be decreased or absent on the affected side. The chest wound will have an audible sucking sound on inspiration. Bubbles often occur around the wound as air escapes through the blood. The actual size of the wound does not give significant indication of the extent of intrathoracic damage. This should be judged by the level of respiratory compromise (Rooney et al. 2000).

Immediate management

This is a potentially life-threatening condition and should be treated in the resuscitation phase of the primary survey. Initial management is relatively simple; it involves maintaining oxygen intake and temporary closure of the chest wound. Oxygen intake is supported by the use of high-flow oxygen via a mask and reservoir bag. If the patient is unable to maintain breathing, artificial ventilation is indicated. The chest wound is covered with a sterile occlusive dressing taped down on three sides to create a flutter valve. During inhalation, the dressing is sucked against the chest wall and acts as a seal, which prevents any further air from entering the pleural space. On expiration, the open side of the dressing pushes away from the patient's skin, allowing air to escape from the pleural space.

A dressing sealed on all sides would result in a tension pneumothorax, as air would enter the pleural space but would have no means of escape. If a tension pneumothorax is suspected, the occlusive dressing should be temporarily removed to allow air to escape (Driscoll et al. 2000).

Any impaled object should not be removed as this significantly increases the risk of respiratory compromise and circulatory collapse. After establishing i.v. access, a chest drain should be inserted through a surgically created hole, not via the wound, to facilitate decompression of the pleural space. Prophylactic antibiotics and anti-tetanus will be necessary. The majority of patients with an open pneumothorax require surgical closure of the wound once their overall condition has been stabilized. It is at this stage that any impaled objects are usually removed.

Massive haemothorax

Haemothorax can result from penetrating trauma or blunt injury where an intercostal vessel or internal mammary artery has been ruptured. A massive haemothorax is usually defined as a rapid accumulation of blood, greater than 1500 ml in the pleural cavity or 200 ml per hour from the chest drain (Feliciano et al. 2001) (see Fig. 7.9).

Assessment

The patient will present with tachypnoea, tachycardia and hypovolaemic shock. Specifically, chest examination will reveal decreased or absent breath sounds on the affected side. On percussion, dullness will be detected over the haemothorax due to the density of blood. Internal jugular veins should be observed; jugular venous pressure (JVP) may be elevated as a result of pressure in the thoracic cavity because of the accumulation of blood, or other associated injury, such as tension pneumothorax or cardiac tamponade. Conversely, neck veins may be collapsed as a result of hypovolaemia.

Immediate management

Initial management is by the simultaneous restoration of blood volume and decompression of the chest cavity. The patient should be given high-flow oxygen via a mask and reservoir bag. Intravenous access using large-bore needles should be established and fluid resuscitation commenced. Once fluid replacement begins, a chest drain should be inserted to drain blood from the thoracic cavity and allow the lung to reinflate. Before a chest drain is inserted, a ruptured diaphragm should be excluded as the cause of reduced breath sounds and dull resonance. This can be done by careful history-taking of the mechanism of injury. A chest drain should always be inserted by blunt dissection, so that any herniated abdominal organs can be felt with a finger prior to the insertion of a drainage tube, thus preventing further injury. Bleeding to the lung parenchyma usually stops once the lung is reinflated because of the drop in pulmonary perfusion (Driscoll & Skinner 2007). An early thorocotomy is indicated if 1500 ml are immediately evacuated; however, some patients who have an initial volume output of less than 1500 ml may require a thorocotomy. This decision is based more on the patient's physiological status than on the rate of continuing blood loss

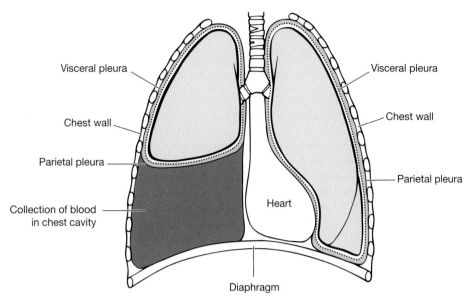

Figure 7.9 Massive haemothorax.

(200 ml/h for 2 to 4 hours) (American College of Surgeons 2004, Feliciano et al. 2001). The patient should ideally have a central venous line placed in order to monitor right-sided cardiac filling pressure.

Flail chest

Flail chest usually results from blunt trauma, most commonly crush injuries (Rooney et al. 2000). It is defined as fractures in two or more adjacent ribs in two or more places, or bilateral detachment of the sternum from costal cartilage, which results in a disruption in the continuity of chest wall movement (Peavey & Newberry 2003). A segment of the thoracic cage loses its bony continuity because of the fractures and subsequently moves paradoxically to the rest of the chest wall. A flail segment results from the fracture of two or more adjacent ribs in two places, therefore disconnecting them from the rest of the thoracic cage (Fig. 7.10).

This paradoxical movement on inspiration reduces tidal volume, and therefore compromises ventilation. While this carries a risk of hypoxia, the primary danger to the patient stems from underlying lung injury. Lung contusion or penetrating injury can cause profound hypoxia, and rib fractures cause significant hypovolaemia, particularly if there is sternal involvement.

Assessment

Rib fractures are extremely painful and the conscious patient will complain of severe chest pain and difficulty in breathing. The patient will be tachypnoeic with

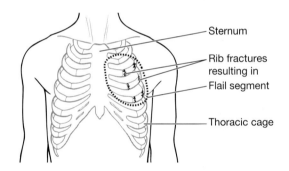

Figure 7.10 Flail chest.

shallow breaths, tachycardic and will show early signs of hypoxia. Examination of the chest usually reveals a paradoxical segment not expanding with the rest of the chest wall on inspiration. Palpation of the area will reveal crepitus and instability of the rib cage. Splinting from chest wall muscular spasm may mask the paradoxical movement, and the diagnosis is not uncommonly delayed until the muscles relax, due to exhaustion or when paralysing drugs are given. The possibility of central flail chest should be particularly considered in patients who have sustained steering-wheel injuries.

Assessment should include careful monitoring for hypoxia. This should include rate and respiratory effort, tachycardia, skin colour, oxygen saturation and arterial blood gases. Arterial blood gas values reflecting respiratory failure aid in diagnosis (American College of Surgeons 2004).

Management

Management involves the restoration of respiratory function. Pain is a significant threat to respiratory function as it reduces respiratory effort, resulting in shallow breathing and reduced tidal volume. In addition, pain inhibits coughing, allowing bronchial secretions to build up, further jeopardizing respiratory function. Adequate pain control is essential to recovery; often the method of choice is an intercostal nerve block, which is performed as part of definitive care.

Both ventilation and perfusion are vital to respiratory function, so initial management should include adequate oxygenation and restoration of circulatory volume. Fluid replacement should be managed carefully, measured by heart rate, capillary refill and urine output. An injured lung is sensitive to underperfusion, which reduces the diffusion rate of oxygen. It is equally sensitive to circulatory overload, which can rapidly cause a raised central venous pressure (CVP) and left ventricular failure.

Unless profound hypoxia is present, many patients with a flail chest maintain their own ventilation, supported with high-flow oxygen via a mask and reservoir bag. The need for mechanical ventilation is determined by respiratory function and the level of hypoxia, not necessarily by the size of a flail segment (see Box 7.9). Continuous positive pressure (CPAP) may be indicated for some patients.

Cardiac tamponade

Cardiac tamponade commonly results from penetrating injury, primarily stab wounds to the chest or upper abdomen (American College of Surgeons 2004). It can also result from blunt trauma if the heart or great vessels have been damaged. Cardiac tamponade can be a rare complication of an expanding, untreated tension pneumothorax which causes mediastinal shift and eventually cardiac compression. Tamponade occasionally results

***

from a myocardial infarction. The pericardium anchors the heart to the mediastinum, diaphragm and sternal wall. The risk of tamponade in trauma occurs because the pericardium is non-elastic and inflexible. This allows the heart to move without causing friction. The heart wall, consisting of myocardium and endocardium, lies beneath the pericardium and forms the muscle needed for cardiac function (see Fig. 7.11).

Cardiac tamponade occurs when injury to the heart or disruption of its blood vessels results in bleeding into the pericardial cavity. Because there is no elasticity in the pericardium, it only requires a small amount of fluid to compress the cardiac wall and chamber. This is primarily because filling capacity is reduced during diastole, and therefore venous pressure is elevated and there is a fall in stroke volume.

Assessment

The mechanism of injury should alert the trauma team to suspect a cardiac tamponade. If a penetrating injury has occurred to the thoracic area, anteriorly, posteriorly or to the left lateral aspect, tamponade should be excluded as part of the primary survey. A patient with cardiac tamponade will be shocked, and therefore assessment of pulse and respiration are important. Specifically, patients will show signs of falling arterial pressure, because of reduced cardiac output, and increased venous pressure, because of cardiac compression. As tamponade worsens, the patient exhibits air hunger, agitation and deterioration in the level of consciousness. Venous pressure can be assessed by venous distension; time should not be spent inserting CVP lines in the initial stages of management (Driscoll & Skinner 2007).

Venous pressure is also influenced by hypovolaemia, and therefore absence of distended neck veins does not exclude cardiac tamponade. Kussmaul's sign, a paradoxical increase in JVP on inspiration (Greaves et al. 2001), may be found with tamponade but is a difficult sign to elicit. The classic diagnostic tool described as Beck's triad is only present in about a third of patients with tamponade, and so should not be too heavily relied upon (Driscoll et al. 1993) (see Box 7.10).

A 12-lead ECG trace is useful. It may indicate damage to myocardium, seen as ST elevation in the affected area. Continuous cardiac monitoring is recommended to detect any rhythm changes, commonly ventricular ectopics.

Management

Similar to all trauma patients, those with cardiac tamponade should be given high-flow oxygen, through a mask and reservoir bag. Initial attempts should be towards circulatory resuscitation to correct hypovolaemia. If

***

Box 7.9   Indications for mechanical ventilation

- Respiratory rate of >30 breaths/min
- Exhaustion
- Falling PaO_2<10.5 kPa on O_2
- Rising $PaCO_2$>6.0 kPa on O_2
- Associated head injuries
- Respiratory rate <10 breaths/min

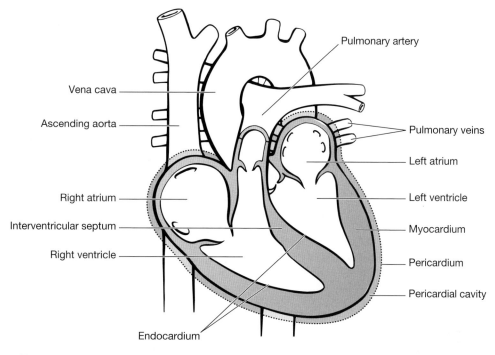

Vena cava

Ascending aorta

Right atrium

Interventricular septum

Right ventricle

Pulmonary artery

Pulmonary veins

Left atrium

Left ventricle

Myocardium

Pericardium

Pericardial cavity

Endocardium

Figure 7.11   The heart.

Box 7.10   Beck's triad

1. *Raised CVP* – due to impaired venous return because of cardiac compression
2. *Hypotension* – low arterial pressure because of poor cardiac output
3. *Decreased, muffled heart sounds* – due to fluid in pericardial cavity

there is no improvement in the patient's condition, pericardiocentesis should be performed to relieve the tamponade. This is a mechanism for draining fluid from the pericardial cavity and reducing cardiac compression. The patient's condition can be improved dramatically by the removal of as little as 20 ml of blood from the pericardial cavity (Rooney et al. 2000).

Pericardiocentesis is performed by inserting a wide-bore cannula, at least 15 cm in length, into the pericardial cavity. This is done 1–2 cm left of the xiphochondral junction at a 45° angle, aiming the needle towards the tip of the scapula. The cannula should be attached to a three-way tap and syringe. Continuous aspiration should take place during insertion.

When blood flows freely into the syringe, the insertion should stop.

Continuous ECG monitoring is imperative during this procedure for a number of reasons. First, if the needle is inserted too far, myocardial irritation (seen as ventricular ectopics on the ECG monitor) or myocardial damage (seen as QRS complexes or ST segment changes) can occur. Should this happen, the needle should be withdrawn gradually until the ECG returns to normal. Second, as blood is removed on aspiration, cardiac decompression occurs and the myocardium expands back into its usual position.

The ED nurse should watch the ECG monitor for signs that the myocardium is touching the cannula. Again, should this occur, the needle should then be gently withdrawn until the ECG returns to normal. Once blood has been withdrawn from the pericardial cavity, the cannula should be firmly taped in position in case further aspiration is required. If blood has clotted in the pericardial cavity, it is impossible to relieve symptoms of tamponade by pericardiocentesis. If the results of pericardiocentesis reveal blood in the pericardial cavity, or if there is a strong clinical suspicion of tamponade, the patient should undergo urgent surgical exploration.

Survival rates from cardiac trauma resulting in tamponade are directly related to speed of definitive surgery (Robertson & Redmond 1994). This is, in part, because a fine balance exists between internal and external pressure during tamponade. Cardiac compression severely compromises circulatory activity and will lead to cardiac arrest if unchecked. However, by reducing cardiac compression, internal cardiac pressure is increased and profound haemorrhage can occur because the tamponade effect is lost. If cardiac arrest occurs, the mortality is linked to the speed at which cardiac bypass can be established; the faster this occurs, the lower is the rate of mortality (Robertson & Redmond 1994). Some EDs recommend emergency thoracotomy in ED should cardiac arrest occur. Survival from this is rare unless cardiothoracic back-up is available and cardiac bypass can be quickly established.

SERIOUS CHEST INJURY

The following injuries can be potentially life-threatening and should be diagnosed as part of the secondary survey and treated definitively (see Box 7.11).

Pulmonary contusion

Pulmonary contusion commonly occurs following a rapid deceleration injury. For example, a restrained passenger in an RTA may come to an abrupt stop on impact, but soft viscera such as the lung remain in motion, causing stretching, tearing and shearing. The resultant bruising and pain cause an insidious onset of respiratory distress, with decreased lung compliance and, rarely, increased airway resistance. It may also occur as a result of blast injuries (Taylor & Dawood 2005).

Assessment
Pulmonary contusion tends to evolve over several hours and signs and symptoms can develop up to 48 hours after the initial injury; therefore the mechanism and the time elapsed can give some clues to pulmonary contusion. It also underlines the importance of regular observation, and of recording and reporting vital signs (Taylor & Dawood 2005, Wyatt et al. 2005). Primarily,

the ED nurse should assess the respiration rate and depth. Patients will classically demonstrate an increasing tachypnoea and increasingly shallow breathing. Initially, the work of breathing is manifested by accessory muscles and intercostal recession. Because ventilation is poor, an imbalance in the ventilation/perfusion ratio occurs. This is demonstrated by a fall in PaO_2; serial arterial blood gas monitoring should take place. The nurse must look for any marks, e.g. abrasions or bruising on the chest wall, following the original injury. These may indicate pulmonary contusion.

Assessment is aided by chest X-ray; contusion usually develops over the first 1–3 days (Greaves et al. 2001) but in severe cases of chest trauma hazy shadowing in the affected areas can be seen within a few hours post-injury (Driscoll et al. 1993). Pulse oximetry and ECG monitoring are also useful.

Management
Management principles entail maintaining respiratory function. High-flow oxygen should be given and the oxygen saturation carefully monitored. Adequate pain control aids respiratory function. Careful fluid balance is imperative to prevent secondary lung damage from pulmonary oedema, as a result of fluid overload, and to ensure fluid replacement is not underestimated; this would cause hypovolaemia and a subsequent reduction in pulmonary perfusion, compounding existing hypoxia.

Indications for mechanical ventilation are shown in Box 7.12.

Blunt cardiac trauma

Blunt cardiac trauma can result in myocardial muscle contusion, valvular disruption or cardiac chamber rupture. This usually results from RTAs and is exemplified by a driver who sustains an impact with the vehicle steering wheel, causing a deceleration injury. It is a

---

Box 7.11   Serious chest injuries

- Pulmonary contusion
- Blunt cardiac trauma
- Aortic dissection
- Ruptured diaphragm
- Airway injury
- Oesophageal rupture

Box 7.12   Indications for mechanical ventilation in patients with pulmonary contusion

- Hypoxia and worsening respiratory function
- Impaired level of consciousness
- Progressive fall in PaO_2
- Progressive increase in $PaCO_2$
- Pre-existing chronic lung disease
- Imminent surgery for associated injuries
- Other systems failure, e.g. renal failure
- Prior to transfer to another hospital

commonly undiagnosed condition, sometimes with fatal consequences. Compression of the heart results in bleeding into the myocardium and ischaemia. The coronary arteries become occluded because of spasm or oedema. The physiological effect of this is similar to a myocardial infarction: the heart becomes ischaemic and, if not treated, necrosis and infarction occurs. Chest pain in patients following blunt cardiac trauma should be assessed like any other cardiac pain. A large percentage of these injuries are overlooked because pain is attributed to chest wall injury, e.g. with rib or sternal fractures.

Assessment

The mechanisms of injury should make the ED nurse suspect a cardiac injury (Dickinson 2004). Blunt trauma is associated with sternal fracture and wedge fracture of the thoracic vertebrae. Assessment should follow the same pattern as the assessment of a patient with a non-traumatic cardiac pain.

Baseline observations should be obtained and the patient should be observed on a cardiac monitor; a 12-lead ECG can be helpful in detecting myocardial damage. It may show a similar pattern to that of an evolving myocardial infarct (see also Chapter 27 [Medical emergencies]). However, myocardial damage can occur without ECG changes. Sinus tachycardia and arrhythmias, such as ventricular ectopics and atrial fibrillation, are indicators of a 'stressed' myocardium.

Management

The priorities for management are to maintain adequate oxygenation and cardiac output. The patient should be given high-flow oxygen through a mask and reservoir bag, and oxygen saturation levels should be monitored. Pain control is important and intravenous morphine is the drug of choice, unless other injuries contraindicate its use. The patient should be managed by giving symptomatic support, i.e. treating dysrhythmias and maintaining blood pressure with drug therapy if necessary.

Aortic rupture

The descending thoracic aorta is particularly susceptible to rupture in rapid deceleration injury. Ninety per cent of patients die immediately (Driscoll & Skinner 2007). Those who survive do so because they have an incomplete laceration near the ligamentum arteriosum. Continuity is maintained by the adventitial layer of the aorta, which contains the haematoma, which has a tamponade effect, preventing massive haemorrhage. Survival depends on rapid diagnosis and surgical repair.

Assessment

The history of deceleration injury should lead the ED nurse to suspect a possible aortic rupture. Because of the tamponade effect, patients with this injury may have lost less than 500 ml of circulating volume, so they may not appear clinically shocked. The patient may complain of chest pain or pain between the scapulae, often described as unrelenting and severe. Other symptoms include dyspnoea and haemoptysis (Peavey & Newberry 2003). If aortic injury is suspected, pulses should be checked in all limbs. Patients with an aortic injury will have higher pulse pressure in upper limbs than in lower limbs. Blood pressure may also vary between arms. Chest X-ray may show a widened mediastinum because of the tamponade effect. Conclusive assessment should include CT scan, angiography and/or transoesophageal echocardiography to show the extent and location of the tear.

Management

Initial management involves stabilizing and resuscitating the patient in preparation for theatre. Definitive management demands rapid surgical repair of the aorta by grafting. Thoracic aortic surgery is carried out at a cardiothoracic centre, so many patients need to be transferred to alternative sites for surgery. Patients should always be intubated prior to transfer and adequate fluid and analgesia should be available. In order to prevent the flimsy adventitial layer from rupturing and leading to fatal haemorrhage, the systemic blood pressure should be kept below 100 mmHg.

Ruptured diaphragm

A ruptured diaphragm can be caused by blunt or penetrating trauma. Generally, penetrating injuries are smaller and less serious; blunt injury, however, can cause large tears. It is uncommon to injure both hemispheres of the diaphragm. The impact of large-scale tearing, particularly rupture to the left side, is that the abdominal viscera herniates into the thoracic cavity. Mortality following a ruptured diaphragm is high, up to 50% (Maddox et al. 1991). These patients often present with a clinical picture similar to a haemothorax, but if a ruptured diaphragm cannot be excluded, diagnosis should be confirmed on X-ray.

Assessment

The mechanism of injury will give a high index of suspicion that a ruptured diaphragm has occurred. This is important because some patients will be asymptomatic, which hampers diagnosis. More commonly, patients will present with respiratory difficulty and tachypnoea due to decreased lung capacity as a result of abdominal contents in the thoracic cavity. In addition to chest pain, patients may complain of dysphagia and dyspepsia because of shifting gastric contents, and shoulder tip pain because of phrenic nerve irritation (Kehr's sign). Chest auscultation will reveal reduced breath sounds on the affected side and bowel sounds may be present. A chest X-ray will complete assessment.

Management
The management priority is to maintain respiratory function. High-flow oxygen should be given via a mask with a reservoir bag. Unless contraindicated because of other injuries, a nasogastric tube should be inserted to decompress the stomach and give symptomatic relief. Chest drain insertion is by blunt dissection because of the risk of rupture to organs such as the liver or spleen. Early surgical repair is the treatment of choice; this minimizes damage to lung tissue from gastric contents if gastric rupture or aspiration has occurred.

Tracheobronchial injuries

Injury to the major airways occurs following both severe blunt trauma and obvious penetrating trauma. Trauma to the major airways is rare, but in the case of blunt trauma it can be difficult to detect. It usually results in some degree of rupture to the airway at one of three anatomical levels.

The larynx
Injury results from RTAs where impact with the steering wheel or dashboard has occurred, or from direct blows from a fist or foot. Attempted hanging can sometimes result in a fractured larynx.

Assessment In addition to pain and dyspnoea, the classic indications of laryngeal damage include hoarseness, crepitus and subcutaneous emphysema around the neck, because of air leaking into tissues.

Initial management entails the establishment and maintenance of a patent airway. Usually a formal tracheostomy is required.

The trachea
Mechanisms of injury are similar to those of laryngeal injury.

Assessment Penetrating injury is usually obvious, but blunt trauma is more difficult to assess, particularly in a multiply injured patient. Respiratory distress is usually the only sign to guide the ED nurse towards an airway injury. The patient may also have haemoptysis if conscious. Obstruction occurs in the airway because of oedema and bleeding.

Initial management is to maintain a patent airway. This normally requires endotracheal intubation. In penetrating injury this can sometimes be achieved through the wound site. Where available, bronchoscopy is useful both to confirm diagnosis and to remove tissue debris and blood. Early surgical repair is required.

The bronchi
The proximal bronchi are anatomically fairly immobile and therefore susceptible to rapid deceleration injury, which results in partial or complete tearing. Patients often have associated lung injuries and the mortality rate is around 30% (Rooney et al. 2000).

Assessment The patient will show signs of severe respiratory distress, have haemoptysis and surgical emphysema. The patient may also have a pneumothorax on the injured side. Bronchoscopy will help to determine the extent of injury.

Initial management is similar to that in tracheal injury, except that oral intubation may be difficult because of oedema. If an adequate airway can be maintained, patients are often managed conservatively. If there is a complete bronchial tear, then surgical intervention is indicated.

Oesophageal injury

Penetrating trauma can cause a rupture to the oesophagus. Oesophageal injury may also be caused by gastric contents creating a tear from inside the oesophagus, often as a result of a blow to the stomach forcing gastric contents up the oesophagus under pressure. The gastric contents then leak into the mediastinum and can erode into pleural cavities.

Assessment
Specific signs include severe pain and shock which is not consistent with other injuries, pneumothorax without fractures, and gastric contents in chest drainage.

Initial management This involves maintaining adequate ventilation, pain control and surgical repair of the oesophagus.

STERNUM, RIB AND SCAPULAR INJURIES

The ribs, sternum and scapula are most commonly damaged by blunt trauma. Such injuries may follow a direct blow to the chest, crushing or rapid deceleration as epitomized by RTAs. Typically, rib and sternal fractures occur on impact with a steering wheel. In comparison with injuries to the scapulae, rib injuries are much more common. Rib fractures are often associated with other injuries and therefore this suspicion should always be borne in mind. A fragment of a fractured rib may pierce the lung, pleura, pericardium or skin. Thus, subsequent complications include pneumothorax and haemothorax. Fracture of the first or second rib and/or scapula often occurs concurrently with serious head, neck, lung, great vessel and spinal cord injury and therefore is of great significance. Lower rib fractures are associated with spleen and liver injuries.

Although rib injuries vary in severity, they are all significant because of the associated pain with chest movement which may cause splinting of the chest and impair ventilation. Furthermore, this may lead to pneumonia and atelectasis. The mechanism of injury, together with chest wall contusions and bruising, should raise suspicion of rib or sternal fractures. The patient may be dyspnoeic and will have pain, localized tenderness, crepitus and deformity. Suitable analgesia to ensure adequate ventilation and deep-breathing exercises are an essential part of the management of fractured ribs. An intercostal nerve block may be used and is often the most effective way of reducing pain and facilitating adequate inspiration.

Since seat-belt legislation was introduced in 1983, an increasing number of patients with seat-belt-related sternal fractures have been reported. As a great deal of force is required to fracture the sternum, underlying injury to the heart and great vessels should be suspected. Monitoring for cardiac dysrhythmias is required for patients with fractured sternum as there may be significant cardiac contusion.

ANALGESIA

Chest injuries cause hypoxaemia directly through lung damage, but also indirectly through reduced chest expansion secondary to pain. Adequate analgesia is therefore essential. The choice of analgesia in trauma care is the use of opiates and these should be used as required in thoracic trauma, remembering that opiates can reduce ventilation and the clearing of secretions.

Local anaesthetic infiltration, e.g. intercostal bupivicaine can be used for extensive rib fractures, effectively blocking the neurovascular bundles in the spaces above and below the fracture sites (Greaves et al. 2001). For long-term relief in patients who are admitted with chest trauma, epidural infusions of local anaesthetic may be used.

CONCLUSION

In the emergency department the main focus for care of patients with chest injury must be to ensure a patent airway, adequate breathing and maintenance of a viable circulation. Essentials of nursing care include early administration of high-flow oxygen, careful monitoring of vital signs and judicious fluid resuscitation. Only when these fundamental elements have been secured can more specific management ensue.

References

American College of Surgeons (2004) *Advanced Trauma Life Support*, 7th edn. Chicago: American College of Surgeons.

Chapman CA (2003) Shock emergencies. In: Newberry L ed. *Sheehy's Emergency Nursing: Principles and Practice*, 5th edn. St Louis: Mosby.

Cole E (2004) Assessment and management of the trauma patient. *Nursing Standard*, **18**(41), 45–51.

Dickinson M (2000) Care of the ventilated patient in A&E. *Emergency Nurse*, **8**(3), 26–33.

Dickinson M (2004) Understanding the mechanism of injury and kinetic forces involved in traumatic injuries. *Emergency Nurse*, **12**(6), 30–34.

Driscoll PA, Grinnutt CL, LeDuc Jimmerson C, Goodall O, eds. (1993) Thoracic trauma. In: Driscoll PA, *Trauma Resuscitation: The Team Approach*. Basingstoke: Macmillan.

Disroll PA, Skinner D (2007) *ABC of Major Trauma*, 4th edn. London: BMJ

Feliciano DV, Moore EE, Mattox KL (2001) *Trauma*, 4th edn. New York: McGraw-Hill

Fitzpatrick J, Mak V (2002) *Injuries and Accidents in London: Too High a Price to Pay?* London: Health of Londoners Programme.

Gallon A (1998) Pneumothorax. *Nursing Standard*, **13**(10), 35–39.

Greaves I, Porter K, Ryan J (eds) (2001) *Trauma Care Manual*. London: Arnold.

Khetarpal S et al. (1999) Trauma faculty and trauma team activation: impact on trauma system function and patient outcome. *Journal of Trauma Injury Infection and Critical Care*, **47**(3), 576–581.

Landon BA, Driscoll PA, Goodall JD (1994) *An Atlas of Trauma Management*. Carnforth: Parthenon.

Maddox P, Mansel R, Butchat E (1991) Traumatic rupture of the diaphragm: a difficult diagnosis. *Injury*, **22**, 299.

Mansour KA (1997) *Trauma of the Chest*. Philadelphia: WB Saunders.

Peavey AA, Newberry L (2003) Thoracic trauma. In: Newberry L ed. *Sheehy's Emergency Nursing: Principles and Practice*, 5th edn. St Louis: Mosby.

Porter K, Greaves I (2003) Crush injury and crush syndrome: a consensus statement. *Emergency Nurse*, **11**(6), 26–30.

Robertson C, Redmond A (1994) *Major Trauma*, 2nd edn. Oxford: Oxford University Press.

Rooney S, Westaby S, Graham T (2000) Chest injuries. In: Skinner D, Driscoll P, Easlam R, eds. *ABC of Major Trauma*, 3rd edn. London: BMJ.

Taylor I, Dawood M (2005) Terrorism: The reality of blast injuries. *Emergency Nurse*, **13**(8) 22–25.

Tortora GJ, Grabowski SR (2003) *Principles of Anatomy and Physiology*. 10th edn. New Jersey: John Wiley & Sons.

Westaby S, Brayley N (1991) Thoracic trauma. In: Skinner D, Driscoll P, Earlan R, eds. *ABC of Major Trauma*. London: BMJ.

Wyatt J, Illingworth R, Robertson C, Clancy M, Munro P (2005) *Oxford Handbook of Accident and Emergency Medicine*, 2nd edn. Oxford: Oxford University Press.

Chapter **8**

Abdominal injuries

Valerie Small

CHAPTER CONTENTS

INTRODUCTION

Abdominal injuries are common in patients who sustain major trauma: approximately one-fifth of all trauma patients requiring operative intervention have sustained an injury to the abdomen (Barry et al. 2003). Unrecognized abdominal injury continues to be the cause of preventable death after truncal trauma (Barry et al. 2003, American College of Surgeons 2004); the resulting mortality rate in patients with abdominal trauma is reported at 13–15% (Emergency Nurses Association 2000).

Identification of serious intra-abdominal pathology is often challenging, as mechanisms of injury often result in other associated injuries that divert attention from potentially life-threatening presentations (Barry et al. 2003, American College of Surgeons 2004). Patients sustaining significant blunt torso injury from a direct blow or deceleration, or a penetrating torso injury, must be considered to have an abdominal visceral or vascular injury (Windsor & Guillou 1999, Barry et al. 2003). Evaluation and stabilization of individuals with traumatic injury utilizing the advanced trauma life support protocols provide a paradigm for patient assessment and management that prioritizes trauma resuscitation, leading to an improvement in quality of care provided by all practitioners involved in the care of patients with trauma (Burkitt & Quick 2002, Sikka 2004).

In this chapter specific issues related to mechanism of injury, patient assessment, physical examination and diagnostic tests will be outlined and nursing care priorities for managing patients with abdominal injuries will be discussed.

ANATOMY AND PATHOPHYSIOLOGY

External anatomy of abdomen

Anterior abdomen

As the abdomen is partially enclosed by the lower thorax the anterior abdomen is defined as the area between the transnipple line superiorly, inguinal ligaments and symphysis pubis inferiorly, and the anterior axillary lines laterally.

Flank

This is the area between the anterior and posterior axillary lines from the sixth intercostal space to the iliac crest. The thick abdominal wall musculature in this location, rather than the much thinner aponeurotic sheaths of the anterior abdomen, acts as a partial barrier to penetrating wounds, particularly stab wounds.

Back

This is the area located posterior to the posterior axillary lines from the tip of the scapulae to the iliac crests. Similar to the abdominal wall muscles in the flank, the thick back and paraspinal muscles act as partial barrier to penetrating wounds.

Internal anatomy of the abdomen

The abdomen has three distinct anatomic compartments – the peritoneal compartment, the retroperitoneal space and the pelvic cavity. The pelvic cavity contains components of both the peritoneal cavity and the retroperitoneal spaces.

Peritoneal cavity

For convenience the peritoneal compartment may be divided into two parts, upper and lower. The upper peritoneal cavity is covered by the bony thorax and includes the diaphragm, liver, spleen, stomach and transverse colon: it is often referred to as the thoracoabdominal component of the abdomen. The diaphragm rises to the level of the fourth intercostal space on full expiration, which allows for injury to abdominal viscera from lower rib fractures and penetrating wounds below the nipple line. The lower peritoneal cavity contains the small bowel, parts of the ascending and descending colon, sigmoid colon and, in women, the organs of reproduction (see Fig. 8.1).

Pelvic cavity

The pelvic cavity is surrounded by the pelvic bones; it contains the rectum, bladder, urethra, prostate gland, iliac vessels and, in women, internal reproductive organs. Examination of the pelvic structures is compromised by the overlying bony framework.

Retroperitoneal space

The retroperitoneal space is the area posterior to the peritoneal lining of the abdomen, and contains the abdominal aorta, inferior vena cava, the pancreas, kidneys, adrenal glands, ureters, duodenum, and the posterior aspects of the ascending and descending colon and the retroperitoneal components of the pelvic cavity. Detecting injuries to the retroperitoneal viscera is difficult and may be delayed due to the obscurity of physical examination and the delay in appearance of signs and symptoms of peritonitis. Diagnostic peritoneal lavage does not sample this space and is therefore an unreliable test for injury to this area of the abdomen (ENA 2000, American College of Surgeons 2004, Sikka 2004).

Mechanism of injury

Many injuries may not manifest during the initial assessment and treatment period, resulting in an undiagnosed or missed injury. The most common errors in the initial assessment of a patient with trauma are an inadequate primary and secondary survey and a low index of suspicion of significant injury. Both of these clinical failures may be attributed to an under-appreciation of and for the mechanism of injury and history of the traumatic episode (Wise et al. 2002, Barry et al. 2003, American College of Surgeons 2004, Sikka 2004).

Missed injury is defined as an injury that is not discovered during the initial evaluation and workup in the emergency department or operating room (Sikka 2004). The incidence of missed traumatic injuries (all injuries) has been broadly estimated to be 1% to 20% in the paediatric population and 1% to 65% in the adult population. More specifically missed intra-abdominal injuries are common and carry an additional risk, as delays in diagnosis are associated with additional surgery with mortality greater than 50% (Buduhan & McRitchie 2000, Connors et al. 2001, Sikka 2004).

Intra-abdominal injuries are classically divided into blunt and penetrating trauma and will be described separately.

Blunt trauma

Blunt abdominal trauma is a leading cause of morbidity and mortality among all age groups (Windsor & Guillou 1999, Barry et al. 2003). Injury to intra-abdominal structures can be classified into two primary mechanisms of injury: compression forces and deceleration forces. Compression or concussive forces may result from direct blows or external compression against a fixed object (lower rim of steering wheel, lap belt, spinal column). Most commonly these crushing forces cause tears and subcapsular haematomas to the solid viscera. These solid viscera, which cannot change shape or stretch, are therefore vulnerable to damage although they are protected by the thoracic skeleton. When great force is applied, they may be crushed between the lower ribs and the anterior vertebral column or the para-vertebral muscles (Porter & Greaves 2003, Better 1999). Fractures of the lower ribs should create a high level of suspicion of associated visceral damage or diaphragmatic injury. Lap-belt marks have been correlated with rupture of small intestine and increased incidence of other intra-abdominal injury (Barry et al. 2003).

Although more commonly injured as a result of penetrating trauma, the pancreas may also be injured by crushing against the anterior spine. These forces may also deform hollow organs and transiently increase intraluminal pressure, resulting in rupture; this is a common mechanism of blunt injury to the small bowel.

Sudden-deceleration injuries may be the result of motor-vehicle trauma or falls from a height. The abdominal organs move at the same speed as the external framework of the body. The external framework may decelerate suddenly, as in the case of a car driver hitting the steering wheel, dashboard and

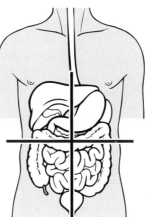

Right upper quadrant

Right lobe of liver
Gallbladder
Pylorus
Duodenum
Head of pancreas
Upper right kidney

Right lower quadrant

Lower right kidney
Cecum
Appendix
Ascending colon
Right fallopian tube (female)
Right ovary (female)
Right ureter
Bladder (distended)

Left upper quadrant

Left lobe of liver
Spleen
Stomach
Left kidney
Body of pancreas
Splenic flexure of colon

Left lower quadrant

Descending colon
Sigmoid colon
Left fallopian tube (female)
Left ovary (female)
Left ureter
Bladder (distended)

(a)

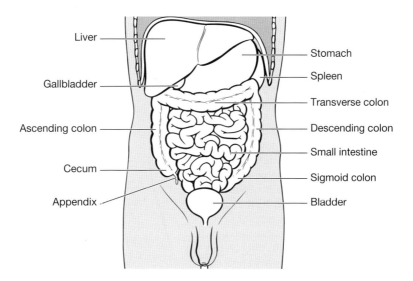

(b)

Figure 8.1   (a): Abdominal contents. (After Stillwell 1996.) (b): Gastrointestinal structures. (After Seidel et al. 1995.)

windscreen during a high-velocity collision. The driver's abdominal organs will continue at the pre-collision velocity, putting strain on or disrupting their points of attachment, until they meet another structure such as the abdominal wall.

Deceleration forces cause stretching and linear shearing between relatively fixed and free objects. Longitudinal shearing forces tend to rupture supporting structures at the junction between free and fixed segments. Classic deceleration injuries include hepatic tear along the ligamentum teres, intimal injuries to renal arteries and injuries to the arch of the aorta. Thrombosis and mesenteric tears can occur as a result of loops of bowel travelling from their mesenteric attachments.

Frequency   The true frequency of abdominal injury due to blunt trauma is unknown. According to the American College of Surgeons (2004), in patients undergoing laparotomy for blunt trauma the organs most frequently injured are the spleen (40%–55%), liver (35%–45%) and small intestine (5%–10%). In addition there is a 15% incidence of retroperitoneal haematoma in patients undergoing laparotomy for this type of injury.

Review of adult trauma databases in the USA reveals that blunt trauma is the leading cause of intra-abdominal injury and that motor-vehicle collisions are the leading mode of injury. Blunt injuries account for approximately two-thirds of all injuries, with a male to female ratio of 60:40. Peak incidence occurs in persons aged 14–30 years (Burkitt & Quick 2002, American College of Surgeons 2004).

Penetrating trauma
Throughout history, humans have created easily concealed personal weaponry designed initially for self-defence. More recently personal weapons are used as a means to steal, murder and create mayhem: personal handguns, spring-loaded stiletto blades, knives and similar weaponry have created an epidemic of violence that is spreading rapidly into all walks of life, affecting people of all ages.

Penetrating injuries are caused as a result of stabbing, accidental impalement, or high- or low-velocity projectiles, such as bullets or debris resulting from blast explosions. Each class of instrument or wounding source is associated with a different injury pattern of tissue damage by laceration or cutting. Abdominal organs are vulnerable to penetrating injuries not only through the anterior abdominal wall but also through the back, flank and chest below the fourth intercostal space, which may result in additional penetration of the abdomen through the diaphragm (Windsor & Guillou 1999, ENA 2000, Barry et al. 2003).

Stab wounds   Stab wounds traverse adjacent abdominal structures and most commonly involve the liver (40%), small intestine (30%), diaphragm (20%) and colon (15%) (American College of Surgeons 2004). Only 33% of stab wounds penetrate the peritoneal envelope, however, and of these peritoneal violations only 50% require intervention (Windsor & Guillou 1999, Barry et al. 2003). Knowledge of anatomic site, number of wounds, and type, size and length of blade will aid in determining the likely path and whether the peritoneum was breached (see Fig. 8.2). Lacerated hollow organs result in haemorrhage and leakage of contained fluids into the peritoneal or retroperitoneal space, resulting in poorly defined and localized somatic pain. Pain radiating to the back or shoulder may provide a valuable clue to the presence of intraperitoneal blood, clots or air. Kehr's sign is described as severe left shoulder pain caused by irritation of the left diaphragm and phrenic nerve, which is induced by laying the patient in a supine position and is indicative of free intra-abdominal blood and clots (Wright 1997,

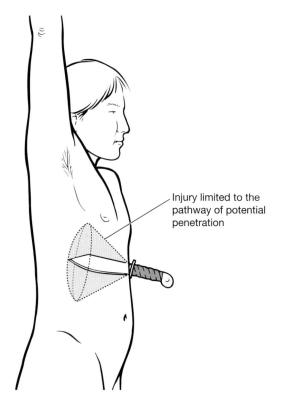

Injury limited to the pathway of potential penetration

Figure 8.2   Path of knife blade penetration in patient. (After McSwain et al. 1996.)

Windsor & Guillou 1999). Ecchymosis around the umbilicus (Cullen's sign) or Grey-Turner's sign, which is described as a bluish discoloration at the lower abdominal flanks and lower back, may appear with retroperitoneal bleeding originating in the kidney or with pelvic fractures. These signs may occur some hours or even days after initial injury but may be observed during nursing assessment in the emergency department (Wright 1997, Blank-Reid 2004).

Gunshot injury Gunshot injuries to the abdomen involve high energies and may damage organs remote from the site of penetration into the abdomen. It is important to establish the type of weapon used, whether handgun, shotgun or rifle, and the distance between the patient and the gun. Gunpowder around the bullet entry site will suggest firing at close range and is usually associated with an increase in injury severity. Up to 95% of gunshot wounds to the abdomen result in visceral injury and require a surgical procedure (Barry et al. 2003). The amount of energy released is proportional to the mass and velocity of the bullet and also depends on the density of tissue involved. A low-velocity bullet from a handgun will release less energy and cause less injury than a high-velocity bullet from a rifle. Similarly, a high-mass bullet will cause more damage than a low-mass bullet of similar velocity. An accurate history

involving the type of weapon used and the range at which it was fired is essential in order to assess the likely magnitude of visceral injury.

A bullet will release its energy in the abdomen in two ways: first, by direct contact with organs in its path. Bullets may take a non-linear path through the abdomen. A simple, straight line connecting entry and exit wounds may not indicate the actual path of the bullet. In cases where there is no exit wound, X-rays will locate the bullet. Second, bullets transfer energy in the form of pressure waves. These pressure waves may disrupt many organs not in the actual path of the bullet. Pressure waves result in cavitation, extending the diameter of injury to many times the actual diameter of the bullet. A low-velocity missile, from a gun travelling at 1000–3000 ft/s, creates a cavity 2–3 times the diameter of the missile (Mattox et al. 2000). High-velocity missiles, i.e. those travelling at more than 3000 ft/s, create a cavity that may be 30–40 times the diameter of the bullet (Dickinson 2004, Revere 2003) (see Fig. 8.3).

Dense, solid viscera are more susceptible to cavitation than hollow organs. The sudden formation of a cavity increases intra-abdominal volume, creating a negative pressure, which may suck debris, such as clothing in through the entry wound resulting in gross intra-abdominal contamination. Gunshot wounds

---

Box 8.1   Diagnostic peritoneal lavage

Indications
Altered sensorium – brain injury, alcohol or drug
    ingestion
Spinal cord injury
Injury to adjacent structures – lower ribs, pelvis,
    lumbar spine
Equivocal physical examination
Prolonged loss of contact with patient anticipated
    (lengthy X-ray studies in haemodynamically
    unstable or stable patient)
Lap belt sign with suspicion of bowel injury

Contraindications
Absolute contraindication
Obvious need for surgery, for instance, due to gunshot
    wound to abdomen
Relative contraindications
Previous abdominal surgery
Pregnancy
Abdominal wall haematoma
Obesity
Distended abdomen

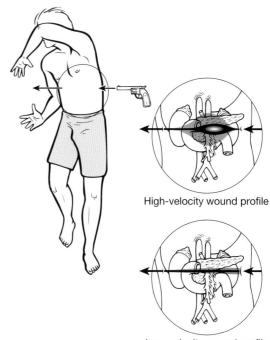

High-velocity wound profile

Low-velocity wound profile

Figure 8.3   Potential injury path of high- and low-velocity bullets. (After Neff & Kidd 1993.)

most commonly involve the small bowel (50%), colon (40%), liver (30%), and abdominal vascular structures (25%) (Barry et al. 2003, American College of Surgeons 2004).

Frequency The frequency of penetrating abdominal injury across the globe relates to the industrialization of developing nations and, significantly, to the presence of military conflicts. The death rate from penetrating abdominal trauma spans the entire spectrum (0–100%), depending on the extent of injury. Patients with violation of anterior abdominal wall fascia without peritoneal injury have a 0% mortality and morbidity rate. An average mortality rate for all patients with penetrating abdominal trauma is approximately 5% (Burkitt & Quick 2002, Barry et al. 2003).

Blast injuries

In general, most blast injuries managed in emergency departments tend to be accidental. They include firework mishaps, unintended occupational or industrial fuel eruptions, and unforeseen mine explosions. In many parts of the world, however, the reality persists of deadly, dormant, non-detonated, military incendiary devices such as land mines and hand grenades. Such devices cause significant numbers of civilian casualties years after local hostilities cease. During wartime, injuries arising from explosions frequently outnumber those from gunshots; many victims are innocent civilians. Blast injuries caused by terrorist bombings are also a growing part of the landscape in which people now live their lives.

The sudden, massive and catastrophic changes of pressure associated with blasts or explosions may damage the air-filled 'hollow' viscera of the gastrointestinal tract. The air within the viscera will transmit the force of the blast equally in all directions, leading to a general disruption or 'bursting' effect (see Fig. 8.4).

Mannion and Chaloner (2005) categorize blast injuries into four categories: primary, secondary, tertiary, and quarternary. A patient may be injured by more than one of these mechanisms.

- A primary blast injury is caused solely by the direct effect of blast overpressure on tissue. Air is easily compressible, unlike water. As a result, a primary blast injury almost always affects air-filled structures such as the lung, middle ear and gastrointestinal (GI) tract. Other injuries include rupture of the eye and concussion without signs of head injury.

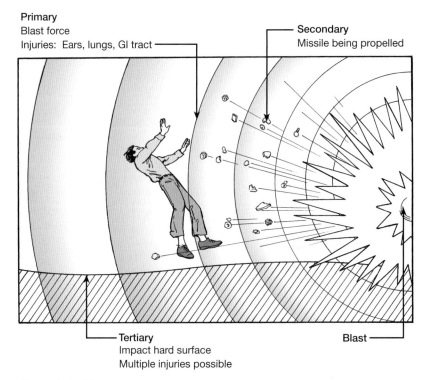

Figure 8.4 Effects of an explosive blast

- A secondary blast injury is caused by flying objects that strike people. Injuries include penetrating ballistic or blunt injuries and eye penetration that can be occult.
- A tertiary blast injury is a feature of high-energy explosions. This type of injury occurs when people fly through the air and hit fixed objects such as walls. Fracture and traumatic amputations and closed and open brain injury are common with tertiary blast injuries.
- Quarternary blast-related injuries encompass all other injuries caused by explosions. For example, the collision of two jet airplanes into the World Trade Centre on 11 September 2001 created a relatively low-order pressure wave, but the resulting fire and building collapse killed thousands (Arnold et al. 2004). The range of injuries from quarternary blasts includes flash, partial and full-thickness burns, crush injuries, closed and open brain injury, asthma or other breathing-related problems from dust, smoke or toxic fumes, angina, hyperglycaemia, hypertension etc. (Taylor & Dawood 2005).

Frequency Internationally the incidence of blast injury is sporadic and infrequent and is dependent on the political (terrorism, occupational health and safety priorities) stability of the region. Mortality rates vary widely and are increased when explosions occur in closed or confined spaces. The presence of tympanic membrane rupture indicates that a high-pressure wave (at least 40 kilopascal [kPa], 6 psi) was present and may correlate with more dangerous organ injury. Table 8.1 provides an overview of explosion related injuries.

ASSESSMENT OF ABDOMINAL TRAUMA

The aim of assessment is to rapidly establish whether an intra-abdominal injury exists, not what the specific injury is. Evidence of intra-abdominal injury mandates urgent surgical exploration of the abdomen, at which time an accurate diagnosis may be made. Assessment is made on the basis of a history, the results of a primary survey, the victim's response to treatment started as a result of that primary survey, a secondary survey including an abdominal examination, and the results of any diagnostic tests such as Focused Assessment Sonogram for Trauma (FAST), Diagnostic Peritoneal Lavage (DPL) or Computed Tomography (CT) scan. The emergency nurse plays a key role in the initial and continuous assessment and monitoring of the injured patient and may be the first member of the trauma team to identify subtle but significant changes in the patient's condition.

History

An accurate history of the events leading to injury is crucial to identifying possible serious intra-abdominal pathology and can direct potential therapeutic priorities. The emergency nurse plays a vital role in gathering and collating information from a number of sources and disseminating that information to members of the trauma team (Cole et al. 2006). Information can be provided by the patient if alert, or by bystanders, police and emergency medical personnel. Pertinent information in assessing the patient injured in a motor-vehicle collision includes the speed of the vehicle, type of collision (frontal or lateral impact, rear impact or rollover), vehicle intrusion into the

---

Table 8.1 Overview of explosion-related injuries (Taylor & Dawood 2005, Centre for Disease Control 2003)

System	Injury or condition
Auditory	Tympanic membrane rupture, ossicular disruption, cochlear damage, foreign body
Eye, orbit, face	Perforated globe, foreign body, air embolism
Respiratory	'Blast lung', haemothorax, pneumothorax, pulmonary contusion or haemorrhage, arteriovenous fistulae acting as sources of air embolism, airway epithelial damage, aspiration, pneumonitis sepsis
Digestive	Bowel perforation, haemorrhage, ruptured liver or spleen, sepsis, mesenteric ischaemia from air embolism
Circulatory	Cardiac contusion, myocardial infarction from air embolism, shock, vasovagal hypotension, peripheral vascular injury, air-embolism-induced injury
Central nervous injury	Concussion, closed and open brain injury, stroke, spinal cord injury, air-embolism-induced injury
Renal	Renal contusion or laceration, acute renal failure due to rhabdomylosis, hypotension, hypovolaemia
Extremities	Traumatic amputation, fractures, crush injuries, compartment syndrome, burns, cuts, lacerations, acute arterial occlusion, air-embolism-induced injury

passenger compartment, types of restraint, deployment of air bag, the patient's position in the vehicle and status of passengers (American College of Surgeons 2004). The history surrounding a patient with penetrating trauma is also important, as it provides clues to the likely injury complex. Clues are gleaned from the injury location and from determination of the associated weapon (e.g. gun, knife) or injury-causing object. The number of gunshots heard, times stabbed, and position of the patient at the time of injury help describe the trajectory and path of the injuring object. Range also is important when assessing gunshot wounds. A careful history that assesses secondary and multi-cavity injuries is vital, as many victims sustain a blunt assault or fall from various heights after sustaining a penetrating trauma (Windsor & Guillou 1999, Barry et al. 2003). See Box 8.2 and Box 8.3.

Blood loss at the scene should be quantified as accurately as possible to help determine transfusion needs. The character of the bleeding (e.g. arterial pumping, venous flow) helps determine whether major vascular

---

Box 8.2 For stabbing or for gunshot injuries impalement

The size, shape and length of the weapon	The type of weapon involved
The number of stabbing attempts made	High/low velocity and bullet size
Blood loss at scene and in transit	Weapon to victim distance
Angle of penetration	Number of shots fired
Height of assailant	
Sex of assailant (males tend to stab upwards)	

(Luckmann and Sorenson 1987)

Box 8.3 Useful information specific to blunt injuries

Motor vehicle speed, or height of fall
Was the victim ejected from the vehicle on impact?
Damage caused to vehicle and position of victim in vehicle
Was the victim restrained by a seatbelt?
The impact configuration

---

injury has occurred. The initial level of consciousness or, for moribund patients, the presence of any signs of life at the scene (e.g. pupillary response, respiratory efforts, heart rate or tones) is vital to determine the prognosis and to guide resuscitative efforts. Particularly important is the patient's response to therapy en route to the emergency department.

PRIMARY SURVEY

The primary survey and resuscitation are examined in detail in Chapter 2 (Trauma life support). Assessment priorities relevant to abdominal trauma are outlined here.

- **Airway maintenance** with cervical spine control.
- **Breathing,** ventilation, and oxygenation: injuries to the diaphragm or penetrating injuries involving the intra-thoracic abdomen and chest may compromise breathing.
- **Circulation** with haemorrhage control: gross external haemorrhage from the abdomen is rare. The abdomen, however, is a potential reservoir for a large volume of occult haemorrhage. Uncontrolled haemorrhage from damaged abdominal organs and vessels will cause hypovolaemia and death. Haemorrhage may remain uncontrolled because it is not detected. Early detection of haemorrhage is therefore essential for survival in any case of abdominal injury. Any hypovolaemia is treated with an intra-venous fluid challenge.
- **Disability:** neurological status.
- **Exposure**: completely undress the patient; care should be taken not to cut clothes across stab or bullet holes as this may destroy crucial forensic evidence. Hypothermia must be prevented by the use of overhead heaters or a warm-air heating system which can be easily controlled and adjusted according to the patient's temperature.
- **Adjuncts to primary survey and resuscitation:** obtain arterial blood gas analysis and ventilatory rate, monitor exhaled CO_2.

The insertion of gastric and urinary catheters is frequently performed as part of the resuscitation phase once problems with airway, breathing and circulation are corrected.

The goal of inserting a gastric tube is to relieve acute gastric dilatation, decompress the stomach before physical examination or performing a diagnostic peritoneal lavage (if indicated) and remove gastric contents, thus removing risk of aspiration (American College of Surgeons 2004). Special consideration should be given in circumstances where there is severe facial trauma or a suspicion of cribiform plate fracture, in which case the gastric tube may be inserted through the mouth.

Similar goals apply to the insertion of a urinary catheter in this phase, such as decompression of the bladder prior to diagnostic peritoneal lavage, in preparation for an abdominal examination and possible surgical entry into the abdomen and to allow monitoring of urinary output as an index of tissue perfusion. Haematuria if present raises a high index of suspicion of genitourinary trauma. Contraindications for urinary catheterization are blood at the urethral meatus, and the presence of a scrotal haematoma, both of which may indicate urethral injury. A disruption to the urethra may require a supra-pubic catheter to be inserted. A urinalysis is carried out on all patients and a urine pregnancy test is indicated in all females of childbearing age (American College of Surgeons 2004).

Radiological examination should not delay patient resuscitation and should be used judiciously. The anteroposterior (AP) chest film and an AP pelvis may provide important information about patients with blunt trauma. A lateral cervical spine X-ray that demonstrates an injury is an extremely important finding and will dictate the patient's management in the secondary survey. Negative or inadequate X-ray does not exclude cervical spine injury and spinal cord protection should continue until further radiological investigation is carried out in the secondary survey.

Diagnostic studies such as diagnostic peritoneal lavage (DPL) and abdominal ultrasound are useful tools for detecting occult intra-abdominal haemorrhage and may be considered at this stage; however, such tests require the skills of an experienced practitioner and may be performed as part of the secondary survey. The indications, advantages and disadvantages of these studies are discussed in further detail in this chapter.

SECONDARY SURVEY

The secondary survey does not begin until the primary survey (ABCDEs) is completed, resuscitation is initiated and the patient is demonstrating normal vital functions (American College of Surgeons 2004). The secondary survey is a head-to-toe evaluation of the trauma patient and includes a complete history and physical examination of all systems and a reassessment of vital signs. A physical examination of the abdomen is performed as part of a complete secondary survey of the patient.

History

The AMPLE history is often useful as a mnemonic for remembering key elements of the history:

A   Allergies, age and alcohol?
M   Medications currently used
P   Past, pertinent medical history
L   Last meal, low temperature?
E   Events/environment related to injury

Physical examination

Abdominal injuries must be identified and treated aggressively; a normal initial examination of the abdomen does not exclude a significant intra-abdominal injury. Close evaluation and frequent re-evaluation of the abdomen preferably by the same observer in conjunction with close monitoring of vital signs is important when dealing with blunt abdominal trauma.

Inspection

The anterior and posterior abdomen as well as the lower chest and perineum should be inspected; injury patterns that suggest a potential for intra-abdominal trauma should raise suspicion (lap-belt abrasions or ecchymosis, steering-wheel-shaped contusions). Obvious abnormalities including distension and asymmetry along with contusions, abrasions, penetrating wounds or exposed viscera should be noted and documented accurately (Blank-Reid 2004, Talley & O'Connor 2006).

Auscultation

Auscultation of the abdomen may be carried out to confirm the presence or absence of bowel sounds; however, this may prove difficult in a noisy emergency department. Auscultation should take place before percussion and palpation because these examinations can change the frequency of bowel sounds. Visceral injury may release blood or enteric contents into the peritoneal cavity, resulting in irritation of the bowel which may produce a paralytic ileus, and thus an absence of bowel sounds. If bowel sounds are heard in the chest it is an indication of diaphragmatic rupture with herniation of stomach or small bowel into the thoracic cavity (ENA 2000, Blank-Reid 2004, Talley & O'Connor 2006).

Percussion

Percussion, or gentle tapping of the abdomen, produces a slight movement of the peritoneum. In the normal abdomen, percussion elicits dull sounds over solid organs and fluid-filled structures such as a full bladder and tympani over air-filled areas such as the stomach. If the peritoneum is injured, or irritated by free fluid released as a result of injury to viscera, this movement will cause pain. This is an unequivocal sign of intra-abdominal injury. Percussion may elicit subtle signs of peritonitis or isolate acute gastric dilatation by producing tympanic sounds or dullness due to haemoperitoneum. Percussion tenderness constitutes a peritoneal sign and mandates further evaluation and surgical consultation (Sikka 2004).

Palpation

Palpation is carried out to elicit and localize superficial, deep or rebound tenderness. The presence of a pregnant uterus, as well as estimation of foetal age, can also be determined at this stage of assessment. Involuntary guarding, rigidity, pain or spasm during palpation indicates peritoneal irritation. These signs may be absent, however, if the patient has competing pain from another injury, a retroperitoneal injury, a spinal cord injury, has ingested alcohol or narcotics or has a decreased level of consciousness.

Log roll and cervical spine immobilization

The patient should be cautiously log-rolled, maintaining cervical spine immobilization. This is necessary for complete assessment of the posterior chest, flank and back. Evidence of penetrating injury, surface ecchymosis, grazing or tenderness over the thoracolumbar spine may indicate possible retro-peritoneal organ injury.

While the patient is in a lateral position, a rectal examination should be performed. Bony fragments felt on rectal examination may indicate a fractured pelvis. Fresh blood in the rectum suggests a disrupted colon or rectum. A high-riding or absent prostate, in the male, may indicate a urethral transection, and contraindicates urinary catheterization. A vaginal examination is necessary in the female patient. Fractures of the pelvis may be discovered by direct palpation, and the integrity of the vaginal wall can be assessed. Examination of the gluteal region which extends from the iliac crests to the gluteal folds should also be carried out. Penetrating injuries to this area are associated with up to 50% incidence of significant intra-abdominal trauma and mandate a search for intra-abdominal injury (American College of Surgeons 2004).

Radiological studies

A lateral cervical spine X-ray, an *anteroposterior* (AP) chest and a pelvic X-ray are the screening radiographs obtained in the patient with multi-system blunt trauma. Abdominal X-rays (supine, upright, lateral decubitus) may be useful in the haemodynamically stable patient to detect extra-luminal air in the retroperitoneum or free air under the diaphragm, both of which mandate urgent laparotomy (American College of Surgeons 2004). The haemodynamically unstable patient with a penetrating abdominal wound does not require radiological screening in the emergency department. An upright chest X-ray is useful in the patient who is haemodynamically stable with penetrating injury above the umbilicus or who has a suspected thoracoabdominal injury. Chest X-ray can detect an associated pneumothorax or haemo-pneumothorax, or isolate air in the peritoneum. Supine abdominal X-ray may be useful to determine the track of a missile or bullet or the presence of retroperitoneal air; however, obtaining an abdominal X-ray is strongly discouraged as it delays more useful investigations (Raby et al. 2005).

Subsequent action

The management of blunt and penetrative trauma to the abdomen that follows the completion of the secondary survey is determined by the results of the physical examination and the circulatory status of the patient, i.e. whether there is any hypovolaemia, and the nature of the response to any fluid challenge measured by frequent recordings of vital signs. All blunt trauma should carry an associated high index of suspicion of intra-abdominal injury. Constant reassessment of the patient is necessary as it may take several hours for symptoms to develop, particularly splenic or duodenal injuries (Eckert 2005).

A three-stage response to abdominal examination exists:

1. **No immediate action – observation only:** a negative abdominal examination with no hypovolaemia. The abdominal examination should be repeated at frequent intervals.
2. **Special diagnostic studies urgently required:** an equivocal or unreliable abdominal examination in a multiply injured patient.
3. **Immediate surgical exploration of the abdomen required:** the need for urgent laparotomy is determined by history, findings on examination, and the results of investigations.

The following indications are commonly used to facilitate the decision-making process and are described by the American College of Surgeons (2004):

- blunt abdominal trauma with hypotension and clinical evidence of intraperitoneal bleeding
- blunt abdominal trauma with positive DPL or FAST
- hypotension with penetrating abdominal wound

- gunshot wounds traversing the peritoneal cavity or visceral/vascular retroperitoneum
- organ eviscerationt
- bleeding from the stomach, rectum, or genito-urinary tract from penetrating wounds
- presenting or subsequent peritonitis
- free air, retroperitoneal air, or rupture of the hemidiaphragm
- contrast-enhanced CT demonstrates ruptured gastrointestinal tract, intraperitoneal bladder injury, renal pedicle injury or severe visceral parenchymal injury after blunt or penetrating trauma.

SPECIAL DIAGNOSTIC STUDIES

If there are early or obvious indications that a trauma patient will be transferred to another facility, time-consuming tests such as diagnostic peritoneal lavage, computed tomography, contrast urologic and gastro-intestinal studies should not be performed (American College of Surgeons 2004).

Diagnostic peritoneal lavage

Diagnostic peritoneal lavage (DPL) was introduced in 1965 (Tumbarello 1998, Schulman 2003) and has been a primary diagnostic method of evaluation of abdomi-nal injury. DPL is a rapidly performed invasive proce-dure that significantly alters subsequent examinations of the patient and is considered 98% sensitive for intraperitoneal haemorrhage (ENA 2000, Schulman 2003). While DPL is a highly sensitive test it lacks spec-ificity for evaluating the severity and identifying the location of the injured organ. It has a complication rate of approximately 1% from mechanical injury to viscera during incision, or during insertion of the catheter (Tumbarello 1998, Schulman 2003). Bleeding from the incision, dissection or catheter insertion can cause false-positive results that may lead to unnecessary lap-arotomy (American College of Surgeons 2004).

It is recommended that the procedure should be carried out by the surgical team caring for the haemo-dynamically unstable patient with multiple blunt injuries. The procedure may also be carried out in haemodynamically stable patients when ultrasound or computed tomography is unavailable (American College of Surgeons 2004).

The preferred procedure involves an open or semi-open technique that is performed in the infra-umbilical area. In pregnant patients or patients with pelvic frac-ture an open supra-umbilical technique is preferred to avoid entering a pelvic haematoma or damaging the enlarged uterus. The procedure is performed under local anaesthetic, with lignocaine and adrenaline to constrict the blood supply to the incised area. A cathe-ter is inserted into the peritoneal cavity through the incision: free aspiration of blood, gastrointestinal contents, vegetable fibres or bile through the lavage catheter in the haemodynamically unstable patient mandates an urgent laparotomy. If gross blood (>10 ml) is not aspirated, lavage is performed with a litre of warmed Ringer's lactate solution (10 ml/kg in a child). Following adequate mixing of peritoneal con-tents with fluid by compressing the abdomen and log-rolling the patient, the effluent is allowed to free drain by gravity and is sent to the laboratory for analysis. A positive test is indicated by the presence of more than 100 000 RBC/mm^3, or more than 500 WBC/mm^3, or a Gram stain with bacteria present (American College of Surgeons 2004).

The indications for carrying out DPL are outlined in Box 8.1.

An absolute contraindication to DPL is an existing indication for immediate laparotomy. The disadvan-tages of DPL include utilizing an invasive technique and requiring the patient to have a gastric tube and indwelling catheter in place to avoid accidental perfo-ration of bladder or stomach. Additional limitations include the inability of DPL to identify retroperitoneal or diaphragmatic injury as well as detecting hollow viscous injuries. The time required for laboratory test analysis and the relative contraindications in patients with prior abdominal surgery, obesity, advanced cir-rhosis of the liver or patients in the third trimester of pregnancy may suggest consideration of other diagnostic tests such as FAST.

Focused abdominal sonography for trauma (FAST)

The use of ultrasound in the evaluation of abdominal injury has been practised since the early 1970s and has grown in popularity as a diagnostic tool in the emergency-department setting particularly since the 1990s (Tumbarello 1998, Schulman 2003, Blaivas et al. 2004, Raby et al. 2005).

Ultrasound can be used to detect with 98% accuracy the presence of haemoperitoneum and visceral injury and it has 98% to 100% specificity in locating the site of injury (Schulman 2003). FAST provides a rapid, non-invasive, accurate and inexpensive means of diag-nosing haemoperitoneum that can be repeated fre-quently (Raby et al. 2005). Even if ultrasonography reveals no obvious aetiology, it can facilitate diagnosis by excluding potentially life-threatening conditions. Emergency abdominal ultrasonography is indicated for the evaluation of aortic aneurysm, appendicitis, and biliary and renal colic, as well as of blunt or penetrating abdominal trauma (Chen et al. 2000, Richards et al. 2002).

The use of FAST is not intended to replace CT or DPL; rather, it is recommended as an adjunct diagnostic tool for rapid screening for potential abdominal injuries during the initial physical examination. It can be performed in the resuscitation room at the bedside while simultaneously performing other diagnostic or therapeutic procedures (Tumbarello 1998, Schulman 2003).

Fast examination

Identification of haemoperitoneum by ultrasound is based upon experience and understanding of abdominal anatomy, therefore specific equipment in experienced hands is a requirement for utilizing such a tool. Current literature recommends that the use of FAST should be limited to trauma surgeons who have completed a special training programme (Schulman 2003, American College of Surgeons 2004).

FAST can demonstrate the presence or absence of pericardial fluid, abdominal fluid, and some parenchymal injuries in a two to three minute examination.

A hand-held transducer is positioned on four key areas to evaluate fluid collection:

- to screen for life-threatening accumulation of pericardial fluid the transducer is placed left of the lower sternum and angled under the costal margin towards the patient's shoulder
- to visualize the spleen and perisplenic area the transducer is placed between the 10th and 11th ribs on the left posterior axillary line
- to evaluate the perihepatic region, the transducer is placed between the 10th and 11th ribs on the right axillary line.
- as blood may accumulate in dependent areas of the abdomen and pelvis, the transducer is placed above the symphysis pubis.

False negatives may result if FAST is performed early on in the patient's care; at least 100 ml of fluid are needed to be detectable on scan (Schulman 2003).

Advantages of FAST include rapid access, quick performance time, non-invasive testing, easy repetition, and no requirement for patient transport (Tumbarello 1998, Eckert 2005). Unlike DPL, ultrasound is capable of locating the injury, testing is not compromised by previous laparotomy or contraindicated in pregnancy and it can be used on patients with clotting disorders. Performance of the test by a trained surgeon or emergency physician eliminates the waiting time for technicians. Reported studies have found that the use of ultrasound has reduced the need for CT

(from 56% to 26%) and DPL (17% to 4%) and reduced overall hospital admission rates by 38% (Branney et al. 1997).

A limitation of ultrasound is in detecting intestinal injury and estimating the amount of haemoperitoneum present. Interpretation of test results may be limited depending on the expertise of the operator and interpreter; it may also be unreliable in patients with obesity, ascites and subcutaneous emphysema. It is important that ultrasound is not used as the single diagnostic tool in evaluating patients with abdominal injury; rather it should be utilized in conjunction with serial physical examinations, DPL, CT scanning and re-evaluation by ultrasound (Tumbarello 1998, American College of Surgeons 2004). The emergency nurse should be aware and anticipate the use of FAST in the early diagnostic phase of trauma patient care and understand the limitations of such a diagnostic test so that continued vital-sign monitoring and vigilance in patient assessment is maintained to avoid missed life-threatening injuries.

Computed tomography

Computed tomography (CT) scanning is a non-invasive radiological examination. It is considered the best method for identifying specific sites and amounts of bleeding, but may miss mesenteric or hollow-organ injury; also some specific injuries to the diaphragm and pancreas may be missed (Schulman 2003). Although CT scanning is the most sensitive diagnostic tool for most abdominal injuries, it is costly and requires time to prepare and execute (Eckert 2005). The patient must be transported to the radiology department, which is contraindicated in the haemodynamically unstable patient. CT may require the administration of intravenous or oral contrast, which can prove problematic where information on allergies is unknown. Additional limitations of CT include inability to perform the scan on an uncooperative patient (American College of Surgeons 2004). See Table 8.2.

SPECIFIC INTRA–ABDOMINAL INJURIES

Diaphragmatic injury

Diaphragmatic injury in blunt trauma is relatively rare. It is estimated that it is seen in 3–5% of all patients with blunt trauma who survive long enough to be admitted to hospital (Symbas & Shields 1987). The diaphragm is integral to normal ventilation and injuries can result in significant compromise. A history of respiratory difficulty and related pulmonary symptoms may indicate a diaphragmatic disruption. The mechanism of diaphragm rupture is related to the pressure gradient

Table 8.2 Comparison of DPL versus FAST versus CT in blunt abdominal trauma (adapted from American College of Surgeons 2004)

	DPL	FAST	CT Scan
Indication	• Provide evidence of bleeding if hypotensive	• Provide evidence of fluid if hypotensive	• Provide evidence of organ injury if BP normal
Advantages	• Early diagnosis • All patients • Performed rapidly • 98% sensitive • Detects bowel injury • No transport required	• Early diagnosis • All patients • Non-invasive • Performed rapidly • Repeatable • 86%–97% accurate • 98%–100% specificity • No transport required	• Most specific for injury • Sensitive: 92%–98% accurate
Disadvantages	• Invasive • Specificity:low • Misses injury to diaphragm and retroperitoneum	• Operator-dependent • Bowel gas and subcutaneous air distortion • Misses diaphragm, bowel and pancreatic injuries	• High cost • Time-consuming • Misses diaphragm and some pancreatic injuries • Transport required

between the pleural and peritoneal cavities. Lateral impact from a motor vehicle collision is three times more likely than any other type of impact to cause a rupture, since it can distort the chest wall and shear the ipsilateral diaphragm (Athanassiadi et al. 1999). Frontal impact from a motor vehicle collision can cause an increase in intra-abdominal pressure, which results in long radial tears in the posteriolateral aspect of the diaphragm, its embryologic weak point. The majority (70–80%) of diaphragmatic injuries occur on the left side, with 20–30% occurring on the right side and 5–10% occurring bilaterally (Shah et al. 1995, Athanassiadi et al. 1999). Diaphragmatic tears do not occur in isolation; patients often have associated thoracic and/ or abdominal injury or a concomitant head or extremity injury. Symptoms and signs of diaphragmatic rupture such as respiratory distress, cardiac disturbances, deviated trachea and bowel sounds in the chest are present in only a minority of patients initially assessed (Symbas & Shields 1987, Athanassiadi et al. 1999). The less-common right-sided ruptures are associated with more severe injuries such as tears of the juxtahepatic vena cava and hepatic veins as well as laceration of the liver. When herniation occurs on the right the liver is always present and the colon occasionally; such injuries result in haemodynamic instability and hypovolaemic shock. Reports on an autopsy series revealed that left- and right-sided diaphragmatic ruptures occurred almost equally; however, the more severe injuries associated with right-sided rupture caused more deaths and thus a lower rate of patient survival until diagnosis

in hospital. The rates of associated injury are: pelvic fractures 40%, splenic rupture 25%, liver laceration 25%, thoracic aortic tear 5–10%. Diagnosis may not be obvious and is made pre-operatively in only 40–50% of left-sided and 0–10% of right-sided blunt ruptures. If diagnosis is not made in the first 4 hours it may be delayed for months or years; thus 10–50% of injuries are diagnosed in a latent phase which occurs as a result of gradual herniation of abdominal contents into the pleural cavity. Diagnosis may be made later still in a third phase which is characterized by bowel or visceral herniation, causing obstruction and/or strangulation of stomach and colon. If herniation causes significant lung compression it can lead to tension pneumothorax, while cardiac tamponade has been described from herniation of abdominal contents into the pericardium (Athanassiadi et al. 1999). The incidence of diaphragmatic injury increases each decade as a result of increased occurrence of high-speed motor-vehicle accidents. Improved survival rates are likely to be due to improvements in pre-hospital and emergency care and earlier recognition and treatment of severe injury.

Duodenum

Duodenal injury is a rare condition and is typically associated with a direct blow to the epigastrium due to a traffic accident or sports injury. Delay in diagnosis is common because the duodenum lies in the retroperitoneum and often combines with other severe injury such as fractures or other organ injury. The incidence of traumatic duodenum injury, however, is lower than other abdominal injury, with reported rates of 3.5–12% (Aherne et al. 2003). Morbidity is more dependent on other associated injuries than on the degree of the duodenal injury. Bloody gastric aspirate or retroperitoneal air on X-ray or abdominal CT scanning will raise suspicion for this injury (American College of Surgeons 2004) and will require further investigation. Treatment is often simple surgical repair but is dependent on the extent and nature of injury to the duodenum and other concomitant injuries.

Solid organ injury

Injuries to the liver, spleen or kidney that result in shock, haemodynamic instability or evidence of continued bleeding remain indications for urgent laparotomy. Isolated solid organ injury in the haemodynamically stable patient can often be managed conservatively but will require evaluation by a surgeon and admission to hospital for observation.

Spleen

Injury to the spleen is most commonly associated with blunt trauma. Fracture of ribs 10 to 12 on the left should raise suspicion of spleen injury which ranges from laceration of the capsule or a non-expanding haematoma to ruptured subcapsular haematoma or parenchymal lacerations. The most serious types of injury are a severely fractured spleen or vascular tear that causes splenic ischaemia and massive blood loss; however, shock and hypotension are present in as few as 30% of patients with splenic trauma (Herman 2003).

Liver

Due to its size and location the liver is the most commonly injured solid intra-abdominal organ (Beckingham & Krige 2001). Severity ranges from a controlled subcapsular haematoma and lacerations of the parenchyma to hepatic avulsion or a severe injury to the hepatic veins. Because liver tissue is very friable and the liver's blood supply and storage capacity are extensive, a patient with liver injury can haemorrhage profusely and may need surgery to control bleeding. The most important decision after initial resuscitation is whether surgery is needed. Computed tomography of the abdomen is useful in haemodynamically stable patients suspected of having a major injury. Patients with large hepatic haematomas or limited capsular tears who have small volume loss may be treated conservatively but require constant observation and repeated examination (Beckingham & Krige 2001).

Genitourinary

Direct blows to the back or flank resulting in contusions, ecchymosis or haematoma are markers for potential underlying renal injury and warrant evaluation of the urinary tract (American College of Surgeons 2004). Contusion is the most common kidney injury and should be suspected in posterior rib fracture or fracture to the lumbar vertebrae. Other renal injuries include lacerations or contusion of the renal parenchyma, the deeper a laceration the more serious the bleeding. Deceleration forces may damage the renal artery: collateral circulation in that area is limited, therefore any ischaemia is serious and may trigger acute tubular necrosis.

Pelvic injury

The pelvis protects the organs within the pelvic compartment, transmits weight from the trunk to the lower limbs and has attachment points for muscles. A stable pelvis can withstand vertical and rotational physiological forces, but either fractures or ligamentous injuries can disrupt pelvic stability. Pelvic blood supply comes primarily from the iliac and hypogastric arteries, which run at the level of the sacroiliac joints. Those arteries are supplemented by a rich associated network, including the superior gluteal artery, which is susceptible to injury in posterior fractures, and the obturator and internal pudendal arteries, which can be injured in fractures of the ramus (Frakes & Evans 2004).

Road traffic accidents cause about 60% of pelvic fractures; most of the remainder result from falls (Frakes & Evans 2004, O'Sullivan et al. 2005). Pelvic fracture is said to contribute to traumatic death but is not the primary cause. For patients with pelvic fracture who die, hypotension at the time of admission is associated with increased mortality (42% vs. 3.4% with stable vital signs), as are head injuries requiring neurosurgery (50% mortality); abdominal injuries requiring laparotomy (52% mortality); concomitant thoracic, urological or skeletal injuries (22% mortality). Survival is poorer for patients with open pelvic fractures and for pedestrians struck by cars (American College of Surgeons 2004, Frakes & Evans 2004, O'Sullivan et al. 2005). Genitourinary injuries are seen in association with 15% of all pelvic fractures. The bladder, rectum and vagina may be punctured by fracture fragments, or the bladder may be ruptured by a direct blow if full of urine. The male urethra that passes through the prostate is relatively immobile; the rest of the urethra passes through the urogenital diaphragm, which is attached to the pubic rami. If the pelvis is fractured, this portion may shear from the rest at the apex of the prostate and the prostate is then displaced upwards. Injuries to the female urethra are rare.

Pelvic fractures can be accurately diagnosed through physical examination but a high index of suspicion for a fracture based on the mechanism of injury is essential. Abrasions, contusions, isolated rotation of the lower extremity and discrepancy in limb length may alert the emergency nurse to the presence of pelvic fracture (Frakes & Evans 2004, Bailey 2005). Gentle compression of the iliac crests is advised to assess for tenderness, crepitus and stability of the pelvic ring. Rocking the pelvis and repeated examination is contraindicated where pelvic fracture is suspected or diagnosed. Repeated examination and excessive or unnecessary movement can aggravate bleeding, displace a fracture or disrupt a pelvic haematoma (American College of Surgeons 2004, Frakes & Evans 2004, Bailey 2005). Immobilization tools and techniques range from applying a sheet wrapped around the pelvis which is pulled tight to external fixation devices which may be inserted by the orthopaedic surgeon in the resuscitation room to limit blood loss. (See also Chapter 5: Skeletal injuries).

ABDOMINAL INJURIES IN CHILDREN

Injury continues to be the most common cause of death and disability in childhood (Rothrock et al. 2000, Wise et al. 2002) and injury morbidity and mortality surpass all major diseases in children and young adults (American College of Surgeons 2004). At least 25% of children with multisystem injury have significant abdominal injury although most are due to blunt trauma, most frequently from motor-vehicle collisions. The priorities of assessment and management of the injured child are the same as in the adult although physically, emotionally, intellectually and socially they differ greatly from adults. Only the differences related to abdominal injuries are considered in this section.

Specific anatomy in children

Children are vulnerable to abdominal injury for a number of reasons. Children are small; therefore any blunt trauma is likely to affect more body systems than in a similar incident involving an adult. The abdominal wall is thin, and offers little protection to its contents. Children have relatively compact torsos with smaller anterior-posterior diameters, which provide a smaller area over which the force of injury can be dissipated. The ribs are more elastic, decreasing protection to the spleen, liver and kidneys. The diaphragm lies more horizontally, lowering and further exposing these organs, which are relatively larger than in adults, with less overlying fat and weaker abdominal musculature (Day & Rupp 2003). The kidneys are also more mobile, and not shielded by perinephretic fat, as in adults. The bladder is superior to the protection of the pelvis, and therefore more vulnerable. Finally, abdominal injuries may cause diaphragmatic irritation and splinting, compromising ventilation (Advanced Life Support Group 1997).

Types and patterns of abdominal injury in children

The majority of abdominal injuries in children are caused by blunt trauma. Penetrating injuries are rare but the hypotensive child who sustains a penetrating abdominal injury requires prompt surgical intervention (American College of Surgeons 2004). Motor-vehicle trauma, bicycle handlebar injuries, falls and non-accidental injury are the most common causes of abdominal injuries (Lam et al. 2001, Day & Rupp 2003). As in adults, the spleen, liver and kidneys are the most commonly injured organs in the child victim of blunt trauma. The mortality of blunt abdominal trauma in children is directly related to the level of involvement: it is less than 20% in isolated liver, spleen, kidney or pancreatic trauma; increases to 20% if the gastrointestinal tract is involved; and increases to 50% if major vessels are injured (Day & Rupp 2003).

Assessment of abdominal trauma in children

The primary survey is carried out as in adults, with the same priorities and aims. An examination of the abdomen is carried out as part of the secondary survey. The examination is the same as that for adults, with the following special considerations. Care should be taken to be gentle on palpation, as any pain will produce voluntary guarding, making assessment difficult. Children swallow air when crying and upset; this produces distension of the stomach, which makes assessment difficult, and may mimic the rigidity and distension found in intra-abdominal injury. A nasogastric or orogastric tube (in infants and patients with maxillofacial trauma) should be placed in the resuscitation phase before abdominal examination (American College of Surgeons 2004). Gastric decompression will facilitate abdominal examination and prevent aspiration of gastric contents if vomiting occurs (Saladino & Lund 2000). A urinary catheter of appropriate size should always be passed, unless contraindicated, in order to decompress the bladder and facilitate abdominal evaluation and close monitoring of urinary output (American College of Surgeons 2004).

Repeated, serial examinations are necessary in children with abdominal trauma because life-threatening abdominal injury may not be apparent upon the initial examination. Severe intra-abdominal haemorrhage in children can be masked by their ability to maintain normal blood pressure with large volume blood loss. Abdominal injury can be obscured by concurrent extra abdominal injury such as head injury, thoracic trauma or fracture of the extremities (Day & Rupp 2003).

Children in whom intra-abdominal injury is suspected on the basis of mechanism of injury or physical examination findings should undergo emergent computed tomography (CT) scanning of the abdomen without waiting for laboratory results.

In the remainder of children (e.g. those with mild to moderate blunt abdominal trauma who are haemodynamically stable, awake, alert and cooperative), laboratory testing can occasionally identify unsuspected injury. The presence of haematuria (>5 red blood cells per high-powered field) or elevation of serum transaminases (ALT >125 U/L or ALT >200 U/L) may be the only indication of intra-abdominal injury in these children.

Diagnostic tests

Abdominal CT is the preferred diagnostic imaging modality to detect intra-abdominal injury in haemodynamically stable children who have sustained blunt abdominal trauma. CT is sensitive and specific in diagnosing liver, spleen and retroperitoneal injuries, which may be managed non-operatively. CT scanning is more frequently used in children because it can evaluate solid organs and the intestines.

Ultrasonography is useful when available for the rapid, early evaluation of children with blunt abdominal trauma who are stable; in such patients it might provide indication for immediate laparotomy (Wise et al. 2002).

The indications for diagnostic peritoneal lavage are the same as in adults; however, the usefulness of the test is questioned in the presence of solid organ injury where little or no peritoneal fluid may be present (Rothrock et al. 2000). Advanced trauma life support protocol suggests that only the surgeon who will care for the injured child should perform the diagnostic peritoneal lavage (American College of Surgeons 2004).

Non–operative management

Surgical intervention is not always warranted for haemodynamically stable children with solid organ injuries. Non-surgical observation of selected solid organ injuries in children is a safe practice that improves patient outcome and resource utilization (Rothrock et al. 2000, Wise et al. 2002). Approximately 90% of children with liver and spleen injuries can be managed non-operatively. In contrast, approximately 50% of children with pancreatic injuries require surgical intervention (Wise et al. 2002). When non-operative management is selected as the treatment option, care must be delivered in a paediatric intensive care facility where staff have the skill to carry out frequent repeated examination and the expertise available to intervene immediately should the child's condition deteriorate (Rothrock et al. 2000).

CONCLUSION

The challenge for nursing the patient with abdominal trauma in the emergency department lies in the rapid stabilization and assessment of the patient leading to early detection of life-threatening abdominal injury.

Training in the systematic assessment and resuscitation of victims of trauma, such as that offered by an Advanced Trauma Nursing Course, or Trauma Nursing Core Course, should be a basic requirement for all emergency nurses.

This training enables emergency nurses to effectively participate as members of the multidisciplinary team, ensuring that a systematic, protocol-driven method of clinical assessment, continuous monitoring and re-evaluation of the injured patient will detect early signs of serious intra-abdominal injury and expedite the need for urgent surgical intervention.

References

Advanced Life Support Group (1997) *Advanced Paediatric Life Support*. London: British Medical Journal Publishing Group.

Aherne NJ, Kavanagh EG, Condon ET, Coffey JC, El Sayed A, Redmond HP (2003) Duodenal perforation after a blunt abdominal sporting injury: the importance of early diagnosis. *Journal of Trauma*, **54**, 791–794

American College of Surgeons (2004) *Advanced Trauma Life Support*, 7th edn. Chicago: American College of Surgeons.

Arnold JL, Halpern P, Tsai MC, Smithline H (2004) Mass casualty terrorist bombings: a comparison of outcomes by bombing type. *Annals of Emergency Medicine*, **43**(2), 263–273.

Athanassiadi K, Kalavrouziotis G, Athanassiou M, Vernikos P, et al. (1999) Blunt diaphragmatic rupture. *European Journal of Cardio-Thoracic Surgery*, **15**, 469–474.

Bailey MM (2005) Staying on your toes when managing pelvic fractures. *Nursing*, **35**(10), 32–34.

Barry P, Shakeshaft J, Studd R (2003) Abdominal injuries. In Sherry E, Triou L, Templeton J eds, *Trauma*. Oxford: Oxford University Press.

Beckingham IJ, Krige JEJ (2001) ABC of diseases of liver, pancreas and bilary system: liver and pancreatic trauma. *British Medical Journal*, **322**, 783–785.

Better O (1999) Rescue and salvage of casualties suffering from crush syndrome after mass disasters. *Military Medicine*, **164**, 366–369.

Blaivas M, Brannam L, Hawkins M et al. (2004) Bedside emergency ultrasonographic diagnosis of diaphragmatic rupture in blunt abdominal trauma. *American Journal Emergency Medicine*, **22**(7), 601–604.

Blank-Reid C (2004) Abdominal trauma: dealing with the damage. *Nursing*, **34**(9), 36–41.

Branney S, Moore E, Cantrill S, Burch J, Terry S (1997) Ultrasound-based key clinical pathway reduces the use of hospital resources for the evaluation of blunt abdominal trauma. *The Journal of Trauma: Injury, Infection and Critical Care*, **42**, 1086–1090.

Buduhan G, McRitchie DI (2000) Missed injuries in patients with multiple trauma. *Journal of Trauma*, **49**, 600–605.

Burkitt, HG, Quick CRG (2002) *Essential Surgery: Problems, Diagnosis and Management*, 3rd edn. London: Churchill Livingstone.

Centre for Disease Control (CDC) (2003) *Explosions and Blast Injuries: A Primer for Clinicians*. Atlanta, CDC.

Chen SC, Wang HP, Hsu HY, et al. (2000) Accuracy of ED sonography in the diagnosis of acute appendicitis. *American Journal of Emergency Medicine*, **18**(4), 449–452.

Cole E, Lynch A, Cugnoni H (2006) Assessment of the patient with acute abdominal pain. *Nursing Standard*, **20** (38), 56–64.

Connors JM, Ruddy RM, McCall J, Garcia VF (2001) Delayed diagnosis in pediatric blunt trauma. *Pediatric Emergency Care*, **17**, 1–4.

Day M, Rupp L (2003) Children are different; pediatric differences and the impact on trauma. In: Czerwinski SJ, Maloney-Harmon PA (eds), *Nursing Care of the Pediatric Trauma Patient*. St Louis: Saunders.

Dickinson M (2004) Understanding the mechanism of injury and kinetic forces involved in traumatic injuries. *Emergency Nurse*, **12**(6), 30–34.

Eckert KL (2005) Penetrating and blunt abdominal trauma. *Critical Care Nurse*, **28**(1), 41–59.

Emergency Nurses Association (2000) *Trauma Nursing Core Course. Provider Manual*, 5th edn. Chicago: ENA

Frakes MA, Evans T (2004) Major pelvic fractures. *Critical Care Nurse*, **24**(2), 18–30.

Herman ML (2003) Gastrointestinal trauma. In: L Newberry, ed. *Sheehy's Emergency Nursing: Principles and Practice*. 5th Edn. St Louis: Mosby.

Lam JPH, Eunson GJ, Munro FD, Orr JD (2001) Delayed presentation of handlebar injuries in children. *British Medical Journal*, **322**, 1288–1289.

Luckman J, Sorenson KC (1987) *Medical-Surgical Nursing*. Philadelphia: Saunders.

McSwain N et al. (1996). *The Basic EMT: Comprehensive Prehospital Patient Care*. St Louis: Mosby.

Mannion SJ, Chaloner E (2005) Principles of war surgery: ABC of conflict and disaster. *British Medical Journal*, **330** (7506), 1498–1500.

Mattox KL, Feliciano DVB, Moore EE (Eds.) (2000) *Trauma*, 4th Edn. New York: McGraw-Hill.

Neff JA, Kidd PS (1993). *Trauma Nursing: the Art and Science*. St Louis: Mosby.

O'Sullivan REM, White TO, Keating JF (2005) Major pelvic fractures: identification of patients at high risk. *Journal of Bone and Joint Surgery*, **87**(4), 530–534.

Porter K, Greaves I (2003) Crush injury and crush syndrome: a consensus statement. *Emergency Nurse*, **11**(6), 26–30.

Raby N, Berman L, deLacey G (2005) *Accident and Emergency Radiology: A Survival Guide*, 2nd edn. Philadelphia: Elsevier Saunders.

Revere CJ (2003) Mechanisms of injury. In: L Newberry, ed. *Sheehy's Emergency Nursing: Principles and Practice*. 5th Edn. St Louis: Mosby.

Richards JR, Schleper NH, Woo B, Bohnen PA, McGahan JP (2002) Sonographic assessment of blunt abdominal trauma: a 4 year prospective study. *Journal of Clinical Ultrasound*, **30**(2), 59–67.

Rothrock SG, Green S, Morgan R (2000) Abdominal trauma in infants and children: prompt identification and early management of life-threatening injuries. Part 1: Injury patterns and initial assessment. *Paediatric Emergency Care*, **16**(2), 106–115.

Saladino RA, Lund DP (2000) Abdominal trauma. In: Fleisher, GR, Ludwig, S, Eds, *Textbook of Pediatric Emergency Medicine*, 4th edn. Philadelphia: Lippincott, Williams and Wilkins.

Schulman CS (2003) A FASTer method of detecting abdominal trauma. *Nursing Management*, **34**(9), 47–49.

Seidel HM et al. (1995) *Mosby's Guide to Physical Examination*. 3rd edn. St Louis: Mosby.

Shah R, Sabaratnam S, Mearns A, Choudhury AK (1995) Traumatic rupture of diaphragm. *The Annals of Thoracic Surgery*, **60**(5), 1444–1449.

Sikka R (2004) Unsuspected internal organ traumatic injuries. *Emergency Medicine Clinics of North America*, **22**(4) 1067–1080.

Stillwell S (1996). *Mosby's Critical Care Nursing Reference Guide*, 2nd edn. St Louis: Mosby.

Symbas PN, Shields TW (1987) Diaphragmatic injuries. In: Shields TW, ed. *General Thoracic Surgery*, 3rd edn. Philadelphia: Lea & Febiger.

Talley NJ, O'Connor S (2006) *Clinical Examination: A Systematic Guide to Physical Diagnosis*, 5th edn. Edinburgh: Churchill Livingstone.

Taylor I, Dawood M (2005) Terrorism: the reality of blast injuries. *Emergency Nurse*, **13**(8), 22–25.

Tumbarello C (1998) Ultrasound evaluation of abdominal trauma in the emergency department. *Journal of Trauma Nursing*, **5**(3), 67–72.

Windsor AC, Guillou PJ (1999) Abdominal trauma. In: Monson J, Duthie G, O'Malley K, eds. *Surgical Emergencies*. Oxford: Blackwell Science.

Wise BV, Spears S, Wilson ME (2002) Management of blunt abdominal trauma in children. *Journal of Trauma Nursing*, **9**(1), 6–14.

Wright JA (1997) Seven abdominal assessment signs *every* emergency nurse should know. *Journal of Emergency Nursing*, **23**(5), 446–450.

Chapter 9

Facial injuries

Elspeth Hair

INTRODUCTION

This chapter deals with facial trauma, highlighting those injuries most commonly identified in emergency departments. It will explain how these injuries are sustained, the treatment and nursing care required and any problems which are likely to arise thereafter.

ANATOMY AND PHYSIOLOGY

The face contains all the special structures and centres for breathing, speech, vision, hearing, mastication and deglutition and ingestion and is highly vulnerable to a wide variety of injuries (Box 9.1; Fig. 9.1). These injuries can often be dramatic and for the patient are frequently disfiguring, leading to considerable psychological damage. Facial injuries often disrupt the appearance and the ability to express emotions. Resultant medico-legal problems may arise if these patients are not handled with the utmost skill and competence.

The diagnosis and treatment of facial fractures depends on the type of injury involved; therefore it is crucial to establish an early clear understanding of the mechanism of injury. Combined with a detailed knowledge of the anatomy and physiology of the injured area and immediate proper care the result for the patient should be one of optimum management.

MECHANISM OF INJURY

Most facial injuries result from blunt or penetrating trauma. Blunt injuries are far more common, including vehicular accidents, altercations, sports-related trauma, occupational injuries and falls. Penetrating injuries include gunshot wounds, stabbings and explosions. Mass, density and shape of the striking object, as well as speed of impact, directly affect type and severity of facial injury. The amount of force required to fracture

Box 9.1 The facial bones

The skeleton of the face is formed by 14 bones including the frontal bones.

Zygomatic – the two bones commonly referred to as the cheek bones

Maxilla – forms the upper jaw, the anterior part of the roof of the mouth, the lateral walls of the nasal cavities and part of the floor of the orbital cavities

Nasal – the paired bones form part of the bridge of the nose. The lower and major part of the nose consists of cartilage

Lacrimal – the two bones are thin and roughly resemble a fingernail in size and shape. They are the smallest bones of the face

Palatine – two L-shaped bones form the posterior portion of the hard palate

Turbinate – two scroll-like bones which project into the nasal cavity. Their function is the filtration of air before it passes into the lungs

Vomer – roughly resembles a triangle in shape and forms the lower and back part of the nasal septum

various facial bones may be classified as high impact (greater than 50 times force of gravity [*g*]) or low impact (less than 50 *g*) (see Box 9.2).

Generally it is accepted that the greater the speed of the vehicle the greater the injury. A history of broken windscreens and damaged dashboards is associated with head and most facial injuries. A bent or collapsed steering wheel should almost certainly make the nurse consider facial or laryngotracheal injuries. In motorcyclists, the necessity for full-face

Box 9.2 Force of gravity (*g*) impact required for facial fracture

High impact
Supraorbital rim: 200 *g*
Symphysis mandible: 100 *g*
Midline maxilla: 100 *g*
Frontal-glabellar: 100 *g*
Angle of mandible: 70 *g*

Low impact
Zygoma: 50 *g*
Nasal bone: 30 *g*

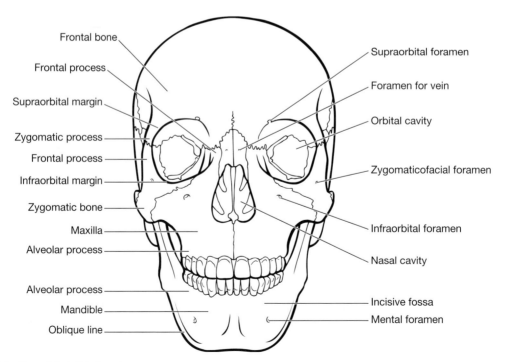

Figure 9.1 Normal facial/skull anatomy.

helmets with correctly mounted chin straps which do not allow the helmet to pivot forwards and fly off is highlighted (Williams 1991).

Inter-personal violence continues to be a source of many emergency department attendances. Studies in the United States, Western Europe and Australia show that, in these areas, the majority of injuries to the facial skeleton occur in males in the 20–30-year-old age group (Allan and Daly 1990). The diagnosis and treatment can often be made more complex as alcohol intoxication plays a major part in many altercations; however, injuries tend to be less severe than those following road traffic accidents (Elder et al. 2004, Magennis et al. 1998, Telfer et al. 1991).

The facial bony structures and sinus cavities have evolved to offer protection to the brain and will collapse under force, expending energy away from the brain. The attachments of facial muscles also assist to expend this energy away by exerting downwards and backwards force to the maxilla. The mandible is often described as one of the strongest bones of the body; however, the condylar necks are frequently fracture sites as they absorb energy forces directed towards the brain. Bony facial injuries are less common in children, representing approximately 10% of cases (Simpson and McLean 1995), because of the resilience and elasticity of their facial tissues. When injury does occur, the pattern differs from adults because the relatively large cranium of the child protects the facial bones.

ASSESSMENT

Maxillofacial trauma is defined as any structural or functional alteration of the bones, nerves, blood vessels or soft tissues of the face that results from accidental or intentional injury (Brown-Stewart 1989). It covers a wide spectrum of disease, ranging from the simple isolated laceration to massive facial trauma with haemorrhage and airway obstruction accompanied by multi-system involvement. While it is usually obvious, bloody and distressing, it is rarely fatal in its own right. Therefore the importance of a systematic examination, as advocated by the Advanced Trauma Life Support principles, cannot be overestimated (American College of Surgeons 2004, Dover 1999).

A thorough history should be obtained, including the cause of the trauma, whether there has been loss of consciousness and whether domestic violence was involved (Hutchinson et al. 1996). Isolated injuries to the maxillofacial skeleton commonly result from an assault. More severe injuries occur after high energy transfer (for example, road traffic accidents or blast injuries) and may be associated with injuries to the head, neck, chest and other body regions (Taylor & Dawood 2005, Hodgkinson 1994).

Initial assessment should involve a rapid but thorough examination of the mouth and throat to identify and eliminate any foreign material. Obstruction may occur instantaneously or slowly, as oedema and bleeding progressively occlude the airway. Upper-airway obstruction is most commonly due to the tongue and foreign bodies, including vomitus, blood, broken dentures, oedema of the area surrounding the epiglottis and more uncommonly injury to the larynx. During unconsciousness tone is lost in the muscles which normally hold the tongue away from the pharyngeal wall. Abnormal or prolonged relaxation of these muscles will allow the tongue to prolapse back, obstructing the upper airway. The nurse must be alert for signs and symptoms of airway obstruction, including agitation, intercostal retractions, dyspnoea, cyanosis, gurgling, stridor and a SaO_2 less than 90% (Henneman et al. 1993).

Intubation of the patient may be inevitable where there is a decreased level of consciousness, and it is often very difficult as the head must be maintained in a neutral position. Performance of non-traumatic intubation is vital, as traumatic insertion causes increased intracranial pressure, which underlines the need to obtain experienced specialist help. The nasopharyngeal route should normally be avoided unless basilar skull fracture has been excluded, thus leaving cricothyrotomy as the method of choice for many patients.

Airway obstruction can be alleviated by manoeuvring the mandible anteriorly, thereby moving the tongue anteriorly (Cicala 1996). This manoeuvre can be accomplished by the chin-lift or jaw-thrust technique. As neither one will compromise a possible cervical spine fracture, both methods should be used in the treatment of trauma patients. While suctioning remains the primary method of clearing secretions, extreme care should be taken not to stimulate the gag reflex or aggravate existing injuries with overactive suctioning techniques. Where appropriate, the fully conscious patient may be allowed to hold their own suction catheter, thereby controlling the build up of secretions and eliminating the risk of over stimulation.

If no airway obstruction is present and the patient is haemodynamically stable, a systematic examination of the head and face can be performed (Box 9.3). Alterations in skin integrity are often readily observable, and their size and location as well as the amount of associated bleeding and surrounding tissue swelling should be determined. Careful inspection and palpation of the scalp should be undertaken for injuries disguised by the hair. The head and face should be palpated for crepitus, bony irregularity,

---

Box 9.3   Assessment of facial injuries

- Adequate airway
- Cervical spine injury
- Bleeding
- Level of consciousness
- Scalp injuries
- Asymmetry of facial structures
- Difficulty in swallowing or talking
- Decreased hearing or tinnitus
- Missing or broken teeth
- Malocclusion of the mandible
- Cerebrospinal leak from eyes, ears, mouth and/or nose
- Visual acuity
- Numbness or tingling on the face

LeDuc Jimmerson and Lomas (1994)

---

tenderness and swelling. Visual acuity and extraocular movements are assessed to detect cranial nerve damage, globe rupture and extraocular muscle injury or entrapment. Diplopia may indicate the presence of an orbital floor fracture (see Box 9.4).

Box 9.4   Examination of eyes following facial trauma

- Visual acuity – can the patient count four fingers? Can he or she read print?
- Limitation of eye movements, diplopia and unequal pupillary levels. If one or more of these is present suspect trauma of the orbital floor and wall with entrapment of periorbital tissues
- Direct, consensual and accommodation reflexes. Examination of these may help detect a rise in intracranial pressure, but be aware of false-positive signs caused by trauma to the globe
- Proptosis (or exophthalmos). This suggests haemorrhage within the orbital walls
- Enophthalmos, the sinking of the eye globe, suggesting fracture of an orbital wall – usually the floor or medial wall
- If periorbital swelling is present, fracture of the zygoma or maxilla should be suspected
- If subconjunctival ecchymosis is present, direct trauma to the globe or a fractured zygoma should be suspected.

(Hutchinson et al. 1996)

The ears and mastoid areas should be inspected for ecchymosis (Battle's sign), lacerations or discharge. Perforation of the eardrum, bloody or serous rhinnorhea or otorrhea, haemotympanum and bilateral periorbital haematomas ('panda eyes') are important findings suggestive of a basilar skull fracture (Criddle 1995). The nose should be examined for alignment, deformity, pain, swelling, septal haematoma, epistaxis and difficulty in breathing. If bleeding and leakage of cerebrospinal fluid are present, an anterior cranial fossa fracture at the cribiform plate should be suspected. Nasal endotracheal or nasogastric tubes should not be passed in case the fracture is further aggravated. Prophylactic sulphonamides or chloramphenicol to prevent meningitis should be prescribed.

Teeth should be examined for fractures, subluxations and avulsions. A tongue blade and good light source can be used to inspect the oral cavity for lacerations. Jaw occlusion should be assessed, checking for pain, malalignment and range of motion.

Because of the location of the seventh cranial (facial) nerve, one or more of its branches are frequently damaged in maxillofacial trauma. Therefore, facial motor and sensory motor function should be assessed before analgesia or anaesthetics are administered. Assessment of the facial nerve includes testing for muscle strength, symmetry and taste sensation on the anterior two-thirds of the tongue (Criddle 1995). Motor function of the facial nerve is checked by having the patient wrinkle his or her forehead, frown, smile, bare the teeth and close the eyes tightly. All three major branches of the trigeminal nerve should also be tested for sensation on each side of the face. Loss of sensation in any one of these areas may imply a fracture in the vicinity of that branch (Fig. 9.2).

Correct positioning of the patient with facial injuries is crucial. After cervical spine injury has been eliminated by clinical examination or lateral cervical X-ray, the fully conscious patient may be allowed to adopt a suitable position for both adequate airway management and comfort. Elevation of the trolley head between 15° and 30° will assist drainage of blood and secretions from the nasopharynx and decrease the amount of blood and secretions from the nasopharynx and decrease the amount of oedema (LeDuc Jimmerson and Lomas 1994).

Soft tissue injuries must be fully inspected. Unexpected foreign bodies are not infrequently found in facial and scalp wounds. Additionally, while extensive superficial lacerations do not usually require a transfusion, there is danger in overlooking the continuous trickle of fresh blood from a puncture wound.

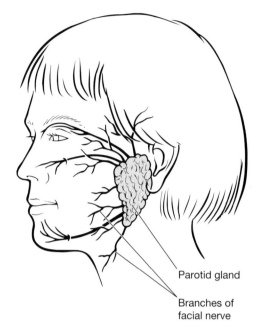

Figure 9.2   Anatomy of facial and trigeminal nerves.

LE FORT FRACTURES

In 1901, Rene Le Fort published the results of his experiments in which he inflicted blows to the heads of 35 cadavers, by striking them with a wooden club and throwing them at the edge of a table. Le Fort fractures is the classification of maxillary fractures commonly used today (Tiner and Luce 1994) (Fig. 9.3). The adult male–female ratio is 3:1; however, male preponderance is reduced to 3:2 in children.

Le Fort I   This can be described as a horizontal fracture through the maxilla and nasal septum, below the level of the malar. This compartment is mobile but produces minimal deformity and will be evidenced by bilateral epistaxis, damage to the dental surface and teeth and crepitus on palpation. Hutchinson (1998) notes that tapping on the teeth produces a brittle sound like the tapping of an empty egg shell.

Le Fort II   The pyramid fracture line passes through the lateral orbital rim, zygomatic arches, roof of the nose and high in the pterygoid plates. This is clinically obvious if displaced, as the 'stove in' face. The middle third of the facial skeleton becomes detached and is usually driven backwards and downwards, thus comprising the airway and producing an open bite. Bilateral subcutaneous haematomas are often present.

Le Fort III   The fracture line passes through the lateral orbital rim, zygomatic arches, roof of the nose and high in the pterygoid plates. It results in complete

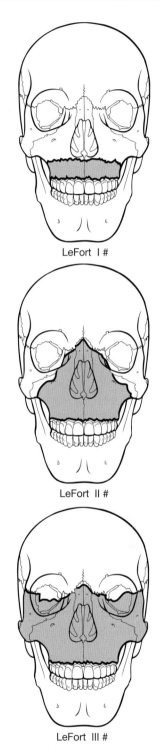

LeFort I #

LeFort II #

LeFort III #

Figure 9.3   Le Fort I, II, III fractures.

separation of the facial skeleton from the cranial skeleton. It is not unusual for patients to sustain different combinations of these fractures, such as a Le Fort II on one side with a Le Fort III on the other. This fracture frequently causes the face to appear long and flat, or 'dish-faced'. Maxillo-facial expertise may be required to make an accurate assessment.

Clinical evidence

Because the force required to create a Le Fort fracture is quite significant, patients with these injuries usually have a history of severe facial trauma. Clinical findings associated with Le Fort fractures include pain, swelling, nasopharyngeal bleeding, flattening and/or elongation of the facial features, tenderness, mobile maxilla and malocclusion – the patient may describe the teeth as feeling different. Anaesthesia of the cheek, caused by damage to the infraorbital nerve, is also a common finding. A cerebrospinal fluid leak may occur in 25–50% of Le Fort II and III fractures (Manson 1984) and indicates the presence of an open fracture.

Patients with Le Fort III fractures, in particular, tend to have massive facial oedema and ecchymosis and occasionally suffer complete airway obstruction secondary to dissection of a haematoma into the palate, pharyngeal wall or tonsillar pillars. Le Fort fractures are frequently associated with mandibular fractures, causing prolapse of the tongue and intraoral haematoma formation (Crumley 1990).

Management

This is initially directed at maintaining the airway, which may be compromised secondary to oedema or haemorrhage. Other causes of obstruction include the accumulation of vomit or other foreign material within the mouth, oedema of the lips, tongue or pharynx resulting from direct trauma, chemical or thermal injuries and instability of the mandible. It may be necessary to pass an endotracheal tube to secure the patient's airway. In extreme cases, where the airway is severely compromised, placing the fingers in the mouth and lifting the soft palate forward may be life-saving. While assessing the airway, the nurse should note the respiratory rate, evaluate breathing patterns and provide supplemental high-flow oxygen (Ritchie 1994).

Conscious patients should be nursed in an upright position with the head well forward (high Fowler's) allowing any fluid to run freely from the mouth, provided no medical contraindications exist, such as C-spine injuries or hypovolaemic shock. Unconscious patients, if not already intubated, should be nursed on their side, allowing fluids to drain unrestricted from the oral cavity.

If a CSF leak is present, anterior cranial fossa and basilar skull fracture should be suspected. Thin, watery, nasal discharge should be considered CSF leakage until proven otherwise and the halo or dextrostix test should be undertaken. Whether there is a CSF leak or not, position, suction and, if required, endotracheal intubation may be satisfactory in securing the airway. Tracheostomy should be considered if the middle third of the face is impacted and cannot be brought forward manually or in the case of uncontrollable postnasal haemorrhage or severe oedema of the glottis.

Because of the potential for the cribiform plate damage in Le Fort II and III fractures with subsequent disruption of the meninges, patients should be instructed not to blow their nose as this may cause contamination of the meninges with nasal secretions, and consequent meningitis (Hutchinson 1998). Prophylactic sulphonamides, such as co-trimoxazole, or alternatively chloramphenicol, may be used to prevent meningitis.

Definitive treatment of Le Fort fractures is usually delayed for several days until the oedema subsides. Nasal and pharyngeal packing may be necessary where severe haemorrhage is present. Wound care should be carried out as soon as possible and facial lacerations should be repaired within 24 hours. Application of ice packs to minimize oedema formation should be considered as soon as practicable. Prophylactic antibiotic therapy should be initiated if CSF leak is suspected or present and adequate analgesia should be administered.

MANDIBULAR FRACTURES

The mandible is a horseshoe-shaped structure suspended from the cranium at the temporo-mandibular joint (Hinchcliffe et al. 1996). The prominent position of the mandible predisposes it to trauma and it may be fractured or displaced as a result of a direct blow to the lower third of the face. After nasal fractures, it is the second most common facial fracture. This may cause a fracture at the site or indirect fracture near the temporo-mandibular joint (see Fig. 9.4). The severity of the fracture may depend upon the mechanism of injury and the dentition of the jaw, as the more teeth there are, the less severe the fracture. Displacement of the fragments depends on the shape of the fracture and the action of muscles. Contra-coup injuries are common in mandibular fractures. A blow sustained on the right mandible frequently results in left mandibular fracture. The majority of mandibular fractures occur in the adolescent or young adult population and are due to interpersonal violence, sports injuries, road traffic accidents and falls (Jones 1997).

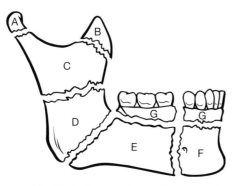

Figure 9.4 Mandibular fracture sites. A: Condyle. B: Coronoid process. C: Ascending ramus. D. Angle. E: Body. F: Symphysis. G: Alveolar process.

Clinical evidence

The importance of correct diagnosis of mandible fractures cannot be stressed enough, particularly in the case of children. If mismanaged or even undetected they may lead to gross asymmetry of growth or ankylosis of the joint. Although clinical manifestations of mandibular fractures will vary depending on the location, assessment usually reveals malocclusion, pain, difficulty in speaking and swallowing, facial asymmetry and decreased range of motion. Bruising of the floor of the mouth is highly suggestive of mandibular fracture. Mandibular injuries are classified as open or closed. Fractures are considered open whenever a communication with either the oral cavity or the skin surface is present.

Evaluation of occlusion is the most important aspect of the mandibular examination. Patients with only mild pain and full range of motion, including lateral motion, a normal bite and no loss of strength are unlikely to have a mandibular fracture (Criddle 1995). Radiographic diagnosis of a fracture is most easily made with a dental panoramic X-ray film, but regular films will detect most fractures. Fractures in the area of the condyles may be visible only on CT scan.

Management

Management of mandibular fractures begins with maintenance of a clear airway as described for Le Fort fractures above, and administration of antibiotics if the fracture is compound, which includes a tooth-bearing area (Roberts et al. 2000). Application of ice-packs or cold compresses to reduce swelling, wound care and repair of oral lacerations to prevent contamination by saliva are also important considerations. Adequate analgesia should be given and the patient prepared for admission to hospital for surgical fixation. This is usually intermaxillary wiring for simple fractures and open reduction with interosseus wiring for more complex fractures. Generally, mandibular fractures will require some sort of jaw immobilization for approximately six weeks to promote both healing and comfort. Fixation is usually delayed until the patient is stable.

ORBIT FLOOR FRACTURES (BLOW-OUT FRACTURE)

Orbital floor fractures result from a sudden increase in intraorbital hydraulic pressure. A high velocity object, such as a ball or fist, that impacts the globe and upper eyelid transmits kinetic energy to the periocular structure resulting in pressure with a downward and medial vector. Smaller objects tend to cause penetrating injuries. The orbital rim is not usually damaged but the bone of the orbital floor gives way under pressure of the eyeball, which can sustain considerable force without rupturing, resulting in the inferior oblique and inferior rectus muscles herniating with some periorbital fat through into the maxillary antrum (see Fig. 9.5).

Clinical evidence

Entrapment of nerves and muscles produce the signs and symptoms associated with this injury. The only evidence of a blow-out fracture may be a 'tear drop' of soft tissue appearing on an X-ray hanging down into the antrum. On examination, enopthalmus, a limited upward gaze, may be detectable. If more than 2 mm of enopthalmus exists, this can create a noticeable imbalance. Most patients present after facial trauma and may describe decreased visual acuity, blepharoptosis, binocular vertical or oblique diplopia. Patients may complain of pain, epistaxis and eyelid swelling following nose blowing.

Wilkins and Havins reported a 30% incidence of a ruptured globe in conjunction with orbital fractures, supporting the notion that a thorough and complete ophthalmic examination is needed. Vision loss may be present in 8% of patients (Tintannalli et al. 1996). Pain, periorbital bruising and subconjunctival haemorrhage are regarded as reliable signs of a blow-out fracture.

Management

Treatment includes the application of cold compresses to reduce oedema formation, antibiotic cover to prevent orbital cellulitis, the administration of analgesia, and vital sign and neurological observation

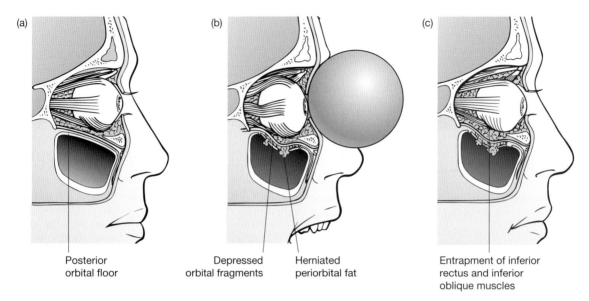

(a)   (b)   (c)

Posterior orbital floor	Depressed orbital fragments Herniated periorbital fat	Entrapment of inferior rectus and inferior oblique muscles

Figure 9.5   Mechanism of injury in blow-out fracture.

recording. To avoid further haemorrhage, the patient should be made aware of the need to avoid blowing the nose. Surgical elevation of the orbital floor may be required after the release of any trapped nerves, usually after 24 hours. As the patient may be acutely anxious about the loss of vision, the nurse should provide reassurance and information about the treatment and care plans.

TEMPOROMANDIBULAR JOINT (JAW) DISLOCATION

Temporomandibular joint (TMJ) dislocations are commonly caused by yawning, chewing or laughing, typically occurring with an audible 'pop' during maximal jaw opening (see Fig. 9.6). Occasionally they are caused as a result of trauma. Although dislocation can be unilateral, it is more commonly bilateral and is always anterior. Many patients with TMJ dislocation have anatomic conditions which predispose them to recurrent episodes.

Clinical evidence

Dislocations of the jaw are relatively easy to diagnose, as the patient will present with a drooling mouth which is propped open, unable to close or move. It is usually very painful and the patient will also find it difficult to speak. If the patient presents with a history of trauma, X-rays should be taken; otherwise they are unnecessary.

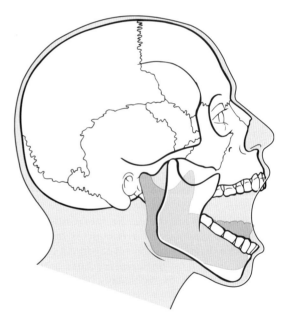

Figure 9.6   Dislocation of the temporomandibular joint dislocation.

Management

The treatment of TMJ dislocation is directed towards relocation of the jaw. Reduction usually requires analgesia and some form of sedation. Short-acting parenteral muscle relaxants, such as diazepam or midazolam, are useful for relaxing jaw spasms and only rarely is there a need to resort to general anaesthesia or open reduction.

In simple disclocations, when the mandibular condyles have been dislocated for less than 2 hours, it may be possible to reduce the condyle into its correct position without any specific medication (Hutchison 1998). Reduction is accomplished by sitting the patient in a chair or on the floor with his or her back to the wall. A physician or nurse practitioner with well-padded thumbs stands directly in front of the patient and places his or her thumbs on the third molars of the mandible with the fingers curled under the symphysis of the mandible. Downward pressure is then applied on the molars with slight upward pressure on the symphysis to lever the condyles downward. As soon as the condyles are past the articular eminence, the strong jaw muscles will cause the mandible to shut suddenly into the normal closed position, hence the need for well-padded thumbs (Amsterdam 1988).

Post-reduction X-rays should be taken if this is the first dislocation for the patient. The patient should be advised to avoid yawning or otherwise stressing the temporomandibular ligaments for several weeks after TMJ dislocation. This will include advice to take a soft diet for several weeks to reduce the risk of further dislocations.

FRONTAL SINUS FRACTURES

Frontal sinus fractures frequently occur as a result of blows to the face, sports injuries and falls on the side of the face. The frontal, zygomatic and nasal bones are affected. They are frequently found to be depressed and can be compound or closed.

Clinical evidence

The patient with a frontal sinus fracture will present with a history of trauma, tenderness and swelling at the site of the injury. Periorbital ecchymosis and severe lateral, subconjunctival haemorrhage are often present. Physical examination is usually hampered by oedema, and these injuries are notorious for appearing insignificant until the oedema resolves (Smith 1991). Related complications, such as eye injuries, supraorbital anaesthesia and CSF rhinorrhoea, may also be present.

Management

This involves wound care and ice packs to reduce swelling. Antibiotic cover will be required if a compound is present. Elevation of the depressed fracture

will be required when the patient's condition is stable. Most zygomatic fractures are significant enough to require open reduction and stabilization with internal wire fixation for 4 to 6 weeks.

NASAL FRACTURES

The nose is the most common site for facial fractures and is frequently associated with other fractures of the middle third of the face. Usually they are the result of blunt trauma because of the prominence and lack of supportive structures. The nasal bones may be displaced laterally or posteriorly depending on the direction of the traumatic force. Traumatic disruption of the nasal bones and cartilages can result in significant external deformity and airway obstruction. The type and severity of nasal fracture are dependent on the force, direction and mechanism of injury (see Fig. 9.7). A small object with a high velocity can impart as much damage as larger objects at a lower velocity. Lateral nasal trauma is most common and may result in the fracture of one or both nasal bones. This is often accompanied by dislocation of the nasal septum off the maxillary crest. Septal dislocation can result in an S-shaped nasal dorsum, tip asymmetry and airway obstruction. Direct frontal trauma to the nose often results in the depression and widening of the nasal dorsum with associated nasal obstruction. More severe injuries may result in comminution of the entire nasal pyramid. If these injuries are not properly diagnosed and corrected, the patient will have a poor cosmetic and functional outcome (Rubeinstein and Strong 2000).

Clinical evidence

Patients with nasal fractures usually present with a history of trauma, oedema, tenderness, ecchymosis and obvious deformity. Periorbital haematoma and subconjunctival haemorrhage may also be present. Epistaxis may or may not be present and is usually minor. It is usually due to bleeding from Little's area and is easily halted by pressure with the thumb for several minutes. It is important to examine the inside of the patient's nose for the presence or absence of a septal haematoma and to observe for CSF rhinnorhea, and indicators of fractures of the cribiform plate (Cantrill 1989).

Management

There is no treatment required for undisplaced fractures; however, the ENT department may wish to see the patient 5–10 days later when any swelling has resolved but before the fracture has united. Conventional packing of the nose may be sufficient, although

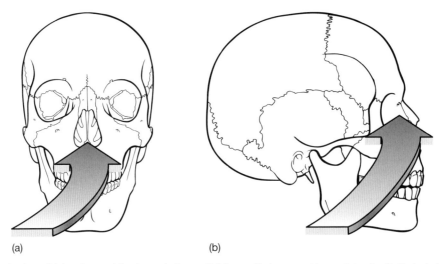

(a)   (b)

Figure 9.7 Mechanism of injury in nasal fractures. A: Tangential forces displace nasal bones laterally, B: Posteriorly directed blows displace fracture fragments into other facial structures. (After Criddle 1995)

a postnasal pack may be required and advice should be sought from an ENT specialist if available.

An X-ray is not essential in diagnosis but is often requested for medico-legal reasons. If haemorrhage has been severe or persistent then vital signs and hae-moglobin level should be checked. For comfort, the patient should be given analgesics and advised to apply a cold compress to the nose.

FACIAL WOUNDS

The face is highly vascular and as a consequence most wounds, even when contaminated, heal well if careful wound management is carried out. Infection is usually rare but haemorrhage can be severe and may result in the patient requiring transfusion. Small puncture wounds that scarcely seem to require suturing may cause life-threatening haemorrhage if they involve an artery such as the facial or superficial temporal arteries.

Wounds should be assessed regularly for blood loss and if there is continued haemorrhage all wounds, however small, should be explored and if necessary blood vessels should be ligated or clipped. Significant haemorrhage can occasionally occur in patients with closed middle-third injuries of the face. This normally presents as a steady flow of blood from the nose and mouth with bleeding into the soft tissues of the face which gradually produces marked facial swelling with skin which is shiny and tense. As road traffic accidents are frequently the cause of facial wounds glass may be present from a shattered windscreen; therefore it is wise to have soft tissue X-rays taken before any attempt is made at wound closure (Reynolds & Cole 2006).

Irregular skin edges should be trimmed, although large areas of skin should not be incised. Dirty abrasions should be scrubbed thoroughly and occasionally general anaesthesia may be required in order to achieve the best result. As facial wounds heal faster than wounds elsewhere, fine monofilament nylon or polypropylene, which causes less tissue reaction, should be used and removed after approximately four days. If required, adhesive strips may be applied when the sutures have been removed. This provides a little extra support and eliminates the risk of scarring caused by suture marks. Repair of complicated wounds may require the skills of an experienced plastic surgeon, and attempts by the inexperienced casualty officer should be avoided whenever possible. Wound care is examined in detail in Chapter 23.

Eyelids

Wounds of the lids frequently occur but are rarely dangerous. The lids, when closed tightly in reaction to a threat, have nearly half an inch (13 mm) of tissue in front of the eyeball, providing adequate cushioning and protection (London 1991). Nevertheless, eyelid wounds caused after a fall or of a penetrating nature may create complications and require meticulous attention, and therefore should be referred to an oph-thalmic or plastic surgeon.

Lips

A blow on the lip can sometimes split it cleanly against the teeth, but if the blow is angled it can cause a shearing of the lip from its attachment to the gum. It is particularly important that perfect alignment of the mucocutaneous junction of the lip is achieved in order to avoid a step resulting in the lip margin (vermilion border). It is possible for injected local anaesthetic to cause distortion of the tissues and the picture may be confused as a result. However, careful attention by an experienced senior doctor or plastic surgeon can produce excellent results.

Infection is common where a penetrating wound is caused by the teeth when both sides of the lip have been involved. It is important that the laceration should be repaired inside and out. Careful examination is required where broken teeth are present to eliminate any fragments which may be retained within the lip.

Eyebrows

Eyebrows should *never* be shaved as they may never regrow properly and can cause unnecessary distress. As in the treatment of the lip, the aim is to achieve perfect alignment. Modern methods include the use of tissue adhesive for many types of wound closure (Davis and Cordeaux 1994). Careful assessment of the type, size and location of wound must take place before any attempt is made, and only those well practised should undertake this task.

Ears

Lacerations involving cartilage will need careful reconstruction, but it should be the skin alone which is sutured, not the cartilage. Avulsion of the pinna is not uncommon as a result of interpersonal altercations. The skin slips and the cartilage is pulled out. If adequate blood supply is retained in the flap which is formed then the cartilage can be tucked back in and the skin sutured.

Haematomas (cauliflower or rugby player's ear) require urgent aspiration, followed by pressure pads bandaged or strapped to press the ear against the head. This procedure may have to be carried out every few days until no re-accumulation of blood occurs, thereby allowing the perichondrium to grow back onto the cartilage. If this is not achieved then it will die and shrivel, resulting in a cauliflower ear.

Rupture of the ear drum can occur from sustaining a blow to the side of the head. After the diagnosis is confirmed the patient should be warned not to allow water into the meatus. The ear should not be packed and no ear drops are required; only referral to an ear, nose and throat clinic is necessary (see Chapter 31 ENT Emergencies).

Teeth

Care must be taken not to miss an inhaled tooth, and if in any doubt an X-ray must be arranged. Lacerations of the lip should be carefully examined for small pieces of broken tooth which may have become embedded there. Tooth sockets which continue to bleed may require packing; this should be done using adrenaline-soaked gauze. Failure to arrest the haemorrhage may result in suturing and/or packing of the socket, with surgical referral to a dentist. If a patient presents with a broken tooth, the ideal storage medium is either milk or the patient's own saliva; however, normal saline is a reasonable substitute. The tooth should not be kept dry or soaked in tap water for any length of time. If the socket is full of blood clot, it should be gently irrigated with normal saline to clear the clot. The tooth should be gripped by its crown the correct way round and re-implanted firmly into the socket. Local anaesthetic may be needed into the local gingival to achieve anaesthesia. The patient may also be fitted with a mouth guard to hold the tooth in place; however, splinting is not necessary unless the tooth is very mobile (Hutchison 1998).

Injuries to inside the mouth and tongue

Theses are most commonly seen in children after a fall, when the teeth penetrate the tongue. Small lacerations can be left untouched and they will heal quickly. Larger lacerations often result in prolonged haemorrhage and can be distressing to both patient and parent. Suturing of the wound is often necessary, especially if the edge of the tongue is involved, causing a flap. Absorbable suture material is often used, thereby reducing the need for a return visit for removal. However, this procedure in children is frequently difficult and occasionally general anaesthesia has to be administered if optimum results are to be achieved.

It is important to examine the patients intraorally for haematoma, especially under the tongue, as this is indicative of a mandibular fracture. The patient or parent should be advised of the need to adopt meticulous oral hygiene care when injury to the tongue or inside the mouth occurs. Antibiotics may be prescribed because of the large amount of bacteria present in the oral cavity.

Fauces

Injury to the tonsillar fossa is often the result of a child falling while holding an object in his or her mouth. As the internal carotid artery is close by and traumatic thrombosis can ensue, this situation should be taken seriously from the outset. The mechanism of injury must be clear before a final conclusion is reached regarding the treatment of cases presenting with this type of injury. The patient should be closely observed for signs of developing retropharyngeal abscess post-injury.

CONCLUSION

All facial injuries should be treated as a head injury; therefore neurological and vital signs should be checked and recorded at regular intervals (see Chapter 4: Head Injuries). Continuous reassurance from both nursing and medical staff will be required due to the distressing nature of the injury. The patient is likely to be very anxious and the nurse will play a major part in the early provision of both physical and psychological care.

Detailed initial assessment of the patient with facial injuries is crucial and will consequently influence the final outcome. Correct airway management is essential and extreme care and continuous monitoring of the patient is imperative if a satisfactory outcome is to be achieved. Severe facial injuries should ideally be managed by an experienced maxillo-facial surgeon if the patient is to receive the best possible care with the best possible outcome.

References

Allan BP, Daly GG (1990) Fractures of the mandible: a 35 year retrospective study. *International Journal of Oral and Maxillofacial Surgery*, **19**, 268–271.

American College of Surgeons (2004) *Advanced Trauma Life Support*, 7th edn. Chicago: American College of Surgeons.

Amsterdam JT (1988) Dental emergencies. In: Rosen P et al., eds. *Emergency Medicine: Concepts and Clinical Practice*. 2nd Edn. St Louis: Mosby.

Brown-Stewart P (1989) Maxillo-facial trauma: implications for critical care. *Critical Care Nurse*, **9**(6), 44–57.

Cantrill SV (1998) Facial trauma. In: Rosen P et al., eds. *In Beaumont Emergency Medicine: Concepts and Clinical Practice*, Vol. 1. 2nd Edn. St Louis: Mosby.

Cicala RS (1996) The traumatized airway. In *Beaumont JL Airway Management Principals and Practice*. St Louis: Mosby.

Criddle LM (1995) Maxillofacial trauma and ear, nose and throat emergencies. In: Kitt S, Selfridge-Thomas J, Proehl JA, Kaiser J, eds. *Emergency Nursing: A Physiologic and Clinical Perspective*. 2nd edn. Philadelphia: WB Saunders.

Crumley RL (1990) Maxillofacial and neck trauma In: Ho MT, Saunders CE, eds. *Current Emergency Diagnosis and Treatment*. Norwalk, Co., Appleton & Lange.

Davis JE, Cordeaux S (1994) Tissue adhesive: use and application. *Emergency Nurse*, **2**(2), 16–18.

Dover MS (1999) Pathophysiology of maxillofacial trauma. In: Alpar EK, Gosling P, eds. *Trauma: A Scientific Basis for Care*. London: Arnold.

Elder RW, Ryan GW, Shults RA, Strife BJ, Swahn MH (2004) Alcohol related emergency department visits among people ages 13 to 25 years. *Journal of Studies on Alcohol*, **65**, 297.

Gerlock AJ, McBride KL, Sinn DP (1981) *Clinical and Radiographic Interpretation of Facial Fractures*. Boston: Little Brown.

Henneman EA, Henneman PL, Oman KS (1993) Ventilation and gas transport: pulmonary, thoracic and facial injuries. In: Neff JA and Stinson Kidd P, eds. *Trauma Nursing: The Art and Science*. St Louis: Mosby Year Book.

Hinchcliffe S, Montague S, Watson R (1996) *Anatomy and Physiology*, 2nd edn. London: Baillière Tindall.

Hodgkinson DW, Lloyd RE, Driscoll PA, Nicholson DA (1994) ABC of emergency radiology: maxillofacial radiographs. *British Medical Journal*, **308**, 46–50.

Hutchinson I, Lawlor M, Skinner D (1996) Maxillofacial injuries. In: Skinner D, Driscoll P, Earlam R, eds. *ABC of Major Trauma*, 2nd edn. London: BMJ Publishing Group.

Jones N (1997) Facial fractures. In: Jones N, ed. *Craniofacial Trauma*. Oxford: Oxford University Press.

LeDuc Jimmerson C, Lomas G (1994) Facial, ophthalmic and otolaryngeal trauma. In: Driscoll PA, Gwinnutt CL, LeDuc Jimmerson C, Goodall O, eds. *Trauma Resuscitation: The Team Approach*. Basingstoke: Macmillan.

London PS (1991) *The Anatomy of Injuries and its Surgical Implications*. Oxford: Butterworth Heinemann.

Manson PN (1984) Maxillo-facial injuries. *Emergency Medicine Clinics of North America*, **2**, 761–768.

Magennis P, Shepherd J, Hutchison I, Brown A (1998) Trends in facial injury. *British Medical Journal*, **316**, 325–326.

Reynolds T, Cole E (2006) *Techniques for acute wound closure. Nursing Standard* **20**(21), 55–64.

Ritchie E (1994) Management of facial fractures. *Emergency Nurse*, **2**(3), 10–15.

Roberts G, Scully C, Shotts R (2000) ABC of oral health: dental emergencies. *British Medical Journal*, **321**, 559–562.

Rubenstein B, Strong EB (2000) Management of nasal fractures. *Archives of Family Medicine*, **9**, 738–742.

Simpson DA, McLean AJ (1995) Epidemiology. In: David DJ, Simpson DA, eds. *Craniomaxillofacial Trauma*. Edinburgh: Churchill Livingstone.

Smith RG (1991) Maxillofacial injuries. In: Harwood-Nuss A, Linden C, Luten RC, Sternbach G, Wolfson AB, eds. *The Clinical Practice of Emergency Medicine*. Philadelphia: JB Lippincott.

Taylor I, Dawood M (2006) The reality of blast injuries. *Emergency Nurse*, **13**(8), 22–25.

Telfer MR, Jones GM, Shepherd JP (1991) Trends in the aetiology of maxillofacial injuries in the United Kingdom. *British Journal of Oral Maxillofacial Surgery*, **29**, 250–255.

Tiner BD, Luce EB (1994) Facial fractures. In: Montgomery MT and Redding SW, eds. *Oral-Facial Emergencies: Diagnosis and Management*. Portland: JBK Publishing.

Tintannalli B et al. (1996) *Emergency Medicine: A Comprehensive Study Guide*. New York: McGraw-Hill.

Williams M (1991) The protective performance of bicyclists' helmets in accidents. *Accident Analysis and Prevention*, **23,** 119–131.

Chapter **10**

Burns

Charlotte Douglas

INTRODUCTION

Despite legislative attempts to improve safety and increase public awareness, patients with burn injuries remain a significant proportion of trauma patients attending emergency departments (EDs) (Herndon 2007). Each year in the UK, it is estimated that 175 000 people visit EDs with acute burn injuries and some 13000 of them need admission to hospital (Dunn 2000). Add to this the number of individuals treated as outpatients and the scale of the problem becomes apparent. Although the chances for survival following the massive trauma of a major burn have improved steadily over the last 25 years, there are still 300 deaths in hospital each year in the UK (Dunn 2000).

The care provided in the first few hours after injury is crucial (Wiebelhaus & Hansen 2001) and without pertinent and urgent treatment the chances of surviving a major burn are greatly reduced. Burn injuries should be thought of as more than 'skin deep': they represent a complicated assault on the body's vital organs and systems. Management of major burn injury must reflect this, and through effective organization and prioritization of care, potentially life-threatening problems can be dealt with successfully, or in some cases avoided in the first instance.

This chapter aims to unravel some of the complexities of burn injury management. Mechanisms of injury with specific first-aid measures, implications of a burn injury in the assessment of airway, breathing and circulation, and immediate psychological care needs will all be covered in detail. The chapter will also consider burn wound management, treatment of more minor injuries and indications for transfer to specialist burns units.

ASSESSMENT

First aid can overlap the initial ED management of burn injuries, especially when first aid has not been commenced at the scene of the incident. It has been proven many times that the decisions and treatment received at the scene, particularly the quality of first aid, often have a profound effect on mortality and morbidity (Dunn 2000). In a stressful situation, confusion often exists over what constitutes safe first aid, particularly for the lay person.

Appropriate action can be summarized as:

- safe removal from the source of the burn – rescuers should be aware of any potential risk or immediate danger from the environment, to themselves, before attempting to remove the casualty
- maintenance of airway
- arresting the burning process by application of cold water to reduce residual heat in body tissues or to remove corrosive substances
- reduction of pain
- protection of damaged skin from desiccation and infection.

During this period it is important to obtain a brief, accurate history of the event (Settle 1995). Establishing what, where, when, why and how injuries happened will enable appropriate, prioritized care to be commenced promptly.

This can be taken from the patient, relatives or ambulance crew (Box 10.1)

The principles of Advanced Trauma Life Support (ATLS), primary and secondary survey, should be applied to the assessment and immediate care of patients with major burn injuries. During the primary survey thorough assessment of the ABCs should be performed.

Box 10.1 Information about patient/incident

- Circumstances of the incident (e.g. explosion, RTA or fire)
- Time of injury, to allow accurate estimation of circulatory fluid loss
- First aid measures undertaken
- Distribution of burns
- Presence of other injuries: fractures, head injury
- Relevant medical history, including tetanus status and current drug therapy

---

Airway and breathing

The first priority in the management of a burn-injured patient is immediate assessment of the patient's airway for patency and maintenance (Jones 2003). Inhalation injury and respiratory complications are two of the leading causes of fatality in the early period following burn injury. The early detection and treatment of airway or breathing problems must be paramount in the patient's overall management. Thermal inhalation (direct heat) and chemical inhalation injuries pose the greatest threat to airway and breathing. A direct heat injury will be evident soon after injury. Unless steam inhalation has occurred, the damage is usually limited to the upper airway. Direct heat injury causes face, neck and intraoral burns and leads to a rapid development of oedema, resulting in complete airway obstruction within hours (Wilding 1990).

Chemical inhalation usually involves the by-products of combustion. The most worrying toxins are those that asphyxiate patients, depriving them of oxygen, carbon monoxide (CO) and cyanide (Jones 2003). The chemicals affect the lower airways, causing alveolar damage, pulmonary oedema and surfactant insufficiency. They reduce the circulatory availability of oxygen because carbon monoxide has a much greater affinity for haemoglobin (Hb) than oxygen, and subsequently induce acidosis. Chemical inhalation should be suspected following a loss of or altered consciousness, history of fire within an enclosed or confined area, the presence of intraoral burns and soot in the mouth, nose and sputum, and where a confirmed history of smoke inhalation exists.

Acute airway obstruction is diagnosed by the presence of dyspnoea, wheezing, hoarseness, stridor, loss of voice and even minimal evidence of laryngeal swelling. Once this has been detected, early intubation is essential to allow effective airway management. If in doubt, intubate; intubation is much more difficult once the patient's airway is swollen.

During the airway assessment, also check for cervical spine injury and take appropriate precautions. If you need to open the airway and you suspect a cervical spine injury, use a combined jaw thrust and spine immobilization manoeuvre. Apply a hard cervical collar if indicated, even if it goes over the burn. (See also Chapter 6: Spinal Injuries).

In less severe cases, where there is no direct evidence of airway involvement, close and careful observations should be continued as symptoms may become apparent over the next 24 to 48 hours (Muehlberger et al. 1998). The ED nurse should not be misled by the apparent mildness of symptoms. This is often an inaccurate indicator of the degree of damage occurring, and the patient's condition should be continually reviewed for increasing shortness of breath, feelings of tightness, wheezing or hoarseness. The patient's chest should be adequately visualized for respiratory effort and bilateral movement. Percussion and auscultation should be performed to determine adequate air entry, and to detect wheezing, signs of pulmonary oedema and lower airway obstruction.

All patients with suspected inhalation injuries should be given high-flow 100% oxygen as soon as possible (McParkland 1999) The administration of high levels of oxygen, via either mask or endotrachael tube, greatly reduces the half-life of carboxyhaemoglobin (COHb) and increases its rate of elimination from the body. This reduces systemic hypoxia. Measuring this can prove difficult in ED because the usual methods such as oxygen saturation monitoring are rendered ineffective as they do not distinguish between oxy- and carboxyhaemoglobin (Wiebelhaus & Hansen 2001). The actual diagnosis of an inhalation injury is often difficult to confirm in the initial stages of care. Investigations include immediate arterial blood gas analysis as a baseline for the evaluation of the patient's pulmonary status, with sequential arterial blood gas measurements to confirm CO elimination (Campbell 2000, Hantson 1997) Oxygen saturation monitoring should not be used until blood gas analysis reveals that COHb concentrations have reached a normal level.

Measurement of COHb and cyanide levels is important, but results are not always immediately available to ED staff. Fibre-optic bronchoscopy is valuable as a secondary investigation to confirm the presence of soot in the lower respiratory tract (Muehlberger et al. 1998). Because of the difficulty in diagnosis, objective observation and reporting of respiratory changes by the emergency nurse provide the subtle indicators needed to decide the treatment needed. Burn injuries result in a significant increase in respiratory tract secretion as part of the histamine response. If the patient has a compromised airway or is intubated, regular suctioning may be necessary to clear the airway of excessive secretions (Swearingham & Keen 1991). Circumferential full-thickness burns to the neck and chest may compromise the mechanism of breathing and necessitate emergency escharotomy (Settle 1995). Chest X-rays are usually obtained, but they do not often show early signs of respiratory problems, although they may highlight other injuries.

Circulation

The patient with major burns will develop severe hypovolaemic shock within 3–4 hours from the time of injury, unless adequate fluid resuscitation measures are initiated (Settle 1995). Damage to the capillary network in the skin leads to loss of water, proteins and electrolytes from the circulation into the interstitial compartment (Hettiaratchy & Dziewulski 2004). There are three reasons for this: wound secretion, evaporation and localized oedema; in severe cases, generalized oedema in surrounding, apparently uninjured, areas also occurs. The oedema occurs because of changes in permeability of capillaries and tissues affected by heat. Fluid consists mostly of dilute plasma, which increases the viscosity of the remaining intravascular fluid and slows or stops blood flow to capillaries. Poor tissue perfusion increases the extent of the burn because of low oxygen (Cook 1997). If this process is left unchecked, severe shock is likely, but given the predictability of fluid loss, the principal aim of care is to anticipate it and compensate with fluid resuscitation (Settle 1995). The greatest amount of fluid loss in burn patients is in the first 24 hours after injury.

Loss of circulating volume always occurs following a major burn injury. Cardiac output is reduced by about a third within the first hour of injury (Cook 1997). Normal compensatory mechanisms allow homeostasis to be maintained initially, but fluid resuscitation is vital if this is to be maintained. Rapid initial transfusion may result in little improvement. It does, however, reduce the impact of a further reduction of cardiac output around 6 hours post-injury. Although haemoglobin becomes more fragile and has a shorter lifespan following a significant burn injury, blood transfusion is not recommended in initial management as it may increase the viscosity of intracellular fluid. Haemolysis will occur in transfused blood, therefore reducing its effectiveness.

Fluid replacement

Intravenous (I.V.) access with large-calibre I.V. lines must be established immediately in a peripheral vein (American College of Surgeons 2004). If possible place two large-bore I.V. devices through unburned skin. If placement of the I.V. cannula is in a burned area, ensure the cannula is correctly and securely inserted into the vein, as swelling will push the hub out and may cause infiltration.

To accurately determine the amount of fluid required, it is necessary to assess the area of body surface damaged by burn injury. The 'rule of nines' (Fig. 10.1) is a convenient tool for a quick initial assessment. The rule of nines cannot be used for children because a child's body has different proportions. The Lund-Browder (1944) assessment guide (Fig. 10.2) enables a more accurate assessment, as it allows for surface area variations with age. If the surface area

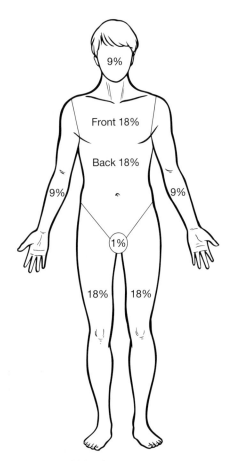

Figure 10.1   Rule of 'nines'.

burned exceeds 15% in adults or 10% in children and the elderly intravenous fluid resuscitation is indicated: over 20% and this resuscitation becomes urgent (Wiebelhaus & Hansen 2001). It is also possible to estimate the patient's likelihood of survival based on the percentage area of body burned (Table 10.1).

Fluid replacement is calculated from the time the burn is sustained, rather than the time resuscitation begins. The most commonly used and favoured resuscitation formula is the Parkland formula, a pure crystalloid formula. It is favoured by the British Burns Association over The Muir and Barclay Formula, which is described for albumin as the resuscitation fluid, because it has the advantages of being easy to calculate and the rate is titrated against urine output.

The Parkland formula

This calculates the amount of fluid required in the first 24 hours. Children require maintenance fluid in addition to this (Table 10.2, Box 10.2).

As stated above, the starting point for resuscitation is the time of injury, not the time of admission. Any fluid already given should be deducted for the calculated requirement.

At the end of the 24 hours, colloid infusion is begun at a rate of:

0.5 ml × (total burn surface area (%) × (body weight (kg)

and maintenance crystalloid is continued at a rate of:

1.5 ml × (total burn surface area (%) × (body weight (kg)

A fluid resuscitation formula can help to reduce inaccuracies in fluid replacement, particularly when assessment has to be made by inexperienced staff, but these formulae only act as a guideline for infusion. Actual amounts of fluid administered should reflect the condition of the patient. The amount of fluid given should be continuously adjusted according to the individual patient's response, to maintain a urinary output of 0.5–1 ml/kg/h (adult) or 1–1.5 ml/kg/h (child) (American College of Surgeons 2004) and other physiological parameters (pulse, blood pressure and respiratory rate).

There is no agreement on the type of fluid which should be used for resuscitating the burn-injured patient. Colloids have no advantage over crystalloids in the initial management to maintain circulatory volume (Heittiaratchy & Papini 2004). In the UK, Hartmann's solution (sodium chloride 0.6%, sodium lactate 0.25%, potassium chloride 0.04%, calcium chloride 0.027%) is the most commonly used crystalloid. Crystalloids are given to supplement that used by metabolic requirements, which tend to increase following injury. In adults, 50 ml/h of sodium base crystalloid should be given to maintain metabolic function. In children, fluid replacement should be titrated by the child's weight (Wilson 1997) (Table 10.2). Colloid use is controversial. However, much protein is lost through the burn wound, so there is a need to replace this: some units introduce colloid after 8 hours, as the capillary leak begins to shut down; others wait 24 hours. Fresh frozen plasma is often used in children and albumin in adults (Heittiaratchy & Papini 2004).

The last step of the primary survey is to look for any obvious disabilities and assess changes in the patient's level of consciousness.

The secondary survey should follow that of the primary. In the secondary survey, expose and examine the patient from head to toe, looking for any minor associated injuries. Care should be

NAME _____   WARD _____   NUMBER _____   DATE _____

AGE _____   ADMISSION WEIGHT _____

LUND AND BROWDER CHARTS

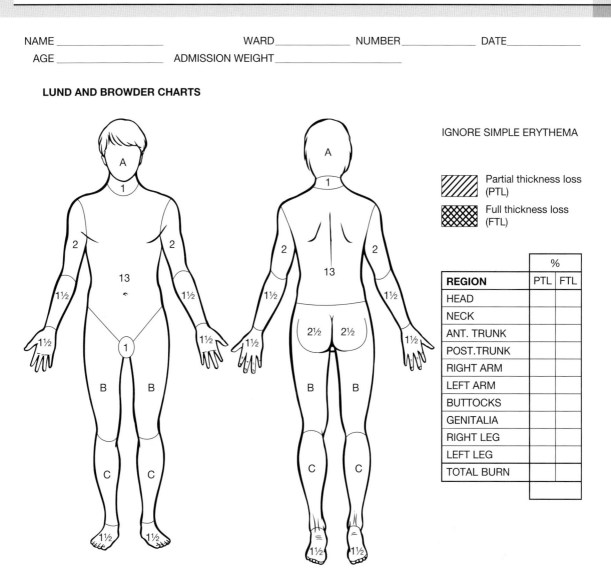

IGNORE SIMPLE ERYTHEMA

Partial thickness loss (PTL)

Full thickness loss (FTL)

REGION	% PTL	FTL
HEAD		
NECK		
ANT. TRUNK		
POST. TRUNK		
RIGHT ARM		
LEFT ARM		
BUTTOCKS		
GENITALIA		
RIGHT LEG		
LEFT LEG		
TOTAL BURN		

RELATIVE PERCENTAGE OF BODY SURFACE AREA AFFECTED BY GROWTH

AREA	AGE 0	1	5	10	15	ADULT
A = ½ OF HEAD	9½	8½	6½	5½	4½	3½
B = ½ OF ONE THIGH	2¾	3¼	4	4½	4½	4¾
C = ½ OF ONE LEG	2½	2½	2¾	3	3¼	3½

Figure 10.2 Lund and Browder (1944) charts.

taken at this stage to prevent hypothermia in an already compromised patient. Obtain an AMPLE history:

Allergies
Medications
Past medical history
Last meal
Events surrounding the injury.

In the resuscitation phase, even seemingly well patients with a major burn should be kept nil by mouth because of the risk of developing paralytic ileus. If this occurs, gastric aspiration via nasogastric

Table 10.1 Statistical values of mortality with age and percentage area of body burned. (From Bull 1971)

Area of body burned (%)	Age (years)								
	0–4	5–14	15–24	25–34	35–44	45–54	55–64	65–74	75+
93+	1.0	1.0	1.0	1.0	1.0	1.0	1.0	1.0	1.0
83–92	0.9	0.9	0.9	0.9	1.0	1.0	1.0	1.0	1.0
73–82	0.7	0.8	0.8	0.9	0.9	1.0	1.0	1.0	1.0
63–72	0.5	0.6	0.6	0.7	0.8	0.9	1.0	1.0	1.0
53–62	0.3	0.3	0.4	0.5	0.7	0.8	0.9	1.0	1.0
43–52	0.2	0.2	0.2	0.3	0.5	0.6	0.8	1.0	1.0
33–42	0.1	0.1	0.1	0.2	0.3	0.4	0.6	0.9	1.0
23–32	0	0	0	0.1	0.1	0.2	0.4	0.7	1.0
13–22	0	0	0	0	0	0.1	0.2	0.4	0.7
3–12	0	0	0	0	0	0	0.1	0.2	0.4
0–2	0	0	0	0	0	0	0	0.1	0.3

0.1 = 10% mortality; 0.9 = 90% mortality.

Table 10.2 Parkland formula for burns resuscitation:

Total fluid requirement in 24 hours =
 4 ml × (total burn surface area (%)) × (body weight (kg))
 50% given in first 8 hours
 50% given in next 16 hours

Children receive maintenance fluid in addition, at hourly rate of:
 4 ml/kg for first 10 kg of body weight *plus*
 2 ml/kg for second 10 kg of body weight *plus*
 1 ml/kg for >20 kg of body weight

---

tube may be necessary to prevent persistent vomiting (Swearingham & Keen 1991). During resuscitation, frequent monitoring is necessary to detect changes and to attempt to maintain the patient's stability. By using several indicators to give a picture of the patient's overall condition, appropriate clinical decisions can be made.

Pulse, respiration and blood pressure   These give an indication of changes to the patient's homeostasis, level of pain and anxiety. Any increase in pulse or respiration rate should be closely monitored and its cause established. Changes to blood pressure are a late sign in most cases of haemodynamic compromise, but monitoring is still valuable.

Altered level of consciousness   This can have a variety of causes, from primary injury to substance abuse, but hypoxia and hypovolaemia should not be disregarded. A sudden onset of restlessness, particularly in children, should be treated with suspicion and other indicators of stability should be checked. Using

the AVPU mnemonic (Alert and orientated, responds to Verbal stimulus, responds to Painful stimulus, Unresponsive) is recommended to determine a child's level of consciousness.

Skin colour   This is used to detect shock, as well as the level of injury to specific areas. A pink skin tone is indicative of a well-perfused patient, whereas pallor indicates arteriole constriction and a blue skin tone indicates venous stagnation consistent with severe shock (Wilson et al. 1987).

Skin and core temperature   This is useful for determining the level of vasoconstriction – the greater the difference, the poorer the level of perfusion. In a well person, this difference is between 18 and 48°C.

Urinary output   Patients with major burn injuries should be catheterized at an early stage, unless specific contraindications exist. Urine output will vary in early resuscitation because of hormones secreted as part of the stress response to injury. As previously stated, adequate fluid resuscitation should yield 0.5–1 ml/kg of body weight per hour (adults). Less than this indicates inadequate resuscitation and large volumes of low-concentration urine indicate overtransfusion.

Central venous pressure   Although this is useful in the monitoring of most cases of major trauma, its value for the burns patient is limited. Changes to CVP are gradual and the risk of infection is high (Copley & Glencorse 1992).

Frequent laboratory analysis of haematocrit level
This gives an indication of the ratio of red cells to plasma volume. An increased haematocrit level indicates a low plasma volume and therefore inadequate fluid replacement.

Box 10.2   Example of Parkland fluid replacement formula

Adult
A 60 kg woman with 20% burn was admitted at 3 p.m. Her burn occurred at 2 p.m.

1. *Total fluid replacement for first 24 hours*
   4 ml × (20% total burn surface area) × (60 kg) = 4800 ml in 24 hours.

2. *50% in first 8 hours, 50% over the next 16 hours*
   2400 ml during 0–8 hours and 2400 ml during 8–24 hours.

3. *Remember to subtract any fluid already received from amount required for first 8 hours*
   Has already received 1000 ml from ambulance services. So need:

   2400 − 1000 = 1400 ml in first 8 hours.

4. *Calculate hourly infusion rate for first 8 hours.*
   Divide amount of fluid calculated in (3) by time left until it is 8 hours **after burn**

   Burn occurred at 2 p.m., so 8-hour point is 10 p.m. It is now 3 p.m., so need:

   1400 ml/7 hours = 200 mls/h from 3 p.m. to 10 p.m.

5. *Calculate hourly infusion rate for next 16 hours*
   Divide figure in (2) by 16 to give fluid infusion rate, so need:

   2400/16 hours = 150 mls/h from 10 p.m. to 2 p.m. next day.

   Remember children need maintenance fluid in addition

Box 10.3   Thermal burns

- **Scalds**
  Injuries from hot fluids, such as tea, bath water, kettles etc., are the most common causes of all burns. Most of these cause skin damage or loss and are extremely painful. Exposure to water at 60°C (140°F) for 3 seconds can cause a deep partial-thickness or full-thickness burn. If the water is 69°C (156°F), the same burn occurs in 1 second. As a comparison, freshly brewed coffee is about 82°C (180°F) (Wraa 1998). Steam can cause deeper injuries because of its heat. Hot fat also causes more severe injury because of its temperature and, usually, a more prolonged contact with skin.

- **Contact**
  The most commonly treated are injuries from contact with hot objects, such as irons, ovens, hot metal or bitumen. Friction contact, e.g. with road surfaces, causes more superficial burn injuries.

- **Flame**
  Ignition of clothing by petrol, barbecues, bonfires, house fires etc. causes severe injury because of the prolonged contact of the source with the patient's skin. Flash burns from lightning or other electrical sources cause brief exposure to very high temperatures and therefore can result in significant injury (Thayre 1995).

Specific burn injuries

Thermal burns

These account for a large percentage of minor burn injuries, and a significant proportion of major burn injuries. They can be subdivided into three groups (Box 10.3, Fig.10.3).

Prehospital management   Remembering the safety of the rescuer, the source of the burn should first be removed, i.e. flames should be extinguished and contact with hot substances reduced. Cold water should be applied to the affected area for approximately 15–20 minutes to dissipate heat and relieve pain. Ice should not be used as it can cause blood vessels to constrict and produce further damage (Hudspith &

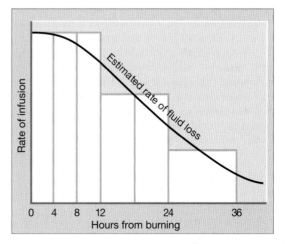

Figure 10.3   Estimated rate of fluid loss (after Bosworth 1997).

Rayatt 2004). Cooling should not exceed 20 minutes because of a significant risk of hypothermia, and the patient should be protected from environmental heat loss. Care should be taken if removing molten clothing, as the risk of devitalizing healthy tissue is high. Adherent material, such as nylon clothing, should be left on. Tar burns should be cooled with water, but the tar itself should not be removed (Hudspith & Rayatt 2004).

Chemical burns

Common injuries occur from contact with acids and alkalines, as well as domestic substances, such as bleach and cleaning agents. The severity of the burn injury will be determined by the type of chemical, its concentration and the length of time it is in contact with the patient's skin (Cook 1997).

Prehospital management The treatment priority lies with removal of caustic chemicals from the patient's skin. After rapid removal of soaked clothing, the patient should be showered by large amounts of running water to dilute and remove the chemical. Dry powders should be brushed off before decontamination with water commences (Wiebelhaus & Hansen 2001). Water has advantages over specific neutralizing solutions. The principal aim of decontamination is to minimize the period of contact between the contaminant and the skin. Time taken searching for particular antidotes leads to deeper levels of injury. More importantly, do not attempt to neutralize a chemical burn; this could cause exothermic reaction and further injury (Wiebelhaus & Hansen 2001). In most cases, adequate dilution reduces the risk of further damage.

Litmus testing of wet skin will indicate acidity or alkalinity, and a neutral buffer solution can be applied, if necessary, once the chemical is diluted sufficiently. In extensive chemical burns, absorption can have systemic effects, including alteration of the blood's acid-base and electrolyte balance, together with renal and hepatic damage (Herbert & Lawrence 1989). Where possible, the identity of the chemical should be established and local poison unit facilities contacted to provide information on specific reactions and antidotes (Settle 1995).

Chemical eye injuries require immediate attention (Glenn 1995). Signs and symptoms include:

- pain
- oedema and irritation of the eyelids
- reddened sclera
- loss of or blurred vision.

Periorbital skin irritation or damage should always increase suspicion of eye problems (Brooks 1989). Alkaline injuries are more serious than those involving acids because they rapidly penetrate the conjunctiva through to the cornea, causing significant long-term damage. In all chemical injuries, the eyes should be irrigated, with water initially and with the eyelids held open, until the contaminant is removed. This can be checked by gently placing litmus paper into the conjuctival sac. Insertion of a buffer neutralizing solution may be necessary to halt the injury process.

Ensure contact lenses are removed prior to irrigation to prevent a film of contaminant remaining between lens and cornea. The use of a local anaesthetic will relieve pain, reduce anxiety and allow easier examination and treatment. Once decontamination has been completed, antibiotic ointments should be prescribed and applied to reduce corneal scarring. All chemical eye injuries must be referred for specialist ophthalmological opinion (Okhravi 1997) (see also Ch. 30).

Electrical burns

These are sometimes more serious than they first appear, as there may be little superficial tissue loss; however, massive muscle injury may be present beneath normal-looking skin. Contact with high-voltage cables can lead to propulsion injuries. Domestic injury, although of lower voltage, can also cause significant damage. The electrical current takes the path of least resistance through the body, usually through the blood vessels, exiting through the earth contact. Small entry and exit points on the skin's surface may belie the amount of damage to the blood vessels, muscles and bone tissue beneath. In addition to direct heat damage caused by the progression of the current injury can be sustained by blood vessel necrosis, severe tetany of muscles, conductivity problems in the myocardium, and the force of propulsive impact, often severe enough to cause bone fractures. These patients often suffer secondary 'flash' burns.

Following electrical injury, cardiac monitoring should be used to detect possible arrhythmias. Depending on the path of the current, a 12-lead ECG should be performed to detect myocardial damage, which may occur at the time of injury or several hours afterwards as myocardial tissue breaks down. In serious cases, where there are ECG abnormalities or a loss of consciousness, 24 hours of monitoring is advised (Hettiaratchy & Dziewulski 2004). Jenkins (2005) suggests that while cardiac dysrhythmias may initially be seen, they may also be delayed for up to 24 hours. These include sinus bradycardia, right bundle branch block and focal ectopic dysrhythmias. Sutcliffe (1998) notes that ST elevation and QT elongation are other non-specific changes associated with severe burns.

Close attention should also be paid to renal function, which will be severely impaired by the release of proteins (myoglobin) from massive tissue breakdown. Hourly urine output should be observed after insertion of a urinary catheter. Darkened urine indicates that myoglobin is present and warrants immediate action to maintain renal function, including intravenous fluid therapy and possibly mannitol to create a high urine output and quickly flush out proteins from the kidneys (Settle 1995).

Cold burns (frostbite)

Although relatively uncommon in the UK, frostbite can be seen in individuals who have had prolonged exposure to extreme cold conditions. Immediate management of the patient concentrates on the monitoring and gradual increase of core body temperature. The extreme cold causes the formation of ice crystals and disrupts cell membranes; vasoconstriction of blood vessels leads to tissue necrosis and an increase in blood viscosity impairs capillary blood flow (Kemble & Lamb 1987). This occurs most commonly on exposed extremities such as fingertips, ear lobes and toes. With superficial frostbite, the frozen part is waxy white and does not blanch or show capillary refilling after mild pressure. The tissue below is soft and resilient on pressure and the affected part is anaesthetic. Rewarming is usually painful, and afterwards the appearance is initially erythematous and oedematous, progressing to a mottled purple colour. Blisters appear, lasting approximately 5–10 days, and eventually dry out leaving a black eschar associated with pain. Demarcation and separation occur over the next month, leaving a delicately epithelialized area which is the site of long-term hypersensitivity.

Deep frostbite occurs when the temperature of a limb is lowered (Morris 1998). The frozen part is waxy white and does not blanch or show capillary refilling after mild pressure. The tissue below is hard and cannot be compressed. The affected part is numb. Rewarming is often painful and afterwards the appearance is usually mottled blue (Mills et al. 1995). Frostbitten areas should be protected from further trauma, quickly reheated in warm water (around 38°C), dried and maintained at room temperature. Thawing frozen tissue is extremely painful, so intravenous analgesia may be given. Heparin therapy may be commenced together with intravenous Dextran 40 to improve peripheral blood flow. Swelling of the whole limb occurs or appears at the demarcation line several weeks later. If necrosis has occurred, the areas are usually allowed to demarcate before amputation surgery is carried out.

Radiation

These are most commonly caused through overexposure to sunlight or sunbeds. The burns are usually superficial but slow to heal due to injury thromboangitis. More serious injury occurs from exposure to nuclear substances or accidents in radiotherapy. Acute radiation syndrome is a symptom complex that occurs following whole-body irradiation. It varies in nature and severity depending on dose, dose rate, distribution and individual susceptibility.

Pre-hospital management Decontamination is necessary in cases of nuclear exposure. If the patient's condition permits, this should be initiated at the scene. Ambulance personnel should wear protective clothing, including rubber gloves and shoe covers. The patient's clothing should be removed and placed in plastic bags and, if possible, soap and water cleansing of exposed skin should be performed. Performing these tasks will minimize contamination of the ambulance and emergency department, most of which are not currently well designed for decontamination patients.

Assessment and management The receiving hospital should be given as much information as possible about the numbers and types of patients involved in a radiation exposure incident, as a decision will need to be made regarding implementation of a full disaster plan versus a limited response. Ideally, contaminated patients should enter the department through a separate, protected entrance. All health care personnel should wear protective, disposable clothing, including surgical gloves and shoe covers. If not already done, the patient should be immediately undressed and washed and all clothing placed in sealed containers labelled 'radioactive waste'. If the patient has open wounds, the surrounding skin should be decontaminated by scrubbing with soap and water. Wounds should be irrigated with copious amounts of saline. The normal principles of wound closure should be followed. No danger to health care personnel should exist if proper precautions are carried out (Markovchick 1992).

Non-accidental injury

Detecting these injuries is important as it is estimated that 3–10% of paediatric burns are due to non-accidental injury (NAI) (Hettiaratchy and Dziewulski 2004). As with other NAIs, the history and the pattern of injury may arouse suspicion.

Assessment and management

Initial treatment of the physical burn injury is paramount. The team should also carry out the following:

- examine for other signs of abuse
- photograph all injuries
- obtain other medical information (from general practitioner, health visitor)
- interview family members separately about the incident to check for inconsistencies and together to observe interaction (Hettiaratchy and Dziewulski 2004).

Any suspicion of NAI should lead to immediate admission of the child to hospital, irrespective of the burn injury, and notification to social services (see also Pre-school children).

BURN WOUND CARE

Initial management of burn wounds

The aims are:

- to limit further damage with appropriate first aid measures
- to assess the depth of injury, in order to determine treatment plan
- to maintain perfusion and protect damaged tissue from desiccation and infection.

Measurement of burn depth

Burns can be divided into two categories: partial- and full-thickness skin damage. Partial-thickness burns are subcategorized into superficial and deep.

Superficial burn injuries   involve skin loss from epidermis only (Fig. 10.4). The dermal capillaries dilate and fluid leaks into the surrounding tissues. This causes increased pressure on intact nerve endings, which results in a reddened painful wound, with good capillary refill. Pain and swelling usually subside within 48 hours and it will heal by epithelialization over a period of about 7 days. These burns usually leave no scarring.!

Deeper partial-thickness burns involve both epidermal and dermal damage of varying depths (Fig. 10.5). Capillary destruction occurs, which results in fluid escaping to form blisters or a shiny wet wound surface. The wound appears less red than a superficial injury and may have some white avascular areas. Nerve supply is sometimes damaged and generally these wounds are less painful than superficial wounds. Sensation is not lost and the patient should be able to distinguish between blunt and sharp. These burns heal by regeneration, usually within 14 days.

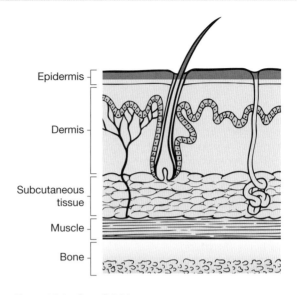

Figure 10.4   Superficial burn.

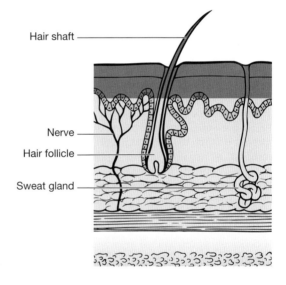

Figure 10.5   Partial-thickness burn.

Full-thickness burns   involve all of the dermal layer and may involve underlying structures such as muscle, tendon and bone (Fig. 10.6). The upper skin layers are destroyed, the wound is avascular and appears white or charred, capillary return is absent, and wound exudate is minimal. Sensation is reduced or absent in full-thickness burns. These injuries heal by granulation. Because of the vascular damage, blood supply is reduced and so necrosis and infection are common. Full-thickness burns often require surgical debridement.

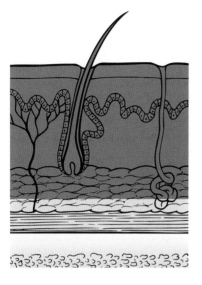

Figure 10.6 Full-thickness burn.

Protection of wound Asepsis is of paramount importance with burn injuries because of the inherent infection risk. Wounds should be cleaned by irrigation with saline. Irrigation reduces the risk of tissue damage when compared with other cleaning methods, and is less painful for the patient. As saline is isotonic, it is unlikely to cause irritation to tissue. Burned clothing, dirt and devitalized tissue should be carefully removed as part of the cleaning process (Copley & Glencorse 1992). Controversy exists over the management of blisters. Although the fluid contained in blisters promotes healing, and the roof of the blister provides an effective cover of protection and, from a practical perspective, many patients find it extremely painful to have a blister de-roofed in the first day or two following burn injury (Cole 2003), it is thought the size and weight of the blister creates a risk of traumatic shearing which can increase the extent of the wound (Collier 2000). To remove this risk, larger blisters should be de-roofed and dead skin removed with sterile scissors (Hudspith & Rayatt 2004). The optimum approach is to aspirate blister fluid, removing the shearing risk and leaving the blister roof in place to act as a natural dressing (Copley & Glencorse 1992).

Exposed wounds have a faster rate of fluid loss than covered wounds (Dziewulski 1992). Wound care should focus on reinstating the functions lost by the destruction of skin, control of body temperature, maintenance of fluid balance and providing a barrier to infection (Collier 2006, Clarke 1992a). For major burn wounds, the replacement of skin functions is the only reason for dressings; they should be simple

and not include creams or lotions. The initial treatment of choice is PVC clingfilm (Allison 2002). It reduces evaporate fluid loss and provides a protective barrier to infection. It is also transparent, allowing continual visual inspection of the wound. Clingfilm can be used next to skin or over wet compresses. It is easy to apply and painless to remove. Clingfilm should not be applied to the face for obvious reasons. The patient needs additional protection against heat loss. It is important to check the patient's tetanus status and administer tetanus toxoid if the patient is not covered. Systemic antibiotics have not proven effective in preventing wound infections (Dziewulski 1992). They should not be used as a prophylactic measure because they increase the risk of resistant bacteria developing (Lawrence 1992).

Pain control

Most patients with burn injuries will experience pain and, after immediate life-saving interventions, pain control should be treated as a priority (Kinsella & Booth 1991). The psychological response to burn injury should not be underestimated when assessing a patient's pain. The euphoria of survival and ignorance or denial of the full impact of injury can result in a transient period of little or no pain. Fear and insight into potential outcomes can also have an effect on the extent and type of pain the patient feels. It is imperative that the ED nurse recognizes psychological influences and uses both pharmacological and psychological methods to achieve pain control.

Assessment of pain should include:

- psychological state
- verbal responses
- facial expression
- mobility
- protecting injured areas
- posture.

It is uncommon for an injury to be solely full-thickness (Settle 1995). It is more likely that the wound will be of mixed depth, and therefore some nerve endings will be intact, causing pain. Pain relief starts with the application of cold water and the burn wound being covered from the air.

Initial treatment in ED can include the use of inhaled nitrous oxide (Entonox) in the conscious patient unless associated injuries prevent this. Nitrous oxide has a rapid effect and gives the patient control over their own pain relief (Toulson 1990). Because it is self-administered, there is an inherent safeguard against overdose.

For major burn injuries, patients should be given small, frequent doses of intravenous opioids until pain relief is achieved (Copely & Glencorse 1992). Intramuscular or subcutaneous routes are inappropriate because of hypovolaemia, which causes reduced peripheral circulation and results in poor absorption of the drug and inadequate pain control. Intramuscular and subcutaneous routes also carry the risk of respiratory or CNS depression. This is because a delayed absorption of the drug takes place as circulation improves. Because this happens rapidly, an overdose effect can occur (Kinsella & Booth 1991).

Assessment of pain should include the observation of non-verbal behaviour, such as facial expressions, distorted posture, splinting and impaired mobility, in addition to verbal responses (Kinsella & Booth 1991). This may also give an indication of other traumatic injuries, especially if the patient has been involved in an RTA, explosion or high voltage injury (Bueno & Demling 1989) (see also Chapter 24).

Escharotomies

Escharotomies are carried out where circumferential full-thickness burns occur around limbs, chest, neck, digits or penis. As oedema develops in the tissue beneath, the relatively inflexible full-thickness injury cannot compensate for the increase in tissue volume and exerts a tourniquet effect. If the increasing pressure is not released at an early stage, usually within 3 hours, ischaemic damage will occur in tissues distal to the burn (Settle 1995). In the case of the chest and neck, the rigidity compromises the expansion of the lungs (Judkins 1992). The procedure is carried out by making longitudinal incisions with a sterile blade through the burned skin to bleeding tissue. The release of tension forces the wound to gape open. An absorbent haemostatic dressing, such as calcium alginate, can be placed into the wounds to arrest bleeding. Because the burns are full-thickness in nature, relatively little analgesia is required (Kinsella & Booth 1990). Although they are an urgent procedure, escharotomies are best done in an operating theatre by experienced staff. Initially, at risk limbs should be observed for signs of impaired circulation, looking at perfusion, capillary refill, temperature and sensation (Molter & Greenfield 1997). Rings, watches, restrictive clothing and tight dressings should be removed and the limbs elevated above heart level to reduce swelling. Controversies surrounding escharotomies are not new and alternatives should be considered in the management of acute burns (Burd et al. 2006).

Psychological considerations

Burn injuries produce highly emotive responses because of their association with loss of life, pain and scarring. The psychological impact can be devastating for the patient, relatives and those required to deal with the aftermath.

The patient

Initial reactions vary, and some patients will exhibit 'shock', bewilderment and disorientation, with an apparent denial of injury linked to internal defence mechanisms to reduce the anxiety associated with severe injury (Blumenfield & Schoeps 1993). Many patients also experience an initial euphoria associated with survival (Copley & Glencorse 1992). Often the significance of injury is not appreciated, particularly where full-thickness damage is involved or where respiratory complications have not had time to develop. Others may be distressed because of pain and anxiety caused by an awareness of the seriousness of their condition (Kinsella & Booth 1991).

Relatives

The fact that the patient is alert, able to talk and not in any great distress can often lead friends and family into a false sense of security, reinforcing a denial that serious injury has taken place (Konigova 1992). For some, the sight of the patient in pain or with facial or hand burns can be very distressing and cause relatives to fear much worse consequences than will actually be the case. Honest, informative support from experienced ED staff is necessary.

Staff

Burn injuries, particularly those as a result of fires, have characteristics that are not shared with other forms of trauma. The smell of burned skin and degree of suffering witnessed, especially where death occurs, can be very upsetting even to experienced staff. Staff support is crucial; however, the nature of support needs to be tangible and flexible in order to respond to individual needs (Regel 1997) (see also Chapter 12).

Transfer to specialist units

Although policies for admission vary, Box 10.4 lists the types of burn injury considered serious enough to warrant specialist attention (NBCR 2001, Bird 1999).

Burns units offer a concentration of resources, in terms of experienced staff and specialized facilities.

Box 10.4   Burn injuries requiring transfer to specialist units. (From Kemble & Lamb 1987)

- **Major burns** – partial- or full-thickness burns involving more than 5% of the total body surface area in babies, 10% in children or 15% in adults.
- **Burns involving inhalation injury**
- **Full–thickness burns** – greater than 2.5 cm in diameter, where skin grafting or flap reconstruction will be necessary to facilitate healing and improve scarring
- **Electrical and chemical burns** – both are often more serious than they at first appear and require specific care
- **Burns involving specific problematic areas** – these include the hands and feet, face, perineum and major joints
- **Burns in those with other problems** – e.g. diabetes, epilepsy, the elderly or where child abuse is suspected

Each unit tends to be highly individualized, with its own protocol for admission. For this reason it is difficult to draw up a definitive etiquette for transferring burn-injured patients. It might, however, be useful to consider the following points when planning a transfer. And remember: *safety is more important than speed.*

Any attempt at transfer must not be considered until the patient is in a stable condition and prepared in such a way that any risk of deterioration in transit is greatly reduced. The airway must be fully assessed and measures must be taken to maintain a patent airway during transfer to reduce the risk of obstruction. An experienced escort, including an anaesthetist where there is airway and respiratory involvement, is essential and the transfer vehicle must be suitably furnished with oxygen, suction and resuscitation equipment. Bird (1999) recommends endotracheal intubation prior to leaving ED. Intravenous access must be established using two wide-bore cannula. Adequate fluid replacement should be commenced and sustained throughout transfer and the patient should be catheterized with accurate measurement and recording before and during transfer. Similar attention must be paid to analgesia. If the patient has suffered electrical injury, myoglobins/haemoglobins in the urine may lead to catheter blockage so should be observed carefully. The patient should be transferred in a warm vehicle, well insulated with blankets, and equipment should have batteries, including spares, sufficient for the journey. Wet dressings are not necessary at this stage (Ellis & Rylah 1990).

Although the initial referral is carried out by medical staff, verbal communication between nursing personnel in the emergency department and receiving burns unit, prior to transfer, is essential. It is worth drawing up a list of local units and their telephone numbers for ease of reference. Confirm with the nurse in charge that a bed is available. Give preliminary verbal information including:

- the name and age of the patient
- relevant medical record
- brief history and time of the incident
- causative agent, petrol, electricity, chemical etc.
- extent, i.e. percentage area involved
- nature of other injuries sustained, particularly any inhalation involvement
- time of accident to commencement of first aid
- time of accident to commencement of fluid resuscitation
- time of departure and estimated arrival time
- whether the patient should be transferred directly to the burns unit or the receiving hospital emergency department.

It is difficult to convey large amounts of complex information by verbal means alone. Therefore, when handing over to burns unit staff, the escorting nurse must have clearly written details, documenting the points outlined above and specifically:

- the patient's clinical observations
- fluid input and urine output, including that during the transfer
- laboratory results, including FBC, U&E, coagulation screen
- blood gas and carboxyhaemoglobin results
- tetanus status
- any medications given
- GP details
- next of kin and relevant social history
- contact name and number of investigating police officers if involved.

Accurate and effective communication improves the continuity of care and allows burns unit specialists to make early decisions about the future course of treatment. It may prove useful to obtain constructive feedback from the burns unit about the transfer procedure and the patient's recovery. This information can be used either to improve the department's future performance or to confirm to those involved that they fulfilled their roles to a satisfactory standard.

Minor burn wound care

Minor burns tend to be classified as those which can be treated on an outpatient basis. The injury usually represents less than 5% of the body surface area and excludes some of the problematic body areas (Duncan & Driscoll 1991) (see Box 10.5).

The patient's social circumstances should be considered and their level of support/aid assessed before a decision to discharge is taken. The initial burn injury causes significant disruption to normal skin function. Heat causes cellular injury, resulting in a breakdown of the skin's protective barrier and a susceptibility to infection. The wound itself is initially controlled by the body's natural inflammatory response. Oedema and exudate are rapidly produced, which can to some extent be minimized by cooling the wound and reducing further cellular damage (Cole 2003).

The area of the injury has three specific parts (Rylah 1992) (Fig. 10.7):

- the zone of necrosis – this is non-viable, or dead, tissue usually found at the centre of the wound
- the zone of stasis – this is the area of the wound which is most vulnerable and potentially salvageable; it consists of viable tissue, but is at risk of ischaemic damage because of reduced tissue perfusion

- the zone of hyperaemia – this is the area immediately surrounding the damage (outermost zone), which is undergoing the inflammatory phase to injury; the tissue itself is undamaged and develops an increased blood flow in an attempt to control the extent of injury.

The healing of a burn wound depends very much on the depth of injury. Superficial and partial-thickness burns involving the epidermis and upper dermal layers will only heal spontaneously by epithelialization and regeneration over a period of 7–14 days. It is this group of injuries which are best treated on an outpatient basis. Deeper partial-thickness burns, with damage to all but the deep dermal layers, will heal much more slowly over a period of 3–4 weeks. Full-thickness burns heal by granulation, a process which can take several weeks or months depending on the size of the injury, its site and the patient's general health and age. This group of patients benefit from referral to specialist units for excision and grafting of wounds.

For those patients who can be discharged, wound care and appropriate advice are paramount. The primary aim is to foster an environment which is appropriate to the healing needs of the wound at a particular stage (see Table 10.3).

Wound cleaning, as discussed above, should be as rigorous for small or minor wounds as for major burns. Differences in management occur in the assessment of wound dressings needed (Edwards 2006).

Box 10.5 Areas of special concern

- Circumferential injury of a limb
- Face
- Eyes
- Ears
- Hands
- Feet
- Perineal injury

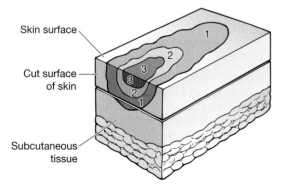

Figure 10.7 Pathophysiology of a burn wound. 1, Zone of hyperaemia; 2, Zone of stasis; 3, Zone of necrosis.

Table 10.3 Stages of wound healing

Stage	Features of healing
Inflammatory (0–3 days)	Initial response to injury causes redness, heat, pain and swelling with copious exudate
Destruction (2–5 days)	Clearing of devitalized tissue and bacteria and development of fibroblasts
Proliferation (3–24 days)	Production of collagen and granulation tissue which fills the wound space. Although it may look 'healed' the wound remains very fragile
Maturation (24 days–1 year)	This focuses on restructuring scar tissue; vascularity decreases and redness fades. The wound area strengthens and by 6 weeks scar tissue has about 50% of the tensile strength of uninjured skin
Contraction (4 days onwards)	Process whereby the wound naturally reduces in size. Usually only occurs in large wounds with considerable tissue loss

Most major injuries will not have their full extent and depth assessed for 48 hours until oedema begins to subside (Pankhurst 1997). For smaller wounds, the aims of burns dressings are to prevent colonization by bacteria, to provide a warm, moist environment for cellular reconstruction, to absorb exudate and to protect the area from further injury.

Dressing care for burns patients may vary according to local policy. However, ED care usually focuses around the inflammatory stage, where copious exudate is present, and the destructive phase where autolysis demands a moist environment. Initially, a multiple layer of paraffin tulle-type dressing, applied under copious padding and bandages, will provide a warm non-adherent, protective dressing for the inflammatory phase. The disadvantage with this method is that, if the dressing soaks through, a tract for infection is created and the patient will need to return to ED for renewal. These types of dressing should be changed at least daily. Antibacterial agents such as silver sulfadiazine cream or an advanced silver dressing such as Acticoat® (Smith & Nephew) are useful in preventing Gram-negative or *Pseudomonas* infections in the initial stages. For the cream to remain effective, it should be reapplied daily for the first 3 days (Holt 1998). The reapplication of the cream and the removal technique, which requires manual cleansing of the wound over exposed nerve endings, are undoubtedly a painful experience. Adequate analgesia for the patient should be considered before and during dressing changes (Varas et al. 2005). In comparison, the benefit of the newer advanced silver dressings is that the often painful dressing changes associated with the cream are avoided as the dressing can be left intact for 3 days. For usage of either product the manufacturer's guidelines should be followed.

After 48 hours, as the wound enters the destructive phase, exudate begins to reduce and the wound benefits from less-frequent dressing changes (Clarke 1992b). Hydrocolloid dressings are most effective for this stage of healing. They provide a warm and moist environment which facilitates autolysis and natural debridement of the wound. For maximum effectiveness, these dressings should be left in situ for 4–7 days depending on the site and extent of the wound. Hydrocolloid dressings are also valuable in the treatment of granulating wounds.

Facial burns. Facial burns should be referred to a specialist unit, unless the injury is simple, e.g.

sunburn. Burns to facial areas should be kept moist with soft paraffin ointment and left exposed. Antibacterial creams should not be used as they can cause skin staining when in contact with oxygen. Ears are the exception to this. Silver sulfadiazine should be applied and the area covered with paraffin tulle and padding. This is because the risk of complications from infection includes ear deformity and internal structural damage.

Hands and feet. One of the treatment priorities is to maintain movement. For this reason, wounds are treated with antibacterial cream and covered with polythene bags or gloves. This allows for observation of the wound as well as movement of digits. Wounds treated in this way require daily dressing changes. Unfortunately, dressings applied to the burnt hand and individual fingers are often bulky (Kok et al. 2006). For further information on wound care see Chapter 23.

Discharge information should include advice about wound care and when to return to ED, but should also include advice on:

- nutrition to promote wound healing
- exercise regimes to restore normal function
- wound progress and scarring.

Psychological support should also be provided at this time, by allowing the patient to express fears or uncertainty about management of the injury as well as to ask any general questions he may have about care.

Conclusion

Caring for a patient with burn injuries represents a multifocal challenge to ED staff. Priorities of care must be with the systematic assessment and implementation of life-saving activities, such as airway management and fluid resuscitation. Protection of burn wounds is imperative if secondary injury and infection are to be prevented. The initiation of wound care and patient education are important for those with minor injuries. All patients need time and psychological support to come to terms with their injury, as even minor wounds create high levels of anxiety about scarring. However, the emergency nurse can do much to alleviate the physical and psychological suffering of the burns patient.

References

Allison K (2002) The UK pre-hospital management of burn patients: current practice and the need for a standard approach. *Burns*, **28**(2), 135–142.

American College of Surgeons (2004) *Advanced Trauma Life Support*. 7th edn. Chicago: American College of Surgeons.

Bird D (1999) Transferring the thermally injured. *Emergency Nurse*, **7**(6), 14–17.

Blumenfield M, Schoeps MM (1993) Psychological reactions to burn and trauma. In: Blumenfield M, Schoeps MM, eds. *Psychological Care of the Burn and Trauma Patient*. Boston: Williams & Wilkins.

Brooks J (1989) Managing eye injuries. *Practice Nurse*, **4**, 451–452.

Bueno R, Demling RH (1989) Management of burns in the multiple trauma patient. In: Maull KI, ed. *Advances in Trauma*, Vol. 4. Philadelphia: Year Book Medical Publishers.

Burd A, Noronha FV, Ahmed K, Chan JYW, Ayyappan T, Ying SY, Pang P (2006) Decompression not escharotomy in acute burns. *Burns*, **32**(3), 284–292.

Campbell A (2000) Hospital management of poisoning in victims suffering from smoke inhalation. *Emergency Nurse*, **8**(4), 12–16.

Clarke JA (1992a) Burns and the burn wound. *Care of the Critically Ill*, **8**(6), 233.

Clarke JA (1992b) *A Colour Atlas of Burn Injury*. London: Chapman & Hall.

Cole E (2003) Wound management in the A&E department. *Nursing Standard*, **17**(46), 45–52.

Collier M (2000) Expert comment on managing burn blisters. *Nursing Times*, **96**(4), 20.

Collier M (2006) The use of advanced biological and tissue-engineered wound products. *Nursing Standard*, **21**(7), 68–76.

Cook D (1997) Pathophysiology of burns. In: Bosworth C, ed. *Burns Trauma: Management and Nursing Care*. London: Baillière Tindall.

Copley J, Glencorse C (1992) The nursing management of burns. *Care of the Critically Ill*, **8**(6), 246–251.

Duncan DJ, Driscoll DM (1991) Burn wound management. *Critical Care Clinics of North America*, **3**(2), 255–267.

Dunn KW (2000) *Standards and Strategy for Burn Care: A Review of Burn Care in the British Isles*. London: National Burn Care Review Committee Report.

Dziewulski P (1992) Burn wound healing: James Ellsworth Laing Memorial essay for 1991. *Burns*, **18**(6), 466–478.

Edwards SL (2006) Tissue viability: understanding the mechanisms of injury and repair. *Nursing Standard*, **21**(13), 48–56.

Ellis A, Rylah LTA (1990) Transfer of the thermally injured patient. *British Journal of Hospital Medicine*, **44**(3), 200–206.

Glenn S (1995) Care of patients with chemical eye injury. *Emergency Nurse*, **3**(3), 7–9.

Hantson P, Butera R, Clemessey JL, Michel A, Baud FJ (1997) Early complications and value of initial clinical and paraclinical observations in victims of smoke inhalation without burns. *Chest*, **111**(3), 671–675.

Herbert K, Lawrence J (1989) Chemical burns. *Burns*, **15**(60), 381–384.

Herndon D (2007) *Total Burn Care*. Philadelphia: Saunders.

Hettiaratchy S, Dziewulski P (2004) Pathophysiology and types of burns. *British Medical Journal*, **328**, 1427–1429.

Hettiaratchy S, Papini R (2004) Initial management of a major burn: assessment and resuscitation. *British Medical Journal*, **329**, 101–104.

Holt L (1998) Assessing and managing minor burns. *Emergency Nurse*, **6**(2), 14–16.

Hudspith J, Rayatt S (2004) First aid and treatment of minor burns. *British Medical Journal*, **328**, 1487–1489.

Jenkins L (2005) Care of the patient with major burns. In: O'Shea RA, ed. *Principles and Practice of Trauma Nursing*. Edinburgh: Churchill Livingstone Elsevier.

Jones R (2003) Smoke inhalation: assessing and managing patients. *Emergency Nurse*, **11**(7), 18–23.

Judkins KC (1992) Burns and respiratory system injury. *Care of the Critically Ill*, **8**(6), 238–241.

Kemble JV, Lamb BE (1987) *Practical Burns Management*. London: Hodder & Stoughton.

Kinsella J, Booth MG (1991) Pain relief in burns: James Laing Memorial essay 1990. *Burns*, **17**(5), 391–395.

Kok K, Georgeu GA, Wilson VY (2006) The acticoat glove: an effective dressing for the completely burnt hand. *Burns*, **32**(4), 487–489.

Konigova R (1992) The psychological problems of burned patients: the Rudy Hermans Lecture 1991. *Burns*, **18**(3), 189–199.

Lawrence JC (1992) Infective complications of burns. *Care of the Critically Ill*, **8**(6), 234–236.

Lund C, Browder N (1944) Estimation of areas of burns. *Surgery, Gynaecology & Obstetrics*, **79**, 352–358.

Markovchick M (1992) Radiation injuries. In: Rose P, Barkin RM, Braen G et al. eds. *Emergency Medicine: Concepts and Clinical Practice*, 3rd edn. St Louis: Mosby.

McParkland M (1999) Carbon monoxide poisoning. *Emergency Nurse*, **7**(6), 18–22.

Mills K, Morton R, Page G (1995) *Colour Atlas and Text of Emergencies*, 2nd edn. London: Mosby-Wolfe.

Molter NC, Greenfield E (1997) Burns. In: Hartshorn HC, Sole MI, Lamborn ML, eds. *Introduction to Critical Care Nursing*, 2nd edn. Philadelphia: WB Saunders.

Morris J (1998) Environmental emergencies. In: Newberry , ed. *Sheehy's Emergency Nursing: Principles and Practice*, 4th edn. St Louis: Mosby.

Muehlberger T, Kunar D, Munster A, Couch M (1998) Efficacy of fibreoptic laryngoscopy in the diagnosis of inhalation injuries. *Archives of Otolaryngology Head & Neck Surgery*, **124**(9), 1003–1007.

National Burn Care Review (2001) National burn injury referral guidelines. In: *Standards and strategy for burn care*. London: NBCR.

Pankhurst S (1997) Wound care. In: Bosworth C, ed. *Burns Trauma: Management and Nursing Care*. London: Baillière Tindall.

Regel S (1997) Staff support on the burns unit. In: Bosworth C, ed. *Burns Trauma: Management and Nursing Care*. London: Baillière Tindall.

Rylah LTA (1992) *Critical Care of the Burned Patient*. Cambridge: Cambridge University Press.

Settle JAD (1995) *Burns: the First Five Days*. Romford: Smith and Nephew.

Sutcliffe AJ (1998) Electrical injuries and the critical care physician. *Care of the Critically Ill*, **14**, 102–105.

Swearingham P, Keen J (1991) *Manual of Critical Care*, 2nd edn. St Louis: Mosby Year Book.

Toulson S (1990) More than a lot of hot air. *Nursing*, **4**(2), 23–26.

Varas RP, O'Keeffe T, Namias N, Pizano LR, Quintana OD, Tellachea MH, Rashid Q, Ward CG (2005) A prospective randomized trial of acticoat versus silver sulfadiazine in the treatment of partial-thickness burns: which method is less painful? *Journal of Burn Care & Rehabilitation*, 26(4), 344–347.

Wiebelhaus P, Hansen SL (2001) What you should know about managing burn emergencies. *Nursing*, **31**(1), 36–41.

Wilding PA (1990) Care of respiratory burns: hard work can bring spectacular results. *Professional Nurse*, **5**, 412–420.

Wilson D (1997) Management in the first 48 hours following burn trauma. In: Bosworth C, ed. *Burns Trauma: Management and Nursing Care*. London: Baillière Tindall.

Wilson GR, Fowler CA, Housden PL (1987) A new burn area assessment chart. *Burns*, **13**(5), 401–405.

PART 3

Psychological dimensions

Chapter **11**

Violence and aggression

Barbara L Neades & Kirsty Jack

INTRODUCTION

Violence and aggression are recognized major hazards for staff within the health care sector. The fields of mental health, learning disability and emergency care, unsurprisingly, report the highest incidence of verbal and physical threats to staff (Health and Safety Commission 1997). The frequent occurrence of violence within the Emergency Department (ED) has been frequently documented (Cembrowicz & Shepherd 1992; Erickson & Williams-Evans 2000; Stirling et al. 2002; James et al. 2006, Luck et al. 2007). While far from, being the only area within the general hospital setting to see a rise in violence, a major stimulus to the Department of Health 'Zero Tolerance' campaign (Department of Health 2000) was the growing level of aggression witnessed within the ED. Although prevention of aggression and violence is the aim, it may not always be possible to stop this occurring in the ED environment. This may be a result of the wide variety of factors that can influence the development of aggression in the ED, some of which are beyond the control of the department.

ED nurses will care for all sorts of human conditions and problems every day of their working lives, most of which will be a result of sudden illness or injury. The nature of these events will produce intense emotions and reactions, some of which will be displayed as aggression. A review of the management of aggression and violence undertaken by the UKCC (2001) suggested that most aggressive incidents within healthcare are not recorded and is therefore it is difficult to measure the problem accurately. Whittington & Wykes (1989) demonstrated that verbal abuse and minor injuries can have a significant effect on the individuals involved, including staff and other individuals who are witnesses or who are involved in an incident. These incidents have a negative impact on the relationship between the professionals and their clients and standard of care provided.

If staff are to attempt to resolve aggression in ED, it is necessary to assess and manage the problem from a holistic and caring viewpoint, maintaining the safety and dignity of everyone involved. This requires the nurse to identify the factors which influence aggression in the ED situation, develop strategies designed to prevent it occurring and managing the aggressive situation effectively when it does occur, protecting the patient, staff and any other individuals involved. This chapter will discuss the problem from these perspectives and offer some suggestions to assist the ED nurse to resolve this increasing difficulty.

WHY AGGRESSION OCCURS IN THE ED

Assessing the source of an aggressive situation in the ED offers particular difficulties to the staff, as there can be a number of factors influencing its development. These include attitudes and responses of staff, the internal state of the individual and the environment of the ED. Standing & Nicolini (1997) argued that the highest risks of violence at work are associated with:

- dealing with the public
- providing care or advice
- working with confused older people
- working with those who have mental health problems
- alcohol or drug misuse
- working alone
- handling valuables or medication
- working with people under stress.

The Royal College of Nursing (1998) noted that many or all of these features are present in the work undertaken by most nurses. Inadequate resources, low staffing levels and inappropriate skill mix also form significant contributory factors. The ED can appear a very hostile and threatening place to a patient or relative in an emotionally charged state. Brennan (1998), in examining the range of theories of aggression and violence, suggested that providing satisfactory definitions or an explanation as to where or how these behaviours originate, is a complex task.

From a psychological perspective, the occurrence of a sudden crisis resulting from a serious illness or accident, with the hurried removal of an individual to an ED, can often trigger strong emotions (Hildegard et al. 1987). These emotions of fear, anxiety, confusion and loss of control often result in stress reactions within the patient or relative and can be displayed in a variety of ways (Farrell & Gray 1992). Many individuals view the ED as an anxiety-provoking and hostile environment. In these situations adrenaline is released and the classical 'fight or flight' response is triggered.

Freud (1932) argued that aggression was an innate, independent, instinctual tendency in humans. Dollard et al. (1939) suggested the hydraulic type model of aggression where he viewed the need to release built-up frustration as a natural event. The suggestion was that when frustration accumulated there was a resultant explosive release displayed as aggression, similar to that of a pressure cooker effect. In contrast, Bandura (1973) identified the way in which children learn aggressive responses, by role modelling what they had observed in adults. Bateson (1980) further argued that an individual is only aggressive when assessed in relation to the other people or surroundings affecting that individual. Other suggest that a major concern was the modelling and frequency of aggression in the media (Berkowitz 1993) and the impact this had on society, especially the impact of violence in films (Gross 1996).

Contributing physiological factors in the development of aggression in the ED include the high consumption or withdrawal from alcohol or drugs (Kaplan and Sadock 1993). Intoxication with these drugs not only reduces the individual's capacity to understand and interpret events but also reduces inhibitory responses in times of stress. Violent incidents in the ED are more likely to occur within the hours of 00.00–07.00, with alcohol being identified as a major cause of violent behaviour (Schnieden & Marren-Bell 1995). This was also a finding of study by James et al. (2006), who noted that assailants were more likely to live in deprived areas.

Other organic reactions seen in acute confusional states, e.g. metabolic disorders, for example, diabetes or hypoxia resulting from respiratory or head-injury problem, may result in altered perceptions for the patient. These alterations in perception may also result in a confused aggressive patient arriving in the ED. When admitting these patients, the nurse may have to utilize very well-developed communication skills in order to make himself/herself understood. In this condition the patient may also experience major problems in perceiving what is happening. The frustration of not understanding can result in aggression as a self-defence mechanism (Taylor & Ryrie 1996).

From a sociological viewpoint, the location of the ED, near to the public street, and with 24-hour access may also attract a number of hostile individuals. Distressed or psychologically disturbed patients often attend EDs aware of the immediate access to medical and nursing care for crisis intervention (RCN/NICE 2005). Their confused or distressed state may also result in aggressive responses to the ED staff (James et al. 2006). The increasing level in society of gang and domestic violence also appears to impact on the occurrence of aggression and violence in the ED (Brantly 1992; Hoag-Apel 1998). Hostility can also be a response to pain, the severity of which often increases with long waits to see medical staff in ED (Wright 1986).

From an organizational perspective the ED itself can also influence the level of aggression displayed by patients and relatives who attend. The frustration that results from unrealistic expectations of the ED service may produce conflict and confrontation between the nurse and the patient or relative. Lack of information and long waiting times for treatment as a result of poor staffing levels can lead to frustration and anger (Jenkins et al. 1998). Poor waiting environments with lack of stimulation have also been suggested as being influential in developing aggression. Judgemental attitudes and behaviours adopted by staff can result in confrontation between the nurse and the patient or relative. Observers highlight how the lack of self awareness of our own responses and behaviours in an aggressive situation can provoke further aggression (Farrell & Gray 1992) and can also lead to non-therapeutic behaviours being adopted by staff (Stuart 1983). These include:

- defensiveness
- condescension
- avoidance.

Other research into aggression and violence suggests that less experienced staff who demonstrated a more authoritarian attitude were potentially more at risk of assault (Breakwell & Rowett 1989). Further studies identify certain characteristics which might be associated with some of assaulted staff, and make them more prone to being assaulted (Lanza et al. 1991). The key element in all these studies is the nurse's ability to communicate in a positive and caring manner with the patient or client. The nurse's verbal and non-verbal communications with the patient or relative are demonstrated to be very important in conveying a caring understanding attitude to an individual in times of stress or crisis, and in averting confrontation or aggression (Vaughan-Bowie 1996). It is acknowledged, however, that it may be difficult for the nurse to mask their underlying negative views on a patient and prevent negative non-verbal cues from being transmitted (Farrell & Gray 1992). Poor staffing of EDs, where there is a considerable workload, may also contribute to an atmosphere of tension. In these conditions, the nurse

may be under pressure to care for a large number of patients at any given time. This lack of time to care for the patient adequately may convey an impression of lack of interest in the patient and relatives, resulting in negative non-verbal cues from the nurse and provoking aggressive confrontations. It is clear therefore that not all aspects of aggression in the ED are preventable, although a number of influential factors do contribute to the occurrence of aggression (Ward 1995). If nurses are to resolve the problem of aggression, a comprehensive review of the preventable factors must be undertaken.

PREVENTION OF AGGRESSION IN THE ED

The environment into which the patient or relative is received can have a major effect on the response to the stressful events experienced. Poor communication between staff and patients on admission and inadequate waiting areas with few or no facilities for stimulation or refreshments can cause frustration in both the patient and relatives. Lack of information and increasing waiting times to see a doctor can often trigger aggressive confrontations between the ED nurse and the patient or relative. Mason and Chandley (1999) suggest that there is a recognized cycle of aggression development which can be divided into three phases (see Fig. 11.1):

- relative norm phase
- pre-aggressive phase
- crisis phase.

When applied to the ED, the relative norm phase could be viewed as the communication and health care information supplied or interventions undertaken on behalf of the patient and relative whilst they wait for treatment or decisions to be made relating to their care. Simple measures that provide the patient or relative with information, such as clear displays of waiting times and comfortable surroundings in which to wait, can relieve the anxiety and tension that may result in aggression. Careful consideration of seating arrangements and decor of the ED can help to reduce stress in those waiting to be treated. Other measures such as providing up-to-date reading material and a TV or radio within the waiting area can reduce the boredom and frustration so often experienced while waiting in the ED. The use of videos or DVDs explaining the ED's organization or providing healthcare information can reduce tension and anxiety in the waiting area. These measures can also be employed to provide health promotion advice to the public. The provision of information is easily the most important issue to stressed relatives and friends, with other

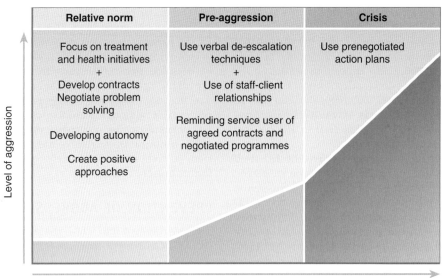

Figure 11.1   The Aggression Cycle (adapted from Mason & Chandley 1999).

environmental factors also impacting on the level of anxiety and frustration experienced by the patient or relative in ED (see Box 11.1).

Box 11.1   Reducing the risk of violence

Environmental factors
- All areas should look clean and welcoming, paying special attention to reception areas
- There should be adequate warmth and ventilation
- Noise should be minimized, e.g. by keeping the TV volume at a comfortable level
- Designated separate smoking areas as appropriate
- Overcrowding as far as possible should be avoided
- Natural daylight and fresh air should be maximized
- Privacy for staff and patients must be provided
- Clear direction signs

Providing a secure environment
- There should be a safe room for severely disturbed people as appropriate
- Consider the weight, size and construction of movable objects
- Allow unimpeded sightlines with access points in sight of staff
- Install alarm, communication and monitoring systems where appropriate
- Clinical areas should be lockable to prevent intruders

The increasing number of nurse triage systems has been invaluable in improving the communication between the nurse and the public in the ED. During triage the patient can be assessed and gain information with regard to the illness or injury and the expected waiting times. This initial assessment allows a relationship to be formed between the nurse and the patient and can provide an opportunity for the nurse to reduce the stress experienced by the patient. Access to the triage nurse keeps patients or relatives in constant communication with their progress through the department, further reducing stress and anxiety (Dolan 1998). The provision of adequate numbers of medical and nursing staff in the ED prevents long waiting times and allows good communication and the development of good patient–staff relationships. Less aggression is usually demonstrated if the patient or relative is satisfied with the level of care provided by the ED and good patient–staff relationships are formulated. This cannot occur in areas where patients and staff are under-resourced and pressured. Dolan et al. (1997) found that the use of nurse practitioners in the ED, which led to reductions in waiting times, also led to a reduction in aggressive incidents at the times when nurse practitioners were on duty. In some inner city EDs it has been necessary, however, to provide increased security measures to limit the risk of aggression to staff. These measures have included the provision of security screens for reception staff, closed-circuit TV cameras, security guards, direct links to police stations via panic buttons and personal attack alarms. Although these measures are not often conducive to conveying a caring, trusting attitude to the public, in some instances they have been required to protect the staff from injury.

MANAGING AGGRESSION IN THE ED

Managing aggression needs to be a planned and organized process. Utilizing the Mason and Chandley (1999) model during the pre-aggression phase, the ED nurse needs to have an awareness of the contributing factors in the development of aggression. In addition, the nurse must also have an ability to spot physical signs of impending aggression in order to measure the potential risk and manage it successfully.

Aggressive outbursts in EDs rarely occur without warning and are almost always preceded by clear indications that the individual is becoming agitated or aggressive. Examination of behaviours immediately prior to an assault suggests that there are often 'normal signs' of impending aggression, both verbal and non-verbal, which if left to go unheeded may result in violent outbursts (Whittington & Patterson 1996). In the patient or relative, these signs include:

- approaching the victim rapidly
- using intrusive gestures
- starting yelling
- prolonged eye contact
- speaking loudly
- invasion of other patients'/staffs' personal space
- frowning
- making threatening gestures.

The ED nurse may not be the intended object of the aggressive individual's outburst, but merely an obstacle in the path of the patient or a vehicle for releasing pent-up emotions. This, however, may be of little comfort to the nurse who experiences an aggressive outburst or who is injured by an agitated patient or relative (Hislop & Melby 2003). The nurse therefore has a responsibility to develop an awareness of the patients' or relatives' emotional status through good communication, in order to prevent potentially aggressive incidents occurring.

Inexperience and lack of skill in some nurses in dealing with aggression may result in their avoidance of the agitated person until a violent situation occurs. Indeed, not all nurses are equipped or able to deal with aggressive or violent individuals. Defusing or de-escalating aggression is a complex process (Morcombe 1999). Self-efficacy is suggested as being a major factor in the success in resolving an aggressive situation (Lee 2001). This perception of ourselves can help guide behaviour and prevent escalation of an aggressive incident. Good verbal communication with the aggressive individual is vital in defusing the situation. A calm, confident, non-threatening but assertive attempt to engage the individual in conversation is viewed as the first step to restoring order to the situation. This low-level approach to communication with the aggressor may prevent them viewing the nurse as the aggressor. Lowe (1992) offers some advice on how to manage the aggressive individual during this important stage:

- inform colleagues prior to your approach
- use confirming messages, expressing the person's worth
- model personal control, and the ability to stay calm during the expression of anger and resentment towards you
- use honesty, expressing your feelings congruently
- if it is safe to do so, suggest a quieter area of the department
- set limits, and clear guidelines, which are consistently exerted
- use structure to let people know in advance what is expected of them
- monitor and learn to recognize patterns of behaviour
- timely and calmly intervene (de-escalation) helping the person to work through their anger, breaking the aggressive cycle
- facilitate expression, allow people to express anger and fear somewhere safely
- use non-verbal skills, avoiding threat, and promoting calm and maintaining openness.

Encouraging the patient to discuss the problem may assist in defusing the tension of the moment. If the aggressive individual is confused or under the influence of alcohol or drugs, the nurse may have to repeat the message several times before being understood. Intoxicated thinking often proceeds by association rather than logic. Key phrases such as 'let us work together' are recommended. Conversely, negative phrases such as 'you're not going to fight or give us trouble' are generally inflammatory, as the patient may associate with the words 'fight' and 'trouble' (Taylor & Ryrie 1996). Nothing will be gained by the nurse responding to the patient or relative negatively, despite the provocation from the aggressor. The nurse should listen carefully to the complaint and attempt to offer an explanation or agree a plan of action with the individual to resolve the situation. The use of solutions which are unachievable and the use of inaccurate information to pacify the individual are to be avoided. When these promises are not forthcoming, aggression is more likely. Self-awareness should also relate to the nurse taking appropriate measures to anticipate potential violence and initiate appropriate behaviours to avoid this. Engaging in communication with large groups of people in an attempt to defuse aggression is not recommended, with aggression being amplified by large groups of people. The aggressive individual should be interviewed in a quiet area, offering privacy and dignity to the patient or relative and allowing them to express the source of their grievance. The approach of the nurse to caring for the aggressive individual is vital in resolving the problem and protecting the nurse from danger of physical injury. Non-verbal communication with the patient via body language is an important factor in reducing tension (Glasson 1993).

The nurse should also be aware of personal space and stand at least two arms' lengths away from the individual, allowing the opportunity and means of escape should it be required. Turning slightly side-on to the person, positioning the feet slightly apart with the body weight evenly distributed will assist in presenting a non-threatening and reasonably protective stance, and offer a useful position to promote a quick escape. Direct eye contact with the individual can also be interpreted as being provocative by the aggressive individual; however, eye contact is an important aspect of communication. It is recommended that staff try to maintain their 'normal' level of eye-contact, and use discreet glances to the aggressor's shoulder area, to create a subtle break in potentially prolonged eye contact. Attentive facial expressions suggest interest to the individual and allow good peripheral vision for the nurse. It is also important for the nurse to be aware of the danger in being trapped in an enclosed area while this conversation is in progress. The nurse should always ensure there is a clear method of exit should it be required. The room where the interview is conducted should be as free as possible of objects which could be used as weapons against the nurse. It is important to bear in mind that all unsecured objects have the potential to be used as weapons. Objects carried by the nurse, such as scissors or pens, can be easily grabbed and used against her/him. Neck chains, ties and an inappropriately draped stethoscope can all quickly become weapons against the nurse. These should all be removed before approaching the individual. In today's society, weapons such as knives and guns can be used by aggressive individuals. The nurse should be aware of suspicious bulges in clothing that may be concealed weapons.

MANAGING THE VIOLENT INDIVIDUAL

Managing the violent individual can be likened to the crisis phase of the Mason and Chandley (1999) model. Many EDs now employ security guards to assist in dealing with violent incidents and issue staff with personal attack alarms to reduce the risks to their person. This support is certainly useful to staff but, if a caring approach is to be adopted for all individuals within the ED, the nurse cannot delegate the responsibility of managing the violent patient or relative to other colleagues. Learning to deal with this challenging and stressful situation is not easy for the ED nurse. The appropriate knowledge and skills must result from a combination of role modelling of good management strategies and education (Paterson & McCormish 1999).

If violence does erupt while the nurse is alone, it is unwise to attempt to restrain the individual. Assistance from other departmental staff, security or local police should be summoned via agreed methods. Until assistance is available, the nurse should make every attempt to avoid physical contact, even if this means there is some damage to property. If assistance is not forthcoming, it is better for the nurse to withdraw to a safe distance and, if possible, observe the individual than to engage that person alone. This can only be done if other patients and staff are not put at risk. If a member of staff is attacked, there should be an attempt made to break away, endeavouring not to put anyone else at risk in doing so. If the situation escalates and restraint is required to contain the aggressive individual, this should be carried out in a coordinated manner with a minimum of three staff.

While some question the use of physical restraint in patient care, Section 19 the Code of Practice for the appropriate application of the Mental Health Act 1983 suggests that there are often valid reasons for using restraint, providing guidance for staff on the response required to care for patients presenting with particular management problems (Department of Health/Welsh Office 1999). They suggest that when approaching an aggressive individual it should be as a member of a three-person team with an identified lead person. Prior to the approach it should have been decided at which point in the response physical restraint is to be used and how this will be signalled by the leader. In addition they offer the following advice on how the aggressive individual should be approached should the crisis point arise:

- ensure that all staff are trained in crisis management
- remain calm and non-threatening in manner, avoiding counter-transference

- assess the person's position and possible mode of attack – adjust response as necessary
- approach safely and gradually – do not be rushed
- move to a side-on position reducing exposure to assault and minimizing the appearance of threat
- one person should be responsible for verbal communication.
- keep talking and negotiating on a non-physical alternative
- do not make promises or make offers which you cannot keep
- provide at least one face-saving opportunity
- the team should all be aware of the safe distance threshold
- if negotiation fails be decisive about reacting as a team
- when the individual is secured, move them to a resting position in a chair, to a trolley or on the floor
- allow the person time to relax
- ensure that only one team member communicates with the person
- use appropriate measures to screen the individual from the rest of the department, maintaining dignity at all times
- when the individual is calm move to a quieter area with less stimulation.

The method of restraint will vary, depending on the incident. There are a variety of systems of physical intervention skills, designed specifically for use in healthcare settings. It is strongly recommended that all staff who may be expected to implement restraint should be fully trained in carrying out these and other related procedures. In any type of restraint, it is essential that the individual being held is not compromised in their ability to breathe adequately. During restraint procedures, one team member must take responsibility for monitoring the individual's airway, breathing and circulation. At no point in any restraint should pressure be applied to the throat, neck, chest, back or abdomen. Physical restraint should be used for the minimum amount of time required to control the situation, and the level of force used should be no greater than that required to achieve safety and control. This may include sedation or observation and counselling of the individual by staff. The decision to release the individual must be made by the team and carried out in a controlled, coordinated fashion to minimize the risk of injury to the violent individual and staff.

At the earliest opportunity, the aggressive individual should be examined by senior medical and nursing staff so that a fuller assessment of the individual's condition may be undertaken. The psychiatric or psychological response of the aggressive individual may help to determine whether they are calm enough to be released, whether they require further intervention, e.g. a psychiatric assessment, or whether they are to be released into the custody of the police. It is acknowledged that in extreme instances the degree of reasonable force necessary to control a violent individual may be of concern to the staff involved. In line with the duty of care to the individual highlighted in the NMC (2002) Code of Professional Conduct, the degree of force should be the minimum required to control the violence in a manner appropriate to calm rather than provoke further violence (Ferns 2005). Staff injured in the attempt to restrain the violent individual must also be reviewed by a doctor at the earliest opportunity and be made aware of their entitlement to criminal injuries compensation, if appropriate.

FOLLOW-UP CARE AFTER AN AGGRESSIVE VIOLENT INCIDENT

In accordance with good professional practice procedures and nursing accountability, any aggressive or violent incidents should be reported to the senior nurse and medical officer and recorded appropriately within the documentation. In recognition of the growing levels of violence in ED, most departments now require completion of an incident form specifically designed to record verbal or physical abuse of the staff. In making the report it is important to provide as much detail as possible about the circumstances of the incident. Analysis of this information may be useful in the prevention of further incidents, safeguarding future ED patients and staff. Box 11.2 identifies some of the information that should be documented following an aggressive

---

Box 11.2 Information to be recorded on the incident form

- When and where the incident occurred
- The names, addresses and status of the people involved
- A brief factual account of the incident, including the main direction of the aggression
- The action taken to resolve the incident
- The names of all additional people bearing professional responsibility
- Observations on the mental state of the aggressive individual involved
- Any injury or damage that occurred
- Any additional comments

or violent event. In addition to the care of the aggressive individual, the ED nurse also has a responsibility for the psychological care of the staff and patients who may have been involved in or witnessed the incident. Distressed staff, patients/relatives should be afforded an opportunity to discuss their fears and anxieties arising from the incident. In some cases following extreme events, post-traumatic counselling may be required by individuals involved in incidents of aggression or violence. It is not a sign of weakness or failure in the ED nurse to admit the need for this support to overcome the trauma of such incidents. Nurses who experience assault or who witness distressing events, either regularly or in a one-off situation, are just as at risk of suffering the effects of post-traumatic stress as any other member of the public (Ward 1995). Critical-incident stress debriefing should also be available for involved members of staff (Whitfield 1994) (see also Chapter 12: Stress and Stress Management).

CONCLUSION

There should be a coordinated approach to dealing with aggression and violence in ED departments, similar to the coordinated approach adopted in dealing with a critically ill patient or a cardiac arrest situation. Planning and resourcing in the prevention of aggression and violence in the ED should, therefore, be as detailed as the planning and resources provided for the prevention of death from cardiac arrest. For this to be achieved there must be a planned policy of response to a violent or aggressive outburst, which is known to all the staff within the department and practised on a regular basis. This policy should include key components such as a risk assessment, prevention strategies, training and frequency of refresher updates for staff, together with acceptable methods of managing violence and aggression (Box 11.3). Education in the factors which may lead to aggression and violence in the ED together with the skills in de-escalation strategies and breakaway techniques are vital for the nurse in ED. Sadly, many education programmes in this area fail to include risk management and prevention strategies within their content. In an attempt to correct this omission this report recommends essential components of any education in this area (Box 11.4).

The purpose of this response must be to control the violent or aggressive outburst as efficiently as possible, thereby minimizing the danger to the aggressive individual, other patients or relatives and to the staff involved. The achievement of this objective has staffing and educational implications for the ED management team. To respond to aggressive or violent incidents in the ED requires the provision of adequate levels of

Box 11.3   Components of the education programme on recognition, prevention and therapeutic management of aggression and violence

Theoretical aspects
- Causes and prevention of violence
- Legal and ethical issues
- Verbal de-escalation techniques
- Barriers to communication, e.g. culture, gender, other disabilities
- Correct application of restraint techniques ensuring prevention of harm to aggressive individual and others
- Post-incident documentation and follow up

De-escalation strategies
- Dealing with space, place and physical distance
- Non-verbal social skills
- Verbal strategies
- Collaborative working

Breakaway techniques
- Escaping holds
- Advice on dealing with armed assaults
- Defending oneself

Restraint techniques
- Restraining hold
- Use of 2–5 person team
- Managing person on the ground
- De-escalation holds
- Negotiating obstacles
- Entry or exit from fixed objects

Adapted from U.K.C.C. (2001).

staff. Failure to provide the staffing levels renders any policy to deal with aggression redundant. The knowledge and skills required by the nurse to deal with such incidents are not commonplace among ED nurses. These skills must be developed through experience and by undertaking specialist training designed to inform the nurse and build confidence in coping professionally with these challenging incidents for the betterment of the staff and patients. Opportunities must be provided for all staff in ED to undertake suitable education programmes and to practise the acquired knowledge and skills regularly. By undertaking these measures, the problem of aggression in ED will not be totally eradicated but the nurse will have the means to deal with the situation in a professional and appropriate manner.

Box 11.4   Topics for trust policies and protocols

- Definition of aggression and violence
- Responsibility for these incidents
- Prevention, identification and management of these incidents
- Response protocol in event of aggressive or violent incident
- Staffing numbers and skill mix to prevent and manage these incidents/supervision for junior or newly appointed staff
- Acceptable methods of de-escalation, breakaway and physical restraint

- Liaison with other healthcare professionals, e.g. psychiatrists
- Liaison with security personnel, e.g. police
- Education and update programmes for all staff
- Reporting procedure in event of these incidents
- Audit of incidents and review dates for policies
- Debriefing and follow up procedures
- Staff support systems in the event of an incident

Adapted from UKCC (2001).

References

Bateson G (1980) *Mind and Nature*. London: Fontana.

Berkowitz L (1993) *Aggression: Its Causes, Consequences and Control*. New York: McGraw Hill.C (1989) Violence and Social Work. In: Archer J, Browne K (eds.) *Human Aggression Naturalistic Approaches*. London: Routledge.

Brantly A (1992) Rising violence in ERs cause hospitals to redesign security. *Modern Healthcare*, **22**(40), 44–46.

Breakwell G, Rowett Bandura K (1973) *Aggression: A Social Learning Analysis*. Englewood Cliffs, New Jersey: Prentice-Hill.

Brennan W (1998) Aggression and violence: examining the theories. *Emergency Nurse*, **6**(2), 18–21.

Cembrowicz SP, Shepard JP (1992) Dealing with difficult patients: what goes wrong? *The Practitioner*, **233**, 486–489.

Department of Health/Welsh Office (1999) *Code of Practice: Mental Health Act 1983*. London: HMSO

Department of Health (2000) *NHS Zero Tolerance Zone*. London: Department of Health.

Dolan B. Waiting Times (editorial) (1998) *Emergency Nurse*, **6**(4), 1.

Dolan B, Dale J, Morley V (1997) Nurse practitioners: role in A&E and primary care. *Nursing Standard*, **11**(17), 33–38.

Dollard J, Doob LW, Miller NE, Mowrer OH, Sears RR (1939) *Frustration and Aggression*. New Haven, CT: Yale University Press.

Erickson J, Williams-Evans S (2000) Attitudes of emergency nurses regarding patient assaults. *Journal of Emergency Nursing*, **26**(3), 210–215.

Farrell GA, Gray C (1992) *Aggression: A Nurses' Guide to Therapeutic Management*. London: Scutari Press.

Ferns T (2005) Terminology, stereotypes and aggressive dynamics in the accident and emergency department. *Accident and Emergency Nursing*, **13**(4), 238–246.

Freud S (1932) *The Complete Psychological Works of Sigmund Freud*. London: Hogarth Press

Glasson L (1993) The care of the psychiatric patient in the Emergency Department. *Journal of Emergency Nursing*, **19** (5), 385–391.

Gross R (1996) *The Science of Mind and Behaviour*, 3rd Edn. London: Hodder and Stoughton

Health & Safety Commission Advisory Committee (1997) *Violence and Aggression to Staff in the Health Services*. London: HSE Books

Hildegard ER, Hildegard R, Atkinson RC (1987) *Introduction to Psychology*. New York: Harcourt Brace Jovanovich.

Hislop E, Melby V (2002) The lived experience of violence in accident and emergency. *Accident and Emergency Nursing*, **11**(1), 5–11.

Hoag-Apel CM (1998) Violence in the Accident and Emergency Department. *Nursing Management*, **29**(7), 60–63.

Jenkins MG, Rocke LG, McNicholl BP, Hughes DM (1998) Violence and verbal abuse against staff in A&E Departments: Survey of consultants in the UK and the Republic of Ireland. *Journal of Accident and Emergency Medicine*, **15**(4), 262–265.

Kaplan HI, Sadock BJ (1993) *Pocket Handbook of Emergency Psychiatric Medicine*. Baltimore: Williams and Williams.

Lanza ML, Kayne HL, Hicks C, Milner J (1991) Nursing staff characteristics related to patients assault. *Issues in Mental Health Nursing*, vol. **12**(3), 253–265.

Lee F (2001) Violence in A&E: The role of training in self-efficacy. *Nursing Standard*, **15**(46), 33–38.

Lowe T (1992) Characteristics of effective nursing interventions in the management of challenging behaviour. *Journal of Advanced Nursing*, **17**, 1226–1232.

Luck L, Jackson D Usher K(2007) STAMP: components of observable behaviour that indicate potential for patient violence in emergency departments. *Journal of Advanced Nursing*, **59**(1), 11–19.

Mason T, Chandley M (1999) *Management of Violence and Aggression for Nurses and Healthcare Workers*. New York: Churchill Livingstone.

Morcombe J (1999) Interpersonal approaches to managing violence and aggression. *Emergency Nurse*, **7**(1), 12–16.

National Audit Office (2003) *A Safer Place to Work: Protecting NHS Hospital and Ambulance Staff from Violence and Aggression*. London: NAO.

Nursing and Midwifery Council (2002) *Code of Professional Conduct*. London: NMC.

Paterson B, McCormish AG, Bradley P (1999) Violence at Work. *Nursing Standard*, **13**(21), 43–46.

Royal College of Nursing (1998) *Dealing with Violence against Nursing Staff: a RCN Guide for Nurses and Managers*. London: RCN

Royal College of Nursing/National Institute for Health and Clinical Excellence (2005) *Violence: The Short-term Management of Disturbed/Violence Behaviour in In-patient Psychiatric Settings and Emergency Departments*. London: RCN

Schnieden V, Marren-Bell U (1995) Violence in the A&E Department. *Accident and Emergency Nursing*, **3**(2), 74–78.

Standing H, Nicolini D (1997) *Review of Workplace Related Violence*. London: HSE Books.

Stirling G, Higgins JE, Cooke MW (2001) Violence in A&E Departments: a systematic review of the literature. *Accident and Emergency Nursing*, (9)2, 77–85.

Stuart G, Sundeen S (1983) *Principles and Practice of Psychiatric Nursing*. St. Louis: Mosby.

Taylor R, Ryrie I (1996) Chronic alcohol users in A&E. *Emergency Nurse*, **4**(3), 6–8.

United Kingdom Central Council for Nursing, Midwifery and Health Visiting (2001) *The Recognition, Prevention and Therapeutic Management of Violence in Mental Health Care*. London: UKCC

Vaughn-Bowie D (1996) *Coping With Violence : A Guide for the Human Services*, 2nd edn. London: Whiting and Birch.

Ward M (1995) *Nursing the Psychiatric Emergency*. Oxford: Butterworth-Heinemann.

Whitfield A (1994) Critical incident debriefing in A&E. *Emergency Nurse*, **2**(3), 6–9.

Whittington R, Wykes T (1989) Invisible Injury. *Nursing Times*, **85**(42), 32

Whittington R, Patterson P (1996) Verbal and non-verbal behaviour immediately prior to aggression by mentally disordered people: enhancing risk assessment. *Journal of Psychiatric and Mental Health Nursing* **3**(1), 47–54.

Wright B (1986) *Caring in Crisis: A Handbook of Intervention Skills for Nurses*. Edinburgh: Churchill Livingstone.

Chapter **12**

Stress and stress management

Heather Josland

CHAPTER CONTENTS

INTRODUCTION

Emergency nursing is generally regarded as stressful. Scenarios that confront emergency staff include patients in severe pain, unpredictability of presentations, trauma victims, dying patients and physically demanding work (Curtis 2001, Cameron et al. 2004). The International Council of Nurses (ICN) recognizes the emotional, social, psychological and spiritual challenges that nurses engage within such complex environments (2000). The intention of this chapter is to provide an understanding of stress and stress management that may assist the ED nurse to cope in a busy and sometimes chaotic environment. Highlighted topics are stress and coping theories, including stressors specific to ED nursing. Contemporary issues contributing to stress take account of workload, nursing shortage, overcrowding, patient expectations and violence. Crucial to this subject is an overview of stress management strategies that includes demobilizing, defusing and debriefing along with emphasis on care and support for ED nurses.

STRESS THEORY

Multiple theories exist on stress and coping in application to physical, cognitive, emotional and behavioural characteristics. Hans Selye (1976) defined stress as the physical body's non-specific response to any demand made on it. The stress response is elicited when an individual perceives a threat to their self, whether real or imagined. Cognitive appraisal of a stressor determines mental as well as physical aspects of emotion. The sympathetic nervous system activates the release of adrenaline and then synthesizes and secretes corticosteroids. The distribution of cortisol into the circulatory system causes raised blood glucose levels, increased heart rate, blood pressure, respirations, peripheral constriction, dilated pupils and a state of arousal or mental alertness (Tortara & Grabowski 2003).

This is what Cannon (1935) called the 'fight or flight response', describing an inbuilt mechanism that enabled our forebears to battle assailants or flee from wild animals. Matsakis (1996) has expanded this to fight, flight or freeze, explaining that contemporary stressors are different from the wild animals or battles facing earlier generations. Immobility or freezing of physical or mental capacities may occur during modern stressful situations. Exhibited behavioural responses of impaired physical or emotional function may include inadequate skills or poor communication.

Selye's (1976) general adaptation system (GAS) is described as alarm where the body attempts to adjust; second, the resistance stage where the body attempts to manage the situation; and third, the exhaustion stage where resources have been drained. Cannon (1935) examined the body's ability to maintain and correct body systems, including regulation of temperature, nervous system, fluid–electrolyte balance and the immune response. Cannon coined the term homeostasis as the body's attempt to re-establish equilibrium. He linked stress to be a cause of disease, explaining that the fight response is the body's attempt towards restoration. When the body faces continued stress, illness can occur. Selye asserted that if illness were a consequence of being *dis* at *ease*, then it would be prudent to utilize preventive measures rather than temporarily patch up or mask disease states (1976).

Exposure to stress is more commonly evidenced by the first and second stages. Selye explained that through recurring experiences individuals learn to adapt and return to a state of homeostasis. He maintained that the ability to adapt to stressful situations and regain homeostasis was an exceptional attribute of humans. McEwen (2000) has identified allostasis as the body's attempt to re-establish homeostasis via a higher or lowered level of physiological function. A continued period of physiological adaptation due to exposure to chronic stress is what McEwen terms allostatic loading. This may be adversely manifested in such disease states as hypertension, neurological or immune dysfunctions. Less commonly, a severe threat or continued demand on individual adaptation resources may result in the third and most damaging stage of the GAS, which is exhaustion.

COPING

In general terms coping refers to the processes or skills used to deal with situations which are out of the ordinary. Some authorities identify coping more readily in the context of crisis or in adjustment to adverse conditions. Wolfe (1950) referred to stress as a process of altered internal dynamics of an individual caused by interaction with external energy from the environment. The person's internal response as they interacted with the environmental pressure was considered by Wolfe to be influenced by prior experiences.

Lazarus's work developed a three-phase approach to stress theory that involved a cognitive process of appraisal, coping and outcome (1966). Primary appraisal consists of the initial evaluation of the stressor and the extent to which the threat is considered to be hazardous. Secondary appraisal considers the availability of coping strategies or resources. Lazarus describes stress as disruption of meaning, while coping is defined as the way in which an individual deals with the disruption.

Subsequently, Lazarus and Folkman (1984) differentiated ways of coping as strategies that are both behavioural and psychological. Efforts to reduce a stressful situation involve action or problem-solving. The direct-action coping method would be to confront or retreat from the perceived threat, while the psychological problem-solving approach would be to reduce stress by reframing the individual's view and response to the stressor. Lazarus and Folkman state that the value of either mechanism determines the effect of the stressor on the individual. Individual style dictates which strategy is applied resulting in outcome. Veranec (2001) adds that factors influencing the stress response consist not only of individual interpretation of the stressor but also of the amount of perceptible support and a person's overall health.

STRESS AND DISTRESS

Perhaps all nurses experience stress in some form, even those who will not admit it. Selye (1976) described eustress as good stress that motivates people to go to work, while distress is the bad stress that can create anxiety and illness through, for example, overwork. Aspects of emergency work necessitate that ED nurses will experience both distress and eustress. Experienced ED nurses may rely on instinct composed of a mixture of knowledge, skills and experience necessary to effectively cope with a variety of situations. Stimuli in the internal environment may arise in terms of thoughts, feelings and physical illness.

Research suggests a vulnerability to adverse effects of stress in a study of Singapore ED nurses. Yang et al.'s (2002) study found ED nurses to have lower levels of lysozome in saliva samples than general ward nurses, correlating with higher levels of perceived stress. Excessive release of glucocorticoids inhibit secretion of immunoglobin A (sIgA) and lysozomes, which both affect immunity levels. This correlated with questionnaires measuring a perceived level of stress scale. Because ED nurses are exposed to significant pressures they should be aware of the signs and symptoms of increasing stress.

SIGNS AND SYMPTOMS OF STRESS

Stress may be observed in colleagues or friends before the affected nurse is actually aware. Stress can subtly influence professional and personal relationships, and is often manifested in forms of physical, emotional, behavioural and mental expression as seen in Table 12.1.

STRESSORS IN ED NURSING

For even the most competent ED nurse, continued exposure to particularly difficult and emotionally draining situations can result in crisis. Key stressors or demands identified in the literature include nursing shortage, workload, overcrowding, violence, shift work, environmental factors, communication problems and burnout (Maslasch 1996). A literature review by Chang et al. (2005) identified common nursing stressors to be

- high work demands with little support
- poor control over workload
- shortage of resources – human and equipment
- excessive duties to perform.

The subject of this review is the implications of stress on the nurse, the organization and the ensuing relationship between role stress and nursing shortages.

Workload, nursing shortage and overcrowding

Workload for ED nurses includes additional stressors, with unexpected numbers and type of patient presentations; rapidly changing status of patients; response to traumatic incidents; and patient violence (Yang et al. 2002). ED nurses have the stress of sudden and unpredictable arrivals of complex presentations without time for preparation. Increasing patient numbers and intensity increase the work of the nurse. The consequences include increased reliance on EDs and lengthening waits (Burt & Schappert 2004, National Audit Office 2004). Chang et al. (2005) blame workload underscored by work stress as the major contributor to the exodus from nursing. Concerns regarding a shortage exist worldwide. According to a study released by the US Department of Health and Human Services, the current shortage of 6% will increase to 20% by 2015, and 29% by 2020 (US Department of Health 2002).

Skill mix

Overcrowding of EDs is acknowledged by Derlet and Richards (2000) to be a critical problem accentuated by staffing and bed shortages, plus increasing patient presentations and severity. Poor skill mix and blocked access to impatient beds can impact heavily on EDs, where competent nurses endure the burden of extra patients while supervising less experienced nurses. Contemporary challenges include a multitude of cultural and language variations that also add to stress with communication difficulties. Iltun (2002) underlines the importance of being aware of one's own values, cultural differences and biases in order to avoid ineffective communication. The underlying danger exists that skill mix with a low ratio of qualified nurses can impact negatively on quality of care and patient expectations.

Patient expectations

Patients have high expectations of health care and an awareness of their rights due to increased information from the health services, media and internet. Newly highlighted successful treatments may be demanded against recommendations of standard procedures

Table 12.1   Signs and symptoms of stress

Mental	Physical	Behavioural	Emotional
Insomnia	Headaches	Distancing	Frequent crying
Poor communication	Fatigue	Cynical	Anxiety
Decreased decision-making	Excessive thirst	Increased ETOH	Frustration
Decreased concentration span	Increased pulse	Increased escape activities	Anger
Memory lapse	Muscle tension	Errors	Depression
Unpleasant dreams	Shortness of breath	Ill temper	Irritability

offered by nurses. Patient rights explicitly stated in The Patient Charter (Department of Health 1995) support them in complaint procedures regardless of whether they are unrealistic or implausible. Nurses can feel unappreciated and disillusioned in their attempts to provide good nursing care. Patients sometimes arrive at ED departments with the expectation they will be seen immediately. Individuals may express opinions that their needs and conditions are the most important and it is their right to do so. Building resentment may be displaced onto the ED nurse who is already feeling frustrated due to inadequate resources.

Violence

Presley & Robinson (2002) argue that prolonged waiting is a possible trigger for violence exacerbated by stress from pain, fear and unpleasant stimuli. Patients and visitors are exposed to noxious smells, sights and sounds in emergency departments. As possible contributors to violence one must also take into account social factors, intoxicants, withdrawal, psychoses, dementias, brain injuries and seizures or post-ictal status. Presley & Robinson advise the ED nurse to manage these through psychological control such as gaining trust or physical control such as ensuring seclusion or restraint through administering prescribed pharmacological sedation (see also Chapter 11: Violence and aggression).

IMPLICATIONS OF STRESS

Patients and families are not usually prepared for managing the intensity of emotions that accompany a traumatic event (ENA 2002). The ED nurse may be expected to deal with a complex mixture of physical, social, emotional and even spiritual patient requirements. The unfortunate consequence of caring for trauma victims or critically ill patients is that the stress can be transferred onto the nurse, often referred to as secondary traumatic stress (Badger 2001, Figley 2002). Some patients or events may connect on a personal level with the nurse, initiating feelings and emotions that would normally be contained. Demands on the nurse may seem insurmountable at times and lead to dissatisfaction and fatigue. ED nurses can face acute and chronic stressors that may accumulate over time from dealing with multiple incidents.

The altruistic nature of nursing lends a vulnerability where attempts to demonstrate high levels of care sprinkled with compassion leave the nurse emotionally and physically exhausted. Consequences of stress can be indicated by cognitive, physical, emotional or behavioural changes. Nurses may experience fatigue,

loss of enthusiasm and energy, sleep disturbance, job dissatisfaction and escape activities such as alcohol or drugs (Spence-Laschinger et al. 2001). A stressed nurse may impose consequences onto patients such as inadequate care, increased waiting times, inattention, impatience and cynicism (Maslach 1996). Poor performance behaviours are indicated by distancing or avoiding the patient, ignoring the patient's feelings, concentrating on equipment instead of the patient, forgetfulness or incompletion of tasks. Maladaptive responses or ineffective coping mechanisms can result in depression and physical illness (Selye 1976).

A study of 43 000 nurses from 700 hospitals in five countries, i.e. England, Scotland, Germany, USA and Canada, identified low morale, job dissatisfaction and burnout as consequences of stress (Aiken et al. 2001). A major concern was reported as inadequate time to complete nursing responsibilities. Inadequate nursing resources were linked to adverse events such as increased patient morbidity and even mortality. Health institutions suffer consequences of stressed nurses revealed by tardiness, absenteeism, errors, workplace conflict, high staff turnover and patient dissatisfaction, all leading to increased cost (Spence-Laschinger et al. 2001). The diversity of ED work, although valued by the nurses, can be difficult to tolerate, especially as it covers such a wide range of conditions and can unexpectedly lead to burnout.

BURNOUT

Maslach (1982) termed the word burnout as an occupational reaction to stress caused by the physical and emotional demands of care for patients. The Maslach Burnout Inventory (MBI) defines the characteristics as emotional fatigue, depersonalization, and feelings of decreased personal worth or accomplishment (1996). The emotional exhaustion was said to be evidenced by a depleted emotional reservoir as occurs under high pressure and patient demands. Depersonalization may occur in the development of negative attitudes towards colleagues or patients. This can lead to workers isolating themselves from others. Poor personal accomplishment can result in self-criticism or feelings of insufficiency. All are indicators for burnout.

Burnout is evident through unrealistic expectations; inflexibility towards change; resentment and suspicion; intolerance; being judgemental; lack of direction or goals; and physical and mental exhaustion, an insensitive attitude towards others, a feeling of being unappreciated, diminished energy, pessimism, inefficiency, increased absenteeism, low morale, low self-esteem and frequent illness (Demerouti 2000 et al.

Iltun 2002, Jackson 2004). Successful coping includes enduring or alleviating stress; upholding worthwhile personal relationships; maintaining self-esteem and value regardless of setbacks; and meeting necessary aspects of stressful duties (Jacobson & McGrath 1983).

Iltun (2002), researching nurse burnout in Turkey, argues that burnout is symptomatic not simply of work stress but of unmanaged stress from excessive demands on workers. The gap between reality and expectations affects nurses' energy levels, job satisfaction and overall health. Iltun found that personal beliefs do play a role in perceived levels of burnout.

In a study using the Maslach Burnout Inventory (MBI), Walsh et al. (1998) showed that lack of staff, pressure of work and patient aggression were the main stressors for ED nurses, coupled with a perceived lack of managerial support and inadequate resources. They found that participants in the study were on the borderline between moderate and high levels of depersonalization, one of the three components of burnout identified by the MBI subscales. They also showed nurses experienced moderate levels of emotional exhaustion. This was reflected in the fact that about half the 134 nurses in the sample reported feeling used up at the end of the day, frustrated by their job and emotionally drained at least once a week.

Accumulation of burnout is insidious, leaving nurses drained, and exhausted with lowered tolerance and immunity Maslach 1982). Maslach warns that burnout leads to impaired work ability. Decreased work satisfaction can spill over to decreased life satisfaction and affect relationships outside of work. Figley (2002) terms this compassion fatigue likened to battle fatigue experienced by soldiers in war-time. Maslach (1982) warns that burnout leads to impaired work ability. Decreased work satisfaction can spill over to decreased life satisfaction and affect relationships outside of work. The fatigue factor influences attitudes that become apparent in unsuccessful communication with colleagues.

Communication problems can create havoc in the already chaotic environment of emergency areas. Burnout is linked with insomnia and escape activities such as increased smoking, alcohol consumption and unhealthy diet (Walsh et al. 1998). Research exploring job satisfaction among nurses and therapists cited stress as a commonly cited reason for absenteeism and emphasized the need for training and support for front-line staff (Webb et al. 2002). Burnout could be considered a potential hazard, with warning signs evident in physical, emotional and behavioural changes (Verarec 2001). This determines a need to encourage a good quality of work life for ED nurses, prevent illness and burnout, enhance patient care and decrease costs to the health provider.

STRESS MANAGEMENT

Critical incident stress (CIS)

Exceptional clinical events have the potential to elicit emotions that are so intense they may impact on the individuals' ability to function during the event or later (Mitchell & Everly 1995). Emotional responses may be suppressed while cognitive functioning allows knowledge and skills to be utilized as the ED nurse manages an airway and draws up drugs in preparation for an emergency intubation. It is after the incident when the patient has left the department that the cognitive subsides and the emotions can then surface, leaving the emergency nurse with a feeling of overwhelming sadness or emotional exhaustion. A more serious condition can occur from significant events or untreated stress in the form of post-traumatic stress disorder (PTSD).

Ochberg (1993) describes PTSD as a catastrophic occurrence that may severely disrupt a person's equilibrium. A study by O'Connor and Jeavons (2003) reported emergency nurses to have higher exposure to critical stress than ward nurses. The most stressful situation for nurses was identified as dealing with the assault or death of a child, while the most frequent was the responding to a sudden arrest. Recognized strategies include defusion, demobilization and critical incident stress debriefing (1997).

Defusion

Defusion may best be described as a short type of crisis intervention. It is intended to bring some psychological closure to the event. This should ideally be carried out before staff leave the shift or within 48 hours (Mitchell 2004). This is an informal talk that allows reflection of thoughts and feelings, often over tea or coffee.

The facilitator maintains a low profile and ensures a safe environment and conditions for the defusing to occur in a healthy manner. In the case of a momentous event, a person trained in debriefing may be required. General rules dictate that only people directly involved in the event are in attendance. Participants are reminded of confidentiality and again support is to be clearly demonstrated. This session is not an evaluation of behaviour, but individuals are encouraged to express feelings and thoughts. Individuals are to be cautioned that some may feel worse when confronting their emotions. It should reduce tension, focus on strengths and skills and assist staff to regain emotional control.

Ideally people will go over the details of the event naturally and spontaneously. Details of other events or other information will not be shared until the entire story has unfolded. Any attempts to curtail disclosure of a critical incident will cause it to emerge later. Time and attention to those involved will on the other hand allow the incident to be laid to rest or ended more appropriately (Wright, 1993).

Demobilization

Demobilization provides staff with a structure to end a duty. While many people end the shift at the same time, some, because of workload or altered shift, may leave at different times. Their needs should not be ignored. Large-scale incidents benefit most from this approach. A room will be needed to hold large numbers of staff. The group should be multidisciplinary. The time is approximately 15 minutes and should be within their working day. It is recommended that it is carried out as soon as possible following the incident.

The team leader should have factual information regarding the whole event from the beginning to the present time. Wright (1993) stresses that all involved people should have obligatory attendance, emphasizing that demobilization is not just for the sensitive or vulnerable or those who think they need it; the whole team must attend to acknowledge that the issue affects everyone. The time may permit questions that enable a clarification of circumstances. Aims of the demobilization are:

- to regain emotional control and cognitive functioning and to reduce tension
- to focus on strengths and skills, to re-evaluate the incident and to receive some factual information
- to begin the recovery process and leave behind some of the stress
- to begin to be educated by the incident.

The difference between a demobilization and defusion is that although they have similar aims, the demobilization is clearly time-limited and focused. Different members of staff will have worked in different aspects of the incident but will generally not be aware of the entire event. For this reason, information regarding the whole incident may be useful.

Information may be given regarding the possibility of adverse reactions after the event. Staff needs may be assessed at this time and advice made available on any required assistance. Demobilization should be ended with thanks extended to every staff member that acknowledges their contribution during a difficult and demanding event. The purpose of the organizational demobilization is to demonstrate support, plan for the immediate future and restore organizational function. A more difficult approach to expedite is that of critical incident debriefing, which permits a deeper exploration of an event.

Critical Incident Stress Debriefing (CISD)

This is a more formal type of debriefing that is expected to be carried out within 24–48 hours after the event. Some authorities recommend that debriefing should be directed only by an experienced person trained in stress management (Mitchell 2004, Human Services Department 1997). The goal of CISD is to assist staff to transfer from a state of high arousal to a state of normalization after a significant event. This time is to permit staff a chance to ventilate feelings such as anger, disappointment or sadness. A possible format for CISD could consist of three 1-hour sessions to be held within two weeks.

Each ED will have their own view on the decided course of action regarding any need or procedure for CISD. Some EDs have teams represented by peer support from all emergency personnel. Interventions were proposed by Mitchell and Everly (1995) to be carried out in seven stages, listed as:

- introductions
- facts
- thoughts
- reaction
- symptoms
- teaching
- re-entry phase.

The first session may cover mainly facts and individual parts in the event. Session two encourages the person or persons to consider thoughts and feelings around the event. The person may be assisted in confronting the more disturbing aspects of the incident. The last session is educational and largely involves natural stress responses and putting strategies in place to avoid further difficulties. This session aims to bring individuals back as much as possible to normal function. Some goals or plan may be established to assist the re-entry.

The rationale behind debriefing is to shed some light around the event, mobilize resources and utilize problem-solving skills that may improve future planning. Support for the individual and group is again paramount. Controversy exists around the proposed benefits of critical incident stress debriefing. Deahl and Bisson (1995) argue that the benefits of debriefing are not scientifically proven. Further research using longitudinal studies is needed to establish proven benefits. A long-term authority on post-traumatic stress disorder, Ochberg (1993) values therapeutic debriefing. Indeed a do nothing' attitude could be considered cruel and may ignore the possibility that a serious incident may induce a strong stress response in a person or persons.

APPROACHES TO SUPPORT AND CARE

Self-support groups

Jackson (2004) cited social support as the most useful coping mechanism for nurses. Groups which meet regularly to discuss cumulative stress have been found to be useful (Wright 1991). Establishing positive support systems at work and home provides effective coping mechanisms. Listening is a basic and simple response and its value should not be underestimated. Talking and sharing with colleagues are well used and caring responses. Trust is imperative, as self-disclosure is involved and insight into the person behind the nursing role will increase the value of sharing (Wright 1992).

Balance and self-care

Maintaining basic health rules of adequate sleep, nutrition, exercise and relaxation or recreational activities outside work will assist the nurse to maintain a healthy sense of balance. Self-care strategies listed by Badger (2000) comprise self-monitoring and reflection, and maintaining realistic goals and expectations. ED nurses cognizant of coping strategies will be able to contribute more meaningfully to care of themselves, their colleagues and ultimately their patients. Jackson's alternative vision for nurses is to create healing communities where a holistic approach enables healing for the mind, body and spirit (Jackson 2004). Her suggestion is for emergency departments to pipe soothing music in the hope of decreasing stress levels. Other suggestions include aromatherapy, massage, reflexology and even art. Jackson assumes that if nurses maintain high levels of wellness themselves, they will be in a position to offer equally therapeutic treatment for their patients. Although idealistic and improbable for most EDs, Jackson's suggestions do remind nurses of the importance of quality time out for self-care.

Education

This book acknowledges the variety of specialities that the ED nurse will encounter, including cardiology, orthopaedics, nephrological emergencies to obstetrical and gynaecological emergencies. Bailey et al.'s (2005) review of literature and survey of nurses revealed a need for health-care organizations to provide education for emergency nurses. ED nurses are expected to have a sound nursing knowledge and skill level encompassing a wide range of medical and surgical conditions. Bailey states that increased knowledge enhances confidence in clinical practice, and produces greater respect amongst colleagues. Possible follow-on effects are stated to be increased job satisfaction, a positive effect on nurse retention and increased patient care and satisfaction.

Education on stress management that encompasses recognition of stressors, stress symptoms and effective strategies to reduce stress may also assist ED nurses. Education and practice for nurses to care for themselves and one another may help build and maintain the resources necessary to offer quality care for others. A desirable goal is for the nurse to regularly update with current trends and practice that will impact positively on patients.

Lastly, evidence suggests that humour is an effective antidote to stress. A study by Wooten (1997) found nurses to have decreased levels of cortisol following laughter training. The important thing is for people to laugh with one another not at one another. Further research is needed to decide on effectiveness of stress-management interventions. The goal is for the ED nurses to harness resources that protect them from burnout and to be in the best position to facilitate quality care of patients, mobilizing the nurse towards healthy adaptation and rewarding interpersonal relationships. Some may argue that the most stressful situations are those which promote the greatest level of satisfaction. This implies then that ED nurses will enjoy adequate levels of eustress that motivate and maintain their commitment to this vital area of nursing.

CONCLUSION

The unique stressors that ED nurses face daily may challenge even the most competent ED nurse. Adrenaline-fuelled efforts to provide good care may be part of the thrill of the work. Nonetheless, it is important for nurses to ensure that they do not expose themselves repeatedly to a state of exhaustion without adequate rest periods. Despite effective coping mechanisms, the continued exposure to pain, suffering, stress and trauma makes the ED nurse susceptible. The literature suggests a need to prevent job stress through encouragement of individual and organizational awareness to address causes rather than symptoms. Departmental policies which address the issues of defusion, demobilization and debriefing make a clear statement that it is the department's philosophy to care for its staff and acknowledge the difficulty of the work. The emphasis is on education that may help emergency nurses recognize signs and symptoms of stress and a range of ways to respond and manage stress effectively. When supported in maintaining their own health within a positive work environment, the ED nurse may possess the necessary resources to facilitate quality health in meeting the wide-ranging needs of their patients.

References

Aiken L, Clark S, Sloane D, Sochalaski J, Busse R, Clarke H, Giovanetti P, Hunt J, Rafferty A, Shamian J (2001) Nurses' reports on hospital care in five countries. *Health Affairs*, **20** (3), 43–54.

Badger J (2001) Understanding secondary traumatic stress. *American Journal of Nursing*, **101**(7), 26–32.

Bailey K, Swinger M, Bard M, Sparrow V, Deegan J, Small K, Janssen R, Naile B, Toschlog E, Sargraves S, Goettler C, Rotondo M (2005). The effectiveness of a specialised trauma course in the knowledge base and level of job satisfaction in emergency nurses. *Journal of Trauma Nursing*, (12)1, 10–15.

Burt C, Schappert S (2004) Ambulatory care visits to physician offices, hospital outpatients departments and emergency departments United States 1999–2000. *Data from the national health care survey.* Centre for Disease Control and Prevention. National Centre for Health Statistics. *Vital Health Statistics*, **13**(157), 1–70.

Cameron P, Jelinek G, Kelly A, Murray L, Heyworth J (2004) Introduction. In: Cameron P, Jelinek G, Kelly A, Murray L, Heyworth J, eds. *Textbook of Adult Emergency Medicine.* 2nd edn. London: Churchill Livingstone.

Cannon W (1935) Stresses and strains of homeostasis. *American Journal of Medical Sciences*, **189**(1), 1.

Chang E, Hancock K, Johnson A, Daly J, Jackson D (2005) Role stress in nurses: review of related factors and strategies for moving forward. *Nursing and Health Sciences*, **7**, 57–65.

Curtis K (2001) Nurse's experience of working with trauma patients. *Nursing Standard*, **16**(9), 33–38.

Deahl MP, Bisson JI (1995) Dealing with disasters: does psychological debriefing work? *Journal of Accident and Emergency Medicine*, **12**(4), 255–258

Demerouti E, Bakker A, Nachreiner F, Schaufeli W (2000) A model of burnout and life satisfaction amongst nurses. *Journal of Advanced Nursing*, **32**(2), 454–463.

Department of Health (1995) *The Patient's Charter.* London: Department of Health.

Derlet R, Richards J (2000) Overcrowding in the nation's emergency departments; complex causes and disturbing effects. *Annals of Emergency Medicine*, **35**(1), 63–68.

Emergency Nurses Association (2002) *Trauma Nursing Core Course Provider Manual*, 4th edn. Chicago: ENA.

Figley C (2002) Compassion fatigue: psychotherapists chronic lack of self care. *Journal of Clinical Psychology*, **58** (11), 1433–1441.

Human Resources Branch Department of Human Services (1997) *Resource Guide for Critical Incident Stress and Debriefing in Human Service Agencies.* Melbourne: Victoria. Government Department of Human Services.

Iltun I, (2002) Burnout and nurses' personal and professional values. *Nursing Ethics*, **9**(3), 269–78.

International Council of Nurses. (2000) Occupational health and safety for nurses. *ICN Position Statement.* Geneva: International Council of Nurses.

Jackson C (2004) Healing ourselves, healing others. *Holistic Nurse Practitioner*, **18**(4), 199–210.

Jacobson S, McGrath H (1983) *Nurses Under Stress.* New York: John Wiley and Sons.

Lazarus RS (1966) *Psychological Stress and the Coping process.* New York: McGraw-Hill.

Lazarus RS, Folkman S (1984) *Stress, Appraisal and Coping.* New York: Springer.

Maslach C (1982) *Burnout, the Cost of Caring: Burnout in Health Professionals*, New Jersey: Prentice Hall.

Maslach C, Jackson S, Leiter M (1996) *Maslach Burnout Inventory*, 3rd edn. Palo Alto CA: Consulting Psychologists Press.

Matsakis A (1996) *I can't get over it: a handbook for trauma survivors*, 2nd ed. Oakland, California: New Harbinger Publication.

McEwen B (2000) Effects of adverse experiences for brain structure and function. *Biology Psychiatry*, **48**(8), 721–731.

Mitchell JT, Everly G (1995) *Critical Incident Stress Debriefing: an Operational Manual for the Prevention of Traumatic Stress Among Emergency Services Workers.* Elliot City: Chevron Publishing Corporation.

Mitchell JT (2004) Characteristics of successful early intervention programs. *International Journal of Emergency Mental Health*, **6**(4), 175–184.

National Audit Office (2004) *Improving Emergency Care in England.* London: NAO.

Ochberg F (1993) Posttraumatic therapy. In: Wilson J and Raphael B, eds. *International Handbook of Traumatic Stress Syndromes.* New York: Plenum Press.

O'Connor J, Jeavons S (2003) Nurse's perceptions of critical incidents. *Journal of Advanced Nursing*, **41**(1), 43–62.

Presley D, Robinson G (2002) Violence and assault in the emergency department. *The Nursing Clinics of North America Emergency Nursing*, **37**(1), 161–169.

Selye H (1976) *The Stress of Life*, 2nd edn. New York: McGraw-Hill.

Spence-Laschinger H, Shamian J, Thomson D (2001) Impact of magnet hospital characteristics on nurses' perceptions of trust, burnout, quality of care, and work satisfaction. *Nursing Economics*, **19**(5), 209–219.

Tortara G, Grabowski S (2003)) *Principles of Anatomy and Physiology*, 10th Edn. New York: Harper Collins.

U. S. Deparment of Health and Human Services. (2002). Projected supply, demand, and shortages of registered nurses: 2000–2020. Health Resources and Services Administration, Bureau of Health Professions. National

Center for Health Workforce Analysis. Rockville, MD: U.S. Government Printing Office.

Verarec E (2001) How to cope with job stress. *Registered Nurse,* **64**(3), 44–46.

Walsh M, Dolan B, Lewis A (1998) Burnout and stress among A&E nurses. *Emergency Nurse,* **6**(2), 23–30.

Webb Y, Stear A, Pettybridge J, Baker R, Elharch G (2002) Nursing the nurses: why staff need support. *Nursing Times,* **98**(16), 36–37.

Wolfe H (1950) *Life Stress and Bodily Diseases.* Baltimore: Williams & Wilkins.

Wooten P (1996) Humour: Antidote for stress. *Holistic Nurse Practitioner* **10**, 49–56.

Wright B (1991) *Sudden Death.* Edinburgh: Churchill Livingstone.

Wright B (1992) *Communication Skills: Skills for Caring.* Edinburgh: Churchill Livingstone.

Wright B (1993) *Caring in Crisis,* 2nd edn. Edinburgh: Churchill Livingstone.

Yang Y, Doh D, Ng V, Lee C, Chan G, Dong F, Goh S, Anantharaman V, Chia S (2002) Self perceived work related stress and the relation with salivary IgA and lysozome among emergency department nurses. *Occupational and Environmental Medicine,* **59**(12), 836–841.

Chapter **13**

Care of the bereaved

Brian Dolan

INTRODUCTION

It is estimated there are some 25 000–30 000 resuscitation attempts in the UK every year (Resuscitation Council 1996). Dealing with the suddenly bereaved in emergency departments is difficult for all staff, no matter how much experience they have. This chapter will consider approaches to the management of sudden death in ED. It will examine the literature surrounding this subject, before exploring the process of care for those who have been suddenly bereaved. It will also outline the care of staff who have cared for the suddenly bereaved.

BACKGROUND

The literature surrounding the subject of sudden death is vast (Royal College of Nursing 2002, Kent & Dowell 2004, Mushtaq & Ritchie 2005). Death is the permanent cessation of all vital functions, the end of human life, an event and a state. Dying is a process of coming to an end: the final act of living (Thompson 1994). Wright (1996) defined sudden deaths as those occurring without warning – the unexpected death. Deaths that result from acute disease, accidents, suicides and homicides fall into this category. It is these sudden deaths that are most frequently encountered in ED.

The Royal College of Nursing (RCN) and British Association for Accident and Emergency Medicine (BAEM) (1995), in the largest study of its kind, considered the facilities in ED departments for the bereaved. A questionnaire was sent to all 267 ED departments in England and Wales to identify the systems, facilities and training provided. Of the 248 (93%) departments that responded, it was possible to estimate that two to three attendances per 1000 new attendances involved relatives who were bereaved following a patient dying in ED. Forty per cent of the departments that responded stated they had two to three deaths per week, with a further 25% having four to five deaths per week. In terms of workload and impact on the average ED, sudden death can be significant for staff as well as for relatives.

The concept of a trajectory of death was developed by Glaser & Strauss (1965, 1968) to refer to the pattern of death. They distinguish between 'quick' and 'slow' dying trajectories. Generally, in ED, the patients have a 'quick' death trajectory, which is unexpected by the family, even when it is the result of a long-standing medical condition, such as heart disease. Lindemann (1944), in a classic study of bereavement, suggested that people who fear the death of a loved one often begin the process of grieving before any loss actually occurs. The acute reactions to loss include an initial period of shock followed by intense emotional pangs of grief. Lindemann identified the following symptoms of normal grief:

- somatic distress, such as feelings of tightness in the throat or chest
- preoccupation with the image of the deceased
- guilt
- hostile reactions
- loss of patterns of conduct.

These symptoms will not be unfamiliar to ED staff who have looked after recently bereaved relatives. Lindemann's work stemmed from a fire at the Coconut Grove night club in 1942 which claimed the lives of 474 people. He found that the fire resulted in a crisis for all individuals closely involved, including staff. Scott (1994) suggested that caring for distressed relatives following a sudden death is perhaps one of the most emotionally draining of nursing interventions. Wright (1996), in a study of relatives' responses to sudden death, found nine common emotional responses identified by nurses as difficult to manage, including:

- denial
- withdrawal
- anger
- acceptance
- isolation
- bargaining
- crying, sobbing, weeping.

It is noteworthy that five of the emotional responses that cause difficulties for ED nurses also correspond with what Kubler-Ross (1973) described as the stages of grief, i.e. denial, anger, isolation, bargaining and acceptance. Kubler-Ross was careful to point out that these stages do not happen in a particular order, and can occur side by side. These stages do not just affect dying patients but, as can be seen above, affect relatives and staff as well.

There is, however, debate regarding the usefulness of identifying emotions in an attempt to define the manifestation of grieving as this may lead people to think of grief in a simplistic way. Thus the theories and emotions attributed to grief should only be used as a guide to inform the possible reactions experienced by those who are bereaved (Davies 1997, Stroebe & Schut 1998, Kent & Dowell 2004). That noted, people experiencing the sudden unexpected death of a loved one are at risk of more pronounced and prolonged grief reactions than those who had been expecting death. There is also a higher morbidity rate among these people in the following two years after the death (Kent & Dowell 2004).

PREPARING FOR RECEIVING THE PATIENT AND RELATIVES

With growing improvements in communications technology, staff are increasingly informed of the impending arrival of critically ill or injured patients by ambulance control or the ambulance crew en route from the scene. This enables staff to prepare the resuscitation room and contact the on-call medical, paediatric and anaesthetic teams as appropriate. In accordance with advanced life-support principles, staff should be designated specific roles for the management of the patient (see also Ch. 2).

The 5–10 minutes' forewarning also serve to mentally prepare staff for the arrival of patients and their relatives. This time can also be used to provide support and guidance for more junior staff about what they might expect. A member of staff should be allocated to receive relatives. This nurse should not have any clinical responsibilities in the management of the resuscitation (see Box 13.1).

When anxious relatives arrive, they should be met by a named link nurse and not be kept waiting around at reception for the department's communications to be established (Li et al. 2002, Purves & Edwards 2005). While the term 'relatives' is used throughout this chapter, it is important to note that in some instances close friends or partners of either sex may be severely distressed and should be handled in the same way as the relatives.

WITNESSED RESUSCITATION

Witnessed resuscitation, the practice of enabling relatives to stay in the resuscitation room while their loved one is being resuscitated, remains controversial

Box 13.1 Principles of best practice when caring for the suddenly bereaved in ED (after Kent & Dowell 2004)

Contacting relatives or friends (see also Box 13.7)
- Communicate by telephone
- Speak to the most significant relative or friend, state own name and position held. If this is not the significant relative, it is important to ascertain where this person can be found
- The caller should state his name, designation and the hospital from which he is calling
- Give the patient's full name
- If there is doubt about the identity of the patient, state it is believed to be this person
- After giving this information, the caller should check that the relative is clear about:
  - Which hospital
  - How to get there
  - What has been said
- The relative should be advised:
  - To get someone to come out to the hospital with them
  - To drive carefully, and preferably get someone else to drive
  - To inform other close relatives or friends where they are heading
- Check understanding
- Records of the time of the call, who made the call, who responded, and how, are important. After a death, some relatives may want to clarify details

Arrival of relatives or friends
- Allocate one support nurse to the family or friends
- Meet them on arrival
- Take relatives or friends to an appropriately furnished private sitting room

Resuscitation
- Inform relatives or friends of the situation, assure them that every effort is being made to save the patient
- Provide an honest update every 10–15 minutes (support nurse)
- Encourage relatives or next of kin to witness resuscitation if they wish

Informing relatives or friends of the death
- Inform relatives or friends promptly of the death, using clear unambiguous language
- Express care and concern, support bereaved relatives and friends whatever their reaction
- Allow time to talk, listen and answer questions

Viewing the body
- Present the deceased person to look as peaceful as possible
- Encourage relatives or friends to see, touch and talk to the deceased person
- Allow time alone with the body
- Allow relatives or friends to participate in the last offices
- Provide the opportunity to see the place of death

The deceased person's belongings
- Fold clothing, place in a specially designed container, avoid plastic clothing bags
- Explain soiled or cut clothes, place a note with clothing stating same

Concluding procedures
- Accommodate cultural or religious rituals
- Discuss organ or tissue donation
- Inform relatives and friends about the post-mortem
- Provide information on arranging a funeral, registering a death and bereavement support groups
- Retain photograph or lock of hair

Follow-up
- Provide a hospital contact number and name of support nurse or doctor
- Ideally provide follow-up care in the week following the death by telephone or written note

(Chalk 1995, Boyd & White 1998, Royal College of Nursing, British Medical Association and Resuscitation Council 2002). A report by the Resuscitation Council (1996) suggested that although many nurses and doctors working in ED departments do not allow relatives to be present in the resuscitation room, the majority of relatives and close friends want to be there. While Dolan (1997) argued that 'enabling witnessed resuscitation is about having enough faith in ourselves as carers to show we are not afraid of others seeing us losing the battle for someone's life', Connors (1996) suggested that the advantages of allowing relatives to be present in the resuscitation room appear to outweigh any potential disadvantages. Box 13.2 and Box 13.3 outline health care professionals' concerns about allowing relatives into resuscitations rooms as well as reasons why relatives should be allowed in the resuscitation room.

Witnessed resuscitation was first documented by the Foote Hospital Michigan, after they introduced

---

Box 13.2 Health care professionals' concerns about allowing relatives in resuscitation rooms

- Family members' uncontrollable grief would disrupt smooth functioning of the resuscitation team
- Family members would become physically involved in the resuscitation attempt
- The team's emotions would be too strongly evoked by family presence
- Fear that some observed action or remark by the medical or nursing staff may offend grieving family members, such as use of humour as a stress reliever (Jezierski 1993)
- Witnessing a resuscitation is an experience that is non-therapeutic and traumatic enough to haunt the surviving family members as long as they live (Osuagwn 1993)
- There would not be enough adequately trained staff to implement a supportive role for all families (Back & Rooke 1994)
- The relatives may become cardiac arrest victims themselves (Osuagwn 1993)
- Fear that allowing observation of the activity and procedures would increase the legal risk (Hanson & Stawser 1992)
- Relatives may feel pressured into attending a resuscitation

---

Box 13.3 Reasons why relatives should be allowed in the resuscitation room

- The relative is able to see rather than being told that everything possible is being done. This comes from the belief that the reality of the resuscitation room is far less horrifying than the fantasy
- The relative is able to touch the patient while she is still warm - to the general public, warm means alive (Connors 1996)
- Relatives can say whatever they need to while there is still a chance that the patient can hear them
- The grieving process is long and hard enough without eliminating any elements that might help adjustment (Martin 1991)
- The family is viewed more as part of a loving family and less as a clinical challenge
- Closer relationships are formed between nursing staff and patient's relatives (Hanson & Strawser 1992)
- Reduces the legal risk as families can see for themselves that no-one is trying to hide anything (Renzi-Brown 1989)
- The relatives feel that they are doing something in a hopeless situation

---

the system in 1982, following two incidents when family members insisted on being present (Hanson & Strawser 1992). They questioned recently bereaved relatives and found that 72% would have liked to have witnessed the resuscitation attempt. As a result, a programme of witnessed resuscitation began; however, there was resistance from many staff members. In an audit 3 years later, staff were questioned about their views and 71% endorsed the practice even though they felt it had incurred an increased stress level.

A UK study by Robinson et al. (1998) found there were no adverse psychological effects among relatives who witnessed resuscitation, all of whom were satisfied with the decision to remain with the patient. The trial was discontinued when the clinical team involved became convinced of the benefits to relatives of allowing them to witness resuscitation if they wished. Psychological follow-up at three and six months found fewer symptoms of grief and distress in the group who had witnessed resuscitation than in the control group. Of the patients who survived none believed that their confidentiality had been compromised.

Witnessed resuscitation is becoming more common and relatives will, in future, increasingly insist on being present. It is already seen as good practice by the working group of the Royal College of Nursing and British Association for Accident & Emergency Medicine (1995) as well as recommended practice by the Royal College of Nursing (2002) and Resuscitation Council (UK) (1996). Nurses should anticipate the changing needs of the community and plan this change carefully. Hampe (1975) found that family members expressed three main needs:

- to be with the dying patient
- to be kept informed
- to know that the dying person was not in pain.

It was also found that the least-supportive measure was to remove the family members from the bedside. Causing those who have been bereaved to feel left out, uninformed and helpless may lead to feelings of anger that can result in unnecessary anger during the grieving process (Wright 1999, Kent & Dowell 2004).

For staff who have, or wish to develop, a witnessed resuscitation policy, Box 13.4 offers guidance on what to say to relatives prior to witnessing a resuscitation. Box 13.5 provides guidance for the team leader, doctors and nurses on how to stop an arrest with relatives present.

Box 13.4   Suggested guidelines for staff on what to say to relatives prior to witnessing a resuscitation

- Relatives should be informed that their loved one is very ill and that at present the heart has stopped, so the doctors and nurses are having to breathe for the patient and artificially make her heart pump by pressing on her chest wall. If there is any signs that the heart is starting to function again, then the team may have to give an electrical shock to try to kickstart the heart again
- Relatives should be informed that the prognosis is very grim and it is very unlikely that their loved one will live. Should the patient come out of this event then the next 24 hours will be critical and there is the likelihood that this event will recur
- Relatives should be given the choice of going into the resuscitation room; they should never be made to feel they must go in
- Relatives should be informed that it is acceptable for them to come in for a couple of minutes at a time and leave whenever they wish
- Relatives should be informed that even though their loved one cannot respond to them it is possible that she might be able to hear them. This information should only be given to relatives who have decided to enter the area

- Relatives should be informed that no more than two to three relatives are allowed into the resuscitation room at any one time, as more might distract or hamper the resuscitation attempt. This number is suggested as it would be very difficult and distressing to the relatives to allow two out of three attending the department into the resuscitation area. The third person would then be lacking in support
- Relatives should be informed that the doctors may ask them to wait outside while some investigations, such as X-rays or invasive procedures, are carried out
- Relatives should be informed that at some point the team will feel that they have done everything possible to regain life, and that unfortunately their loved one is going to die. When this decision has been reached, the carer should say something like, 'We're going to stop soon, we've tried everything and nothing is helping'
- Before all attempts have ceased, the team should try to accommodate the relatives and give them the opportunity to be able to get close to their loved one to say 'goodbye' etc.

Box 13.5   Guidance for team leader, doctors and nurses on how to stop an arrest with relatives present

- The relatives must be supported by an experienced trained nurse, and this must be this nurse's only role. The relatives should have been informed before entering the scene that the prognosis is very poor and that the chances of successful resuscitation are very slim
- The decision to stop resuscitation should be made quietly. All staff involved should be consulted and, if feasible, the relatives should be included in this
- The team leader with the help of the support nurse, will inform relatives that the resuscitation attempt has failed and that they are about to stop
- Gradually, one by one, staff should leave the scene, those with no active involvement leaving first. The

team leader should stay to support the relatives and nurse looking after them. When most of the staff have left, the staff member carrying out cardiac massage should stop and leave quietly. The anaesthetist should then turn off the ventilator and cardiac monitor and, when possible, remove the ET tube, stop all i.v. lines and then leave the area
- When ready, the nurse should then escort the relatives out of the area and follow the local bereavement guidelines
- The team leader will talk to the relatives in the relatives' room, answering any questions that may arise. The support nurse should still be with the relatives
- All staff should be involved in the debriefing

BREAKING BAD NEWS

For relatives who are waiting in the 'sitting room' or 'relatives' room', it should be sensitively decorated, bright and well lit (see Box 13.6). Frequent updates on the patient's condition are important. The link nurse should liaise with staff in the resuscitation

room to maintain communication between the relatives and the resuscitation team. Concise terms such as 'critical', 'serious', 'good' and 'fair' appear to be reasonably understood by lay and professionals alike.

In the event of cessation of resuscitation, if relatives are not present when the patient dies, or if they arrive after the death, staff will have to break the news to

Box 13.6   Facilities for the bereaved in the emergency department

In the room there should be:

- Comfortable, domestic chairs and sofas. In recognition of people with special needs, for example, the elderly, appropriate furniture should be provided
- Tissues
- Ashtrays
- A telephone with direct dial access for incoming and outgoing calls
- Telephone directories
- A washbasin, with soap, towel, mirror and freshen-up pack
- TV/radio available, but not prominent
- Hot and cold drinks should be available. A fridge and kettle point enable independence, and are convenient for staff. A non-institutional tea/coffee set should also be available
- Toys and books should be available

them. McLauchlan (1996) suggested that breaking bad news has to be tailored to the situation and particular relatives; however, the following principles apply:

- On leaving the resuscitation room, the breaker of bad news, who is usually a doctor but may also be a nurse, should take a moment to gather his composure. Removal of plastic aprons, stethoscopes around the neck and other obviously clinical paraphernalia is recommended.
- It is important to confirm that the correct relatives are being addressed. It can be a simple but traumatic mistake to inform the wrong people of the death of a relative.
- On entering the relatives' room, it is important for the nurse and doctor to introduce themselves. Sitting down to talk with relatives gives the impression that the bearers of bad news are not in a rush to leave.
- During the interview, it may be helpful and natural to touch or hold the hand of the bereaved relative(s). While various social and cultural factors may influence the appropriateness of this, if it feels appropriate then it probably is right.
- Getting to the point quickly is important.

When providing information and answering questions, keep it honest, direct and simple. Phrases like 'dead' and 'died' should be used as they are unambiguous. Giving the news thoughtfully and showing

concern will enable the relatives to understand the event as reality.

- If a language barrier exists, attempt to obtain a translator from outside the family and prepare the translator. If a family member is the only translator, it is important to acknowledge how difficult a task it is to hear bad news about a loved one and to explain the news to someone else.
- Euphemisms should be avoided at all costs. Table 13.1 outlines phrases that should not be used when breaking bad news.
- After breaking the bad news, allow time and silence while the facts sink in, re-emphasizing them if appropriate. Sometimes, just listening to someone who is distressed, or sitting in silence with them, witnessing their grief, may be the most important service a nurse or doctor can provide for someone who is bereaved (Casarett 2001).
- Be prepared for a variety of emotional responses or reactions. Some may appear unmoved, while others will sob and wail. These reactions are not the fault of the bearer of bad news, but are a reaction to the news itself.
- Offer the relatives the opportunity to view the deceased.

Communication is a dynamic, complex and continuous exchange (Winchester 1999). Frequently, however, the person communicating the bad news feels that it has been done badly. In a health profession which still sees death as a failure, this is not surprising, especially when it is compounded with the powerful feelings evoked by sudden death. Thayre & Hadfield-Law (1995) noted that, when preparing to give bad news, it is essential that the nurse is aware that increasing urbanization, advances in medical technology and skills, and the declining size and importance of the extended family have all

Table 13.1   Phrases to be avoided when breaking bad news

What is said	What the relative may understand
We have lost him	He has gone missing in the hospital
She has passed on	She has been transferred to another ward
He has slipped away	He has sneaked out of the department
She has suffered irreversible asystole	Nothing!

decreased people's experience of close death. In addition, changing cultural and religious practices mean that nurses may not always be aware of family needs in this respect. It is also important to stress that when breaking bad news the medical facts are less important than the compassion shown to relatives.

Telephone notification

Where possible, telephone notification of bereavement should be avoided as it can cause acute distress to the receiver as well as to the person delivering the news. Wright (1993) noted that the feelings of a person receiving information over the telephone frequently include the following:

- 'They knew more than they said'
- 'I am not sure what they said'
- 'It cannot be as bad as they say'
- 'I am not sure what they want me to do'
- 'It does not make sense'.

Fears of the individual giving information over the telephone may include:

- 'I hope I have identified and am speaking to the right person'
- 'What if they collapse when I tell them, and they are alone?'
- 'Panic may prevent them hearing me'
- What will I say if they ask me outright if their relative is dead?'
- 'People just should not hear this over the phone'.

Thayre & Hadfield-Law (1995) suggested that information given over the telephone should be in small units. Following the shock of bad news, people tend to respond only to simple questions or instructions and may be slow to take in involved explanations. Jones & Buttery (1981) found that relatives only rarely asked over the telephone whether their loved one was dead. Box 13.7 outlines the information that should be given to those who ring or are contacted about death or critical illness of a relative.

VIEWING THE BODY

The opportunity to see the dead person should always be offered and gently encouraged (Haas 2003). While some well-meaning friends or relatives may discourage this act, it is an important part of accepting the reality of the situation and can facilitate grieving and ease feelings of guilt after sudden death (Vanezis & McGee 1999). Jones & Buttery (1981) found that relatives of sudden-death victims who spent time with the body in the ED concluded that the viewing process was helpful.

Box 13.7   Information to give to relatives over the telephone

- Clear, concise communication is vital
- The caller should state his name, designation and the hospital from which he is calling
- If this is not the significant relative, it is important to ascertain where this person can be found
- Give the name of the ill or injured person and her condition
- If there is doubt about the identity of the patient, tell the relative it is believed to be this person
- After giving this information, the caller should check that the relative is clear about:
  - which hospital
  - how to get there
  - what has been said
- The relative should be advised:
  - to get someone to come out to the hospital with them
  - to drive carefully, and preferably get someone else to drive
  - to inform other close relatives or friends where they are heading
- Records of the time of the call, who made the call, who responded, and how, are important. After a death, some relatives may want to clarify details

---

The environment in which the relatives view the body should be made as non-clinical as reasonably possible. Monitors should always be switched off. Drips and invasive treatment aids, such as ET tubes, catheters and cannulae, should be removed. Before allowing viewing, blood should be wiped from the patient's body, eyes should be closed and a blanket should cover the patient up to the upper shoulder. Leaving the deceased person's arm(s) over the covers and respectful washing of the face and combing of the hair should be done before relatives attend. Religious insignia can be added as appropriate. Sufficient chairs should be available for relatives to sit down. Reluctant or unwilling family members should be reassured that viewing is a highly personal decision and that a decision *not* to view the deceased person may be best for many people.

When the dead person is disfigured or mutilated, the relatives' wishes are paramount. Gentle, honest explanations beforehand can inform the relatives' decision about whether they wish to see the dead person (Davies 1997). The relatives should be encouraged to touch, hold, kiss, hug or say goodbye to their loved one. When speaking of the dead person, use the person's name, 'him,' or 'her', but never 'body' or 'it'.

Warn the family that the patient may look different from their expectations. Unless there are suspicious circumstances and the police wish to remain with the body, the relatives may also like to be left alone with the body and must be given permission to stay as long as they wish or as is practically possible (Morgan 1997).

ORGAN DONATION

Body organs and tissues, such as the kidneys, heart, liver, pancreas and corneas, may be donated by the patient for availability for transplant. There is, however, a great shortage of organs for transplant, which continues to limit transplant efforts, and the demand is growing at a much greater rate than the supply (Wilkinson 2000). The usage of potential organs from emergency departments is very low. Sweet (1996) noted that there are two types of donor of organs and tissues for transplantation. First, there are the 'beating-heart' donors, who constitute either those who have been declared brain dead – i.e. where respiratory and circulatory functions are maintained solely by mechanical ventilation – or those who are living, who can only donate kidneys and bone marrow. If they fit the criteria, brain-dead donors can be multi-organ donors, i.e. their organs and tissues can be used in transplantation. Second, there are the 'non-beating-heart' donors, where death with cessation of circulatory and respiratory function has occurred. This is the type of donor usually found in ED. Wellesley et al. (1997) noted that the organs that can be donated from ED include corneas, heart valves and, in certain departments, kidneys. For heart valves there must be no congenital valve defect, no systemic infection, no hepatitis B or C, and the donor must not be HIV-positive. For corneas, there are even fewer contraindications: no scarring of the cornea, no infection in the eye and no invasive brain tumours. Both organs are very successfully transplanted, with at least 85% success for corneas and even higher for heart valves, due to the absence of rejection problems.

Consent from the coroner may be a limiting factor to tissue retrieval in ED. Unless a doctor is prepared to sign a death certificate to state that a patient died of natural causes then the coroner must give consent prior to removal of any organ or tissue, as stated in the Human Tissue Act 2004.

Many nurses believe relatives should not be approached about organ donation in ED, feeling that they have been through enough (Coupe 1990). However, a recent small-scale study by Wellesley et al. (1997) highlighted that 27 (72.9%) of the 37 recently bereaved respondents to a questionnaire would not

have minded being asked about organ donation following a sudden death. They suggested that the subject could be broached by having leaflets in the room where relatives are given the bad news, as a way of introducing this delicate subject and providing more information. They believe the interview with bereaved relatives needs to be carried out sensitively by senior nurses, registrars or, in some cases, the consultant, who have been appropriately trained and who have access to staff support within the ED (see also Ch. 38: Law).

LEGAL AND ETHICAL ISSUES

Contact with the coroner's officer may occur in the ED or in the home when the notification of the death and identification of the body are established. It is important to distinguish between a coroner's officer who gathers and records details related to the death, e.g. by attending postmortems, and the coroner, usually a doctor or lawyer, who responds to the results of the details by concluding on the circumstances of the death and reaching, if necessary, a verdict at inquest.

Scott (1995) suggested that relatives are often devastated by the news of the death and that these feelings are intensified at the thought of the purposeful mutilation of the body at autopsy. In fact, the autopsy is a legal requirement for most deaths that occur in ED (see Box 13.8). This information needs to be conveyed to patients in a dignified, sensitive way.

Controversy exists over whether personal possessions, and in particular jewellery and precious metals,

---

Box 13.8 Criteria for investigation of a death by a coroner

The coroner is a doctor or lawyer responsible for investigating death in the following situations:

- The deceased was not attended by a doctor during the last illness or the doctor treating the deceased had not seen her after the death or within 14 days of the death
- The death was violent or unnatural or occurred under suspicious circumstances
- The cause of death is not known or is uncertain
- The death occurred in prison or in police custody
- The death occurred while the patient was undergoing an operation or the patient did not recover from the anaesthetic
- The death was caused by an industrial disease

should be given to relatives. Should relatives wish to remove any rings or special belongings, they should be enabled to do so. Legally, a witnessed signature is sufficient to corroborate the act of handing over or retaining property and this may be obtained from another nurse, doctor or coroner's officer (Cooke et al. 1992). Clothing should be carefully folded and itemized along with any other possessions such as jewellery and money. The nurse should seek permission from the family to dispose of badly damaged clothing. This should be recorded in the patient's notes.

SUDDEN INFANT DEATH SYNDROME

This issue is addressed in detail in Chapter 15.

STAFF SUPPORT

Cudmore (1998) believes that ED nurses are 'at risk' of developing post-traumatic stress reactions because of their exposure to traumatic events as a routine part of their job, which for most people would be outside the range of human experience. Walsh et al. (1998) argued that if stress is the main cause of burn-out, then understanding coping mechanisms is the key to minimizing the problem. Coping strategies employed by those working with trauma include the following:

- suppressing emotions and feelings
- mutual staff support
- promoting a sense of unreality
- mental preparation for tasks
- feeling competent and capable
- regulating exposure to the event
- having a sense of purpose
- humour.

Box 13.9 outlines the effects of traumatic events on carers. The following are methods that staff working with dying people can use to improve their coping skills:

- the encouragement of personal insight to understand and acknowledge one's own limits
- a healthy balance between work and outside life
- the promotion of a team approach to care
- an ongoing support system within work and outside work
- for those working in isolation, continuing guidance and support, from peers and superiors

(Defusion, demobilization and critical incident debriefing skills for staff are discussed in detail in Ch. 12.)

Box 13.9   The effects of traumatic events such as failed resuscitation attempts on carers

- **Emotional effects** – anxiety, depression, anger, guilt, irritability and feelings of helplessness
- **Cognitive effects** - memory/concentration changes, nightmares, intrusive thoughts and imagery
- **Behavioural effects** - alters use of drugs, alcohol, nicotine, caffeine etc., social withdrawal and loss of interest in usual activities
- **Relationship effects** - changes in work, social, intimate and sexual relationships through irritability, inability to share feelings, isolation and conflict of loyalty between work and home
- **Somatic effects** - changes in sleeping and eating habits, altered energy levels, an increase in accidents and physical health problems
- **Motivational effects** - viewing life from a different perspective, often as more tenuous. Values may be reoriented to less materialistic ones

---

CONCLUSION

Sudden death, by whatever cause, is a stressful and distressing event for staff as well as for patient's relatives. While ED departments may be geared towards saving lives, death should not be seen by staff as a failure. No matter how confident or experienced the practitioner, it is never easy to tell relatives or friends that a loved one has died (Kendrick 1997). In relation to the needs of relatives, Dolan (1995) argued that:

> '... in so many respects, it seems worth the effort and distress of the trip to know that everything that could be done was done. The tacit transfer of responsibility from patient and family to health carers highlights that while caring costs, our compassion must never get sacrificed as the cost of our caring.'

This chapter has highlighted the process of care for those who have been suddenly bereaved. Within an ageing society, it is likely that more people will require the resuscitative efforts of ED staff; however, many will not survive. Their relatives are particularly vulnerable in this traumatic situation and require the nurse to advocate for them at this time, enabling them to witness the resuscitation if they wish and receive the news of death with compassion and understanding. For ED personnel, training and ongoing support will enable them to deal with the challenges of caring for such vulnerable people. The unexpected end of one person's life is the beginning of someone else's grief. ED nurses are in a key position to enable a relative's last memory of a loved one to become a lasting memory of compassionate support and care.

References

Boyd R, White S (1998) Does witnessed cardiopulmonary resuscitation alter perceived stress levels in Accident and Emergency staff? *Journal of Accident and Emergency Medicine*, **15**, 109–111.

Casarett D et al. (2001) Life after death: a practical approach to grief and bereavement. *Annals of Internal Medicine,* **134**(3), 208–215.

Chalk A (1995) Should relatives be present in the resuscitation room? *Accident and Emergency Nursing*, **3**(2), 58–61.

Connors P (1996) Should relatives be allowed in the resuscitation room? *Nursing Standard*, **10**(44), 44–46.

Cooke MW, Cooke HW, Glucksmann EE (1992) Management of sudden bereavement in the accident & emergency department. *British Medical Journal*, **304**, 1207–1209.

Coupe C (1990) Donation dilemmas. *Nursing Times*, **86**(27), 34–36.

Cudmore J (1998) Critical incident stress management strategies. *Emergency Nurse*, **6**(3), 22–27.

Davies J (1997) Grieving after a sudden death: the impact of the initial intervention. *Accident and Emergency Nursing*, **5**(4), 181–184.

Dolan B (1995) Drama within a crisis – relatives in the resuscitation room. *Journal of Clinical Nursing*, **4**(5), 275.

Dolan B (1997) Editorial. Underlining compassion in casualty. *Emergency Nurse*, **5**(2), 1.

Glaser BG, Strauss AL (1965) *Awareness of Dying*. Chicago: Aldine Press.

Glaser BG, Strauss AL (1968) *Time for Dying*. Chicago: Aldine Press.

Haas F (2003) Bereavement care: seeing the body. *Nursing Standard*, **17**(28), 33–37.

Hampe SO (1975) Needs of the grieving spouse in a hospital setting. *Nursing Research*, **24**, 113–120.

Hanson C, Strawser D (1992) Family presence during CPR: Foote Hospital Emergency Department's nine-year perspective. *Journal of Emergency Nursing*, **18**(2), 104–106.

Human Tissue Act (2004) London: HMSO.

Jezierski M (1993) Foote Hospital emergency department: shattering a paradigm. *Journal of Emergency Nursing*, **19**(3), 266–267.

Jones WH, Buttery H (1981) Sudden death: survivors' perceptions of their emergency department experience. *Journal of Emergency Nursing*, **7**(1), 14–17.

Kendrick K (1997) Sudden death: walking in a moral minefield. *Emergency Nurse*, **5**(1), 17–19.

Kent H, McDowell J (2004) Sudden bereavement in acute care settings. *Nursing Standard*, **19**(6), 38–42.

Kubler-Ross H (1973) *On Death and Dying*. New York: Macmillan.

Li S et al. (2002) Helpfulness of nursing actions to suddenly bereaved family members in an accident and emergency setting in Hong Kong. *Journal of Advanced Nursing*, **40**(2), 170–180.

Lindemann E (1944) Symptomatology and management of acute grief. *American Journal of Psychiatry*, **101**, 141–148.

McLauchlan CAJ (1990) Handling distressed relatives and breaking bad news. *British Medical Journal*, **301**, 1145–1147.

McLauchlan CAJ (1996) Handling distressed relatives and breaking bad news. In: Skinner, D, Driscoll P, Earlam R, eds. *ABC of Major Trauma*, 2nd edn. London: BMJ.

Martin J (1991) Rethinking traditional thoughts. *Journal of Emergency Nursing*, **17**(2), 67–68.

Morgan J (1997) Introducing a witnessed resuscitation policy to ED. *Emergency Nurse*, **5**(2), 13–17.

Mushtaq F, Ritchie D (2005) Do we know what people die of in the emergency department? *Emergency Medicine Journal*, **22**, 718–721.

Osuagwn CC (1993) More on family presence during resuscitation. *Journal of Emergency Nursing*, **19**(4), 276–277.

Purves Y, Edwards S (2005) Initial needs of bereaved relatives following sudden and unexpected death. *Emergency Nurse*, **13**(7), 28–34

Resuscitation Council (1996) *Should Relatives Witness Resuscitation?* London: Resuscitation Council.

Robinson SM, Campbell-Hewson GL, Egelston CV, Prevost AT, Ross SM (1998) The psychological impact on relatives of witnessing resuscitation. *Lancet*, **352**(9128), 614–617

Royal College of Nursing and British Association for Accident and Emergency Medicine (1995) *Bereavement Care in A&E Departments: Report of a Working Group*. London: RCN

Royal College of Nursing (2002) *Witnessed Resuscitation*. London: RCN

Royal College of Nursing, British Medical Association and Resuscitation Council (2002) *Decisions Relating to Cardiopulmonary Resuscitation: A Joint Statement from the British Medical Association, Resuscitation Council (UK) and the Royal College of Nursing*. London: BMA.

Scott T (1994) Sudden death in A&E. *Emergency Nurse*, **2**(4), 10–15.

Stroebe M. Schut H (1998) Culture and grief. *Bereavement Care*, **17**(1), 7–11.

Sweet A (1996) Organ donation and transplantation. *Emergency Nurse*, **3**(4), 6–9.

Thayre K, Hadfield-Law L (1995) Never going to be easy: giving bad news. *Nursing Standard (RCN Nursing Update supplement)*, **9**(50), 3–8.

Thompson D (1994) Death and dying in critical care. In: Burnard P, Millar B, eds. *Critical Care Nursing*. London: Baillière Tindall.

Vanezis M, McGee A (1999) Mediating factors in the grieving process of the suddenly bereaved. *British Journal of Nursing*, **8**(14), 932–937.

Walsh M, Dolan B, Lewis A (1998) Burnout and stress among A&E nurses. *Emergency Nurse*, **6**(2), 23–30.

Wellesley A, Glucksmann EE, Crouch R (1997) Organ donation in the accident and emergency department: a study of relatives' views. *Journal of Accident and Emergency Medicine,* **14**, 24–25.

Wilkinson R (2000) Organ donation: the debate. *Nursing Standard*, **14**(28) 41–42.

Winchester A (1999) Sharing bad news. *Nursing Standard*, **13**(26), 48–52.

Wright B (1993) *Caring in Crisis*, 2nd edn. Edinburgh: Churchill Livingstone.

Wright B (1996) *Sudden Death: A Research Base for Practice*. Edinburgh: Churchill Livingstone.

Wright B (1999) Responding to autonomy and disempowerment at the time of a sudden death. *Accident and Emergency Nursing*, **7**(3), 154–157.

Chapter **14**

Psychiatric emergencies

Barbara Warncken & Brian Dolan

CHAPTER CONTENTS

INTRODUCTION

It is estimated that 1–2% of patients presenting to an emergency department (ED) require a formal mental-state assessment (Andrew-Starkey 2004). A psychiatric emergency is any disturbance in the patient's thoughts, feelings or actions for which immediate therapeutic intervention is necessary (Kaplan & Sadock 1993). The reasons most frequently given by patients for emergency psychiatric visits include (Gillig et al. 1990):

- a need to talk things over so decisions can be made
- to help get control over themselves
- treatment for 'nerves'
- to obtain or adjust medications.

People who come to ED range from those with specific requests for help to those who are brought in against their will for reasons they do not understand. In either case, the patient or carers may believe that the patient is no longer able to maintain coping abilities at his usual level of functioning.

The reasons why many of these patients attend ED are multifactorial. A primary reason, however, is the deinstitutionalization of the mentally ill, due to the introduction of psychotropic medication in the 1950s and the changing focus on treatment and rehabilitation within the community. As a consequence, for many in society, their only access to health care is through ED (Ambrose 1996).

For the ED nurse who deals with various life-threatening emergencies on a routine basis, these needs may not appear to be true emergencies; however, it is a crisis that brings the psychiatric patient to the ED and the nature and degree of a crisis are defined by the person experiencing it. It is also to be seen as an opportunity, because prompt and skilful interventions may prevent the development of serious long-term disability and allow new coping patterns to develop (Aguilera 1998).

AETIOLOGY OF MENTAL ILLNESS

It is recognized that genetic, biological and biochemical dyscrasias play a significant role in the causes of major psychiatric illness. It is therefore difficult to discuss psychiatric disorders as having a purely organic or functional basis. However, for the purpose of this chapter, organic disorders will be considered as those disorders that have a grossly identifiable and potentially reversible physiological cause, such as endocrine and metabolic disorders, neurological causes and drug-induced states. Functional disorders will be considered as those disorders without a grossly identifiable physiological cause.

ASSESSMENT OF PSYCHIATRIC PATIENTS IN ED

The goals of ED psychiatric evaluation are to conduct a rapid assessment, including diagnosis of any underlying medical problems, to provide emergency treatment and to arrange appropriate disposition (Greenstein & Ness 1990). These goals will be hampered by various obstructions and restrictions, such as time and space, departmental milieu, inability to obtain a history from a disturbed or distressed patient and experience of staff. Information collected must be concise and methods of assessment flexible enough to take into consideration the patient's and the unit's needs. Relevant details must be documented, as they may be the only recorded evidence of symptoms displayed by the patient in the acute phase. This forms the baseline for the management and treatment plan. Records are also important for medicolegal reasons. The nurse should make full use of any information source available, such as family, escorts, ambulance personnel, community staff, police, hospital notes and other staff who may know the patient from previous attendances or admissions. Once an assessment is made, the patient should be given the appropriate triage category employed by the unit, e.g. Manchester Triage guidelines (Mackway-Jones et al. 2005).

History

History is usually initiated by the triage/assessment nurse, who must speedily determine the urgency of the crisis for which the person is seeking care and his capacity to wait. The nurse at this time has to determine how much of a risk the patient poses to himself and to others, such as violent tendencies,

suicide, self-mutilation, impaired judgement, etc. The history should include:

- reason for attendance
- history of presenting illness
- past general medical/psychiatric history
- social history
- family history.

The triage/assessment nurse may be the patient's first contact with the healthcare system, and an attitude of acceptance, respect and empathy, with a desire to help, should be conveyed to the patient. This first contact may significantly influence the patient's acceptance of emergency care and his receptivity to future treatment. Ward (1995) suggested the following as a reasonable focus to begin with:

- What does the patient want?
- Who is in danger?
- What has caused this behaviour?

And, if the patient is already known:

- What has happened in previous situations like this?
- What did this mean to the patient the last time it happened?

Mental state examination

Examination of the mental state in psychiatry is analogous to the physical examination in a general medical or surgical practice (Andrew-Starkey 2004). At a minimum the nurse should note:

- Appearance and general behaviour – especially if the patient is disturbed and no history is available. Assess the state of the patient's clothes, cleanliness, facial expression and reaction to the interviewing clinician. Describe motor behaviour, impulse control, orientation, eye contact, attention/concentration, posture, memory.
- Mood – blunting/flattening of affect, agitation, hypomania, diurnal mood variation (depressed in the mornings, but feeling brighter in the evenings or vice versa), sleep pattern, appetite, weight loss/gain.
- Speech and thought – this assessment should include form and content of speech, rate and rhythm, anxieties, suicidal/future references, evidence of formal thought disorder, thought broadcasting, thought insertion, pressure of speech, ideas of reference, delusions (for glossary of terms see Box 14.3).
- Abnormal perceptions and related experiences – hallucinations, derealization, depersonalization.

- Cognitive state – if an organic diagnosis is suspected, a more formal and detailed examination is required.
- Insight and judgement –does the patient recognize that he is ill and in need of assistance? Is he able to make rational judgements?
- Impulse control – is the patient capable of controlling sexual, aggressive or other impulses? Is he a potential danger to himself or others? Is this as a result of an organic mental disease or of psychosis or chronic character traits?
- Physical assessment – a complete physical assessment is required to rule out a physical cause. This will include neurological observations, BM stix, glucose, U&Es, FBC, LFT(DAX), thyroid function tests, ECG etc.

Formulating and agreeing a nursing and medical management framework of aims and objectives are important, i.e.:

- main features of presenting complaint
- physical examination and consultation
- investigations undertaken
- provisional and differential diagnosis, e.g. organic cause, acute functional psychosis (schizophrenia, affective states), neurosis, personality disorders
- any immediate intervention taken.

If admission is not recommended or required, the ED nurse should be aware of local services and agencies that the patient may be referred to, such as:

- chemical dependency/detox services
- outpatients
- crisis telephone numbers
- day hospital facilities
- social services
- facilities available for the homeless
- hostels
- ethnic-minority advisory groups
- interpreters
- rape-counselling centres
- needle exchanges
- sexual health and associated conditions services
- police/probation officers.

ACUTE ORGANIC REACTIONS

Frequently, acute organic reactions present to ED as psychiatric emergencies when the aetiology is unknown and there is loss of behavioural control (Box 14.1). The most consistent symptom of an acute organic reaction is impairment in the consciousness, worsening symptoms at night, and good pre-morbid personality.

Box 14.1   Causes of acute organic reactions

- Trauma
- Infection
  Local
  - cerebral abscess
  - meningitis
  - encephalitis
  - syphilis
  - cerebral malaria
  General
  - systemic infection
  - septicaemia
  - typhus
  - typhoid
- Cerebrovascular
  - cerebrovascular accident
  - transient ischaemic attack
  - subarachnoid haemorrhage
  - subdural haemorrhage
  - hypertensive encephalopathy
  - systemic lupus erythematosus
  - cervical arteritis
- Epilepsy
- Tumour
  - primary secondary metastatic effects
- Organ failure
  - renal, cardiac, hepatic, respiratory
- Anaemia
- Metabolic
  - U&E imbalance
  - acid-base imbalance
  - uraemia
- Endocrine
  - hypo/hyperthyroidism,
  - hypo/hyperparathyroidism, hypopituitarism
  - hypo/hyperglycaemia
- Deficiency disorders
  - thiamine, nicotinic acid, folic acid, vitamin B_{12}
- Toxic causes
  - drug overdose
  - alcohol withdrawal
  - lead, arsenic, carbon monoxide/ disulphide, mercury

Nursing and medical management

A treatment plan, both nursing and medical/psychological, will be based on the cause and presenting behavioural disturbance. If possible, medication should be withheld, as this may mask or distort neurological signs, unless the patient's presenting behaviour warrants it.

A physical examination should be performed on all patients presenting with a psychiatric crisis in order to rule out common physical illnesses that mimic psychiatric disorder (see Box 14.2). People with mental health problems have a higher morbidity rate for physical illness than the general population, so their physical symptoms and complaints need to be taken seriously and investigated (Gournay & Beadsmore 1995). Diagnostic tests to confirm or rule out physical conditions masking psychiatric disorders or vice versa should be performed as necessary.

ACUTE PSYCHOTIC EPISODE

Psychotic patients experience impaired reality testing as they are unable to distinguish between what is real and what is not. Their thought processes are often disordered and often characterized by hallucinations, delusions, ideas of reference, thought broadcasting and thought insertion (Kaiser & Pyngolil 1995) (see

---

Box 14.2   Organic illnesses or conditions that mimic psychiatric symptoms

- Thyrotoxicosis
- Hypoparathyroidism
- Hypoglycaemia
- Phaeochromocytoma
- Carcinoid syndrome
- Brain tumours or bleeding
- Head trauma
- Seizure disorders, such as, epilepsy
- Drug ingestions or poisoning
  - amphetamines
  - hallucinogens
  - lead poisoning
  - steroid toxicity
  - atropine
- Myxoedema
- Cushing's syndrome
- Porphyria
- Hyperparathyroidism
- Addison's disease
- Systemic lupus erythematosus
- Carcinoma

Box 14.3). It is essential that the ED nurse is able to differentiate between a psychosis with an organic cause, e.g. delirium, and a functional psychosis, e.g. schizophrenia. Psychotic patients may present to ED on an emergency basis when it is:

- an acute psychotic episode, first presentation
- the exacerbation of a chronic state
- a long-term problem where the patient is requesting admission, support or medication
- a catatonic excitement/stupor.

Schizophrenia

There are circumstances, as mentioned above, where patients with schizophrenia may present as an emergency to ED. Schizophrenia is the commonest form of pyschosis and, while it can develop at any age, it most commonly starts in late adolescence and early twenties. It has a prevalence of approximately 1% worldwide and highest in inner cities (Boydell et al. 2003).

Clinical features

Clinical features will depend to a certain extent on the type of schizophrenia – paranoid, hebephrenic, simple or catatonic. The distinction between subtypes will be based on a full assessment and is less relevant in ED.

The 'first rank' symptoms of schizophrenia are rare in other psychotic illnesses, e.g. mania or organic psychosis. The presence of only *one* of the following symptoms is strongly predictive of the diagnosis of schizophrenia:

- auditory hallucinations, especially the echoing of thoughts, or a third-person 'commentary' on one's actions, e.g. 'Now he's taking his jacket off'
- thought insertion, removal or interruption – delusions about external control of thought
- thought broadcasting – the delusion that others can hear one's thoughts
- delusional perceptions – i.e. abnormal significance for a normal event, e.g. 'The sun shone and I knew it was a sign from God'
- external control of emotions
- somatic passivity – thoughts, sensations and actions are under external control (see Box 14.3).

These acute symptoms may be superimposed on those of a chronic illness, e.g. apathy, impaired social network etc. Personal hygiene in the psychotic patient is frequently neglected. He may be incontinent and have a poor diet intake.

Long-term patients frequently attend ED as a 24-hour walk-in service for requests of admission, social support or medication. Often these patients are in need of reassurance and support. If the delusions or hallucinations are a re-emergence in a long-term patient, the

Box 14.3 Acute psychotic episode symptoms

- Ideas of reference
    Referring to him in their gestures, speech, mannerisms

- Delusions, delusional mood
    A fixed false idea or belief held by the patient which cannot be corrected by reasoning

- Hallucinations
    Apparent perception of external object not actually there involving any of the special senses, e.g. visual, auditory, third person auditory, voices arguing, commenting, commanding, gustatory, tactile, olfactory

- Disorder of experience of thought
    Thought insertion: patient believes others are inserting, placing thoughts into his mind
    Broadcasting: person believes his thoughts are being broadcasted and that all are aware of what he is thinking
    Blocking: interruption of a train of speech as a result of the person losing his train of thought

- Experience of passivity
    A delusional feeling that the person is under some outside control and therefore must be inactive

- Disturbance of speech
    Tangential speech: a style of speech containing oblique or irrelevant responses to questions asked, e.g. the person will talk about world hunger when asked about his breakfast
    Poverty of content: restriction of speech, so that spontaneous speech and replies to questions are brief and without elaboration
    Word salad: a characteristic of schizophrenia – a mixture of words that lack meaningful connections

- Emotional disturbance
    Emotional flattening: without normal 'highs' or 'lows' of feelings
    Inappropriate affect: incongruous responses to situations, e.g. laughing at hearing sad news

- Motor disturbance
    Excitement; bizarreness, in response to hallucinations; stupor

patient may be referred to outpatients for adjustment of medication. It is important to ensure that the patient's consultant and community team are aware of his attendance and changes, and that appropriate referrals are made.

Kaiser & Pyngolil (1995) suggested that the following therapeutic principles be used in guiding the ED nurse caring for patients who are experiencing distortions in thought content and perception (which are often associated with great fear):

- Attempt to establish a trusting relationship. The nurse should reassure the patient that she wants to help and that the patient is in a safe place and will not be harmed.
- Attempt to determine whether there was a precipitating event that triggered the psychotic episode. If so, evaluate it accordingly.
- If an organic, reversible cause is identified, reassure the patient that his feelings and thoughts are temporary.
- Minimize external stimulation. Psychotic people may be having trouble processing thoughts and often hear voices. By decreasing external stimulation, the nurse may decrease sensory stimulation to which the patient may be responding.

- Do not attempt to reason, challenge or argue the patient out of his delusions or hallucinations. Often these patients need to believe their delusions in order to decrease their anxiety and maintain control.
- The nurse should not imply that she believes the patient's hallucinations or delusional system in an attempt to win his trust. Statements to the effect that the nurse does not hear these things the patient is hearing but is interested in knowing about them are recommended.
- Do not underestimate the significance of a patient's psychotic thoughts. They are very real to the patient, and he cannot just 'put them aside'.
- Unless restraint is required, physical contact with psychotic patients or sudden movements should be avoided, as they may induce or validate the patient's fears.

Puskar & Obus (1989) suggested the following questions be asked when assessing a possibly schizophrenic patient:

- Do your thoughts make sense to you?
- Do you have ideas that come into your head that do not seem to be your own?

- Do you worry about what other people think about you?
- Do you think other people know what you are thinking?
- Do you hear your own thoughts spoken out loud?
- Do you sometimes feel that someone or some outside influence is controlling you, or making you think these things?

Once an organic cause has been ruled out, admission from ED will generally be required if the patient is disturbed, suicidal/homicidal or experiencing command hallucinations telling him to harm himself. The prognosis with schizophrenia varies widely, as with any chronic disorder. Approximately 15–25% will recover completely from an acute episode of psychosis, 10% will have ongoing severe problems and the remainder have a fluctuating course with reasonable function. There may be suicidal ideation; about 10% of patients with schizophrenia will commit suicide within 5 years of the onset of their illness and about 30% of people with schizophrenia attempt suicide at least once. Male patients and those who are unemployed, socially isolated, or recently discharged from hospital are most at risk (Doy et al. 2006).

Depression

Depression is a period of impaired functioning associated with depressed mood and related symptoms, including sleep and appetite changes, psychomotor changes, impaired concentration, fatigue, feelings of hopelessness, helplessness and suicide (Kaplan & Sadock 1993). Although estimates vary, approximately 20% of women and 10% of men will suffer from depression at some point in their lives. Community surveys indicate that 3–6% of adults are suffering from depression at any one time (Merson & Baldwin 1995). While it is a condition that can affect any individual at any time of life, Barker (1999) suggests that it is most prevalent in the working age population. The prevalence is approximately 2–3 times higher in women than men (Weissman et al. 1996).

Clinical features
Clinical features may include many of the following: depressed mood and affect; feelings of hopelessness, helplessness and worthlessness; guilt and inappropriate self-blame; suicidal ideation; decreased energy and activity; agitation/stupor; psychomotor retardation; anorexia; weight loss; and early morning wakening/difficulty getting to sleep. In more severe cases the patient may have somatic delusions and/or auditory hallucinations.

Nursing and medical management
Kaplan & Sadock (1993) proposed the following guidelines for evaluation and management of depression in ED:

- Treat any medical problems that may have resulted from suicide attempts or gestures.
- Maintain a safe environment for the patient.
- Rule out organic and pharmacological causes of depression.
- Make an assessment of the severity of depression to determine the patient's disposition.

It is important to convey an attitude of compassion, empathy and understanding to the depressed patient (Moore & McLaughlin 2003). It is also worth reassuring the patient that depression is reversible. However, it is pointless attempting to talk the patient out of depression as he cannot snap out of it any more than he could snap out of a diabetic coma. The patient's social networks should be identified and mobilized where appropriate. The patient should be placed in a safe room, especially if he is at high risk of suicide. The room should be free of any objects which can be used to self-harm, e.g. glass, telephone cords etc. The patient will need admission if he is suicidal, stuporous, hyper-agitated or lacks social support. Referral to the psychiatric outpatient department or other services should be arranged if the patient does not require admission, and his GP and/or community psychiatric nurse (CPN) should be informed of the attendance at ED. The outlook for depression varies with the severity of the condition. For major depression approximately 80% of people who have received psychiatric care for an episode will have at least one more episode in their lifetime, with a median of four episodes. The outcome for those seen in primary care also seems to be poor, with only about a third remaining well over 11 years and about 20% having a chronic course (Anderson et al. 2000).

Antenatal and postnatal mental health problems

Mental disorder during pregnancy and the postnatal period can have serious consequences for the mother, her infant and other family members. ED nurses may be the first contact the pregnant woman may have with services in both the antenatal and postnatal periods. The assessing nurse should ask questions about past or present severe mental illness including schizophrenia, bipolar disorder, severe depression and psychosis in the postnatal period. Any previous treatment by a psychiatrist or specialist mental health team and whether there is a family history of mental illness.

The assessing nurse should also ask the following two questions to identify possible depression:

During the past month, have you been bothered by feeling down, hopeless or depressed?

During the past month, have you been bothered by having little interest or pleasure in doing things?

If the woman answers yes to both the initial questions- the nurse should consider the following question:

Is this something you feel you need or want help with?

NICE Guidelines (2007).

Women requiring psychological treatment should be referred for co-care between obstetric and mental health services and should be seen for treatment normally within 1 month of initial assessment. This is because of the lower threshold for access to psychological therapies during pregnancy and the postnatal period arising from the changing risk-benefit for psychotropic medication at this time.

In the postnatal period, the patient may present with:

- acute organic reaction
- affective psychosis
- schizophreniform psychosis.

Affective puerperal disorder episode. Problems may range from 'the blues' to a clinical depression severe enough to require admission.

Puerperal psychosis. Symptoms may occur within 2 weeks to approximately 9 months following the birth of a child. Postnatal depression is common; it has been estimated to affect 13% of women in the first year following the birth of their child, which equates to 70 000 women annually in the UK (Warner et al. 1996). There may be clouding of consciousness, perplexity, delusions and hallucinations.

Management

If after assessment in ED the patient can be managed on an out-patient basis, adequate home support should be initiated and the presenting complaint treated as appropriate. Generally, patients presenting with puerperal psychosis or severe clinical depression will require admission from ED, and arrangements should be made for both mother and baby. Medication in ED will need to be selective to prevent drugs being prescribed which are secreted in breast milk if the mother is breast-feeding. Although some cases of postnatal depression last less than three months, 30–50% may last for more than six months. If a mother develops postnatal depression in her first pregnancy, then she is at a 30% risk of recurrence with subsequent pregnancies.

Hypomania/mania/acute or chronic mania

Hypomania is the term used to describe a syndrome involving sustained and pathological elevation of mood, accompanied by other changes in function, such as disturbances of physical energy, sleep and appetite. Mania is a similar syndrome in which the patient additionally holds delusional ideas, i.e. he is psychotic (Merson & Baldwin 1995). The patient who frequently attends ED does so when he has become too disruptive for family life. He may have a history of mania or depression, with his behaviour becoming increasingly disruptive over a few days. As a result, if mania is not controlled, the patient is at risk of harming himself or others. Drugs such as steroids and amphetamines may also trigger mania.

Clinical features

The key component of manic disorders is a persistent elevation of mood. However, these feelings of euphoria and elation may vacillate with feelings of irritability and hostility. The patient may experience racing of thoughts and pressure of speech and it may be very difficult to sustain conversations with patients in a manic state due to the constant pressure of bubbling and exciting ideas. Grandiose delusions are common and can lead to dangerous activities by the patient; for instance, he may believe he (and others) can fly and want to jump off a building. Such patients are therefore at high risk of suicide or homicide and should be assessed accordingly.

Nursing and medical management

Nursing care of these patients must centre on protecting them and others from injury while measures to control mania are instituted. If the patient has a history of mania, he is likely to be prescribed lithium carbonate. This is a metallic salt, identified as controlling mood swings in the 1970s. It has the ability to stabilize mood, thus reducing the possibility of elation and severe depression. If the patient has had two or more episodes of mania in 5 years or less, it is likely he is on lithium therapy, and the levels and dosage may require adjustment as necessary (Dinan 2002). Lithium toxicity usually occurs at greater plasma concentration levels of 1.5 mmol/L Li$^+$, although it can occur at therapeutic levels (0.4–1.0 mmol/L Li$^+$). Toxic levels may result from deliberate overdose, inappropriate usage or non-compliance. It can lead to electrolyte disturbance through water loss, diarrhoea, vomiting and polyurea. Early symptomatology also includes nausea, sweating, tremor and twitching. With plasma concentrations above 2.0 mmol/L (severe overdosage), symptoms displayed include convulsions, oliguria/renal failure and hypokalaemia. ECG changes (inverted/flat T wave) may also be present. Lithium should be stopped and urea and electrolytes checked. The patient should be admitted and haemodialysis or peritoneal dialysis may be required. In acute overdose much higher serum concentrations may be present without features of toxicity, and measures to increase urine production are necessary.

The manic patient requires patience in handling and tolerant, tactful, kindly authority to make it as restful and unstimulating as is reasonably possible. It is essential to make appropriate arrangements to provide close observation and to protect the patient from danger and over-exhausting himself. As this kind of close observation can be quite exhausting for staff, one-to-one nurse contact is advised, with each nurse taking turns for a maximum of 30 minutes each. The ED nurse must provide fluids and snacks of high calorific value for this patient, in order to reduce the risk of dehydration and hypoglycaemia.

Management of a manic patient outside hospital is only possible when the patient is sufficiently insightful to comply with treatment and where there is considerable and dependable informal support (Merson & Baldwin 1995). Admission to hospital is usually indicated.

Bipolar disease

This is a major mental illness characterized by mood swings, alternating between periods of excitement and an overwhelming feeling of sadness, misery, gloom and despondency. Management in ED is directed towards presenting symptoms.

ANXIETY STATES

Anxiety is an emotional sense of impending doom, a mental sense of unknown terror or fear of losing one's mind (Kaiser & Pyngolil 1995). The patient may present to ED when symptoms are no longer tolerable or when there is a marked deterioration in ability to carry out day-to-day activities. Patients may also present with panic attacks.

Clinical features

Anxiety is characterized by both psychological and physiological features (Merson & Baldwin 1995):

- Psychological symptoms and signs
  - apprehensiveness
  - unfounded worrying
  - fearfulness
  - inner restlessness
  - irritability
  - exaggerated startle response
- Physiological features
  - autonomic in origin; e.g. palpitation, breathlessness, epigastric discomfort, diarrhoea and urinary frequency
  - musculoskeletal, e.g. tension, stiffness and tremor.

Patients may be brought to ED with an acute anxiety attack, exhibiting signs associated with sympathetic nervous system stimulation, such as tachycardia, palpitations, sweaty palms and hyperventilation. This change in respiration can produce serious biochemical changes due to the lowering in blood CO_2 levels that occurs with overbreathing. This in turn upsets the pH balance, making the blood more alkaline, which in turn upsets the calcium balance, causing muscle spasm (tetany) and tingling in the fingers. There is a characteristic carpopedal spasm of the fingers and abdominal cramps that are associated with hysterical hyperventilation. Their effect is to make the patient even more anxious and therefore more likely to hyperventilate. The solution is to reassure the patient and encourage him to use a rebreathing bag to increase the CO_2 levels to normal as he rebreathes exhaled CO_2. After about 15 minutes, the respiratory rate will be back to normal and the muscle cramps will resolve (Walsh and Kent 2001).

Tachycardia is a common feature of anxiety attacks; however, in attempting to rule out organic causes of anxiety, it should be noted that tachycardia in patients experiencing anxiety attacks usually does not exceed 140 beats/minute, whereas in paroxysmal supraventricular tachycardia the heartbeat is usually above 140 beats/minute. In addition, supraventricular tachycardia is more likely to respond to vagal stimulation than tachycardia due to anxiety.

Nursing and medical management

The patient may respond to explanation, reassurance and a feeling of security. Admission may be required to break the cycle; if medication is required, 10 mg diazepam i.v. is usually given. If admission is not required, the aim should be for symptomatic relief and psychological support. Reassure the patient and allow him to discuss problems at his own pace. Arrange follow-up appointments for further treatment as appropriate.

ALCOHOL–RELATED EMERGENCIES

Around 90% of adult population drink alcohol at some time, 28% of men and 11% of women exceed safe levels of consumption, 1–2% of the population have alcohol problems and there are 200 000 dependent drinkers in the UK (Ashworth & Gerada 1997). Every year, the adverse effects of alcohol consumption lead to an estimated 1.2 million assaults, result in 150000 hospital admissions and cost the NHS £1.7 billion (Smith & Allen 2004, Bellis et al. 2005).

Alcoholic patients may present with a variety of problems:

- intoxication
- withdrawal states – delirium tremens
- morbid jealousy
- alcoholic hallucinations
- physical consequences of alcohol abuse, e.g. tuberculosis, GI bleed.

It is dangerous and unrealistic to attempt to conduct a satisfactory psychiatric interview when someone is intoxicated. While this may occasionally leave ED staff feeling frustrated, on-call psychiatrists or community psychiatric nurses (CPNs) will rarely attend ED while the patient is intoxicated on the grounds that no meaningful psychiatric interview can take place. Clinical management of patients with alcohol intoxication is often confounded by the potentially disruptive and violent behaviour associated with intoxication.

Alcohol is a central nervous system (CNS) depressant. Measures of alcohol are described in units, with one unit being equal to half a pint of ordinary beer, one standard glass of wine or one-sixth of a gill of spirit (a pub measure) at 40% alcohol concentration. Blood alcohol concentration (BAC) is a measure of the amount of alcohol (mg) present in the bloodstream (per 100 ml), with a standard unit containing approximately 15 mg of alcohol. As with any drug, the effect of a certain dose will vary with the physical and psychological condition of the user (Kennedy & Faugier 1989). Degrees of intoxication may be classified as mild, moderate or severe.

Mild intoxication occurs in individuals with a BAC of up to 80 and is usually achieved with between one and five units. The typical reaction in an emotionally stable person is a feeling of warmth and cheerfulness accompanied by impairment of both judgement and inhibition. Apart from an increased susceptibility to accidents and the risk of post-intoxication headache and mild gastritis there is negligible health risk from a single episode of intoxication at these levels.

Moderate intoxication occurs in individuals with a BAC of between 80 and 150, who will exhibit a loss of self-control, slurred speech, double vision and memory loss. This is usually achieved with doses of up to 10 units. These symptoms are similar to those of raised intracranial pressure, diabetic hypoglycaemia and drug overdose. These and other possible aetiologies must therefore be excluded prior to such behaviour being ascribed purely to alcohol intoxication.

Accurate assessment and diagnosis of a patient's condition at this level of intoxication may be confounded due to alcohol's desensitizing effect on pain response and its disruption to levels of consciousness. Other health problems from this level of intoxication include vomiting, severe gastritis, pancreatitis, hepatitis and interactions with medication and/or existing medical problems (Taylor & Ryrie 1996).

A BAC of between 200 and 400 leads to sleepiness, oblivion and coma, with possible cough reflex depression and airway obstruction from vomit or tongue. Such patients require constant neurological observation and may well require airway and cardiovascular support.

With a BAC of more than 400, death from severe CNS depression, particularly respiratory depression, is possible. Full emergency resuscitation with endotracheal intubation and cardiovascular support may be necessary. Stomach lavage should be considered with extreme caution since chronic alcohol abuse may result in peptic ulceration and/or oesophageal varices. In very severe alcohol poisoning, some patients may require transfer to intensive care units for haemodialysis or haemoperfusion. A BAC of over 600 is usually fatal and is generally only achieved by ingestion of large amounts of spirits.

Nursing management

Due to the behavioural component of moderate intoxication, these patients have the potential to become uncooperative, disruptive and violent, making assessment and treatment very difficult. Ballesteros et al. (2004) recommend a variety of behavioural management techniques which ED staff may employ in such situations. As with any patient, a friendly interest and recognition as a person are essential. Staff are also advised to pace their interactions to suit the impaired cognitive processing of the patient, allowing him to comprehend what is required or suggested. Intoxicated thinking often proceeds by association rather than logic. Key words such as 'let us work together' or involving the patient in actions such as helping with dressings is recommended. Conversely, negative phrases such as 'you're not going to fight or give us trouble' are generally inflammatory, as the patient may associate with the words 'fight' and 'trouble'. In addition, adopting a non-authoritarian but confident manner, acting calmly and quietly, separating opposing groups and removing the injured person from his accompanying friends are valuable approaches.

Levels of intoxication are not static but exist on a time continuum line in relation to blood concentration of the drug. Alcohol is metabolized at approximately one unit or 15 mg of blood alcohol per hour, which is slower than most people drink alcohol. Nurses should therefore be aware that patients can move rapidly from mild to life-threatening intoxication while in the ED as they absorb previously ingested alcohol and/or drugs. Conversely, the aforementioned behavioural problems associated with moderate intoxication may follow treatment for the physical effects of severe intoxication.

The easiest way to determine risk levels is to ask patients how much they drink. While there is a general belief that people are reluctant to accurately disclose their drinking patterns, there is good evidence to suggest this is not so and that information on the whole is sufficiently truthful (Watson 1996). Information should be sought in a sensitive but matter-of-fact way when asking about other lifestyle factors such as diet and smoking. Patterns of consumption are also important since a man who drinks 21 units on 1 or 2 days a week is likely to experience different problems from someone who drinks as much, but in smaller amounts, on a more regular basis.

A more subjective approach to assessment, which provides information on an individual's experience of his alcohol use, is the CAGE questionnaire, which includes the following four questions:

- Have you ever had to Cut down your alcohol intake?
- Have you ever become Annoyed with the amount of alcohol you drink?
- Have you ever felt Guilty about how much alcohol you drink?
- Have you ever used alcohol as an Eye-opener in the morning?

A positive response to two or more of these questions is considered to indicate an unhealthy attitude towards drinking which warrants some form of intervention (Kennedy & Faugier 1989).

Management of acute alcohol intoxication, the identification of potential problem drinkers and the provision of brief interventions do not require the skills of the specialist practitioner. Some basic knowledge and specific nursing actions are necessary, which may be employed as part of standard ED service provision; however, there is evidence to suggest that the profession, while acknowledging its role in the detection and management of alcohol-related problems, often fails to address such issues adequately (Watson 1996).

MUNCHAUSEN'S SYNDROME AND MUNCHAUSEN'S SYNDROME BY PROXY

This is characterized by a patient frequently and repeatedly seeking admission, usually travelling to out-of-area ED units. Munchausen's syndrome and Munchausen's syndrome by proxy are characterized by a person simulating physical or mental illness, either in himself or, in the case of Munchausen's by proxy, in a third person, e.g. a child. The carer, usually the mother or both parents, fabricates symptoms or signs and then presents the child to hospital. There is an overlap with other forms of child abuse (see also Ch. 16).

The symptoms are supported by a plausible history and convincing physical signs. Motivation derives from a desire for attention. Physical examination may reveal multiple scars. Walsh (1996) identified five broad types of presentation by patients with Munchausen's syndrome:

The acute abdominal type   These patients will manifest acute abdominal symptoms and swallow objects, including safety blades and safety pins, in order to obtain the surgery and hospitalization they crave. Nuts, bolts, coins and other paraphernalia are also swallowed. In well-documented cases, individuals have obtained well over 100 admissions and laparotomies in double figures.

The haemorrhagic type   This presentation is characterized by complaints of bleeding from various orifices. One eye-watering approach is for the patient to insert a coat hanger or needle into the penis, causing trauma and bleeding to the urethra. The positive test for haematuria, along with proclaimed symptoms of renal colic, usually lead to an injection of the desired analgesic agent. Presentations of haemoptysis and haematemesis are also lent further credibility by self-inflicted wounds to the back of the tongue with needles or razor blades.

The neurological type   This type of the syndrome is characterized by patients presenting with convincing (and not so convincing) epileptic fits or complaints of migraine. Men more frequently present with pseudo-fits than women. The practice of sternal rubs and squeezing the nail bed with a biro smacks of punishment and cannot be condoned under any circumstances. A more humane and equally effective means of assessing a pseudo-fit is to gently stroke the eyelashes in an unsuspecting 'unconscious' patient. It is difficult for them not to reflexively flicker their eyes, an action which would not occur in the genuinely unconscious patient (Dolan 1998).

The cardiac type   Here, the patient will present with a classic, textbook display of central chest pain, sometimes described as cardiopathia fantastica (Mehta & Khan 2002). Many such patients will be aware that i.v. diamorphine is administered for cardiac-related chest pain, hence their behaviour.

The psychiatric type   In some instances, patients will imitate various forms of mental illness in order to gain admission to psychiatric units and hospitals.

Clinical features and management

The diagnosis is generally not apparent at first presentation, although characteristic features may be noticeable in retrospect:

- The patient may be unwilling to provide significant personal details, such as an address or that of the next of kin.
- Patients may claim to be in transit and offer elaborate and seemingly implausible explanations for their movements (pseudologia fantastica).
- The presentation of symptoms may be classical, reflecting careful rehearsal – leading to retrospective opinions among professionals that symptoms were 'too good to be true'.
- There may be signs of recent i.v. sites or cut-downs. Multiple abdominal scars should rate a very high probability of Munchausen's, especially if the first two points are present.
- The patient's manner and behaviour, especially when he thinks he is not being observed, give cause for suspicion (Walsh 1996).
- The patient may have significant links with the health-care profession, either through family connections or a paramedical occupation or as a result of prolonged hospital stays earlier in life (Merson & Baldwin 1995).

Management within ED is usually difficult due to time restrictions on obtaining a full history. The patient/carer, when confronted with the fictitious nature of the symptoms (his own or a third person's), usually discharges himself. Communication with other ED units and mobilization of services are required, e.g. the health visitor or GP.

SUICIDE AND DELIBERATE SELF-HARM

Suicide occurs when a person knowingly brings about his own death. There are approximately 4000 suicides in England and Wales each year, equivalent to one death every two hours, and it is the third most common cause of death in people aged 15–30 (Crawford 2001). In England the death rate from suicide is 8.6 deaths per 100 000 population. The majority of suicides continue to occur in young adult males – that is, those under 40 years. In relation to women of the

same age, younger men are more likely to commit suicide. The peak difference is the 30–39 age group, in which four males commit suicide to each female. The average ratio between men and women of all ages is almost three male suicides to each female. Once people pass 50 years of age, the ratio stabilizes at around 2.5 male suicides to each female (CSIP/NIMHE 2006a). Among those with mental health problems, suicide is the single largest cause of premature death; 10% of people with psychosis will ultimately kill themselves, two-thirds within the first 5 years (Wiersma et al. 1998). Around the time of emerging psychosis young females have a 150-times higher and young males a 300-fold higher risk for suicide than the general population (Mortensen 1995, CSIP/NIMH 2006b).

Deliberate self harm (DSH), formerly known as parasuicide, is a non-fatal act of self-injury or the taking of substances in excess of the generally recognized or prescribed therapeutic dose. The incidence of self-harm, of which 90% of cases involve self-poisoning, now accounts for 100 000 admissions to hospital per year, making DSH the most common reason for acute medical admission among women aged under 60 (Crawford 2001).

Although potentially lethal drugs are regularly consumed, the overall hospital mortality rate is less than 1% (Valladares 1996). Ryan et al. (1996) noted that there is a significant association between suicide and previous attendance at ED with deliberate self-harm. It is now commonly held that those who commit suicide and those who undertake acts of deliberate self-harm are two distinct groups (Vaughan 1985). Box 14.4 outlines the high-risk factors associated with suicidal behaviour; Box 14.5 highlights Beck's suicide scale, which has been used to identify the seriousness of suicidal intent; and Boxes 14.6 and 14.7 provide assessment tools of suicidal ideas and risk (Hughes & Owens 1996).

The risk of suicide is increased by a factor of 100 compared with that in the general population where there is both a recent history of deliberate self-harm and persistent, distressing suicidal ideation. Many of the suicide intent scales depend on the balance between lethality and rescuability (Pritchard 1995). Lethality is the medical danger to life; methods such as shooting and jumping from a high building have high lethality values, whereas a tranquillizer overdose will have a lower lethality value. Conversely, someone who takes an overdose of tranquillizers and alcohol and then disappears into the sea has a low likelihood of rescuability. The person who is drunk and attempts to take a large number of tablets in front of their partner has a high likelihood of rescue. The

Box 14.4   High-risk factors associated with suicidal behaviour

Demographic factors
- Adolescence or older than 45 years
- Male
- White
- Protestant
- Separated, divorced or widowed
- Living alone
- Unemployed

Antecedent life circumstances
- Previous suicide attempts
  - recent attempt(s) with serious intent
  - previous attempt(s) with resultant physical or mental sequelae
  - previous attempt(s) that did not effect desired response(s)
- Family history of suicide or suicide attempts
- Inadequate or unavailable support systems
- Major life changes
  - major losses, e.g. spouse, job, money
  - major illness (of self or others)

Psychiatric conditions
- Depressive illnesses
- Alcoholism
- Schizophrenia

Box 14.6   The assessment of suicidal ideas: progressively specific questions

- How do you see the future?
- Do you ever feel hopeless, like giving up?
- Do things ever seem so bad that you feel you cannot go on?
- Have you ever wished you could go to sleep and not wake up?
- Have you ever thought of doing anything to harm yourself?
- Have you made any plans for that?
- Have you done anything about it?

Box 14.7   Assessing suicidal risk following deliberate self-harm

- What happened before and during the self-harm event?
- Did the patient intend to die?
- Does the patient still intend to die?
- Does the patient have a psychiatric disorder?
- What are the patient's problems?
- What are the patient's resources for dealing with this crisis?

Box 14.5   Beck suicide risk scale (Beck et al. 1974)

Preparation
- Act planned in advance
- Suicide note written
- Action in anticipation of death, for example, writing a will

Circumstances of the act
- Patient was alone
- Timed such that intervention was unlikely
- Precautions taken against discovery

Sequelae of the act
- Did not seek help
- Stated wish to die
- Stated belief that the act would be proven fatal
- Sorry the act failed

overall level of intent depends on the balance between lethality and rescuability (Jones 1995).

Obtaining a history from a patient following a suicide attempt is frequently very difficult. The patient may also give false information to avoid embarrassment. A patient has the right to refuse treatment, and any treatment which is enforced on a patient is considered assault or battery (Dimond 2004). Under common law, treatment can be given without the consent of the patient in cases of necessity: circumstances in which immediate action is required and necessary to preserve life or prevent a serious or immediate danger to the patient or others. The treatment or physical restraint used must be reasonable and sufficient only to the purpose of bringing the emergency to an end. Medical treatment should be administered under the specific direction of a medical practitioner (Hughes & Owens 1996). This duty is imposed by statute and the NMC Code of Professional Conduct (2004) and is underpinned by the principles of civil law relating to negligence, including the Mental Capacity Act 2005 (Gertz et al. 2006).

The feelings of ED staff towards patients with self-inflicted injuries appear to be predominantly negative (Stockbridge 1993, Celenza 2004). Ward (1995) recommends that the nurse seeks to make sense of the patient's behaviour from the patient's point of view, rather than the nurse's. The key to a successful nurse/patient relationship lies in establishing a positive rapport from the initial assessment. A strategy for achieving this was suggested by Burnard (1990) in relation to interviewing technique. He proposed the acronym 'SOLER' to remind the interviewer of the following:

- sit squarely opposite the patient, not behind a desk, and avoid distraction.
- open positioning, feet apart and palms resting on thighs.
- lean forward towards the client.
- eye contact – show attention and give feedback. This helps to establish a relationship. No staring or glaring.
- relax – tension or fidgeting may convey impatience or lack of interest.

This position helps to make the nurse appear warm and empathetic. By adopting this strategy the nurse should be able to dissociate herself from prejudicial feelings, and the patient is more likely to feel accepted and worthwhile.

If the patient is determined to be at continued risk, the nurse should not leave him alone. If the patient is considered to be at high risk and is not willing to accept hospitalization, involuntary admission will be necessary. If doubt exists, caution should be exercised and admission arranged.

Self-mutilation

Destructive acts against the self, such as putting a fist through a window and wrist cutting, may occur as behaviour secondary to personality problems. Patients are usually in their 20s or 30s and may be single or married. Most patients who cut themselves have a history of self-injury. The wrists, arms and thighs are common sites, and instruments such as razor blades, knives, broken glass or mirrors may be used. The wounds are usually relatively superficial and the patient may describe how the act brings relief of tension and depersonalization. Patients who self-mutilate tend to have low self-esteem but the lethality of the intent is usually low.

Nursing management

Treatment in ED should revolve around immediate care of the injury, evaluating the risk of suicide,

protecting the patient from further self-harm and assisting in crisis resolution (Repper 1999). Patients who attend regularly following acts of deliberate self-harm may leave staff feeling frustrated and hostile towards them. However, such beliefs and attitudes must not be allowed to interfere with the care of the patient. The environment of care should be supportive and non-confrontational for patients who deliberately self-harm, and care should be delivered non-judgementally. Given the degree of aggression which is channelled internally into acts of deliberate self-harm, the ED nurse should also exercise caution when caring for these patients as the aggressive tendencies exhibited may be directed towards staff. Referral to appropriate agencies, such as community psychiatric nurses (CPNs), is encouraged so that the patient can ventilate and discuss feelings and explore other ways of coping more appropriately (McElroy & Sheppard 1999, Perego 1999, Brookes & Leach).

INDIVIDUAL AT ODDS WITH SOCIETY (SOCIOPATHY)

Sociopathy refers to a group of well-defined anomalies or deviations of personality which are not the result of either psychotic or any other illness. Numerous theories have been put forward as to why this disorder should develop (Bowlby 1965, Cleckly 1967).

The patient may present to ED with depression, suicidal gestures, abuse of drugs, alcohol and sex, or as a result of aggressive and violent behaviour and lack of impulse control, etc. Management requires a complete history to be taken to exclude epilepsy, hypoglycaemia or any other acute organic reaction. Treatment is directed at managing the presenting condition with a firm and consistent approach. Reference to mental health teams is as appropriate.

VIOLENT PATIENTS

Violence or threats of violence may be associated with a variety of disorders, e.g. psychosis, chemical intoxication, sociopathy, etc., or with a specific situation, such as lack of communication. The nurse should be alert for violence, particularly if the patient has a previous history of violent behaviour or poor impulse control, if he has been brought in by the police or if he is verbally or physically threatening.

There are several management points in ED:

- Always manage the patient with the required number of staff to do so appropriately and beware of uniform limitations.
- Be familiar with the alarm/security system.

- If entering a room, do so letting a colleague know where you are. See the patient in a non-isolated room and leave yourself and the patient an exit.
- Maintain a quiet, calm but firm approach. Avoid any contact which may be misinterpreted.
- Monitor both your own and the patient's reactions.

Management

If circumstances allow, try to establish whether a psychiatric disorder is present: is the patient demanding; is conscious level fluctuating? If a psychiatric disorder is present, assess the need for admission and suitability of facilities available. Give medication as appropriate

If no clinical reason for admission is elicited and the patient remains disruptive, security and/or the police should be contacted (see also Chapter 11: Violence and Agression).

LEARNING DISABILITY CLIENTS AND MENTAL HEALTH PROBLEMS

Patients with learning disabilities may present with:

- self-mutilation
- depression
- schizophrenia
- anxiety.

The patient should be assessed as appropriate and a history taken from the escort. If admission is not required, referral to local learning-disability services and social services may be required to provide an emergency service. If behaviour is disturbed and the patient requires medications, low doses of neuroleptics should be given because of susceptibility to side-effects (see also Chapter 32: People with Learning Disabilities).

ELDERLY CLIENTS PRESENTING TO ED WITH MENTAL HEALTH PROBLEMS

Psychiatric emergencies arising 'de novo' or superimposed upon dementia include:

- acute confusional states
- mania – usually a history of bipolar disease is present
- depression and deliberate self-harm
- paranoid disorder.

In healthcare for the elderly, the decision as to whether to admit a patient is usually made after careful assessment. Ideally, problems presented by the elderly client will be assessed by the healthcare for the elderly team (mental health) on a domiciliary visit. In reality, elderly patients may be referred or present directly to the ED. Therefore the nurse must be alert to social admission. Dementia per se is not a sole reason for admission.

Assessment should be directed towards:

- evidence of an acute organic reaction, such as recent confusion, disorientation etc.
- in the absence of an acute organic reaction, whether mental illness is present, e.g. clinical depression, paranoid psychosis
- strength of family support, if any; respite need
- whether behaviour is disturbed.

If admission is necessary, the appropriate team should be contacted. If immediate treatment is required, medication should be limited to low doses, particularly if there is evidence of renal or hepatic improvement (see also Chapter 21).

CHILD AND ADOLESCENT PSYCHIATRY

Children and adolescents will present to ED as emergency referrals. The ED nurse should be familiar with the procedure to contact the duty child and adolescent mental health team and management should be discussed with them. Any child or adolescent present with psychiatric pathology should be taken as seriously as any other age group and managed according to the presenting condition.

Common psychiatric presentations include:

- chemical abuse
- suicidal behaviour/deliberate self-harm
- depression – reactive and endogenous
- early schizophrenia
- adolescent behavioural disorders
- eating and nutrition disorders.

Management

- Assess, treat and admit as appropriate
- Referral to child psychiatric team
- Support and reassurance for the patient and family
- Institute appropriate follow-up.

PATIENTS ATTENDING ED WITH EATING DISORDERS

The most common of these are:

- anorexia nervosa
- bulimia nervosa
- compulsive eating/food addiction – severe overweight.

Patients with eating disorders may present to ED with problems such as osteoporetic fractures, collapse, infection, dehydration, oedema, cardiac failure, fatigue, cyanosis, bradycardia, hypotension, weight loss, obesity, hypoglycaemia, hypocalcaemia/kalaemia, infertility, amenorrhoea, constipation and vomiting, or may be referred by dental practitioners for dental problems. In addition, they may present with agitation, depression or acopia.

Management

Treatment is aimed at the presenting symptoms and includes a complete physical work-up. Admission in the acute phase is usually required. In ED, basic nursing care as well as care of malnutrition/dehydration needs to be addressed.

SOCIAL PROBLEMS

Some people tend to use ED as a crisis walk-in clinic, e.g. someone who has become acutely disturbed or who is blamed as the cause of a crisis and is brought to ED as the patient (Brookes & Leach 2004). Although these incidents may not be true psychiatric emergencies, ED is seen as a 24-hour emergency unit, when no other help or assistance is perceived to be available. The presence of an impartial observer and environment may enable the patient and his family/carers to discuss the problems for the first time. Referral to agencies for follow-up is required, e.g. to counselling services in general and/or for specific needs, such as HIV, rape, social worker or probation officer.

Other social problems that may present to ED are those people searching for a trolley, bed, shelter or food, often with no apparent psychiatric or medical illness. These patients can be very difficult or manipulative and require limit-setting and firm handling. The opportunity to discuss problems may help but the nurse should attempt to clarify what type of assistance the person requires and be familiar with telephone numbers of agencies able to help, such as crisis centres, social security, local hostels, emergency social workers, etc.

ACUTE STRESS REACTION

This is a common, normal response to an unwanted situation and may last days to weeks and may be triggered by exposure to a traumatic event. It may develop into a more severe disorder such as simple/complex post-traumatic stress disorder (PTSD). Simple or complex PTSD can manifest itself both physically and mentally and may present with a variety of symptoms that usually appear within 6 months of the traumatic event and/or co-morbidity e.g. alcohol/chemical dependency, sleep problems, fear and anxiety, tearfulness, sadness, helplessness, anger, irritability, guilt, concentration/memory problems, body pains, avoidance/numbness and unpleasant intrusive thoughts/flashbacks/nightmares and hyper vigilance.

The onset of a stress response is associated with specific physiological actions in the sympathetic nervous system, both directly and indirectly through the release of epinephrine and to a lesser extent norepinephrine from the medulla of the adrenal glands. The release is triggered by acetylcholine released from pre-ganglionic sympathetic nerves. These catecholamine hormones cause an immediate physical reaction by triggering increases in heart rate and breathing, peripheral vasoconstriction or vasodilatation (see Chapter 22: Physiology for practice). In ED, management will depend on presenting symptoms and referral for cognitive behavioural therapy may be appropriate (NICE 2006) (see Chapter 12: Stress and Stress Management).

IATROGENIC DRUG–INDUCED PSYCHOSIS

Non-specific psychosis may occur, including mania, delirium, schizophreniform psychosis or depression in patients on maintenance therapy for a physical condition, e.g. Cushing's syndrome. If a patient's condition precludes reducing the dose of medication, antipsychotics can be administered concurrently to control symptoms.

Psychotropic drugs have served to revolutionize the treatment and care of the mentally ill. However, these drugs can also have side-effects which may require management in the ED. All antipsychotic agents may produce acute dystonias, akathisia, parkinsonism, and akinesia.

Acute dystonia

Symptoms usually occur 1 hour to 5 days after commencement of antipsychotic medication, especially with high-potency neuroleptics such as haloperidol or trifluperazine. Dystonic reactions are prolonged tonic contractions of muscle groups. When the muscles of the neck, tongue and jaw are involved, this is called torticollis. Torticollis combined with contractions of the extraocular muscles, whereby the eyes are rolled upwards with the head turned to one side, is called occulogyric crisis.

Although these muscle contractions can be very frightening for the patient, they can usually be easily reversed with the intramuscular administration of 2 mg of benztropine mesylate or 10 mg of procyclidine. The nurse should stay with the patient and provide reassurance that the reaction can be reversed usually within 5–20 minutes of injection.

Akathisia

Symptoms of akathisia usually occur within 2–3 months of commencement of medication. The patient complains of an inability to sit still, pacing and fidgeting. While this is not an emergency, it can be distressing for the patient and be mistaken for agitation associated with the patient's primary disorder. Antiparkinsonian agents such as benztropine mesylate provide relief.

Akinesia

Akinesia is an extrapyrimidal reaction characterized by signs and symptoms of decreased motor activity. The patient experiences fatigue and muscle weakness. It can easily be controlled with an anti-parkinsonian agent (Kaiser & Pyngolil 1995).

MONOAMINE OXIDASE INHIBITORS (MAOIs)

MAOIs inhibit monamine oxidase, therefore causing an accumulation of amine neurotransmitters. The metabolism of some amine drugs and tyramine found in some foods may cause a dangerous rise in the blood pressure. MAOIs also interact with opiates, lithium and tricyclic antidepressants. The danger of interaction persists for up to 14 days after treatment with MAOIs is discontinued.

Hypertensive crisis may occur if MAOIs are taken in combination with:

- amphetamines
- appetite suppressants
- dietary amines, cheese, marmite, broad beans, chocolate, bananas, Chianti wine, whiskey, beer, caffeinated tea or coffee
- proprietary cold and allergy remedies containing sympathomimetics, e.g. adrenaline, phenylephrine.

Hypertensive crisis is characterized by the sudden onset of severe throbbing headache, nausea, vomiting and dizziness. The patient's blood pressure can be as high as 350/250 mmHg, and chest and neck pain, palpitations and malignant hyperthermia, the usual cause of death in patients experiencing hypertensive crisis, may occur.

Nursing and medical management

Hypertensive crisis is an emergency, and therefore the patient's vital signs should be monitored closely and 12–15 L of oxygen administered via a tight-fitting reservoir mask. Intravenous phentolamine 5–10 mg should be given to reduce the patient's blood pressure and repeated as necessary. Supportive measures include forced diuresis, and therefore urine output should be monitored. Hypertensive crisis should resolve 1–3 hours after initiation of treatment.

Rare but potentially life threatening adverse drug reaction that results from intentional self-poisoning, therapeutic drug use or inadvertent interactions between drugs. It is a consequence of excess serotonergic activity in the central nervous system and peripheral serotonin receptors. This excess serotonin activity produces a specific spectrum of clinical findings which may range from barely perceptible to being fatal.

There is no laboratory test for serotonin syndrome, so diagnosis is by symptom observation and the patient's history. It may go unrecognised as it may be mistaken for a viral illness, anxiety, neurological disorder or worsening psychiatric condition.

Symptoms are often described as a "clinical triad of abnormalities":

Cognitive effects; mental confusion, hypomania, hallucinations, agitation, headache, coma.

Autonomic effects; hyperpyrexia, shivering, sweating, fever, hypertension, tachycardia, nausea, diarrhoea, late stage presentation may include rhabdomyolysis, metabolic acidosis, seizures, renal failure and disseminated intravascular coagulation.

Somatic effects: Muscle twitching (myoclonus/clonus), hyperreflexia, and tremor.

There is no antidote to the condition itself and management involves removing the precipitating drug and the initiation of supportive therapy (control of agitation, autonomic instability, hyperthermia) and the administration of serotonin antagonists.

The clinical features of neurolpetic malignant syndrome and serotonergic syndrome are very similar, thus making diagnosis very difficult. Features that classically present in narcoleptic malignant syndrome that are useful for differentiating the two syndromes are: Fever and muscle rigidity.

CONCLUSION

Psychiatric emergencies present a particular challenge to ED nurses as they may be a result of physical or functional disorders and increasingly present for the first time to EDs for initial management. There has been a recent increase in the number of liaison psychiatric nurses working within the ED. Among other responsibilities, referrals may be made to them for assessment of patients attending the ED with non- life threatening deliberate self-harm injuries. They also have a major role in the assessment and management of behaviourally disturbed patients who are referred to the ED or are self-referrals. They have particular skills on advising on the management of psychotic or suicidal patients and can advise the ED team appropriately. This chapter has considered the more common psychiatric emergencies and identified a range of interventions for nurses to employ when caring for these distressed and frequently distressing patients. Recognizing and understanding these emergencies will help the nurse meet the challenges of psychiatric emergency care in ED.

References

Aguilera D (1998) *Crisis Intervention: Theory and Methodology*, 8th edn. St Louis: Mosby.

Ambrose K (1996) Mental health care in A&E: expanding nursing roles. *Emergency Nurse*, **4**(3), 16–18.

Anderson IM, Nutt DJ, Deakin JF (2000) Evidence-based guidelines for treating depressive disorders with antidepressants: a revision of the 1993 British Association for Psychopharmacology guidelines. *British Journal of Psychopharmacology*, **14**(1), 3–20.

Andrew-Starkey S (2004) Mental State Examination. In: *Textbook of Emergency Medicine* (2nd edn) (eds Cameron P, Jelinek G, Kelly AM, Murray L, Brown AFT, Heyworth J). Edinburgh: Churchill Livingstone.

Ashworth M, Gerada C (1997) ABC of mental health. Addiction and dependence – II: Alcohol. *British Medical Journal*, **315**(7104), 358–360.

Ballestero J, Gonzales-Pinto A, Querejeta I, Arino J (2004) Brief interventions for hazardous drinkers delivered in primary care are equally effective in men and women. *Journal of Addiction*, **99**(1), 3–20.

Barker P (1999) Therapeutic nursing of the person in depression. In: Clinton M, Nelson S, eds. *Advanced Practice in Mental Health Nursing*. Oxford: Blackwell Science.

Beck AT, Morris JB, Beck A (1974) Cross-validation of the suicidal intent scale. *Psychological Reports*, **34**(2), 445–446.

Bellis MA, Hughes K, McVeigh J, Thomson R, Luke C (2005) Effects of nightlife activity on health. *Nursing Standard*, **19**(30), 63–71.

Bowlby J (1965) *Child Care and the Growth of Love*. Harmondsworth: Penguin.

Boydell J, Van Os J, Lambri M, Castle D, Allardyce J, McCreadle RG, Murray RM (2003) Incidence of schizophrenia in south-east London between 1965 and 1997. *British Journal of Psychiatry*, **182**, 45–49.

Brookes JG, DS (2004) Crisis intervention in the emergency department. In: *Textbook of Emergency Medicine* (2nd edn) (eds Cameron P, Jelinek G, Kelly AM, Murray L, Brown AFT, Heyworth J). Edinburgh: Churchill Livingstone.

Burnard P (1990) *Learning Human Skills: an Experiential Guide for Nurses*. Oxford: Heinemann.

Care Services Improvement Partnership/National Institute for Mental Health in England (2006a) *National Suicide Prevention Strategy for England: Annual Report on Progress 2005*. London: Care Services Improvement Partnership.

Care Services Improvement Partnership/National Institute for Mental Health in England (2006b) *10 High Impact Changes for Mental Health Services*. London: Care Services Improvement Partnership.

Celenza A (2004) Deliberate self harm/suicide. In: *Textbook of Emergency Medicine* (2nd edn) (eds Cameron P, Jelinek G, Kelly AM, Murray L, Brown AFT, Heyworth J). Edinburgh: Churchill Livingstone.

Cleckly B (1967) *The Mask of Sanity*. New York: Basic Books.

Crawford M (2001) Psychological management following deliberate self harm. *Clinical Medicine*, **1**(3) 185–187.

Dimond B (2004) *Legal Aspects of Nursing*, 4th edn. Hemel Hempstead: Prentice Hall.

Dinan TG (2002) Lithium in bipolar mood disorder. *British Medical Journal*, **324**(7344), 989–990.

Dolan B (1998) The hospital hoppers. *Nursing Times*, **94**(30), 26–27.

Doy R, Blowers EJ, Sutton E (2006) The ABC of Community Emergency Care: 16 mental health. *Emergency Medicine Journal*, **23**, 304–312.

Gertz R, Harmon S, Laurie G, Pradella G (2006) Developments in medical law in the United Kingdom in 2005 and 2006. *European Journal of Health Law*, **13**, 143–158.

Gilig P, Dumaine M, Hilard JR (1990) Who do mobile crisis services serve? *Hospital and Community Psychiatry*, **41**, 804–805.

Gournay K, Beadsmore A (1995) The report of the clinical standards advisory group: standards of care for people with schizophrenia in the UK and implications for mental health nursing. *Journal of Mental and Psychiatric Nursing*, **2**, 359–364.

Greenstein RA, Ness DE (1990) Psychiatric emergencies in the elderly. *Emergency Medicine Clinics of North America*, **8**, 429–441.

Hughes T, Owens D (1996) Management of suicidal risk. *British Journal of Hospital Medicine*, **56**(4), 151–154.

Jones L (1995) Assessing suicide risk in A&E. *Emergency Nurse*, **2**(4), 7–9.

Kaiser J, Pyngolil MJ (1995) Psychiatric emergencies. In: Kitt S, Selfridge-Thomas J, Proehl JA, Kaiser J, eds. *Emergency Nursing: a Physiologic and Clinical Perspective*, 2nd edn. Philadelphia: WB Saunders.

Kaplan HI, Sadock BJ (1993) *Pocket Handbook of Emergency Psychiatric Medicine*. Baltimore: Wilkins & Wilkins.

Kennedy J, Faugier J (1989) *Drug and Alcohol Dependency Nursing*. Oxford: Heinemann Nursing.

Mackway-Jones, K Marsden J, Windle J (2005) *Emergency Triage*, 2nd edn. Oxford: Blackwell Publishing.

McElroy A, Shepherd G (1999) The assessment and management of self-harming patients in the accident and emergency department: an action research project. *Journal of Clinical Nursing*, **8**(1), 66–72.

Mehta NJ, Khan IA (2002) Cardiac Munchausen syndrome. *Chest*, **122**(5), 1649–1653.

Merson S, Baldwin D (1995) *Psychiatric Emergencies*. Oxford: Oxford University Press.

Moore K, McLaughlin D (2003) Depression: the challenge for all healthcare professionals. *Nursing Standard*, **17**(26), 45–52.

Mortensen PB (1995) Suicide among schizophrenic patients: occurrence and risk factors. *Clinical Neuropharmacology*, **18**: S1–S8. Suppl. 3.

National Institute of Health and Clinical Excellence (2006) *Computerized Cognitive Behaviour Therapy for Depression and Anxiety*. London: NIHCE.

Nursing and Midwifery Council (2004) *Code of Professional Conduct: Standards for Conduct, Performance and Ethics*. London: Nursing and Midwifery Council.

Perego M (1999) Why A&E nurses feel inadequate in managing patients who deliberately self-harm. *Emergency Nurse*, **6**(9), 21–27.

Pritchard C (1995) *Suicide – The Ultimate Rejection?: A Psychosocial Study*. Buckingham: Open University Press.

Puskar KR, Obus NL (1989) Management of the psychiatric emergency. *Nurse Practitioner*, **14**, 7, 9–10, 12, 14, 16, 18, 23, 26.

Repper J (1999) A review of the literature on the prevention of suicide interventions in accident and emergency departments. *Journal of Clinical Nursing*, **8**(1), 3–12.

Ryan J, Rushdy A, Perez-Avilla CA, Allison R (1996) Suicide rate following attendance at an accident and emergency department with deliberate self harm. *Journal of Accident and Emergency Medicine*, **13**, 101–104.

Smith C, Allen J (2004) *Violent Crime in England and Wales*. Home Office: London.

Stockbridge J (1993) Parasuicide: does discussing it help? *Emergency Nurse*, **1**(2), 19–21.

Taylor R, Ryrie I (1996) Clinical management of acute and chronic alcohol use in A&E. *Emergency Nurse*, **4**(3), 6–8.

Weissman M M, Bland R C, Canino G J, Faravelli C, Greenwald S, Hwu H-G, Joyce P R, Karem E G, Lee C-K, Lellouch J, Lepine J P, Newman S C, Rubio-Stipec M, Wells J E, Wickramaratne P J, Wittchen H-U, Yeh E-K (1996) Cross-national epidemiology of major depression and bipolar disorder. *Journal of the American Medical Association*, **276**, 293–299.

Valladeres P (1996) Comparing clinical management of overdoses. *Emergency Nurse*, **4**(1), 6–8.

Vaughan P (1985) *Suicide Prevention*. Birmingham: PEPAR.

Walsh M, Kent A (2001) *Accident & Emergency Nursing: A New Approach*, 4th edn. London: Butterworth Heinemann Ltd.

Walsh M (1996) *Accident & Emergency Nursing: A New Approach*, 3rd edn. London: Butterworth Heinemann Ltd.

Ward M (1995) *Nursing the Psychiatric Emergency*. Oxford: Butterworth-Heinemann.

Warner R, Appleby L, Whitton A, Faragher B (1996). Demographic and obstetric risk factors for postnatal psychiatric morbidity. *British Journal of Psychiatry*, **168**(5), 607–611.

Watson H (1996) Minimal interventions for problem drinkers. *Journal of Substances Misuse for Nursing, Health and Social Care*, **1**(2), 107–110.

Wiersma D, Nienhuis FJ, Slooff CJ, Giel R (1998) Natural course of schizophrenic disorders: a 15 year follow-up of a Dutch incidence cohort. *Schizophrenia Bulletin*, **24**, 75–85.

PART **4**

Life continuum

Chapter 15

Infants

Donna McGeary

INTRODUCTION

Parents often bring their baby to the emergency department (ED) because it offers 24-hour access to advice and healthcare. To the nurse, this may not always seem appropriate; however, if a therapeutic relationship is to be established with the family, nurses must learn to see the problem through the parents'/carers' eyes as well as from a professional perspective. Some families experience problems in accessing health care, particularly within inner cities and areas of ethnic diversity (Bedford et al. 1992). A number of factors could account for this. Knowledge about health-care provision of out-of-hours GP services affects parents' decision-making, as does the workload and availability of the GP or health visitor. The proximity of an emergency department to patients' homes also influences uptake of facilities.

Parental anxiety plays a large part in determining appropriate action in accessing healthcare. Social isolation makes decision-making more difficult, as does inexperience, for instance, a first baby. These groups of carers are more likely to use ED for the support and advice once offered in the extended family structure. It is important for nurses to remember that many parents bring their baby to ED because they have assessed their baby's condition and have actively decided that ED or hospital care is needed.

ASSESSMENT

Whatever the parent or carer's reasons for choosing the ED for their baby, the emergency nurse should attempt to meet the family's needs by aiming to establish a rapport during the initial assessment. This helps to reduce parental anxiety and fretfulness in the baby, and prevents some of the tensions that hinder assessment and subsequent treatment. The nurse should approach the family in a calm and confident way. A crying baby at 3.00 a.m. may seem trivial or 'inappropriate' to staff who are knowledgeable professionals, but to parents who are tired, anxious and inexperienced it is a frightening and emotional time.

Initial assessment allows the nurse to collect information about the infant's condition and factors leading to admission. Parents' fears and anxieties can be explored. Honest, informative communication can provide a realistic view of waiting times, and help parents understand the likely treatment of their baby. This enables them to begin to trust the nurse and believe the care they have sought will be effective. Parent/carer cooperation relies on the formation of therapeutic relationships. Sometimes the emergency nurse is, in fact, caring for a well infant whose parents/carers are anxious or concerned. Effective care from the emergency nurse can go a long way towards meeting the needs of these families.

DEVELOPMENT OF THE NORMAL INFANT

For an emergency nurse to accurately assess and care for an infant, he or she must be aware of babies' expected development milestones at various ages. Developmental tables are a useful guide to infant development (Table 15.1).

The accurate assessment and recognition of a seriously ill child or injured infant means the nurse must rely on parents or carers to give an accurate history of the presenting complaint. At this stage, it is useful to clarify who is accompanying the infant. The confidence and cooperation of the parent or carer should be sought by allowing them to express concerns and disclose information about the infant's health problems. It is important for the assessing nurse to check information: for example, if the parent/carer says the infant has a rash the nurse should look at it to determine its relevance, or if a parent/carer says the infant is sleepy, the nurse should handle the infant during the initial assessment.

The assessment of young infants is also complicated by many factors (Box 15.1). The first several weeks of life are a period of tremendous developmental change, making a three-week-old infant very different from an eight-week-old infant, who in turn is different from a 12-week-old infant. During the first four weeks of life, for instance, many activities, such as sucking, eye-opening and grasping are reflex in origin and can persist even in the face of serious diseases (Zukin et al. 1998).

Encourage the parent or carer to stay with the baby and where possible get the adult to hold the baby on her or his lap. This has the dual benefit of making the baby feel more secure because of familiarity (Bernado et al. 1990) and helping the parent/carer to retain some control over the proceedings. The nurse should speak in soft tones and avoid sudden movements, so the baby is less likely to become distressed. Accurate assessment of infants is dependent on gaining trust and cooperation, and this approach can optimize the process. For example, an infant can only focus on one thing at a time: successful assessment can therefore be aided by distraction;

Table 15.1 A brief outline of developmental milestones

Age	Stage of development
4–6 weeks	Smiles to social stimuli
2 months	Smiles and vocalizes when talked to
	Eyes follow moving person/object
3 months	Holds a rattle when placed in hand
	Turns head to sounds on level with ear
5 months	Laughs aloud
	Pulled to sit – no head lag
	Able to reach and grasp objects
6 months	Sits on floor with support
	Rolls prone to supine
	Begins to imitate, for example, cough
	Held in standing position puts weight on legs
9 months	Crawls on abdomen
	Stands holding onto furniture
10 months	Waves good-bye
	Helps parent/carer when being dressed, for example, by holding arms for coat
	Pincer grip used to pick up fine objects
12 months	Walks holding onto furniture or with one or two hands held
	Speaks two or three words with meaning

Box 15.1 Assessment of the infant

- Rapid cardiopulmonary assessment – ABC
- Length of current illness
- Symptoms and additional circumstances surrounding the illness/injury
- Immunization status
- Medical problems
- Prescribed medication/over-the-counter medication
- Known allergies
- Feeding and sleeping patterns
- General demeanour and condition should be assessed
- Interaction/response to accompanying adult

for example, diverting the infant's attention with a toy can make taking an axillary temperature easier (Morcombe 1998). It may be worth involving play specialists at this stage to help with distraction techniques. It is worth remembering an infant may be crying loudly and in obvious distress, but the disinterested, lethargic and quiet infant is always a cause for concern.

Vital signs

Normal parameters for an infant's vital signs change with age; therefore knowledge of normal ranges at specific ages is necessary in order to detect abnormalities (see Table 15.2). Table 15.3 shows the anatomical and physiological differences in children as a basis for signs and symptoms.

Airway and breathing

The anatomy of an infant's airway differs significantly from that of an adult or older child (Gilbert et al. 1993, Advanced Paediatric Life Support 2001). The tongue is proportionately bigger in the mouth, thus increasing the risk of oral obstruction. Babies are obligatory nose breathers and become distressed when their nose is blocked with mucus secretions or a foreign body. The upper airway is smaller and narrower than that of an older person; therefore they are more quickly distressed. Respiratory obstruction can occur as a result

Table 15.2 Vital signs in infants.

Age (months)	Average weight (kg)	Normal BP	Heart rate	Respiratory rate
1	4	60–90/45–60	120–160	30–60
3	5	74–100/50–70	120–160	30–60
6	7	74–100/50–70	120–160	30–60
9	9	74–100/50–70	120–160	30–60
12	10	80–112/50–80	90–140	24–40

Table 15.3 Anatomical and physiological differences in children as a basis for signs and symptoms

Respiratory
- The tongue and the pharyngeal are softer and relatively larger when compared to the size of the oral cavity
- Small amounts of mucus, blood or oedema may occlude the airway because of its smaller diameter
- Infants for the first few months of life are obligatory nose breathers. Any nasal obstruction can cause respiratory distress
- The trachea is shorter, increasing the possibility of intubation of the mainstream bronchus
- The chest wall in infants is more pliable because the sternum and ribs are cartilaginous. A significant force may result in an injury to an underlying structure without concomitant fracture

Cardiovascular
- Infants can compensate for a 25% blood loss by increasing the heart rate and peripheral vascular resistance, which maintains a normal systolic blood pressure; therefore, blood pressure is an unreliable indicator of shock
- Tachycardia is one of the first signs of shock but can also be caused by many other factors, including agitation.
- The circulating blood volume of an infant is approximately 90 ml/kg. Small blood loss can stimulate compensatory mechanisms

Temperature regulation
- A greater ratio of body surface to body mass and less subcutaneous tissue for heat insulation means infants have a less effective thermoregulatory mechanism. Infants and small children lose a significant amount of heat through their heads.

Other characteristics
- The anterior and posterior fontanelles are open in infants
- The head is heavier and larger in relation to the rest of the body, predisposing the infant/child to head and neck trauma
- The cranium is thinner and more pliable
- The liver is more anterior and less protected by the ribs
- The kidneys are more mobile and not protected by fat
- The bones of the extremities are more pliable and resilient to injury

(ENA 2000)

of oedema, mucus, blood or constriction (Chameides 1990).

Stridor is a high-pitched inspiratory noise, which can be created by minimal oedema or obstruction but acts as an indicator of imminent respiratory distress. Infants have less respiratory reserve, despite a greater oxygen uptake, because of their faster metabolic rate. Poorly developed intercostal muscles and cartilaginous ribs do not aid the increased activity of breathing during illness. As a result, infants will develop respiratory distress more quickly. Grunting is produced by exhalation against a partially closed laryngeal opening (glottis). It requires considerable effort and is a sign of severe respiratory distress.

It is important that infants presenting with a history of respiratory difficulty are assessed carefully. Estimates of respiratory rate are frequently inaccurate (>20%) in clinical practice in both adults and children, but especially in infants if they are awake and agitated (Simoes et al. 1991). Parents or carers may hold important clues to the cause of perceived or actual respiratory problems. The nurse must be able to listen, reduce the parents/carers fears and rapidly assess the physiological state of the infant's respiratory function (Table 15.4).

Circulation

Every infant and child attending ED should be thoroughly and continually assessed, using a structured rapid cardiopulmonary assessment. Blood volume in a child is 80 ml/kg, with total blood volume much less than in an adult. Loss of one cup of blood in a 10 kg child is equivalent to blood loss of almost 1 litre in an adult. A child responds to increased cardiac output with tachycardia. Tachycardia may initially increase cardiac output during periods of distress; however, prolonged tachycardia of more than 200 beats/min for infants and 170 beats/min for children causes decompensation and decreased cardiac output. While tachycardia is an initial response to physiological compensation, bradycardia is a more ominous sign as it indicates a loss of normal compensatory mechanisms and the onset of decompensated shock. Close attention to heart rate and rhythm, skin signs, capillary refill time and mental status is the key to

Table 15.4   Paediatric differences in airway, breathing and circulation

Factor	Nursing considerations
Airway	
Large tongue	Airway is easily obstructed by tongue; proper positioning is often all that is necessary to open the airway
Smaller diameter of all airways (in a 1-year-old child, tracheal diameter is less than child's little finger)	Small amounts of mucous or swelling easily obstructs the airways; child normally has increased airway resistance
Cartilage of larynx is softer than in adults; cricoid cartilage is narrowest portion of neck	Airway of infant can be compressed if neck is flexed or hyperextended; provides a natural seal for endotracheal tube
Breathing	
Sternum and ribs are cartilaginous; chest wall is soft; intercostal muscles are poorly developed; infants are obligate nose breathers for first 4 weeks of life; increased metabolic rate (about twice that of an adult); increased respiratory demand for oxygen consumption and carbon dioxide elimination	Infant's chest wall may move inward instead of outward during inspiration (retractions) when lung compliance is decreased; greater intrathoracic pressure generated during inspiration; anything causing nasal obstruction can produce respiratory distress; respiratory distress causes increased oxygen demand, as does any condition that increases metabolic rate, such as fever
Circulation	
Child's circulating blood volume is larger per unit of body weight, but absolute volume is relatively small; 70–80% of a newborn's body weight is water, compared to 50–60% of an adult body weight, about half of this volume is extracellular	Blood loss considered minor in an adult may lead to shock in a child; decreased fluid intake or increased fluid intake or increased fluid loss quickly leads to dehydration
Increased heart rate, decreased stroke volume; cardiac output is higher per unit of body weight	Tachycardia is the child's most efficient method of increasing cardiac output if the heart rate is greater than 180–200 beats/min

(After Cosby 1998)

early recognition of compensated shock. Gentle pressure should be applied to the forehead or sternum for five seconds and released and observed for capillary refill. A refill time of >2 seconds indicates poor perfusion, although this may be influenced by a number of factors, particularly cold. Capillary refill should be recorded serially to monitor the response of any measures undertaken to improve circulatory status and is recognized as a better indicator of tissue perfusion than systolic blood pressure (Salter & Maconochie 2005).

Cardiopulmonary failure may be present in any child with respiratory distress, cyanosis or impaired conscious level or in those who suffer severe trauma. The ED nurse should develop expertise and skills to identify subtle changes in a child's condition in order to correlate them into a meaningful picture (see Table 15.4).

Disability

Parents are often the first to recognize decreased levels of consciousness, often stating their infant to be 'not acting normal'. An accurate history from parents is important and it is important to ask about trauma, previous medical problems, ingestions, and signs and symptoms of infection. Evaluation of the history and level of consciousness can be enough to classify the child's condition as an emergency. An altered level of consciousness in any child is an emergent condition. Signs of an impaired conscious level include drowsiness, difficulty to arouse, agitation, failure to recognize or interact with parents and failure to respond to stimuli. A rapid assessment of conscious level can be made using the AVPU scale, that is Alert (fully responsive), Verbal (patient makes response when spoken to), Pain (patient only responds when mild pain inflicted) and Unresponsive (when patient does not respond to either pain or voice). A child who only responds to pain or who is unresponsive has an equivalent Glasgow Coma Scale of 8 or less. Metabolic considerations are also crucial, particularly in relation to derangement of blood glucose levels, so in addition to the ABCs, the emergency nurse should always remember 'DEFG' – 'don't ever forget glucose'.

THE CRITICALLY ILL INFANT AND CHILD

Cardiopulmonary arrest in infants and children is seldom a sudden event and rarely due to a primary cardiac event. It is often the end result of progressive deterioration in respiratory and circulatory function. It usually results from a period of hypoxia and acidosis, which has been caused by respiratory and/or circulatory failure (Bruce-Jones 1994). If pulseless cardiac arrest occurs the outcome is bleak. Early recognition and treatment to prevent cardiopulmonary arrest is fundamental to successful resuscitation. Thus cardiopulmonary arrest can often be prevented if the clinical signs of respiratory failure and shock are recognized promptly.

Paediatric primary and secondary assessment

Primary assessment consists of evaluation of ABCs and neurological status. The primary survey should include assessment of respiratory effort, skin colour and temperature, and heart rate and quality and level of consciousness. Secondary assessment consists of vital interventions and a head-to-toe survey (Box 15.2).

Respiratory rate

The infant and young child's respiratory muscles are not well developed, so the diaphragm plays an

---

Box 15.2   Primary assessment

- Rapid cardiopulmonary assessment – ABC
- Observe the baby's respiratory rate
- Look at skin colour; is the baby pink, pale, or cyanosed; is the colour different centrally and peripherally?
- Listen to breathing; is there stridor, wheezing or grunting?
- Look at chest movements; are they equal on both sides, is there intercostal recession; is the baby using shoulders and head bobbing to aid respiratory effort; is there nasal flaring?
- Check pulse; is it within normal ranges; is the baby tachycardic or bradycardic; what is the pulse pressure?

- Is the baby pyrexic?
- Avoid distressing the baby - usually the parent or carer can hold the infant as they have often found the position most comfortable for the baby. This is usually semi-upright.
- Determine the infant's responsiveness - does he or she react to stimulus from the nurse; is he or she interacting with the parent/carer; is the baby aware of his or her surroundings?
- Is the baby easily distracted, upset, irritable, fretful, restless, floppy or unconscious?
- Is a blood glucose test indicated?

essential role in breathing. Observation of the rise and fall of the abdomen is the best method for assessing respiratory rate in patients less than two years old. As respiratory rates are often irregular in small children, the rate should be carefully assessed for a full minute. A neonate has a normal respiratory rate from 30–40 breaths/min, which slows as the child grows older. A resting rate faster than 60 breaths per minute is a sign of respiratory distress in a child, irrespective of age (Cosby 1998). Other clinical signs of distress include nasal flaring, use of accessory muscles, recession, grunting, stridor and wheezing.

Skin perfusion and temperature

The skin colour and temperature should be consistent over the trunk and limbs; however, when assessing the patient consider the ambient temperature. Decreased skin perfusion can be an early sign of shock. Clinical signs of poor perfusion include peripherally cool skin, pallor, mottling and peripheral cyanosis. Capillary refill time is also useful in assessing perfusion. The sternum or forehead are preferred sites (Maconochie 1998) as ambient temperatures can affect peripheral sites. Sufficient pressure to cause the skin to blanch should be applied for five seconds and the length of time for normal colour to return recorded (Castle 2002).

Heart rate and blood pressure

Increases in pulse rate, poor peripheral perfusion and delayed capillary refill are reliable signs of circulatory failure but blood pressure is particularly unreliable (Castle 2002). Sinus tachycardia is a common presentation in most unwell, anxious children. Further assessment will be needed to determine and treat the cause. Bradycardia in a sick child is a pre-terminal sign, however, and indicates imminent cardiopulmonary arrest. Decreased perfusion to extremities results in weak peripheral pulses. Vital signs should be documented as part of the baseline assessment. Children in early shock may have a normal blood pressure reading initially because of ability to compensate. A dropping blood pressure is a serious sign warranting immediate intervention as a child can lose a significant amount of blood before the blood pressure decreases (Hazinski 1992). A normal range for blood pressure can be estimated by the following equation: (Age $\times 2$) $+80$ = Estimated normal systolic blood pressure.

Management priorities

Using a structured approach, such as Paediatric Advanced Life Support (PALS), the ED nurse must determine the relevance of the clinical signs found

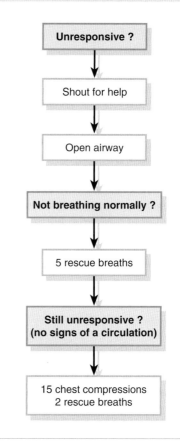

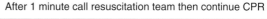
After 1 minute call resuscitation team then continue CPR

Figure 15.1 Paediatric basic life support.

and prioritize further management. The child should be categorized as:

- in cardiopulmonary failure
- in definite respiratory failure/shock
- in potential respiratory failure/shock
- stable

Paediatric Basic and Advanced Life Support interventions may be required (see Fig. 15.1 and Fig. 15.2).

PAEDIATRIC ADVANCED LIFE SUPPORT

Establish basic life support (Resuscitation Council UK 2005). Oxygenate and ensure the provision of positive pressure ventilation with a high inspired oxygen concentration. Attach a defibrillator or monitor and monitor the cardiac rhythm. Check the pulse; for an infant feel for the brachial pulse on the inner aspect of the upper arm; for a child feel for the carotid pulse in the neck, taking no more than 10 seconds. Assess the rhythm on the monitor as being:

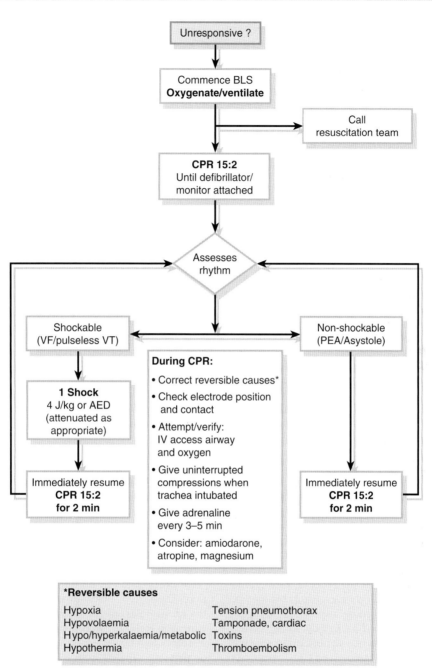

Figure 15.2 Paediatric advanced life support.

- non-ventricular fibrillation (non-VF) or non-pulseless ventricular tachycardia (non-VT) (asystole or electromechanical dissociation)
- ventricular fibrillation (VF) or pulseless ventricular tachycardia (VT).

In general, disorders of rate and rhythm in the paediatric population are relatively benign. Heart rates are much more rapid and QRS complexes are narrower. The underlying mechanism, treatment and ultimate prognosis of the paediatric dysrhythmia are dependent on the structural aspects of the heart and its conduction system and less dependent on pre-existing coronary artery disease (Toepper & Hakim 1998). Non-VF/VT is the most common presenting dysrhythmia. It is usually due to hypoxia and associated acidosis following a period of respiratory or cardiac failure. This leads to a profound bradycardia which results in asystole, although pulseless electrical activity (PEA) is also common (Castle 2002). PEA and asystole can be due to a number of potentially treatable causes such as:

- hypoxia
- hypovolaemia
- hyper/hypokalaemia
- hypothermia
- tension pneumothorax
- tamponade
- toxic/therapeutic disturbances
- thromboemboli
  (Resuscitation Council (UK) 2005b).

The treatment of non-VF/VT is effective ventilation using high concentrations of oxygen and administration of adrenaline/epinephrine 10 µg/kg (0.1 ml of the 1:10000 solution) by the intravenous, intraosseous or endotracheal route (100 µg/kg). Four minutes of basic life support at a rate of 15 chest compressions to 2 ventilations should be carried out between doses of adrenaline, with the monitor checked every two minutes to confirm asystole/PEA. Repeating the cycle at least twice more is encouraged to aid the circulation of drugs and the correction of hypoxia and acidosis. Consider the use of other medications and treat reversible causes.

VF/VT is less common in paediatric life support but the nurse must always be aware of the possibility of treating this arrhythmia rapidly and effectively. Place the defibrillator paddles on the chest wall; one just below the right clavicle, the other at the left anterior axillary line; for infants, when using this method of monitoring, it may be more appropriate to apply the paddles to the front and back of the infant's chest. Defibrillate the heart with one defibrillation shock at 4 J/kg followed by two minutes of CPR. After two minutes pause briefly to check the monitor. If VF/VT is still present a second shock at 4 J/kg should be delivered followed by a further two minutes of CPR. Adrenaline (10 µg/kg) should be given immediately before the third shock. After a further two minutes of CPR pause briefly to check the monitor. If the rhythm is still VF/VT, a dose of amiodrone (5 µg/kg) should be given followed by a fourth shock. Continue giving shocks every two minutes with a dose of adrenaline before every other shock (ALSG 2006).

There are various causes of VF/VT in children but drug overdose, hypokalaemia and hypothermia should be actively considered (Resuscitation Council (UK) 2005b).

CAUSES OF RESPIRATORY DIFFICULTY

Inhalation of foreign body

Inhalation of a foreign body (FB) should always be considered if a baby presents with a sudden onset of cyanosis, stridor or choking. This is more common in toddlers than infants (Cantrill 1993). Timely treatment will prevent severe complications. The Heimlich Manoeuvre or abdominal thrusts are not recommended in infants as they may cause intra-abdominal injury (APLS 2001). Blind finger sweeps to remove foreign bodies may convert a partial obstruction of the upper airway to a total obstruction, as the foreign body can pass from the upper part of the larynx to obstruct the airway completely at the level of the cricoid cartilage (Salter & Maconochie 2005).

Infants with total airway obstruction should be placed prone with their head being well supported by the operator and five back blows should be given in rapid succession to relieve the obstruction. If this is not successful, place the infant supine on a firm surface and give five chest thrusts (Resuscitation Council 1997).

Bronchiolitis

Bronchiolitis is the most common lower respiratory tract infection in infants (Agency for Healthcare Research and Quality 2003) and around 90 per cent of cases are attributed to the respiratory syncytial virus (RSV) (Barkin & Rosen 1994). It is most prevalent in winter and is the most frequent cause of pneumonia in infancy (Dinwiddie 1990). Bronchiolitis is often precipitated by an upper respiratory tract infection. The virus causes an inflammatory response in the bronchioles, thus causing constriction of the airway. The resultant secretions begin to accumulate, as exudate cannot be easily expectorated because of damage to ciliated cells. This results in impaired gaseous exchange (McFarlane 1992).

Infants present with a three to five day history of 'runny nose', cough and low grade pyrexia worsening over a period of a few days. This leads to irritability, poor feeding and eventually to dehydration and respiratory distress (Barkin and Rosen 1994). Initial assessment will reveal an infant with dyspnoea and tachypnoea, and an expiratory wheeze. There may be signs of respiratory distress with intercostal recession, use of accessory muscles and nasal flaring.

Infants under six months, or those born prematurely, are at greatest risk of respiratory failure or apnoeic episodes (Wolfram 1992). Infants with chronic lung, cardiac, or neuromuscular conditions are also at risk of RSV infection (Garzon et al. 2002).

Nursing interventions include reassurance of parents/carers and maintenance of a calm environment. The infant should be given oxygen by the least distressing route – via nasal cannulae or a facemask, blowing close to the infant. Pulse oximetry will indicate the effectiveness of the treatment and a SaO_2 of less than 95% is found to be the single best predictor of severe bronchiolitis although a low SaO_2 is not always apparent (Darr 1998). Nebulized beta antagonists can be effective bronchodilators (Sanchez et al. 1993). The emergency nurse should carefully monitor the infant's respiratory function. If the infant responds well to nebulizers, tachypnoea reduces and the infant is feeding, it is appropriate for parents/carers to continue care at home in most cases. They should, however, be advised to return if the infant's condition worsens or the infant is reluctant to feed. High-risk children who should be hospitalized include those younger than three months and those with a preterm birth, cardiopulmonary disease, immunodeficiency, respiratory distress, inadequate oxygenation (Prassaad Steiner 2004) or if the infant is lethargic, dehydrated, not feeding or there has been suspicion of apnoea.

Feeding is an important landmark in the severity of bronchiolitis. As dyspnoea increases the infant becomes fatigued, and the effort required to feed and maintain respiration is too great. At this stage the infant begins to demonstrate signs of respiratory distress. Young babies do not have a great fluid reserve and can become rapidly dehydrated. This results both from the reduced fluid intake and from increased insensible loss due to tachypnoea. These infants may require IV fluid replacement and in severe cases mechanical ventilation (Barkin & Rosen 1994). Infants with suspected bronchiolitis should be nursed away from other babies and stringent cross-infection measures should be employed as RSV is particularly contagious (Hay 1996).

THE FEBRILE INFANT

After breathing difficulties, fever is the most common reason for seeking medical care for a child (Armon et al. 2001). Fever represents a normal physiological response that may result from the introduction of an infectious pathogen into the body and is hypothesized to play a role in fighting and overcoming infections. However, at initial presentation, 5% to 22% of all febrile children lack definitive symptoms or signs that point to an affected organ or lead to a diagnosis, thus making it difficult to distinguish between a minor febrile illness and one that is life-threatening (Park 2000, Pantell et al. 2004). Therefore, all infants presenting to the ED complaining of fever/temperature should be thoroughly assessed at triage. Fever is shown by a rectal temperature of 38°C (100.4°F) or higher. Hyperpyrexia, that is, a temperature above 41°C (105.8°F), is an uncommon but serious problem, with approximately 20% of children experiencing convulsions (Surpure 1987). A concise but detailed history of the illness should be taken, gathering the following information:

- sequence of events
- accompanying symptoms such as vomiting
- fluid intake and output
- present medications and regularity including dosage of anti-pyretics
- immunization status.

Nursing activities should include:

- airway, breathing and circulation
- observe skin circulation, colour and rashes
- weight
- assess general handling and alertness as the infant is undressed
- distraction therapy helps in ascertaining whether the infant is either hot and miserable but responsive, or acutely ill
- a newborn with a temperature less than 36°C axilla should have a BM stick recorded.
- place a urine pad in situ for specimen collection.

A large study undertaken in the United States identified the factors associated with a high risk of bacteraemia/bacterial meningitis in infants

- age ≤ 30 days
- higher temperatures
- ill appearance
- abnormal cry
- abnormal WBC count (Pantell et al. 2004).

For this reason it is important not to dismiss an infant as being well if he/she is apyrexic. Check when antipyretics were last administered and ensure that the infant's temperature is within normal acceptable range; however, it must be noted that there is no correlation between fever reduction with antipyretic medication and the likelihood of serious bacterial infection (ACEP 2003). Check heart rate, skin colour and capillary refill to ensure the baby is truly apyrexic, and not peripherally shut down, septic or in shock. One of the most common reasons for pyrexia in infants attending ED is a simple viral illness and these often do not need medical intervention. The most important intervention from the nurse is discharge advice to the parents about temperature control and the use of antipyretic drugs such as paracetamol or ibuprofen in those older than six months. It is useful to support this advice with written instructions for parents.

FEBRILE CONVULSIONS

Febrile convulsions are seizures that occur in a child with a febrile illness. They are common, but usually benign events occurring in infants, toddlers and young children. Witnessing a convulsion is, however, extremely distressing for parents. Approximately 2–4% of all children are affected (Waruiru & Appleton 2004, Ling 2000). The seizures are generalized of tonic-clonic nature, usually lasting less than 10 minutes and complete recovery usually occurs within one hour (Valman 1993). The onset of a febrile convulsion is often the first sign that an infant is unwell, as seizures usually occur near the onset of a fever rather than after prolonged fever (Brunner & Suddarth 1991). The peak incidence occurs between 8 and 20 months; febrile seizures are uncommon after 5 to 6 years (Zukin et al. 1998).

A comprehensive review of the literature by Armon et al. (2003) identified the conditions usually associated with febrile convulsions. In order of decreasing frequency these are:

- viral infections
- otitis media
- tonsilitis
- urinary tract infection
- gastroenteritis
- lower respiratory tract infection
- meningitis
- post-immunization.

Infants who arrive in the emergency department still convulsing obviously need urgent assessment and intervention. Maintaining a clear airway and providing adequate oxygenation are the first priorities. Clothes should be removed and temperature recorded. Rectal administration of anticonvulsants and antipyretics should be considered, although there is no evidence that antipyretics reduce the risk of subsequent febrile convulsions in at-risk children (El-Radhi & Barry 2003). Rectal diazepam at 0.5 mg/kg produces an effective blood concentration of anticonvulsant within 10 minutes (Valman 1993). Most febrile convulsions are self-limiting, but if an anticonvulsant has been used careful monitoring of the infant's respiratory function and blood pressure should be observed until an adequate conscious level is regained.

As most infants will arrive 'post-ictal', respiratory function and temperature should be assessed and antipyretics administered if necessary. Parents and carers need a lot of support and reassurance that febrile convulsions do not harm the child and they are not the same as epilepsy. They may also be advised that although epilepsy can develop later, it is rare, developing in only one in 100 children who have had two or more convulsions. Immunization is still advised after a febrile convulsion, even if, as rarely happens, the febrile convulsion followed an immunization (Waruiru & Appleton 2004).

Infants with simple febrile seizures may be discharged after appropriate fever control has been achieved, although many paediatricians will admit a child for 24 hours observation following a first convulsion. Before discharge parents need to be advised about temperature control at home, and shown how to manage any further convulsions. Children at high risk of recurrences of febrile seizure (i.e. complex features of febrile convulsions, family history of febrile convulsions, age less than 1 year, low grade fever at the onset of febrile convulsions) develop recurrences in at least 80% of cases, while those without these risk factors rarely develop recurrences (El-Radhi & Barry 2003).

MENINGITIS

Meningococcal disease is one of the most important medical emergencies, demanding early diagnosis and prompt treatment with effective therapy (Boyne 2001). Meningitis in infancy has serious consequences, with 2% of those who survived the acute attack in one large study of 1880 children with meningitis dying before the age of 5 years (Bedford et al. 2001). The long-term consequences can even be seen where the behaviour of teenage children who had meningitis in infancy is worse than that of control children who did not have infantile meningitis when rated by parents and teachers (Halket et al. 2003). Peak incidence is between 3 and 12 months, although the mortality remains above other age groups until around the age of two years, when numbers fall (Wilson & Lilley 1994). Meningitis is a consequence of inflammation of the meninges, and is most commonly caused by infective agents such as viruses and bacteria. Bacterial meningitis is spread between people by droplet infection, whereas some viral infections can be found in other agents such as polluted water (Kumar & Clark 1990). Common causes of bacterial meningitis are *Streptococcus pnuemoniae*, *Neisseria meningitides* and *Haemophilus influenzae*, the latter being reduced by the introduction of the Hib vaccine in childhood immunizations.

While viral meningitis is rarely severe and children tend to make a rapid complete recovery (Davison & Ramsey 2003), bacterial meningitis in infants is a paediatric emergency. In the newborn, it has a mortality of 25% (Kelnar 1995). Early recognition and treatment are vital; any delay in recognition can prove catastrophic for the infant. The disease has a rapid onset and, left undiagnosed, death may occur in less than 48 hours. One aid to recognition is the use of cascade protocols for detecting meningitis; however, it should always be considered in any infant with unexplained pyrexia or illness. Protocols for the management of bacterial meningitis will aid rapid treatment once suspected; these should be agreed with the paediatric department and made readily available to ED staff. The nurse will usually be the first person to assess an infant; therefore accurate and thorough recordings are vital. Pyrexic, lethargic infants should always be fully assessed. Signs and symptoms of bacterial meningitis are given in Box 15.3

Infants with suspected meningitis require immediate urgent care. If a petechial or purpuric rash is present deterioration will be rapid. The rash is distinctive and easily identifiable as it will not diminish or blanch on pressure. Skin with a mottled pale appearance can be a sign of shock and sepsis.

Box 15.3 Signs and symptoms of bacterial meningitis

Non-specific signs and symptoms
- Drowsiness
- Irritability
- Off feeds
- Distressed when handled
- Vomiting
- Pyrexia

Specific signs and symptoms
- Neck stiffness
- Tense bulging fontanelle
- Purpuric or petechial rash
- Mottled appearance
- Hypothermic

Late signs and symptoms
- High pitched moaning cry
- Reduced level of consciousness/coma
- Neck retraction/arched back
- Shock
- Widespread haemorrhagic rash

If symptoms are vague or suggestive of possible early meningitis a rapid septic screening should be performed. This should include: strict monitoring of vital signs including respirations and blood pressure, physical examination for obvious sources of infection, for example, ears or upper airway, blood analysis and culture, urine microbiology and lumbar puncture. Intravenous access should be established and fluid administration commenced at an appropriate rate for the infant's weight and physical condition. Rapid administration of antibiotics can be life-saving, and it is recommended that these are administered prior to the sometimes lengthy process of lumbar puncture.

A lumbar puncture is performed to detect the presence of bacteria in the cerebrospinal fluid. While there is some debate about the merits of undertaking a lumbar puncture in an infant with petechial rash, as it adds very little in terms of diagnosis and carries a high risk of making the haemodynamically unstable infant worse, nevertheless, whether the decision is to perform a lumbar puncture or not, antibiotic treatment should not be delayed (Bashir et al. 2003). The administration of antibiotics immediately prior to lumbar puncture rarely alters the cerebrospinal fluid enough to interfere with interpretation or detection of bacteria (Bernardo & Schenkel 1995). Lumbar puncture is contraindicated if raised intracranial pressure is suspected, as it enhances the risk of producing cerebral herniation. For the lumbar puncture to be performed the infant is placed in the lateral decubitus position, on his/her side, with the knees drawn up to the abdomen and the neck flexed forward. The infant's shoulders and hips are kept perpendicular to the examination trolley throughout the procedure (Fig. 15.3). The infant should be attached to a cardiac monitor and respiratory effort should be watched closely during the procedure, as critically ill infants are at risk of cardiopulmonary arrest. Holding the infant in the necessary position for lumbar puncture increases this risk; therefore the procedure should be carried out with care and vigilance (Bernardo & Schenkel 1995) (Fig. 15.3).

This assessment period is obviously distressing for parents. During the septic screening and particularly when performing invasive investigations, it is important to explain the nature of these procedures and give the parents the option to stay with the infant or leave. This will prevent unnecessary anxiety and allow the parents to remain actively involved should they wish.

In most cases of bacterial meningitis a broad-spectrum cephalosporin (cefotaxime or ceftriaxone) is the most appropriate empirical choice in children over 3 months old. These cover *Neisseria meningitides*, *Streptococcus pneumoniae* and *Haemophilus influenzae*, and

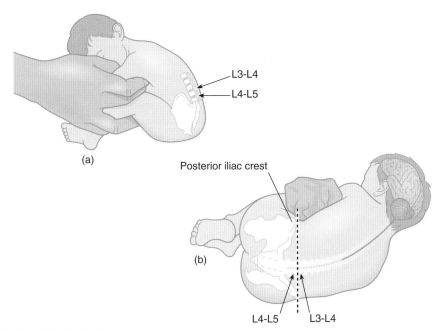

Figure 15.3 Baby in position for lumbar puncture.

penetrate CSF well. Ampicillin should be added in young infants (less than 3 months old) to cover *Listeria monocytogenes* (El-Bashir et al. 2003). Depending on the causative organisms, prophylactic treatment may also be required for the immediate family. The ED nurse should ensure this is not overlooked and where possible should facilitate its prescription by medical staff. The public health department should also be informed.

DEHYDRATION IN INFANTS

Dehydration occurs when fluid loss exceeds fluid intake over a period, leaving the body in negative fluid balance. It is a consequence of many illnesses in infancy, particularly those involving the gastrointestinal tract. It is also the main cause of fever during the first week of life (Tiker et al. 2004). Initial assessment should include a history from the parent/carer leading up to ED attendance, including changes in feeding pattern, what the infant has taken in the last 24 hours, whether the baby is off feed, or appears more thirsty. Is there a history of vomiting, diarrhoea, or constipation? What is the urine output like? Has there been obvious weight loss?

Physical assessment of the infant should include:

- airway, breathing and circulation
- is the infant obviously dehydrated, with dry mucous membranes, absent tears and saliva, poor

skin turgor, sunken eyes, or depressed anterior fontanelle?

The percentage of body water in an infant is greater than that of an older child or adult, thus dehydration in infants is more rapid in onset and potentially more serious. It is paramount to accurately assess the degree of dehydration to determine the treatment regime, although it is worth noting that a baby who is seriously dehydrated may continue to feed well, so feeding should not be used as an indication of well-being (Dwight & Collier 2001). Dehydration can be classified as mild (<5%), moderate (5–10%), or severe (>10%) (Cincinnati Children's Hospital Medical Center 2002, McVerry & Collin 1999) (see Table 15.5).

The fluid deficit can be calculated by the formula: Percentage dehydration × weight × 10; for example a 10 kg infant who is 10% dehydrated has a total fluid deficit of 1000 ml, to be replaced over 24 hours (APLS 2001). If moderate or severe dehydration is present intravenous fluid therapy should be commenced. In the case of mild dehydration, oral fluid replacement should be attempted unless specific contraindications exist. Oral rehydration solutions (ORS) are an easily metabolized fluid and electrolyte replacement and significantly reduce admission rates from the emergency department (Boyd et al. 2005). If the infant does not tolerate oral fluid, because of poor feeding or vomiting, he/she may be admitted for fluid

Table 15.5   Degree of dehydration in infants

Sign	Mild	Moderate	Severe
Increased pulse	−	+	+
Rapid respiration	−	+/−	+
Hypotension	−	+/−	+
Dry mucous membrane	+/−	+	+
Reduced skin turgor	+		+
Sunken eyeballs	−	+	+
Depressed anterior fontanelle	−	+	+
Urine output	Reduced	Oliguria	Oliguria/anuria
Blood pH (usually tested in moderate to severe dehydration)	7.40–7.30	7.30–7.00	<7.10

replacement. If the infant is discharged parents should be advised about fluid maintenance and monitoring. The use of clear fluids often needs to be stressed to parents, who are worried about their baby being hungry if they are not taking milk feeds.

FAILURE TO THRIVE

This is a general descriptive term applied to poor growth in early life (Wells 2001). The weight of the infant falls below that expected for the gestational and post-natal age (Brunner & Suddarth 1991). In the first few months of life, one-third of infant energy intake is diverted to growth, whereas by one year of age this proportion has dropped to less than 5% (Wells & Davies 1998). These infants have a history of failure to gain weight, and loss of subcutaneous fat or muscle mass. Undernutrition is strongly implicated and most children with failure to thrive have been found to be substantially underweight for height, although the degree of underweight is not always obvious, even to experienced clinicians (Wright 2000). Children with a history of failure to thrive have been found to have clinically and statistically significant behavioural deficits and consistently depressed scores in cognitive, neurological and psychomotor development (Perrin et al. 2003).

Failure to thrive is not often the primary reason for emergency department attendance. Parents may bring their baby because of related symptoms such as lethargy, weight loss or poor feeding; similarly they may be unaware of a development problem. Initial recognition of failure to thrive often relies on the familiarity of the nurse with normal infant development. The actual intervention will depend on the severity, and the social circumstances surrounding attendance. Although abuse or neglect was previously viewed as the primary cause of non-organic failure to thrive, in practice there is no evidence for it in the vast majority of cases. However, while deliberate neglect is rare, accidental neglect could be considered to include mothers who do not provide the optimum response to infant needs; therefore management of the condition will still often involve addressing parental behaviour (Milan et al. 2004, Wells 2001). Hospital admission is not always indicated; empowering parents to care for their baby at home is often more appropriate. Adequate community support is imperative: the health visitor and the family's GP should be informed.

THE VOMITING INFANT

Vomiting is a common symptom of many presentations of infants in ED. The most common cause of vomiting is acute gastroenteritis. Other infections include urinary and respiratory tract infections, ear infections and tonsillitis. Poor feeding techniques or excessive feeding may also lead to vomiting.

Assessing the infant with vomiting

- airway, breathing and circulation
- record birth weight and present weight.
  As a general rule infants double their birth weight by 5–6 months and triple their weight by one year
- urine output
- bowel actions.

Management

Management of infantile vomiting should focus on correcting fluid deficits as well as definitive treatment of the underlying cause. Most well hydrated infants with a self-limiting problem can usually be discharged home with appropriate advice regarding feeding.

Gastroenteritis

Acute gastroenteritis is a clinical syndrome characterized by the onset of diarrhoea and/or vomiting
which is often accompanied by fever (Khatib 1986).
Acute gastroenteritis lasting less than 10 days is one
of the most common medical illnesses of childhood
(McVerry and Collin 1999). Parents bring their child
to ED in varying stages of ill health, the majority of
which can be managed at home. An accurate history
should be taken to rule out chronic illness. The following information should be gathered:

- when the illness commenced
- diet and fluids taken
- episodes of vomiting since onset
- episodes of diarrhoea since onset
- urine output
- relevant medical history
- note any recent visits abroad
- prescribed medication or over the counter
  medication.

The priority is to assess for dehydration (see
Table 15.5). Vital signs should be recorded and oral
rehydration should be initiated to replace the fluid loss
and assess tolerance. Small amounts of clear fluid, preferably oral rehydration solution, should be given at frequent intervals. Most infants with a gastrointestinal
infection can be treated at home with oral rehydration
but infants less than 6 months and those living in poor
social conditions are particularly vulnerable and may
require hospital admission (Wharton et al. 1988).

Gastro–oesophageal reflux

Asymptomatic, infrequent reflux of gastric contents is
physiological. Reflux is most common in young
infants, who effortlessly regurgitate milk over parents, furniture and carpets. While the vast majority
remain well, infants may present with failure to gain
weight or weight loss, feeding problems or anaemia
(Meadow & Newell 2002). Gastro-oesophageal reflux
can also result in recurrent pulmonary disease due
to the acid erosion.

Intussusception

Intussusception is a telescoping of a portion of the
intestine. The onset is sudden and typically occurs
in males aged 3–8 weeks (Brown 2002). It causes
severe intermittent attacks of screaming and abdominal pain, often with associated drawing up of the legs,
vomiting and pallor. The infant is irritable or lethargic
with paroxysms of colicky pain. Diarrhoea is mucous-
laden and blood-stained 'red currant jelly' stools are

passed. An infant presenting with this history should
be seen as a matter of urgency; however, classic symptoms are absent in up to half of babies with intussusception (Barkin & Rosen 1994). If an infant presents with an
unaccountable change in behaviour, listlessness or
altered level of consciousness intussusception should
be suspected.

The infant with intussusception is extremely unstable; therefore, intravenous access should be established and referral to a paediatric surgeon should be
swift. Intussusception can be diagnosed on X-ray in
some patients, or with ultrasound scan, but barium
enema is both diagnostic and therapeutic in up to
75% of cases, particularly when early intervention
occurs (Stephenson et al. 1989). During this procedure
close monitoring of the infant's vital signs are necessary, as shock and perforation of the bowel are potential side-effects. If a barium enema does not result in a
reduction of the intussusception surgery is indicated
as a matter of urgency.

Pyloric stenosis

Pyloric stenosis is a disorder that usually becomes
apparent during the first few weeks of life, although it
can go undiagnosed for as long as six months. It occurs
in 1 in 150 boys and 1 in 750 girls (Meadow & Newell
2002). There is progressive hypertrophy of the pylorus
causing partial or total obstruction of the pyloric
sphincter. Typically, the infant has poor weight gain
or weight loss due to the projectile vomiting that occurs
after feeds. The infant is excessively hungry and shows
a willingness to feed immediately after vomiting. This
can be very distressing for parents, particularly those
caring for their first baby. Many parents blame their
feeding technique, and careful intervention from ED
staff is needed to establish diagnosis and reduce
feelings of anxiety or guilt the parents may have.

Pyloric stenosis does have a familial incidence so
parents of a second or subsequent baby may already
suspect what is wrong, and come to ED seeking confirmation and action from staff. The infant may or may not
be dehydrated on attendance but this largely depends
on the duration and severity of the stenosis. A test feed
is indicated to help establish diagnosis. As the stomach
fills, waves of peristalsis become visible until the infant
vomits. These babies will be admitted to hospital and
undergo surgery once rehydrated and stable.

THE INJURED INFANT

The infant is totally dependent on his or her parents/
carer, and accidents that occur to infants are a reflection of this fact (Mead & Sibert 1991). As the infant
develops, his or her mobility increases together with

a growing susceptibility to injury. Constant supervision of infants is not always possible. Parental behaviour and education can help reduce the serious consequences of injury.

Assessment of the injured infant

Parents are often distressed and anxious, and may feel guilty or responsible for the infant's injury. Assessment, therefore, needs to be done carefully if a therapeutic relationship is to be established. The following information should be collected;

- time elapsed since injury
- was the accident witnessed?
- cause and mechanism of injury
- accident environment or whether indoors or outdoors
- examine wound/injury
- analgesia
- relevant medial history, immunization status, medications.

This assessment gives the nurse an insight into the history leading to injury and the family dynamics and should highlight any areas of concern relating to the family's psychosocial set-up, as well as determining the actual severity of the injury. ED nurses must remain vigilant for possible or evident non-accidental injuries (see also Chapter 16: Pre-school Children). The majority of injuries to infants are minor, requiring a one-off visit to ED. On discharge, written advice to support nursing and medical intervention should be given.

HEAD INJURIES

These injuries normally occur when the baby is dropped, or has fallen. The risk of head injury following a fall is likely as infants have relatively large heads in proportion to their bodies. Most head injuries are minor and the majority of infants recover uneventfully; however, head injuries remain a significant cause of death among infants. A non-mobile infant may fall from a height such as parents' arms, a bed or a baby chair put on a work surface. As injury severity correlates with the distance fallen, CT scanning should be considered (NICE 2003). Skull fractures are relatively common in these cases, whereas injuries in toddlers tend to be caused by tripping over and are generally benign (Davies 2003) (Box 15.4).

Scalp signs may include lacerations or haematomas. Small, firm haematomas are generally benign, even if quite prominent. Larger, 'boggy' haematomas are highly indicative of underlying fracture. A thorough history of events prior to admission should be obtained – this will give an indication of the degree of trauma. No infants or children presenting with head injuries that require imaging of the head or cervical spine should be transferred to the community until assessed by a clinician experienced in the detection of non-accidental injury. Information collected is outlined in Box 15.4.

Box 15.4   Assessment of head injured infant

- Was the accident witnessed and how long ago did it occur?
- Were there external forces involved, such as RTA, trauma to head by moving object, or a fall from one surface to another?
- What surface did the infant fall onto, for example, linoleum floor, pavement, carpeted floor?
- How was the infant immediately following the accident – did he/she cry immediately, lose consciousness, or fit?
- Has the infant vomited? Infants often vomit as a normal reaction to a stressful event; vomiting more than three times is considered significant
- Is he/she drowsy or unrousable? Sleeping is an automatic response to injury for an infant, particularly if the time coincides with a normal sleep time, or if the infant is in an environment with rhythmic noise or movement, such as a car. For drowsiness to be significant the child must have reduced movements during sleep, or be slow to respond to stimuli which would normally wake him/her. Parents can often be the best judges of this as they are used to their baby's sleep pattern. Emotion can, however, render the parent/carer less objective.
- Establish any relevant medical history, immunization status, and medications.
  Physical assessment of the infant's condition should include;
- Airway, breathing, circulation
- Examination of the scalp for evidence of injury, lacerations, or haematomas.
- Palpate for tenderness, bony deformity and check the anterior fontanelle
- Observe the nose and ears for evidence of bleeding or fluid leak
- Examine the infant for any other injuries

Treatment for most infants attending with head injury revolves around observation and advice to parents, but nurses must be able to detect and act on findings indicative of a more serious injury. Advice should include advising the parents or carers to bring the infant back to the emergency department if there is poor feeding, persistent crying, vomiting more than once or drowsiness (see also Chapter 4: Head Injuries).

CHILD PROTECTION

While child protection issues span the whole of childhood, this issue is addressed in detail in Chapter 16.

SUDDEN INFANT DEATH SYNDROME

This is undoubtedly one of the most traumatic and emotionally devastating events ever to happen to a family. One baby in every 1500 live births dies suddenly and unexpectedly between the ages of one week and two years; however, the rate has fallen from 0.55 cot deaths per 1000 live births in the UK in 2000 to 0.43 per 1000 live births in 2004. During the period 2000–2004, 89% of all sudden infant deaths in England and Wales occurred among babies aged less than six months. Fifty-nine per cent of sudden infant deaths in England and Wales occurred among boys, while boys comprised 51% of all live births (figures refer to the period 2000–2004). Since the launch of the Reduce the Risk campaign in England and Wales in 1991, the number of babies dying of cot death has fallen by around 75%. Cot death is the leading kind of death in babies over one month old – claiming more lives than meningitis, leukaemia, other forms of cancer, household and road traffic accidents put together (FSID 2005, Meadow & Newell 2002, APLS 2001).

Sudden infant death syndrome (SIDS) remains a mystery but is more common in winter months among boys and babies of low birth weight, with the peak incidence being four weeks and four months, in homes where the infant shares a bed with the parents, in urban rather than rural areas, and in homes which are socially and economically deprived, and it occurs usually during sleep, which gives rise to it sometimes being called 'cot death'. The infants' mothers also tend to be younger and to smoke (Meadow & Newell 2002). Half of all babies who die of SIDS have had a recent upper respiratory tract infection. A common scenario is one where the infant is found dead a few minutes or hours after being put to rest in his or her cot.

Box 15.5   Prevention of SIDS

Back to sleep
  Avoid sleeping prone
Not too hot, light bedclothes
  16–20°C overnight, head exposed, no hat
Feet to foot
  Baby's feet touching foot of cot
Smoke free zone
  Avoid smoking in pregnancy and in the home
Avoid bed-sharing
  Maternal bed smoking plus bed-sharing is associated with a 33% increase in incidence of SIDS
Prompt medical advice
  If unwell, feverish or less responsive

(Meadow & Newell 2002, Mitchell 1992)

Suffocation, electrolyte imbalances, mineral deficiencies, cardiac dysrhythmias, infection, anaemia, seizures, hyperthermia, hyperthyroidism, upper airway obstruction, congenital abnormalities and occult trauma are but a few of the possible explanations for sudden infant death. Although these factors may play a role in a small number of what appear to be SIDS deaths, the majority of these deaths remain unexplained (Gausche 1992). The infant who has suffered a cot death experiences irreversible cardiac and respiratory arrest. See Box 15.5 for advice on prevention of SIDS.

Initial response

Active resuscitation may already have been initiated by paramedics or parents; the infant is assessed quickly while resuscitation continues.

The main objectives of management in the accident and emergency department are:

- to check whether there is any prospect of survival, and to carry out resuscitation as appropriate
- to provide support for the family
- to collect evidence that might help determine the cause of death
- to ensure compliance with the law and the meeting of forensic requirements (Foundation for the Study of Sudden Infant Deaths 2002).

Parents should be given the choice whether they wish to stay with the baby during resuscitation or wait in a relative's room close by. Whichever the parents decide, an experienced nurse should accompany them. This nurse must ensure that the parents are fully informed of what is happening with their baby, particularly to explain procedures that may look alarming, such as cutting off clothes or intubation. It is essential the parents are not given false hope; this can easily be done inadvertently by using phrases such as 'it will be all right'. If other siblings or children have been brought to hospital with the parents, it is often appropriate for them to be looked after by a suitable person away from the immediate resuscitation area or in a relative's room; ED staff must be guided by the parents' wishes about this.

The emergency nurse accompanying the parents should try to obtain a brief history of the infant's age, general health, development and events leading up to the incident, including the circumstances of how the infant was found and when or if resuscitation was initiated. Find out the names of the people who have come with the baby and their relationship to him/her. A calm, unhurried manner will usually help in getting this information, given that the atmosphere will be fraught and tense. The nurse should establish whether the parents would like spiritual support and if required contact the appropriate religious leader.

The doctor or resuscitation team leader, whenever possible in consultation with the parents, should decide how long it is appropriate to continue attempts at resuscitation. It is usual to discontinue resuscitation if there is no detectable cardiac output after 30 minutes (including any resuscitation prior to arrival). Break the news of the infant's death to the parents, avoiding the use of euphemisms. When informing the family, it is important the words 'death' or 'died' are used. This avoids any potential misconceptions and finalizes what has happened. For many younger parents, this may be their first experience of a close bereavement; it is important to explain the coroner's duty to investigate all sudden deaths. Parents should be told they will be asked to make a statement and that the coroner's officer or police may visit their home and may take the baby's bedding for examination to help establish the cause of the death. This is routine procedure and it is important to stress that this does not mean anybody will be blamed or that an inquest will necessarily be held. Staff should take care when cutting off or removing the infant's clothing, as the police may also want this. The nurse caring for the parents should stay with or be available to the family up until they leave the department.

A physical examination should be carried out as soon as resuscitation has been completed or abandoned, and should be done by an experienced paediatrician. An immediate careful record should be made, including the use of a body chart when relevant. Features to be recorded include the following:

- the baby's general appearance, state of nutrition and cleanliness
- the weight, freshly measured, without clothes or equipment, and position on centile chart
- rectal temperature
- marks from invasive or vigorous procedures, such as venepuncture or cardiac massage
- rashes and other skin conditions
- any other marks on the skin, including bruises and abrasions, with an estimate of their age
- appearance of the retinae
- any lesions in the mouth (allowing for effects of intubation)
- any signs of injury to the genitalia or anus (Foundation for the Study of Sudden Infant Deaths 2002).

Continuing care

Ensure that a quiet area is made available for the family to spend time with their baby to say goodbye. New clothes in a range of suitable sizes in which the baby can be dressed before viewing, including a shawl, a nappy and a bonnet, should be available. Never hurry the parents or relatives to see the baby or go home. Acknowledge that families may remain in the department for a considerable amount of time. The nurse must be patient and offer reassurance that fault cannot be attributed to anything or anyone, especially to those whose care the infant was in at the time of the incident. If possible take a photograph of the baby and obtain a lock of hair; take foot- and handprints although parents may not want them at this time but may be grateful later (Osborne 2000, RCN and BAEM 1995). If the mother is breast-feeding she will need immediate advice on suppression of lactation. If the baby was a twin, recommend immediate admission of the surviving twin, with the mother, for monitoring and for investigation of possible metabolic disorders.

Discharge advice and information

Provide written information on what will happen next, as little of what is said may actually be heard by the grief-stricken parents or family. The family should be offered either the Foundation for the Study of Sudden Infant Deaths (FSID) or the hospital's own guidelines for EDs on unexpected infant deaths as well as information about the patient liaison officer, who can offer guidance on funeral arrangements etc.

A folder of relevant information should be provided, which should include: contact details for paediatricians designated for cot death; phone numbers of coroners, and of local religious leaders; information on different cultural practices with regard to death and bereavement; information about the procedure for death registration and for inquests; a list of local funeral directors; details of support agencies, including the national and local services offered by FSID; and copies of FSID's leaflet 'When a baby dies suddenly and unexpectedly'. The GP and health visitor should be informed as soon as possible. Between one and three months after the death, the parents should be offered an appointment to see a revelant consultant in order to explain the medical facts and after support (RCPCH, 2007).

Staff grief

The impact of a baby's death on staff is enormous. Staff should be trained in how to deal with a family whose baby is brought in moribund or dead. The training should be concerned mainly with communication skills, such as the breaking of bad news, sympathetic listening, responding to questions, nonverbal communication and dealing with anxiety, grief and anger. It should also include awareness of different cultural attitudes. Time must be made for critical incident debriefing (Cudmore 1998). Staff dealing with the family need to acknowledge their own grief. Crying or brief withdrawal is an acceptable reaction.

CONCLUSION

This chapter has outlined some of the more common and distinctive infant complaints that may present in the emergency department. Some important and useful considerations of infants presenting in ED may be noted. The infant's presenting complaint should be addressed together with the family as a whole unit. Always consider the infant's home and social circumstances when assessing and treating injuries or ailments. Parental anxiety may be a major manifestation of presenting infants.

Parents often feel guilty and or inadequate about their baby's injury or illness, especially when they are acutely unwell or seriously injured. Parents may not be familiar with the hospital environment and they may feel helpless, lost and anxious. Discharge advice must be given clearly and in a language suitable for the parents' understanding and wherever possible this should be supported by written information. Community services, particularly the family's health visitor, should be informed of any concerns and can assist the family after discharge. Thorough assessment is essential at all times to ensure the infant's safety, comfort and quality care. Emergency nurses are the key carers and the formation of a therapeutic relationship with the family is invaluable.

References

ACEP [American College of Emergency Physicians] (2003) Clinical policy for children younger than three years presenting to the emergency department with fever. *Annals of Emergency Medicine*, **42**, 530–545.

ALSG [Advanced Life Support Group] (2006) *Advanced Paediatric Life Support: The Practical Approach.* Manchester: ALSG.

Advanced Paediatric Life Support (2001) Third edn. The Advanced Life Support Group. London: BMJ Publishing.

Agency for Healthcare Research and Quality (2003) *Management of Bronchiolitis in Infants and Children.* Summary, Evidence Report/Technology Assessment: Number 69. Rockville, MD, Agency for Healthcare Research and Quality.

Armon K, Stephenson T, Hemingway P et al. (2003) An evidence and consensus based guideline for the management of a child after a seizure. *Emergency Medicine Journal*, **20**(1), 13–20.

Armon K, Stephenson T, Gabriel V, MacFaul R, Eccleston P, Werneke U, Smith S (2001) Determining the common medical presenting problems to an accident and emergency department. *Archives of Disease in Childhood*, **84**(5), 390–392.

Barkin RM, Rosen P (eds) (1994) *Pulmonary Disorders* In: *Emergency Pediatrics: A Guide to Ambulatory Care*, 4th edn. St Louis: Mosby.

Bedford HE, Jenkins SM, Shore C, Kenny PA (1992) Use of an east end children's accident and emergency department for infants: a failure in primary health care. *Quality in Health Care*, **1**, 29–33.

Bedford H, de Louvois J, Halket S, Peckham C, Hurley R, Harvey D (2001) Meningitis in infancy in England and Wales: follow up at age 5 years. *British Medical Journal*, **323**(7312), 533–537.

Bernardo LM, Schenkel KA (1995) Pediatric medical emergencies. In: (eds Kitt S, Selfridge Thomas J, Proehl JA and Kaiser J). *Emergency Nursing: A Physiologic and Clinical Perspective* 2nd edn. Philadelphia: WB Saunders Company.

Boyd R, Busuttil M, Stuart P (2005) Pilot study of a paediatric emergency department oral rehydration protocol. *Emergency Medicine Journal*, **22**(2), 116.

Boyne L (2001) Meningococcal infection. *Nursing Standard*, **16**(7), 47–53.

Brown AFT (2002) *Accident and Emergency: Diagnosis and Management.* London: Arnold.

Bruce-Jones J (1994) PALS: paediatric resuscitation. *Emergency Nurse*, **2**(1), 7–9.

Brunner LS, Suddarth DS (1991) *The Lippincott Manual of Paediatric Nursing* 3rd edn. London: Chapman and Hall.

Castle N (2000) Paediatric resuscitation: advanced life support. *Nursing Standard* **17**(11), 47–52.

Chameides L (1990) *Textbook of Paediatric Advanced Life Support*. Dallas: American Heart Association and American Academy of Paediatricians.

Cincinnati Children's Hospital Medical Center (2002) *Evidence Based Clinical Practice Guideline for Children with Acute Gastroenteritis (AGE)*. Guideline 5. Cincinnati: Cincinnati Children's Hospital Medical Center.

Cosby C (1998) Pediatric emergencies. In: *Sheehy's Emergency Nursing: Principles and Practice* (4th edn.) (ed. L Newberry). St Louis: Mosby.

Cudmore J (1998) Critical incident stress: management strategies. *Emergency Nurse*, **6**(3), 22–27

Darr C (1998) Asthma and bronchiolitis In: *Emergency Medicine: Concepts and Clinical Practice* (eds-in-chief R Rosen and R Barkin). St Louis: Mosby.

Davies FCW (2003) *Minor Trauma in Children*. London: Arnold.

Davison KL, Rasmay ME (2003) The epidemiology of acute meningitis in children in England and Wales. *Archives of Disease in Childhood*, **88**, 662–664.

Dinwiddie R (1990) *The Diagnosis and Management of Respiratory Disease*. Edinburgh: Churchill Livingstone.

Dwight O, Collier J (2001b) *Gastroenteritis in Infants and Young Children*. Leicester: National Patients' Access Team.

El Bashir H, Laundy M, Booy R (2003) Diagnosis and treatment of bacterial meningitis. *Archives of Disease in Childhood*, **88**(7), 615–620.

El-Radhi AS, Barry (2003) Do antipyretics prevent febrile convulsions? *Archives of Disease in Childhood*, **88**(7), 641–642.

Emergency Nurses Association (2000) *Trauma Nursing Core Course*, 5th edn. Chicago: ENA.

Foundation for the Study of Infant Deaths (2002) *Sudden Unexpected Deaths in Infancy: Suggested Guidelines for Accident and Emergency Departments*. London: FSID.

Garzon LS, Wiles L (2002) Management of respiratory syncytial virus with lower respiratory tract infection in infants and children. AACN Clinical Issues: Advanced practice in Acute and Critical Care. *Emerging Infections*, **13**(3), 421–430.

Gausche M (1992) Sudden infant death syndrome. In: *Emergency Medicine: Concepts and Clinical Practice* (eds P Rosen et al.). St Louis: Mosby Year Book.

Gilbert EG, Russell KE, Deskin RW (1993) Stridor in the infant and child. *AORN Journal*, **58**(1), 23–43.

Halket S, de Louvois J, Holt DE, Harvey D (2003) Long term follow up after meningitis in infancy: behaviour of teenagers. *Archives of Diseases in Childhood*, **88**, 395–398.

Hampson-Evans D, Bingham R (1998) Paediatric advanced life support. *Care of the Critically Ill*, **14**(6), 188–193.

Hazinski M (1992) *Nursing Care of the Critically Ill Child*. 2nd edn. St Louis: Mosby.

Hay P (1996) Care of the infant with bronchiolitis. *Emergency Nurse*, **4**(3), 19–22.

Kelnar CJH, Harvey D, Simpson C (1995) *The Sick Newborn Baby* (3rd edn.). London: Baillière Tindall.

Khatib H (1986) Acute gastroenteritis in infants. *Nursing Times*, **82**(17), 31–32.

Kumar PJ, Clark ML (1990) *Clinical Medicine* (2nd edn.). London: Baillière Tindall.

Ling SG (2000) Febrile convulsions: acute seizure characteristics and anti-convulsant therapy. *Annals of Tropical Paediatrics*, **20**(3), 227–230.

Maconochie I (1998) Capillary refill time in the field – it's enough to make you blush! *Pre-Hospital Immediate Care*, **2**, 95–96.

McFarlane K (1992) Caring for the infant with RSV infection. *Paediatric Nursing*, **4**(8), 10–12.

McVerry M, Collin J (1999) Managing the child with gastroenteritis. *Nursing Standard*, **13**(37), 49–53.

Mead D, Sibert J (eds) (1991) *The Injured Child: An Action Plan for Nurses*. London: Scutari Press.

Meadoow R, Newell S (2002) *Paediatrics*. Oxford: Blackwell Science.

Milan S, Lewis J, Ethier K, Kershaw T, Ickovics JR (2004) The impact of physical maltreatment on the adolescent mother – infant relationship: mediating and moderating effects during the transition to early parenthood. *Journal of Abnormal Child Psychology*, **32**(3), 249–261.

Mitchell EA, Aley P, Eastwood J (1992) The national cot death prevention program in New Zealand. *Australasian Journal of Public Health*, **16**, 158–161.

Morcombe J (1998) Reducing anxiety in children in A&E. *Emergency Nurse*, **6**(2), 10–13.

National Meningitis Trust (1992) *Meningitis Factsheet*. London: National Meningitis Trust.

NICE (2003) *Head Injury: Triage, Assessment, Investigation and Early Management of Head Injury in Infants, Children and Adults*. Clinical Guideline 4. London: National Institute of Clinical Excellence.

Osborne M (2000) Photograph and mementoes: the emergency nurse's role following sudden infant death. *Emergency Nurse*, **9**(7), 23–25.

Pantell RH, Newman TB, Bernzweig J, Bergman DA et al. (2004) Management and outcomes of care of fever in early infancy. *Journal of American Medical Association*, **291**(10), 1203–1212.

Park JW (2000). Fever without source in children: recommendations for outpatient care in those up to 3. *Postgraduate Medicine*, **107**(2), 259–266.

Perrin E, Frank D, Cole C et al. (2003) *Criteria for Determining Disability in Infants and Children: Failure to Thrive*. Rockville, MD: Agency for Healthcare Research and Quality.

Prassaad Steiner R (2004) Treating bronchiolitis associated with RSV. *American Family Physician*, **69**(2), 325–332.

Resuscitation Council (UK) (2005a) *Paediatric Basic Life Support*. London: Resuscitation Council (UK).

Resuscitation Council (2005b) *Paediatric Advanced Life Support*. London: Resuscitation Council (UK).

Royal College of Nursing and British Association for Accident and Emergency Medicine (1995) *Bereavement Care in A&E Departments*. London: RCN.

Royal College of Nursing (1990) *Nursing Children in the Accident and Emergency Medicine Departments*. London: RCN.

Royal College of Paediatrics & Child Health (2007). *Report of the Intercollegiate Committee for Services for Children in Emergency Departments*. London: Royal College of Paediatrics and Child Health.

Salter R, Maconochie I (2005) Paediatric emergencies. In: *Principles and Practice of Trauma Nursing* (ed. RA O'Shea). Edinburgh: Elsevier Churchill Livingstone.

Sanchez I, Dekoster J, Powell R (1993) Effect of racemic epinephrine and salbutomol on clinical score and pulmonary mechanics in infants with bronchiolitis. *Journal of Paediatrics*, **122**(1), 145–151.

Simoes E et al. (1991) Respiratory rate: measurement of variability over time and accuracy at different counting periods. *Archives of Disease in Childhood*, **66**(10), 1199–1203.

Stephenson CA et al. (1989) Intussusception: clinical and radiographic factors influencing reducibility. *Pediatric Radiology*, **20**, 57.

Surpure JS (1987) Hyperpyrexia in children: clinical implications. *Paediatric Emergency Care*, **3**, 10–12.

Tiker F, Gurakan B, Kilicdag H, Tarcan A (2004) Dehydration: the main cause of fever during the first week of life. *Archives of Disease in Childhood Fetal and Neonatal Edition*, **89**(4), F373–F374.

Toepper WC, Hakim SN (1998) Cardiac disorders. In: *Emergency Medicine: Concepts and Clinical Practice* (eds-in-chief R Rosen and R Barkin). St Louis: Mosby.

Valman HB (1993) Febrile convulsions. *British Medical Journal*, vol. **306**, 1743–1745.

Waruiru C, Appleton R (2004) Febrile seizures: an update. *Archives of Disease in Childhood*, **89**(8), 751–756.

Wells J, Davies P (1998) Estimation of the energy cost of physical activity in infancy. *Archives of Disease in Childhood*, **78**, 131–136.

Wells J (2001) Failure to thrive. *Primary Health Care*, **11**(6), 41–49.

Wharton BA, Pugh, RE, Taitz LS, Walker-Smith JA, Booth IW (1988) Dietary management of gastroenteritis in Britain. *British Medical Journal*, **296**, 450–452.

Whitfield A (1994) Critical incident debriefing in A&E. *Emergency Nurse*, **2**(3), 6–9.

Wilson M, Lilley M (1994) Meningitis in childhood. *Paediatric Nursing*, **6**(7), 23–26.

Wolfram PW (1992) Asthma and bronchiolitis In: *Emergency Medicine: Concepts and Clinical Practice* (eds P Rosen, RM Barkin et al.), 3rd edn. St Louis: Mosby Gilbert.

Wright C (2000) Identification and management of failure to thrive: a community perspective. *Archives of Disease in Childhood*, **82**, 5–9.

Zukin DD, Grisham JE, Saulys A (1998) Fever in children. In: *Emergency Medicine: Concepts and Clinical Practice* (eds P Rosen et al.). St Louis: Mosby Year Book.

Chapter 16

The pre-school child

Julie Flaherty & Brian Dolan

INTRODUCTION

It is widely accepted that approximately 3.5 million children attend emergency departments (EDs) each year. In some inner city areas 60% of child attendees will be under the age of 5 years. As many as 4 out of 5 children attend with minor injuries, with 1 in 5 attendances resulting from parental concern about acute illness (Department of Health (England) (DoH) 2004). Findings from the Children's National Service Framework (NSF) 2004 (DoH 2004) indicate that 70% of children attending rural emergency departments have accidental injuries and in inner city EDs 70% of attendees are for acute medical illness. Boyle et al. (2000) found that the numbers of children attending as a proportion of the local childhood population had increased, while the proportion of children admitted had declined from 56% to 32%.

In the younger age group 1 child per 1000 of the population is in hospital with acute illness on any given day (DoH 2003a). Only a small percentage, less than 0.25%, of all children attending ED will require a paediatric intensive care bed.

Changing patterns of illness in children have shown a decrease in many of the acute presentations to ED. This is due in part to revision of immunization programmes, and the introduction of new technology such as CT scanning. Near patient testing with rapid results in ED have also helped speed up diagnosis and clinical management plans. Health promotion and early preventive measures have improved management of some children's conditions such as asthma. However, there is an increase in recognition of emotional/behavioural problems across childhood, including deliberate self-harm and harm to others (DoH 2003a).

Between 1 and 4 years a child's physical and mental development is very rapid, with 50% of the child's mental capacity developed before the age of 5 years (Brain & Martin 1989). Coupled with substantial leaps in acquisition of language and multi-skills, such quick development can prove the danger for unsuspecting parents/carers. It can come as a surprise when the child is first able to scrabble up the stairs and reach up to a work surface or has the strength to pull over a chair. Pre-school children usually arrive in accident and emergency as a result of accidental injury. The visit to ED is often a child's first experience of hospital, thus making the whole incident doubly traumatic. Young children have insatiable curiosity about their surrounding environments, creating greater vulnerability by being generally unaware of the imposing dangers. The challenges of climbing furniture, stairs, the opening of all manner of containers, sampling even the most unpalatable of agents all increase the likelihood of a small child suffering falls, minor injury and poisoning (Mead & Sibert 1991).

Parents and carers have their own anxieties, which can in turn increase the anxiety of the child. Parents often feel incredibly guilty about accidents and injuries that their children suffer. These anxiety feelings often overwhelm parents so much so that they are less aware of the child's need for support and re-assurance.

Parents/carers frequently experience a lack of confidence in their judgement when their child is ill (Kia 1996). This uneasiness often stems from fears that their child might have meningitis. Parents/carers want to be on the safe side, want a professional diagnosis and to know that there is nothing seriously wrong.

Parents/carers remain anxious and concerned, having to manage their sick child at home even after reassurance. In situations like this it has been shown that parents/carers do not know how to contact health services when their child has not improved (Neill 2000). It has been shown that in seeking advice, parental assessment of severity of illness and the subsequent need for admission to in-patient units correlates with that of the doctors and likelihood of significant diagnosis at discharge (MacFaul et al. 1994).

With a still-developing immune system the onset of illness is often rapid in pre-school children, leading to a speedier deterioration of the child's general condition. Young children do not have an adult's resilience to withstand heat, fluid and electrolyte loss. They are, however, better able to cope with these metabolic changes than babies. An ED nurse needs to know the normal activity and physical development in children of pre-school age, in order to effectively assess their condition and initiate care. This chapter will consider normal childhood development and some of the common reasons for ED attendances within this age group.

NORMAL DEVELOPMENT

The child in the age range of 3 months to 1 year is termed an infant; 1 to 3 years a toddler; and 3 to 4 years a pre-school child (Brunner & Suddarth 1991). In the context of this chapter all children above the age of 1 will be considered pre-school children. The pre-school child, unlike the infant, has begun to develop his own identity. From about the age of 2 the child discovers that he can control what happens around him; motor skills develop rapidly and a child able to walk, run, climb and jump uses the newfound skills to explore his environment. The child strives for autonomy and self-esteem. However, he also needs to know the safety limits of behaviour in a given environment. For example when climbing the stairs with a parent the child may feel good because of the praise for his achievement, but this needs to be tempered so the child is aware that it is not good to climb over the stair gate and attempt to climb the stairs alone.

Pre-school children perceive the world differently from adults. Children of this age begin to demonstrate the concept to intelligence (Lowe 1985). They display various thinking processes, which are important to consider when a child is trying to explain the reason for deeds and events. The 2-year-old is egocentric and will perceive that he is the centre of his world, being unable to identify with anybody else's point of view. The child may believe that it is he who is responsible for events which we know to be out of his control. Children often perceive illness and injury as a punishment for something they did or failed to do (Eiser 1985).

Throughout this pre-operational phase of development memory and imagination are developing rapidly. There is a tendency to mix fact with fantasy and a belief that the child's thoughts can control events. There is an intuitive, magical quality to their thoughts (Hall & Elliman 2003).

THE CHILD UNDER STRESS

The pre-school child is more vulnerable and traumatized when separated from his parents than at any other age. Bowlby (1953), in his famous study *Child Care and the Growth of Love*, shows how a child suffers maternal deprivation when separated from his significant carers, the male or female person who supplies love, care, protection and comfort (Lowe 1985).

Since then, many seminal reports have confirmed the importance of keeping parents and child together (DoH 2004, Ministry of Health 1959). This is particularly important in ED where events leading to attendance will have caused some stress (see Box 16.1). Effective nursing interventions at this early stage can

> **Box 16.1 Categories of children's worries (Vistintainer & Wolfer 1975)**
>
> - Physical harm or bodily injury in the form of discomfort, pain, mutilation and death
> - Separation from parent or absence of trusted adult
> - A strange unknown environment
> - Uncertainty about limits and expected acceptable behaviour
> - Loss of control, autonomy and competence

do a lot towards developing a rapport with the child and family, and to alleviate stress and fear. Acknowledging the child's suffering and putting it into context using toys or pictures can be helpful, as is prompt pain relief. Parental input from the outset is essential not only to reduce stress and induce normality in the child but also to reduce stress in the parents/carers themselves. Encouraging parents/carers to undress their child and to help them with the examination as well as to be there to give reassurance to their child reinforces the parents' importance in the treatment and helps to allay their fears.

It is easy in circumstances following an accident for the parents to feel inadequate or lose confidence in their own ability. This must be addressed in ED constructively and without proportionate blame, to enable the parents to support their child. Reassurance, information and what the parents/carers can do to help their child should be clearly communicated. Poor handling of parents in ED can have a long-term effect on both the child and the family's recovery (Mead & Sibert 1991).

The environment in which a child is cared for has come under much scrutiny in recent years (Bentley 2004, National Audit Office 2004, RCPCH 1999). Facilities for children are best provided in an environment away from adult patients. Children should have their separate waiting area geared towards their needs with appropriate toys, books, television, video and electronic games. Treatment areas should also be child-oriented not only in décor and furnishings but also in equipment so time is not wasted hunting for appropriate items such as child-size blood-pressure cuffs or pulse oxy-sensitivity probes. The RCPCH (1999) recommends that children should be cared for in an audio-visually separate ED department.

COMMUNICATING WITH CHILDREN

A key factor in reducing stress and relieving anxiety is the way by which we communicate with the child and family. The value of effective communication is not only dependent on the nursing staff but also on the multi-disciplinary team. Good communication is the basis of forming a trusting relationship with the child and family. With a pre-school child the use of non-verbal communication in the way that we express ourselves is equally important as speech. Children of this age might appear shy, withdrawn or outgoing. Whatever impression they give, they will have an awareness of facial expressions, gestures, eye contact, watching and waiting in anticipation. This should be borne in mind when communicating with children; get down to the child's level, as towering above them is intimidating. Address the child by their name, talking in a soft tone, and bring the level of conversation to things that are familiar to the child, such as the topic of a television programme or TV characters.

Children should be kept informed in a meaningful manner about their care and what will happen next. With parental help boundaries for behaviour can be set which in turn help the child who feels out of control with what is happening. The ED nurse's attitude should be family-oriented when dealing with children. Parents are often under a great deal of stress, feel guilty and are very anxious. These negative emotions can have a profound effect on the child. The parents need reassurance and a chance to relay their fears and guilt to the nurse (Bentley 2004).

A critical attitude from nursing and medical staff will only reinforce the guilt and inadequacy the parent is likely to experience. An anxious parent will make the child feel anxious. Keeping the parent informed and building the bond between the family and staff will help the child (Maller et al. 1992).

UNDERSTANDING ILLNESS

To a young child illness is remote and viewed as an external process. There is a tendency to believe this has something to do with magic or is a punishment. Pre-school children do not fully understand internal body processes. In this pre-operative phase (Piaget 1990), children are only just developing their thought processes in relation to internal body organs. They have little concept of where internal organs lie, other than the heart, which lies in the middle of their chest and is used for loving and caring. When talking with pre-school children they often describe tummy ache and at the same time point to their head or equally they will say they have headache and point to their tummy. A child of this younger age is concerned with external injury and very often frightened of seeing blood, small cuts and marks. The external aspect of his environment such as light, equipment, uniforms and noise will affect the child much more than an explanation of what is going on in his/her body. Play is a very important aspect of the child's care and is at the very centre of a healthy child's life (Webster 2002). Children can express fear and anxiety through play so a playful environment will help reduce stress and anxiety. Watching a child play gives a fair assessment of social and multi-skills. Playing with children during examination and assessment will help the child understand treatment and procedures. Dolls and teddy bears come in very useful when trying to demonstrate what is about to be done to a child. Through play children are able to learn both the sensory and concrete information they need in preparation for some clinical procedures.

ASTHMA

It is estimated that about 3.4 million people in the UK have asthma symptoms that require treatment (European Respiratory Society and European Lung Foundation (ERS & ELF) 2003). The rate for children is one in seven (1.5 million) and for adults one in 25 (1.9 million) (ERS & ELF 2003). Asthma is acknowledged to be the most common long-term childhood condition. Trends in mortality in children show little improvement over the last decade. Regardless of medical advances and technological improvement in asthma management confidential enquiries into asthma deaths have often indicated that the fatality could have been avoided if there had been better preventive measures, better recognition and help in avoiding delay during the final attack and in receiving earlier emergency care. Younger children with asthma are particularly vulnerable because they rely on others to react to the severity of their condition and to act on their behalf. Children in the 0–4 year age range have the most frequent health consultations with their GP and out-of-hours services for asthma conditions.

When a young child attends ED with breathing difficulties, it is important that he/she is not unnecessarily distressed any further. Practical steps to prevent distress include not separating the child from the parents or carer, behaving in a calm and friendly manner, and assessing the child promptly in an appropriate environment. If a child does become overly upset, the extra energy and oxygen needed when crying can be enough to turn a moderate asthma attack into a severe one.

Assessment

The overall clinical picture is developed from the combination of history, physical assessment and clinical investigations. If the child has obvious breathing difficulty, oxygen and nebulized bronchial dilators should be commenced immediately, prior to detailed history-taking from the parents/carers. Children under the age of five cannot adequately use a peak flow meter so PEF is not recommended for this age group. Questions which should be asked in establishing a history of the event and the child's general health are given in Box 16.2.

Physical assessment

Observing the child's respiration is the most reliable indicator of his condition. The respiration rate and depth should be established first as this correlates to the severity of asthma. An increase in the work of breathing is demonstrated by the use of accessory muscles (best noted by palpating neck muscles) and nasal flaring (British Thoracic Society & SIGN 2005). Intercostal and sternal recession is an indication of moderate to severe respiratory difficulty. As the child's ability to speak is an indication of respiratory function, the nurse should know if the child can speak in full sentences using more than a few words or not at all. Parents are invaluable in assessing difficulties in the child's normal pattern of speech, as ability to converse varies with this age group.

A rise in the pulse rate can be indicative of increasing hypoxia but must be considered within context. If the child is upset, pyrexial or on beta agonists such as salbutamol, a tachycardia would be expected. That noted, increasing tachycardia generally denotes worsening asthma; a fall in heart rate in life-threatening asthma is a pre-terminal event.

Although wheezing is a classic symptom of bronchospasm, it is unreliable in detecting the severity of an episode. At assessment, any audible wheeze or wheeze on auscultation should be recorded and used as baseline. It is important to remember that if air is not being moved effectively in and out of the lungs,

---

Box 16.2   Establishing history of asthma attack

- How long has this episode lasted?
- Is the child getting better or worse?
- What medication has been given prior to ED attendance and what was the effect?
- Is there an identifiable trigger to the episode?
- Is the child on regular medication? If so, what is it?
- Has the child had previous serious asthma episodes requiring steroids or hospital?
- How frequent are the asthma symptoms?
- Does the child have any other illness?

no wheeze will be present. Peak flow measurement is considered an important indication of the severity of an asthma episode; however, Scullion (2005) notes that young children can also be confused by the exhalation method required to use a peak flow meter. Exercise testing, by getting a child to run around for about six minutes, may therefore be more suitable for younger children (Price et al. 1999). Peak flow measurement should therefore only be attempted in children who have previously and regularly used a peak flow meter.

Pulse oximetry is one of the most useful diagnostic aids in the under-five age group. It is non-invasive and the monitor can be a distraction for the child. Pulse oximetry will identify reductions in oxygen saturation, which may not be obviously clinical. The lower the oxygen saturation, the more severe the impact of the attack on the child, so it is important to ensure oximetry reading is accurate. Poor contact, excessive movement and temperature of the child's skin can all affect the accuracy of the reading. The ED nurse can check the validity of the oxygen reading by matching the peaks of recording, bleeps or monitored pulse rate to the child's actual pulse rate.

These should be the same if the oxygen saturation level is to be considered accurate. In severe asthma arterial blood gases should be measured and act as an indication of the level of respiratory distress and possible need for artificial ventilation. If response to treatment is poor, a chest X-ray should be considered to exclude specific localized aetiology such as pneumothorax.

Management

In cases of life-threatening asthma (Box 16.3) these children need immediate high-flow oxygen via a non-rebreathing mask, and a nebulized beta agonist such as salbutamol. Preparation should be to establish i.v.

access for the administration of medications. Children in this age group both deteriorate and respond to treatment rapidly. The nurse must be vigilant for any changes and equipment should be at hand for intubation and ventilation.

Rapid oxygen therapy and nebulized bronchial dilators should be commenced and in cases of severe asthma (Box 16.4) an oxygen saturation of at least 95% should be the aim (BTS & SIGN 2005). It is important not to distress the child unnecessarily as this significantly increases the work of breathing. Intravenous access should be considered particularly if the child does not respond rapidly to nebulizer therapy.

Compliance with treatment is crucial to the successful management of this group of children. It is important to be calm and to keep the parents/carers informed of treatment plans to enable them to assist in the care of their child. Initial management involves inhaled bronchial dilators (short-acting and long-acting) and cortical steroids are the drugs of choice. The administration of beta agonists such as salbutamol 2.5 mg is the first-line treatment for acute asthma and they can be given by a variety of devices. For the mild to moderate asthma a spacer with mask can be ideal for the younger age group. However, with moderate to severe asthma it is advisable to use a nebulizer. It is important that the nurse explains what is being done first and uses toys and play where appropriate. Alternative devices such as mouthpiece nebulizer can be more successful. If the child is very upset it is sometimes better to get a parent to hold the nebulizer by the child's mouth than to increase the level of distress by attaching the mask to the child. If the child responds well to nebulizer treatment, he should be detained in ED for at least two hours post nebulizer to ensure that the response is not transient. If the response is not maintained, the child should be admitted for nebulizer and further observation.

When planning the discharge of a young child from ED it is important that parents understand and

---

Box 16.3   Life-threatening asthma signs

- Silent chest on auscultation
- Oxygen saturation less than 85% on air
- Reduced respiratory effort with marked use of accessory muscles and severe recession
- Hypotension
- Unable to speak
- Exhaustion
- Reduced level of consciousness or confusion
- Coma

Box 16.4   Severe asthma signs

- Agitated
- Respiratory rate over 50 breaths/min
- Intercostal recession
- Oxygen saturation less than 90%
- Pulse >130
- Only able to say odd word – nods in response to questions

are happy with ongoing treatment plans. Although a child may appear well after a nebulizer therapy for an acute episode of asthma the small airways obstruction can persist for several days. Parents must be able to administer supportive therapy at home. Many devices exist to assist young children in the inhalation of bronchial dilators. Spacers are commonly used for children under the age of five (BTS & SIGN 2005). These create an enclosed space between an aerosol inhaler and the child's mouth allowing him to work at his own pace without the need for hand-breathing coordination which an aerosol would demand. The child can be taught to take five long exaggerated breaths from the spacer for each actuation of the aerosol into the spacer (BTS & SIGN 2005).

The early use of steroids for acute asthma can reduce the need for hospital admission and prevent a relapse in symptoms after initial presentation. A short course of oral steroids can speed up the race for recovery from an acute episode of small airways obstruction. Prednisolone for three days is recommended for children who have not responded to regular home treatment over a period of 24 hours or more prior to ED attendance.

Children regularly on inhaled steroids may also benefit from this boost. As well as advice on drug therapy, it is important that parents and carers are able to detect their child's worsening condition and know when and where to seek help (Box 16.5 for moderate asthma signs). Parents/carers should be advised to return to emergency department if:

- respiratory rate increases
- recession becomes apparent
- the child is using accessory muscles to breath
- the ability to speak deteriorates
- the positive response to inhale bronchodilators reduces
- the child becomes agitated and is not behaving as normal for a child

Follow-up should be arranged for all children discharged from ED; this can usually be done via the child's usual GP or regular asthma clinic.

Box 16.5 Moderate asthma signs

- Alert and oriented
- Tachypnoea
- Able to speak normally
- Audible wheeze

ACUTE LARYNGOTRACHEOBRONCHITIS (VIRAL CROUP)

With pre-school children having, on average, between six and eight respiratory infections a year (Lissauer & Clayden 2001), recognition of symptoms of respiratory illness is one of the most common reasons that parents seek medical attention for their children (Kline 2003).

Croup is a broad term used to describe an infection, usually viral in nature of the upper airway and vocal chords. Symptoms include a barking cough that sounds like a seal, low-grade fever and hoarseness. With severe croup a harsh, high-pitched stridor may be heard when the child breathes in. The stridor is made worse by crying, agitation and coughing. It is most common between six months old and four years (Kelsey & McKewing 2006). Croup most commonly occurs in damper weather of late autumn, winter and early spring. Typically the symptoms are worse between 6 p.m. and 6 a.m. and peak around the second or third night.

Pathophysiology

Croup encompasses a range of upper respiratory inflammations, mostly viral in nature. The most common source is acute laryngotracheobronchitis caused by the parainfluenza virus. This inflammation spreads through the bronchus and results in:

- mucosal oedema
- inflammation of the subglottic area
- increased mucus production, which can affect the entire respiratory tract.

The increase in mucus together with the pharyngeal irritation results in the hoarse cough. Obstruction to airflow through the upper airway causes stridor and difficulty in breathing, and can progress to hypoxia. Hypoxia with mild obstruction indicates involvement of the lower airway, where obstruction causes ventilation perfusion mismatching. Later, hypercapnia occurs as hypoventilation progresses with obstruction (Dykes 2005). Less common symptoms of croup are highlighted in Box 16.6.

History

The ED nurse can quickly put together a picture of viral croup by asking the parents/carers about the lead up to attendance such as:

- duration
- symptoms – are they worse at night?
- is the child drinking?
- is the child talking normally?
- past medical history.

Box 16.6   Less common symptoms of croup

- Inhalation of a foreign body, which has become lodged in the laryngeal region. This should be considered in all cases of stridor, as inhalation is often witnessed in small children
- Tonsilitis can present with stridor or hoarse cough when there is tonsillar enlargement often associated with glandular fever
- Angioneurotic oedema resulting from an acute anaphylactic reaction
- Bacterial: trachetis is an unusual cause of croup but has a high mortality rate if not treated. These children look toxic, like those with epiglottitis, but are differentiated by their croupy cough. Intubation and antibiotic therapy are required promptly
- Diphtheria is uncommon in the UK but should be considered in children with croup symptoms who have not been immunized against diphtheria

The nurse can expect to find a history of illness worsening over several days. Viral croup usually starts with a coryzal illness (common cold) and is followed after 48/72 hours by a sudden and often frightening onset of stridor and barking cough. At this stage children are commonly brought to ED. Unlike epiglottitis, children with croup are able to drink, although they complain of a sore throat. The ED nurse should expect these children to be able to talk but their voices will have varying levels of hoarseness. Significant past medical history is uncommon but previous airways disease or recurrent croup should be noted.

Physical assessment

Assessment of the child in ED should focus on determining the degree of threat to the respiratory function. The work of breathing should be assessed in terms of the child's colour, level of consciousness, respiratory rate, use of accessory muscles, nasal flaring and intercostal recessions. The degree of stridor is significant; the nurse should know whether the stridor is inspiratory, which usually indicates a supraglotic cause, or expiratory, which usually comes from the trachea. In severe cases inspiratory and expiratory stridor may be present. The loudness of the stridor is not an indication of its severity (Morton & Phillips 1996), but loudness of stridor often influences the degree of anxiety. It is important to establish whether stridor is present at rest or only when the child becomes agitated or exerts him or herself.

Heart rate should be regularly monitored. Tachycardia, particularly if it coexists with agitation, restlessness or altered consciousness, is associated with increase in hypoxia. Oxygen saturation should be measured in children with increased respiratory rates and tachycardia and saturation levels below 95% should be treated with oxygen therapy. By assessing a child with viral croup the ED nurse would expect to find a clinical picture of moderate fever, with a child unwell for a few days with a sudden onset of harsh dry and a barking cough. The child will usually be active, but irritable and easily upset. The key to successful management lies with accurate assessing and responding to the level of respiratory compromise. Clinical investigations, such as blood tests and chest and neck X-rays, do little to alter the management plan and much to increase the child's distress and anxiety. For this reason investigations of this nature should not form part of the initial management (Box 16.7).

The child should always be nursed in the position that is most comfortable for him. This is usually semi-upright, cradled in his parent's or carer's arms. As anxiety and psychological distress have a detrimental effect on respiratory function, every effort should be made by the ED team to keep the child calm and accommodate his wishes.

Having assessed the severity of the croup, the first line treatment is dexamethasone 0.15 mg/kg orally (Geelhooed et al. 1996) followed by an adrenaline nebulizer 5 ml 1 in 1000. This is best administered by a parent holding the nebulizer in front of the child, as face masks and mouth pieces can be frightening and considerably increase the child's distress. Adrenaline acts both as a bronchodilator and suppresses histamine, thereby reducing mucous secretions and relieving airway obstructions. The effects of adrenaline

Box 16.7   Priorities in treatment of croup

- Rapid and accurate assessment of airway impairment
- Keep the child calm. Nurse in a comfortable position; involve parents/carers
- Give nebulized adrenaline 0.5 mg/kg of 1:1000 preparation up to 5 ml maximum
- Give nebulized steroids – dexamethasone 150 mg, 600 mg single dose
- Maintain hydration
- Monitor oxygen saturation levels; intubate if child has unresolved, worsening hypoxia

nebulizers are relatively short-acting, lasting approximately two hours. Reassessment should take place shortly after the adrenaline nebulizer. Should the child's condition be worsening then a repeat adrenaline nebulizer 5 ml 1 in a 1000 should be administered while preparations for intubation are under way. However, if the child is showing signs of improvement then a further assessment should be taken 30 minutes post-nebulizer. If the child continues to improve they should be admitted to an in-patient children's unit. For mild to moderate croup dexamethasone 0.15 mg/kg orally would be given and continuous assessment should take place. Should the child be seen to be improving, discharge home with advice and children's community nursing support would be advisable. A child who is no better and remains stable should be admitted at this stage to a children's in-patient unit.

Children should have oxygen saturation levels monitored and there should be vigilant observation for clinical signs of hypoxia. In children who are not clinically hypoxic, oxygen therapy is considered unnecessary and sometimes unhelpful as it makes the child distressed. Hypoxia in children with croup is usually a late sign and should be treated seriously. It usually indicates a need for medical intervention in airway management and in the case of a fatigued child intubation is often necessary. All children with clinical hypoxia should be nursed in high-dependency or resuscitation areas and appropriate airway maintenance should be available.

Hydration is an important and sometimes overlooked area of care in the child with croup: many are reluctant to drink because of a painful throat and some, particularly younger children, find it difficult to take fluids because of dyspnoea. Parents should be encouraged to give frequent small amounts of clear fluid where possible. This not only prevents dehydration, but also helps to reduce tenacity of secretions. If a child is too short of breath to take fluids or is clinically dehydrated intravenous fluid replacement should be considered after initial symptoms have been relieved. Antibiotics are not considered useful as croup is predominantly of viral origin.

Criteria for admission

All children with moderate to severe croup should be admitted for observation. This can be determined by poor or transient response to treatment, persistent stridor at rest, oxygen saturation level below 92% and any degree of hypoxia. Admission should also be considered for any child who is clinically dehydrated. Some social circumstances should be examined when making a decision to admit or discharge

the child. If the family live a long distance from healthcare facilities or do not have transport admission should be considered.

Discharge advice

If, after a period of observation, the child is considered well enough to be discharged, the parents/carers should be given clear advice on home care, which should be supported with written information. The advice should include the following:

- stay with the child and observe the breathing pattern, as a worsening obstruction will not always wake the child from sleeping
- if croup returns look after the child in a warm humidified environment, such as a steamy bathroom, such as with a hot shower running for five to ten minutes
- if there is no improvement or the child worsens return to ED.

EPIGLOTTITIS

Aetiology

Epiglottitis is a bacterial infection caused by *Haemophilus influenzae* type b (HIB) and is a relatively uncommon but life-threatening condition. Unlike laryngotracheobronchitis, it has no winter peak of incidence, nor is it more common in the evening or at night (see Table 16.1). It can occur at any time of the day, throughout the year. People of all age groups are at risk of contracting epiglottitis but it is most common in the age group two to seven years old. The incidence of epiglottitis has steadily declined since the HIB vaccine became routine in childhood immunization programmes.

Pathophysiology

Epiglottitis is a serious life-threatening condition because *Haemophilus influenzae* infection causes a rapid inflammatory infection in the epiglottis, vallecula, arytenoids and aryepiglottic folds; the tissues swell downward and over the glottic opening, making breathing difficult.

Assessment

History
Obtaining an accurate history from parents/carers is imperative, as physical examination of the child is restricted when epiglottitis is suspected. Duration of the child's illness is an important factor in determining the likelihood of epiglottitis. Illness is rapid

Table 16.1 Differentiation of croup from epiglottitis

Symptom	Croup	Epiglottitis
Age	6 months – 3 years	2–5 years
Season	Winter	All year
Worst time of day	Evening/ night	Any time
Aetiology	Parainfluenza virus	*Haemophilus influenzae*
Onset	Over days	Over hours
Proceeding illness	Yes	No
Fever	<38.50°C	>38.50°C
Sore throat	Sometimes	Yes
Drooling	No	Yes
Cough	Harsh barking	No
Stridor	Inspiratory and expiratory	Soft expiratory
Voice	Hoarse	None
Wheeze	Often present	None
Position	Varied, active	Upright with neck extended

in onset, with respiratory symptoms occurring in a matter of hours. Despite this, other foci of infection are common with epiglottitis, usually otitis media or lymphadenitis. Because of the urgent need for treatment, the ED nurse should simultaneously perform a physical inspection of the child if epiglottitis is suspected. This should differentiate between inhalation of a foreign body and epiglottitis. Additionally, croup is a common misdiagnosis in young children; however, patients with epiglottitis do not have the distinctive, barking cough that patients with croup have.

Physical assessment

It is vital that the child's throat is *not* examined because any irritation increases the inflammatory responses and increases epiglottic swelling, often resulting in complete airway obstruction. Distressing the child also increases the risk of airway obstruction. For theses reasons, assessment is a hands-off visual activity. Children with epiglottitis usually prefer to sit up leaning forward, often with their neck extended forwards and their elbows on their knees, the so-called tripod position. This allows the maximum use of their compromised airway. Most children will have a soft inspiratory stridor without an associated cough. Most children are reluctant to speak but those who do usually have a muffled voice. Drooling is a strong indication of epiglottitis because swallowing is painful, due in part to a sore throat (Tanner et al. 2002).

The child usually has significant pyrexia in excess of 38.5°C. Stridor is frequently present.

Management

If epiglottitis is suspected the most important action is to summon specialist help. The child's epiglottis needs to be examined under anaesthesia in theatre and an artificial airway established in a controlled environment. While waiting for this the ED nurse should keep the child and parent/carers calm, ensuring that the child is in the most comfortable position for him and is given oxygen if possible. This is best achieved by sitting the child on the parent's lap and getting the parent to hold the mask near the child. If the child is upset by oxygen therapy then it should not be pursued.

As any child with epiglottitis is at risk of airway obstruction at any time the ED nurse should always have equipment available to establish artificial ventilation; because of the position and degree of swelling of the epiglottis intubation in emergency can be extremely difficult. It is often necessary to perform a cricothyroidotomy. Once an artificial airway has been successfully established and the child is haemodynamically stable, other investigations and definitive management can take place, usually in the paediatric intensive care unit. This includes blood screening and cultures, the initiation of antibodies and maintenance of hydration.

ACCIDENTAL INJURY

More accidents happen in the home than elsewhere and children under the age of five are the most vulnerable. In 2002, 477 500 children under the age of five needed hospital treatment and around 120 children died as a result of home accidents (RoSPA 2006). Falls account for the majority of non-fatal accidents, while the highest number and proportion of deaths, 46%, are due to house fires (Office for National Statistics 2002).

The causes of accidents involving pre-school children are varied. Young children are vulnerable because they rely on their parents to provide a safe environment for them and to keep a careful watch on them while they explore and play. The role of the ED nurses is not just associated with treatment; they are also in a position to help educate the public and prevent further accidents occurring. Despite all these opportunities, comparison of the home accident statistics for 1999 and 2002 indicates that despite the increased awareness and health promotion and a commitment to prevent home accidents the overall incidence of home accidents continues largely unabated (RoSPA 2006).

Aetiology of accidental injury

The factors that increase a child's risks of accidental injury are similar to agents that may increase the incidence of non-accidental injury. A child from a working-class background (social class V) is more likely to be killed accidentally than those from a professional family (RoSPA 2006). Environmental stress in the family such as illness, shortage of money and paternal tension leads to an increase in the incidence of childhood accidents.

In emergency departments, the main focus of care has traditionally been to diagnose and treat the child's injury. Nurses are very good at providing parents/carers with information about how to look after the child's injury at home, but less good at actively engaging in health promotion.

Timely intervention by ED staff can prevent further accidents and ease the impact of family tension or stress. This intervention may be in the form of actual advice on accident prevention or referral to other professionals. Most emergency departments have visiting liaison services and are able to communicate information to the family's own health visitor by telephone or by fax. The health visitor also has the advantage of knowing the family and can follow up ED attendances of pre-school children under the age of five with supportive information and active accident prevention. Parents respond better to familiar health visitors who can give one to one advice. By visiting the family home the health visitor can identify and discuss specific hazards.

ACCIDENTAL POISONING

In 2002, of the 31 500 children under the age of 15 who attended hospital after suspected poisoning, over 26 000 were under five years old (CAPT 2004). Accidental poisoning has a higher incidence in families with existing stresses such as illness, pregnancy or recent birth, absence of one parent, a house move or anxiety/depression in a parent. The most commonly digested poisons are childhood medicines such as paracetamol elixir or cough mixture, oral contraceptives and vitamin supplements. Household products such as detergents, bleach, disinfectant, perfume and cosmetics are also commonly ingested. See Boxes 16.8, 16.9 and 16.10. RoSPA (2006) have suggested that the provision of a secure cupboard within the home should be provided as part of the built-in provision of any new homes that are built. The best location for the cupboard would be within the kitchen at a height of 1.5 metres above floor level so that smaller children cannot gain access.

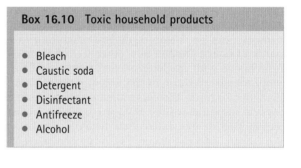

Box 16.8   Non-toxic agents

- Most cosmetics – beware of alcohol in perfumes
- Non-leaded paint
- Inks
- Most antibiotics
- Vitamins
- Oral contraceptives

Box 16.9   Toxic drugs

- Paracetamol
- Salycilate and aspirin
- Tricyclic antidepressants
- Narcotics
- Iron

Box 16.10   Toxic household products

- Bleach
- Caustic soda
- Detergent
- Disinfectant
- Antifreeze
- Alcohol

Assessment

History

Establishing a clear history can often prove challenging for the ED nurse. Parents and carers and the child are very often distressed and the information may be scanty. The nurse must try to find out:

- what has been taken – the container is a useful aid to active ingredients
- how much has been ingested – the container will give useful clues to the amount left, as will the appearance of the child if spillage is possible
- parents and carers should be asked about spillages at home
- description of child's behaviour or symptoms since ingestion: vomiting is of a particular significance as it reduces the likelihood of absorption

- any pre-existing illness should be noted as should any medication the child is currently taking: unless clear evidence to the contrary exists the ED nurse should assume and treat the child as if he has ingested the maximum amount of poison available

The majority of children who have ingested the common poisons noted above will show no immediate physical signs. As a baseline the following should be established:

- respiration rate and depth
- pulse and circulatory status
- consciousness level
- pupil size and reaction
- skin condition evidence of irritation/burn particularly around or in the mouth
- weight of the child.

Clinical management

Specific management of a poison can be aided by gaining specialist advice from a regional poisons unit or via Toxbase. Common principles of care exist: for most poisonous substances information and clinical management can be easily downloaded from specialist advice centres.

Gastric lavage has limited effectiveness in children because of the small size of tube used. For this reason it is not recommended except in varying consciousness levels when gastric emptying is considered essential. In those circumstances, intubation and anaesthetic cover are essential before insertion of the gastric tube takes place.

In the majority of cases of accidental poisoning, the potential toxicity is low and therefore enforced emesis is considered unnecessary. In these cases activated charcoal is used as a binding agent to absorb toxins. A single dose of activated charcoal in most cases should be given within one hour of ingestion. The dose by weight is calculated at one gram per kilogram or a dose by age 25 to 50 grams (RCPCH 2003). Because of the risk of aspiration charcoal should never be given in the absence of a gag reflex or where there is impaired consciousness unless the airway is first protected by an ET tube.

The majority of children who have ingested these substances do not need gastric evacuation or observation and can be safely discharged home. Parents should be constructively offered advice and support, as many will have found the child's accidental poisoning very distressing.

Children who have ingested large amounts of paracetamol-based substances or aspirin should have their blood checked four hours after ingestion for serum paracetamol or salycilate while the child is waiting in the ED. If levels are normal the child can be discharged home. Ingestion of tricyclic antidepressant is the commonest cause of death in children with accidental poisoning (Morton & Philips 1996). Such children should have continuous cardiac monitoring, as cardiac dysrhythmia is common and cardiotoxicity is often the reason for mortality.

With narcotic drugs, clinical symptoms are similar with all types of opiate drug and the nurse should suspect ingestion of narcotics if the child has pinpoint pupils. Sometimes an accurate history can be difficult to obtain, particularly if the drug is an illegal substance. Narcotic drugs often cause respiratory depression for several hours after ingestion and have a sudden onset. If the child shows signs of respiratory depression or is unconscious intravenous naloxone should be given. Children should always be admitted following narcotic poisoning.

Iron/alcohol ingestion

Although used as dietary supplement, an excess of iron is extremely toxic. It causes severe gastric haemorrhage. Any symptoms the child may have should be treated on admission; IV access should be established at an early stage and fluid resuscitation commenced if necessary. Intramuscular desferrioxamine (30 mg/kg) should be given, and may be necessary over a 24 hour period depending on the severity of symptoms.

As a general rule emetics should not be given as a first-line treatment; milk can be given. Advice specific to the substance should be sought from the poison centre. Young children accidentally ingest alcohol in drinks or in perfumes/aftershave. Small amounts of alcohol can result in hypoglycaemia in children. A blood sugar level should be established and intravenous dextrose-based fluids given to the child if the child is significantly intoxicated or hypoglycaemic. Drowsy or unconscious children need airway management and close observation. Alcohol needs time to be excreted from the body and care in the emergency department revolves around maintaining homeostasis during this time. Once the child is alert and aware of his surroundings he can be discharged. Parents should be advised to increase the fluid intake over 12 hours after discharge and return if the child shows signs of gastric discomfort. If the parent/carer offers a history inconsistent with the child's condition or offers no explanation of poisoning the possibility of deliberate poisoning by a parent or a third party should be considered. It is often difficult to establish deliberate poisoning conclusively but a long and vague medical history of the child and frequent hospitalization may raise suspicions.

TRAMPOLINE INJURIES

Figures produced by the Royal Society for the Preventions of Accidents (RoSPA) for 2002 showed 11 500 people attended ED after injury while trampolining, of whom 4200 were children under the age of 15. Trampoline accidents usually occur when more than one person is using the trampoline at the same time. The younger the child the more vulnerable they are to injury: this is in part due to their low body weight (RoSPA 2005).

Young children should always be supervised when using trampolines even though it has been acknowledged that more than half of trampoline accidents occur while under supervision from parents or carers. Only one child at a time should be on the trampoline. Due to the smaller size of the pre-school child, accidents often happen because two or more smaller children are using the trampoline at a time, which may result in collision and unnecessary falls. Trampoline accidents happen when children try different stunts such as somersaults, bouncing at the sides of the trampoline, jumping off the trampoline sustaining limb injuries or crouching underneath the trampoline and equipment. Limb injuries are most common, with neck and head injuries being the most serious.

CYCLING INJURIES

Cyclist casualties in 2004 showed that cycling accidents increase as children grow older and peak at around 16 years old. In 2004, 34 children died through injuries sustained while cycling. A further 724 children were seriously injured and 4780 children were slightly injured (Child Accident Prevention Trust 2006).

Causes of cycling injury include doing tricks, riding too fast or ineffective braking. Injury patterns include head injuries ranging from fatal skull fractures and brain damage to minor concussion cuts and grazes. Chest and abdominal injuries are much less frequent but are more often serious. The pre-school child often sustains cuts, bruises and grazes from falls from their cycle while learning to cycle. Often pre-school children have cycling accidents when stabilizers are removed from the cycle, but the child is not fully co-ordinated or proficient at cycling.

SAFEGUARDING CHILDREN

The protection of children is everyone's business (Department of Health 2003b). Whether working directly with children and young people or with adults whose lives impact on children, a health professional can make all the difference. In the past 30 years no fewer than six major child-protection cases have hit the national headlines in the United Kingdom (Parton 2004), the most recent of these being the Victoria Climbié inquiry. Victoria was brought to England by her father's aunt in March 1999. She was brought from her native country on the Ivory Coast with great hope that she would receive a better education and a better life in England. Tragically within 10 months at the age of 8 years Victoria died of appalling and sustained abuse. Yet during that 10 months there were no fewer than 12 occasions when local services had the opportunity to protect her but failed to do so. Indeed, Lord Laming's (DoH 2003c) report provided some 108 recommendations for improving the child-protection system, with 22 recommendations related to the acute sector. Emergency services were one of the many areas criticized by Lord Laming.

Victoria's case is by no means unique. Reviews and enquiries into the cases where children have been let down by services identify the same concerns. Lessons learnt indicate that child protection is about doing simple things better and adopting a common-sense approach. Most importantly, sharing information is paramount, as are acting when in doubt and having clear pathways of communication. The NMC (2004) Code of Professional Conduct states that all nurses have a duty and personal responsibility to act in the best interests of the child or young person, and to inform and alert appropriate personnel if they suspect a child is at risk or has been abused.

On three separate occasions Victoria attended two emergency departments. On each of the visits there were suspicions that Victoria was suffering from non-accidental injury. However, despite the emergency medicine clinicians referring Victoria to the senior paediatric team, documentation of her injuries and communications to senior staff and doctors of concern for Victoria were inadequate. Within 10 days of this first emergency-care episode Victoria attended a second ED with severe scalds to the scalp from boiling kettle water. Again, the examining doctor acknowledged the strong possibility that the injuries were non-accidental. Nobody ever asked Victoria any questions in relation to her injuries, how they happened and the circumstances around the incident.

Within months, in a final visit to an ED, Victoria's temperature being only 27°C, her injuries too numerous to be recorded, she was transferred to paediatric intensive care with severe hypothermia and multi-system failure, where she died the next day. Victoria had 127 separate injuries to her body and she was unable to straighten her legs due to contraction from scarring and being kept in a confined space. There was a complete failure by health-care clinicians, despite all the clinical evidence, to record information comprehensively, to record and share concerns and to record completed actions that these concerns had prompted. Worst of all, nobody noticed when things were not being done.

Lord Laming identified five key messages from the Victoria Climbié inquiry. These were:

- communication
- written documentation
- working with each other
- training
- recognition of child abuse.

It may be that a child is seen just once and yet the record of the event could help to save a life. Victoria had no fewer than five 'unique' hospital reference numbers. Often it is only when many apparently unrelated factors are pieced together that practitioners can identify a case of child abuse. Good record-keeping is always factual, clear, accurate, accessible and comprehensive. Write down all observations and discussions as they happen, include details of communications with other healthcare agencies notified. Seek guidance from trust policy and senior colleagues, liaising with a designated named child protection nurse, always dating and timing any actions. Confidentiality must not be confused with secrecy. Information should always be shared on a 'need to know' basis when it is in the best interest of the child. The intercollegiate committee services for children in emergency departments, recommends that all staff whether clinical or non-clinical must receive training in safe guarding children appropriate to their posts (RCPCH 2007).

The legislative framework for child protection is enshrined in the Children's Act (Department of Health 1989) and the Children (Scotland) Act (Scottish Office 1995) alongside the formal response of the Victoria Climbié inquiry (Department of Health 2003c): both promoted partnership working. This includes inter- and intra-agency working, children and families and the independent and voluntary sector. The main focus of Every Child Matters (Department for Education and Skills 2004) identifies five key areas for measurement;

- be healthy
- stay safe
- enjoy and achieve
- make a positive contribution
- achieve economic wellbeing.

To this end, each local authority has to develop its own children and young people plan. The plan should set out and prioritize actions for achievements of the five key areas. The statutory requirement to have such a plan will ultimately identify the positive impact in safeguarding and making a better place for children.

Prevalence

In 2002, there were 27 800 children on the child protection register, more males than females; 39% were considered to be at risk due to neglect, 16% due to physical abuse, 17% due to emotional abuse and 11% due to sexual abuse. About 80 children die each year from abuse or neglect in England and Wales (Department of Health 2002). There are currently over 30 000 children on the child protection register, yet this represents only a fraction of the total number of children at risk as most cases of child abuse go unreported (NSPCC 2003).

First-born children are more likely to be affected and it is not uncommon to find one child is abused while other siblings are free from abuse. Young children of pre-school age are more at risk because they cannot seek help. Most children are abused by a parent; but in this context a not uncommon scenario is a co-habitant living in the house who is not the child's biological parent. Statistically, the younger the parents the more likely it is that they will abuse their children. Child abuse is also seen across all layers of society. The acknowledgement that child abuse exists and is quite common is an important start for emergency department staff; however, in order to enable detection the nurse needs to keep an open and enquiring mind. It is also worth noting that children who are subjected to maltreatment are unlikely to have one type of abuse (Browne 2002) (see Box 16.11).

Physical

Most commonly physical abuse is inflicted on the child under the guise of punishment or when an adult loses control. It usually involves violence, often of a short duration but repetitive. Physical abuse includes poisoning and suffocation. A study of non-accidental drownings found that there were no cases of

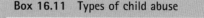

Box 16.11   Types of child abuse
<ul><li>Physical</li><li>Neglect</li><li>Emotional</li><li>Social</li><li>Sexual</li></ul>

accidental bath drowning over the age of 18 months, and in all cases over this age the child drowned due to abuse or epilepsy (Kemp et al. 1994). Equally, Barber & Sibert (2000) suggest that it is very rare for children over the age of 3 years to present with non-accidental bruising or fractures, in contrast to accidental causes. Besharou (1990) notes that deliberately inflicted burns can be distinguished by their severity and area. For instance, burns resulting from deliberate immersion in hot water have distinct lines around them and no splash marks (Joaghim 2003, Besharou 1990). In the absence of a clinical or plausible accidental explanation, these types of injuries are highly suggestive of abuse.

Neglect

Neglect is the persistent and severe failure to provide love, care, food, shelter or the physical circumstances to allow for normal development (Box 16.12). It also includes wilfully exposing a child to any kind of danger. Neglect can lead to failure to thrive, manifest by a fall away from initial centile lines in weight, height and head circumference, which is why repeated growth measurements are crucially important in primary care. Signs of malnutrition include wasted muscles and poor condition of skin and hair. It is important not to miss an organic cause of failure to thrive; if this is suspected, further investigations will be required.

Emotional abuse

Emotional abuse is the persistent emotional ill-treatment of a child such as to cause severe and persistent adverse effects on the child's emotional development. It may involve conveying to children that they are worthless or unloved, inadequate, or valued only in so far as they meet the needs of another person; having age or developmentally inappropriate expectations imposed on children; causing children frequently to feel frightened; or the exploitation or corruption of children (DoH 2003b). All abuses involve some emotional ill-treatment. Iwaniec (1997) argued that parents and carers who persistently criticize, shame, threaten, humiliate, induce fear and anxiety and who are never satisfied with the child's behaviour and performance (and do so deliberately) are emotionally abusive and cruel. Children suffering from emotional abuse may be withdrawn and emotionally flat. One reaction is for the child to seek attention constantly or to be over-familiar. Lack of self-esteem and developmental delay are again likely to be present.

Sexual abuse

This is discussed in a separate section further on.

Persistent rejection or neglect can lead to the child failing to thrive and can affect the child's stature. Common physical and non-physical indicators of child abuse are given in Box 16.13.

The parents

The vast majority of child abuse involves at least one of the child's parents. Approximately one-third of parents who were abused as children are at risk of abusing their own children. As abused children, they may have been subjected to marked negative

---

Box 16.12　Common indicators of child neglect (Sheridan 2003)

Physical indicators
- Poor hygiene and/ or clothing that does not protect a child from weather
- Chronic signs of malnutrition and dehydration
- Poor oral hygiene or untreated dental problems
- Failure to receive immunizations
- Child abandonment
- Delays in seeking prompt medical care for an acute injury or illness
- Failure to give child a prescribed medication, which results in the child developing more severe symptoms
- Failure to thrive in infants

Emotional and behavioural indicators
- Delay or absence of age-appropriate behaviours, especially in infants and young children
- Constant hunger
- Poor personal hygiene
- Lethargy in the absence of illness
- Social withdrawal or depression
- Relentless attention-seeking behaviour
- Minimal response to painful medical interventions
- Suicidal ideation or attempts
- Poor state of clothing
- Emaciation
- Untreated medical problems
- No social relationships
- Compulsive scavenging

Box 16.13   Common indicators of child abuse (Sheridan 2003)

Physical indicators
- Alterations in skin integrity
- Abrasions to palms, elbows, or knees from being pushed down
- Burns resulting from:
  cigarettes and cigars
  curling tongs, clothes iron
  chemicals
  friction – being dragged in the ground
  immersion in hot liquid or 'dunking' injury patterns
  splashes
- Bite marks – human are crest-shaped
- External genitalia lacerations or abrasions
- Vaginal bleeding, discharge or infections
- Penile bleeding, discharge or infections
- Rectal bleeding, discharge or infections
- Patterned bruises such as from a whip, belt or other implement
- Bruises in various stages of healing

Alterations in musculoskeletal system
- Multiple fractures
- Fractures in various stages of healing
- Spiral or midshaft fractures of long bones
- Fractured ribs – uncommon in young children
- Skull fractures

Neurological impairment
- Acute onset of paresis
- Post-concussion symptoms
- Intracranial haemorrhage
- Visual impairment resulting from retinal detachment

Non-physical indicators
- Conflicting histories obtained from parent(s) or adult (s) and child regarding the nature of the child's injuries
- Children who are not allowed by the parent(s) or adult (s) to verbalize a history despite the fact that they are developmentally and chronologically old enough to do so
- A history given by the parent(s) or adult(s) that does not fit the nature of the presenting injuries
- Children who display fearful body language, e.g. guarding when a sudden movement is made
- A delay in bringing the child to ED for treatment of an injury or illness that indicates abuse or neglect

reinforcement and an inability to get their needs met, little practice in problem-solving, and no basis for trusting others. As a consequence they may lack empathy with their children as little was directed towards them and a self-perpetuating cycle then begins (Tercier 1992). The parents may present as hostile or exhibit a lack of concern or guilt or may show a lack of interest or disturbed interaction with the child and seem more interested in their own problem than the child's: for example, how they are going to get home. That noted, it is important to acknowledge the crisis and distress that investigation and intervention cause to the child and family and that there may be conflicting interests between the needs of the child and those of the parents; however, it is also important to stress that under the Children Act (DoH 1989) the child's welfare is paramount.

The child

These children have a number of characteristics that predispose them to victimization. They are often the unwanted child of unplanned pregnancies, illegitimate births, and the opposite sex from that desired by the parents, born in periods of crisis or from a former relationship. The children themselves may have problems that make them difficult to rear, being poor feeders, or with challenging behaviours, abnormal sleep patterns, excessive crying and hyperactivity. The child may present as passive, withdrawn and uncomplaining during dressings, or may present hyperactive, angry or rebellious behaviour. There may be obvious signs of neglect.

Management of suspected child abuse

Every emergency department should have an agreed procedure for the management of suspected child abuse and nurses need to be acquainted with this procedure. All such cases of suspected abuse should be reported to senior medical staff and consultant paediatricians for further investigation and intervention where necessary. Suspicions of child abuse start at initial assessment; an astute nurse will pick up discrepancies in the history of the incident, incompatibilities between the alleged mechanism of injury and the actual injury, and the usual interactions between the child and his carer (Saines 1992). All life-threatening conditions must be given immediate attention; however, while the nursing care and treatment of the child's physical needs remain paramount, the emotional needs of the child must also be addressed.

When clinicians are suspicious of child abuse they have a duty to inform the parents of the need to inform and notify a child protection agency. Local guidelines for child protection should be followed and the child and family should be supported and cared for in a private but safe area during their stay in ED (DoH 2003b).

The health workers attitude can have a great impact on the child. It is imperative that the health carer appears non-judgemental and is not disgusted by findings or revelations. These should be handled with diplomacy to prevent a difficult situation from becoming inflamed; however, it should be acknowledged that abused cases of any kind could foster feelings amongst staff of hostility and anger towards the alleged perpetrators; nevertheless, for nursing to be effective, staff must control these feelings. Team leaders and members should monitor each other's emotional and physical well-being and provide support for those who appear to be affected by an incident (Cudmore 1998).

Careful documentation is critical in cases of suspected child abuse. For the nurse taking a history, the single most important factor is the history of the incident as told by the child. It is important to write exactly, or as closely as possible, any allegations of abuse or neglect, noting who made them and who was present. The veracity and accuracy of information recorded should be exact.

Evidence

No child should be discharged into the custody of parents or carers if staff feel there is a risk to the child's health and welfare. Where parents are unwilling to co-operate the protection of the Children Act DoH (1989) may need to be applied to bring an Emergency Protection Order. In most instances, however, where non-judgemental approaches are used and open communication prevails parental agreement will be forthcoming.

Consent for photographs should be sought before any photographs of injuries as they may play an important part in subsequent legal proceedings as well as providing valuable clinical evidence.

Sanders and Cobly (2005) note that there is a 'culture' of under-reporting of suspected non-accidental injury in children in emergency departments, which is largely to do with the fact that a significant proportion of medical and nursing staff receive no formal training in identifying potential indicators of child abuse and because they have no rapid access to a paediatric opinion. Additionally, bureaucratic and inter-professional barriers to accessing confidential information about children from social services registers also lead to long delays in the ability of clinicians to obtain a rapid assessment of each suspected case of abuse.

The reforms arising out of Lord Laming's inquiry into the death of Victoria Climbié, who died of abuse at the hands of her aunt and her aunt's partner, present an ideal opportunity to encourage clinicians to be alert to the possibility of Non-accidental injury (NAI) and address the current culture of under-reporting (DoH 2003c). The recommendations from this report are reshaping the way child protection cases are managed and have influenced the children's national service frameworks (DoH 2003c, Welsh Assembly Government 2004).

SEXUAL ABUSE

This occurs when dependent, developmentally immature children are forced to participate in sexual activity. Although sexual abuse may occur at any age peaks tend to occur between the 2 to 6 years and 12 to 16 years (Tercier 1992). Perhaps the most difficult area of abuse to detect in ED is sexual abuse, primarily because sexually abused children often display no physical signs and it is therefore necessary to be alert to the behavioural and emotional factors that may indicate abuse.

Various degrees and forms of sexual abuse include molestation, touching or fondling of the child's genitalia, masturbation of the perpetrator by the child, combination of oral-genital contact, attempted or actual anal or vaginal intercourse, exhibitionism, voyeurism and exploitation of children in the preparation of pornographic materials. Sexual abuse differs from other forms of child abuse in that it is not used as a form of punishment. However, while violence is seldom a factor, coercion and threats are common (Tercier 1992). Hobbs & Wynne (2001) suggest that physical abuse and sexual abuse are thought to be closely related; however, the two can occur independently of each other. This relationship is based on power: the threat of physical abuse gives the perpetrator the power to ensure the compliance of the child and allows them to guarantee that the child keeps the sexual abuse a secret (Chudleigh 2005).

Sexual abuse may present to ED staff in a number of different ways:

- physical complaints: for example, abdominal pain, urinary tract infection, per rectum and per vaginal bleeds
- parental accusations; this should always be taken seriously where one parent or carer accuses another
- request by the child for help; children do not fabricate stories of sexual activity

- physical abuse; children who have been physically abused may present with evidence of sexual abuse; careful examination may reveal trauma or infection
- emotional or psychological problems; these may present as bed-wetting, night terrors and developmental regression
- sexually transmitted diseases; any sexually transmitted disease in a child should be considered evidence of sexual abuse until proven otherwise.

Management

The management of children who are suspected of being sexually abused is similar to that for child abuse. Establishing rapport and trust is critical, using language that is appropriate for the child's age and development stage: it is important to stress that children have short attention spans and therefore a prolonged interview will not be tolerated. Children must be constantly reassured that it is all right to share their secrets with the nurse and for this reason it is best to interview the child away from the family members, even those not initially believed to be involved in the abuse or neglectfulness (Sheridan 1995). Once there is significant indication that sexual abuse may have occurred, arrangements should be made for physical examination to be carried out by an experienced paediatrician. It may be appropriate for a forensic doctor to be present to save the child being repeatedly examined. At this stage the social services and police should be involved. A professional colleague should be present, however, and responses should be recorded verbatim.

A number of key facts need to be established in gaining a history of sexual abuse. These are presented in Box 16.14.

All too often ED staff do not hear the outcomes of particularly difficult cases such as suspected child sexual abuse. It is good practice to promote inter-disciplinary team meetings for a period review and updating of such cases to provide feedback, support and opportunities to further improve protocols.

FABRICATED ILLNESS

Fabricated illness in babies and children by a parent/carer is often referred to by any number of different terms, most commonly Munchausen's syndrome by proxy (MBP), factitious illness by proxy or illness induction syndrome (DoH 2004). It was Professor Roy Meadows (1977, 1997) who first described Munchausen by proxy (Box 16.15). However, in 2001, following continuing contention regarding the existence, application and definition of the term MBP and many complaints by parents/carers claiming to be falsely

---

Box 16.14   Sexual abuse history

- Date and time of assault
- Place of assault(s)
- Number of people involved and relationship to abused
- Physical characteristics
- Use of restraints
- Use of sexual aids
- Use of lubricants, powders or other chemicals
- Statements made during assault
- Use of photographs or videotaping
- Removal of locks of hair or other 'artefacts'
- Form of assault, i.e. vaginal, anal or oral intercourse
- Occurrence of ejaculation
- Oral manipulation of breasts or other body parts
- Use of condom
- Bath, douche or clean mouth after assault
- Last bowel movement and last urination
- Last menstrual period, if appropriate
- Use of contraceptive pill or IUD, if appropriate
- Use of tampons or pads, if appropriate

---

accused of child abuse, the Department of Health developed guidance for child protection professionals attempting to give credibility and validity to MBP and introduced the new term 'fabricated illness' (DoH et al. 2004). Munchausen by proxy is now the term reserved for the disorder whereby there are two elements, one indicating a behaviour in the parent/carer for a particular self-serving psychological need and secondly a diagnosis in the child who has been harmed by the parent/carer (Schreier 2002).

Fabrication of illness or illness induction should be considered whenever a baby or child presents with unusual signs and symptoms that are not easily explained physiologically. The fabrication of illness is usually manifested in one of three ways:

- induction of illness or injury by a variety of means
- falsification of signs and symptoms which may include fabrication of past medical history
- falsification of specimens of bodily fluids, falsification of hospital record charts, letters and documents.

The variety of diseases mimicked or produced is alarmingly diverse and limited only by the parent's imagination and insanity. The child, who is usually under 5 years old, is most commonly presented with problems related to one body system such as blood in urine or recurrent seizures. The illness story is

---

Box 16.15   Characteristics of Munchausen's Syndrome by Proxy (Meadow 1982)

- Persistent or recurrent illnesses that cannot be explained or are very unusual
- Laboratory results or physical findings that are at variance with the general health of the child
- Symptoms that only occur when the child is in the presence of the caretaker
- A caretaker who appears overly attentive, with prolonged visiting or living in with the child in the hospital
- Standard treatments that are not tolerated, e.g. i.v. lines that always come out, vomiting of medications
- A caretaker who does not seem as concerned about the child's illness as the medical or nursing staff
- A caretaker with previous medical experience or education
- Atypical episodes of seizures, near-miss SIDS or SIDS, apnoeic or cyanotic episodes occurring only in the presence of the caretaker and which do not seem to respond to standard therapy
- A history of multiple resuscitations in a child with no recognizable cardiopulmonary abnormalities

List of behaviours exhibited by carers with parenting responsibilities (Quality Protects DFES 2004)

- Deliberately inducing symptoms in children by administering medicines or other substances, or by means of suffocation
- Interfering with treatments by overdosing, not administering, or interfering with medical equipment
- Obtaining specialist treatments or equipment for children who don't require them
- Exaggerating symptoms, causing professionals to undertake investigations and treatments which may be invasive, are unnecessary and therefore harmful and possibly dangerous
- Claiming the child has symptoms which are unverifiable unless obviously directly, such as pain, frequency of passing urine, vomiting, or fitting, claims result in unnecessary investigations and treatments which present secondary physical problems
- Alleging psychological illness in a child

---

related consistently by the carer, who in 90% of cases is the child's natural mother. Events relating to the illness episode only start in her presence. While ideal parenting behaviours may be demonstrated, the mother is often inappropriately calm in relation to the gravity of the child's illness.

Fabricated illness is a very serious business, and can be difficult to detect. McClure et al. (1996) found that 6% of children died as a direct result of extreme fabricated illness, with 12% requiring paediatric intensive care. Up to 35% of children from reported incidents suffer major physical problems as a result of the abuse, with as many as 50% children experiencing long-term morbidity. Child welfare concerns arise when things just don't seem to add up (Box 16.16).

It is possible that there is any number of explanations for any of these circumstances and each will require careful consideration. When concerns are such that a positive explanation for the child's presentation is that of fabricated illness then referral to a senior paediatrician and social services should be made.

One must remember that personal information about the child and family held by professionals is subject to a legal duty of confidence and should not be discussed inappropriately without the consent of the subject. Notwithstanding this, the law of disclosure of confidential information is necessary to safeguard children in the public interest: that is, the public interest in maintaining confidentiality (DoH et al. 2004). Without exception children are entitled to the same duty of confidence as adults.

Box 16.16   Child welfare concerns (Quality Protects DFES 2004)

- Reported signs and symptoms found on assessment are not explained by any medical condition the child might be suffering from; or
- Physical examinations and results of diagnostics do not explain symptoms and signs on examination; or
- There is an inexplicably poor response to prescribed medication and treatment; or
- New symptoms are reported on resolution of previous ones; or
- Reported symptoms and found signs are not observed independently of the carer; or
- The child's normal, daily life activities are being curtailed beyond what might be expected for any known medical disorder from which the child might be suffering

Despite the understandable feelings of anger and frustration of clinical staff in these situations, the need for non-judgemental care remains paramount, as is the continuing need for vigilance to safeguard children. Support and debriefing should be made available for staff, including all the multidisciplinary team who have been involved in the care of abused children and who have been affected by fabricated or induced illness (Dolan 1998).

CONCLUSION

Children of pre-school age are more likely than others to attend for emergency treatments, because of their vulnerability to accidents and illness. Emergency departments can be developed to become more child-oriented, helping to reduce children's anxieties.

The emergency nurse should appreciate the importance of supporting and reassuring a child's family.

Through helping them, the nurse will help the child and increase their cooperation. It is important that professionals working with children have fundamental knowledge of normal development stages, both physiological and cognitive, enabling the consultation to be pitched at the appropriate level for the child and family.

A trip to the emergency department is usually the young child's first experience of hospital. Every effort should be made to make the experience as little traumatic as possible. Avoid separation from parents/carers, explain simply what is wrong, and if and how it can be amended in a language that is easily understandable to the child. On this first visit to the hospital, it is the emergency nurses' responsibility to ensure the experience is as positive as can be.

References

Barber MA, Sibert JR (2000) Diagnosing physical child abuse: the way forward. *Postgraduate Medical Journal*, **76**, 743–749.

Bentley J (2004) Distress in children attending A&E. *Emergency Nurse*, **2**(4), 20–26.

Besharou D (1990) *Recognising Child Abuse: A Guide for the Concerned*. London: Free Press.

Bowlby J (1953) *Child Care and the Growth of Love*. London: Penguin.

Boyle R, Smith C, McIntyre J (2000) The changing utilisation of a children's emergency department. *Ambulatory Child Health*, **6**, 39–43.

Brain J, Martin MD (1989) *Child Care and Health for Nursery Nurses*. 3rd edn. Cheltenham: Stanley Thornes and Hulton.

British Thoracic Society (BTS) and Scottish Intercollegiate Guidelines Network (SIGN) (2005) *British Guideline on the Management of Asthma: A National Clinical Guideline*. Edinburgh: BTS/SIGN.

Browne K (2002) Child abuse: defining, understanding and intervening. In: Wilson K, James A (eds) (2002) *The Child Protection Handbook*. 2nd edn. Baillière Tindall.

Brunner LS, Suddarth DS (1991) *The Lippincott Manual of Paediatric Nursing*. 3rd edn. London: Harper and Collins.

Child Accident Prevention Trust (CAPT) (2004) *Poisoning Factsheet*. London: CAPT.

Child Accident Prevention Trust (CAPT) (2006) *Children's Road Crashes Factsheet*. London: CAPT.

Chudleigh J (2005) Safeguarding children. *Paediatric Nursing*, **17**(1), 37–42.

Cudmore J (1998) Critical incident stress management strategies. *Emergency Nurse*, **6**(3), 22–27.

RJ Davies PM, Meadow SR, Sibert JR (1996) Epidemiology of Munchausen's by proxy, non-accidental poisoning, and non-accidental suffocation. *Archives of Diseases in Childhood*, **75**, 57–61.

Department for Education and Skills (2004) *Every Child Matters*. London: The Stationery Office.

Department of Health (1989) *The Children Act*. London: HMSO.

Department of Health (2002) *Referrals, Assessments, and Children and Young People on the Child Protection Registers, England: 2001/2002*. London: Department of Health.

Department of Health (2003a) *The Ill Child Module Ambulatory Care Sub Group Children's National Service Framework*. London: Department of Health.

Department of Health (2003b) *'What to do if you're worried a child is being abused'*. London: Department of Health.

Department of Health (2003c). *The Victoria Climbié Inquiry: Report of an inquiry by Lord Laming. Cmnd 5730*. London: The Stationery Office.

Department of Health (2003d) *Getting the Right Start: National Service Framework for Children*. London: Department of Health.

Department of Health (2004) *The National Service Framework for Children, Young People and Maternity Services*. London: Department of Health.

Department of Health, Home Office, Department of Education and Skills, Welsh Assembly Government (2004) *Safeguarding Children in which Illness is fabricated or induced*. London: Department of Health.

Dolan B (1998) The hospital hoppers. *Nursing Times*, **94** (30), 26–27.

Dykes J (2005) Managing children with croup in emergency departments. *Emergency Nurse*, **13**(6), 14–19.

Eiser C (1985) *The Psychology of Childhood Illness*. New York: Springer-Verlag.

European Respiratory Society/European Lung Foundation (2003) *European Lung White Book The First Comprehensive Survey on Respiratory Health in Europe*. Huddersfield: The Charlesworth Group.

Geelhooed GC (1996) Sixteen years of croup in a West Australian teaching: effects of routine steroid treatment. *Annals of Emergency Medicine*, **28**(6), 621–626.

Hall D, Elliman D (2003) *Health for all Children*. 4th edn. Oxford: Oxford University Press.

Hobbs CJ, Wynne JM (2001) *Physical Signs of Child Abuse*. London: WB Saunders.

Iwaniec D (1997) *The Emotionally Abused and Neglected Child*. Chichester: John Wiley.

Joaghin V (2003) Working together for child protection in A&E. *Emergency Nurse*, **11**(7), 30–37.

Kelsey J, Mckewing G (2006) Respiratory illness in children. In: Glasper A, Richardson J, eds. *A Textbook of Children's and Young People's Nursing*. Edinburgh: Churchill Livingstone Elsevier.

Kemp A, Mott AM, Sibert JR (1994) Accidents and child abuse in bathtub submersions, *Archives of Diseases in Childhood*, **70**, 435–438.

Kia J (1996) Parents difficulties and information needs in coping with acute illness in pre-school child: a qualitative study. *British Medical Journal*, **313**, 987–990.

Kline A (2003) Pediatric respiratory distress. *Nursing*, **33**(9), 58–63.

Lissauer T, Clayden G (2001) *Illustrated Textbook of Paediatrics*. Edinburgh: Mosby.

Lowe GR (1985) *The Growth of Personality from Infancy to Old Age*. Harmondsworth: Penguin.

McClure et al. (1996).

MacFaul R, Glass EJ, Jones S (1994) Appropriateness of paediatric admissions. *Archives of Disease of Childhood*, **71**, 50–58.

Maller D, Harris PJ, Whatley L, Taylor J (1992) *Nursing Children: Psychology, Research and Practice*, 2nd Edn. London: Chapman and Hall.

Mead D, Sibert J (1991) *The Injured Child: An Action Plan for Nurses*. London: Scutari.

Meadow R (1997) *ABC of Child Abuse*, 3rd Edn. London: British Medical Association.

Meadow R (1977) Munchausen Syndrome by Proxy. The Hinterlands of Child Abuse. *Lancet*, **2**, 343–345.

Ministry of Health (1959) *The Welfare of Children in Hospital (The Platt Report)*. London: HMSO.

Morton R, Phillips B (1996) *Accident and Emergencies in Children*, 2nd Edn. Oxford: Oxford University Press.

National Audit Office (2004) *Improving Emergency Care in England*. London: NAO.

National Society for the Prevention of Cruelty to Children (NSPCC) (2003) *Facts and Figures about Child Abuse*. London: NSPCC.

Neill SJ (2000) Acute childhood illness at home: the parents' perspective. *Journal of Advanced Nursing*, **31**(4), 821–832.

Nursing and Midwifery Council (2004) *Code of Professional Conduct: Standards for Conduct, Performance and Ethics*. London: Nursing and Midwifery Council.

Office for National Statistics (2002) *Mortality Statistics; Injury and Poisoning: England & Wales*. London: Office for National Statistics.

Parton N (2004) From Maria Colwell to Victoria Climbié: reflections on public inquiries into child abuse a generation Apart. *Child Abuse Review*, **13**, 80–94.

Piaget J (1990) *The Child's Conception of the World*. New York: Little Fields Adams.

Price D, Ryan D, Pearce L et al. (1999) The AIR Study: asthma in real life. *Asthma Journal*, **4**(4), 74–78.

Royal College of Paediatrics and Child Health (1999) *Accident and Emergency Services for Children: Report of a Multidisciplinary Working Party*. London: Royal College of Paediatrics and Child Health.

Royal College of Paediatrics and Child Health (RCPCH) (2003) *Medicines for Children*. London: RCPCH.

Royal College of Paediatrics and Child Health (RCPCH) (2007).

Royal Society for Prevention of Accidents (RoSPA) (2006) *Accidents to Children: Can the Home Ever be Safe?* Birmingham: ROSPA.

Royal Society for Prevention of Accidents (RoSPA) (2005) *Leisure Safety Information: Trampoline Safety*. Birmingham: RoSPA.

Saines J (1992) A considered response to an emotional crisis; A&E nurses role in detecting child sexual abuse. *Professional Nurse*, **8**(3), 148–152.

Sanders T, Cobley C (2005) Identifying non-accidental injury in children presenting to A&E departments: an overview of the literature. *Accident & Emergency Nursing*, **13**(2), 130–136.

Schreier H (2002) Munchausen by Proxy defined. *Paediatrics*, **110**(5), 985–988.

Scottish Office (1995) *Scotland's Children: A Brief Guide to the Children (Scotland) Act (1995)*. Edinburgh: The Stationery Office.

Scullion J (2005) A proactive approach to asthma. *Nursing Standard*, **20**, 9, 57–65.

Sheridan MS (1995) The descent continues: An updated literature review Munchausen's syndrome by proxy. Child Abuse & Neglect. *The International Journal*. **27**(4), 431–451.

Tanner K, Fitzsimmons G, Carrol D, Flood TJ, Clark JE (2002) *Haemophilus influenzae* type b epiglottitis as a cause of acute upper airways obstruction in children. *British Medical Journal*, **325**(7372), 1099–1100.

Tercier A (1992) Child abuse. In: Rosen P, Barkin RM, Braen G et al. eds. *Emergency Medicine: Concepts and Clinical Practice*, 3rd Edn. St. Louis; Mosby Year Book.

Visintainer MA, Wolfer JA (1975) Psychological preparation for surgical pediatric patients: the effect on children's and parent's stress responses and adjustment. *Pediatrics*, **56**(2), 187–201.

Webster A (2002) The facility role of the Play Specialist. *Paediatric Nursing*, **12**, 7 pp.24–27.

Welsh Assembly Government (2004) *NSF for Children, Young People and Maternity Services*. Cardiff: Welsh Assembly Government.

Chapter 17

Age 5 to puberty

Anita Tyler

INTRODUCTION

This chapter considers reasons for emergency department (ED) attendance by children between the ages of 5 and 13 years. While this age range is somewhat arbitrary, especially in the context of the decreasing age of puberty, for the purposes of this chapter it will be used as a chronological benchmark between pre-school children and adolescence. Some of the more common injuries and conditions occurring in this age group will be considered, with particular reference to a child's development and the need for a suitable environment and a family-centred approach.

Children's school years are proposed as the best years of their lives, but unfortunately they are also a very dangerous time. Each year one in five children attends an emergency department and one in 10–15 children will be admitted to hospital (Department of Health 2005). Death in childhood is most prevalent during the first year of life, while the fewest deaths occur between the ages of 5 and 14. Of these deaths trauma and neoplasms are the biggest killers (Advanced Life Support Group 2001, NICE 2005). The number of deaths from trauma in this age group has decreased dramatically since 1991: this may be due to an increase in safety awareness or an increase in paediatric resuscitation courses.

Children's deaths following injury are most commonly road traffic accidents (RTAs) followed by drowning, suffocation, fire and falls (Mead & Sibert 1991). About 10 000 children are permanently disabled annually as a result of accidents (Morton & Phillips 1996). However, the figures do not show the real impact an accident can have on both the child and the extended family. The cost can be enormous in both physical and emotional terms.

CHILD DEVELOPMENT

Children are involved in different types of accident according to their stage of development. At 5 years of age children run confidently, although they frequently fall. As they progress from infant to junior to secondary school, balance and coordination improve, as does their dexterity. Children in this age group become more aware of their bodies and subsequently may be self-conscious during examinations.

Piaget's theory of the development of causal reasoning (Piaget 1983) demonstrates a systematic progression in children's understanding of illness: this is linked to Piaget's four stages of cognitive development.

sensori-motor	birth – 18 months
pre-operational	18 months – 7 years
concrete-operational	7 years – 11 years
formal-operational	11 years – adult

The pre-operational stage is dominated by the perception and direct experiences, while illness concepts are related to phenomenism and contagion. Phenomenism occurs in the younger children in this stage, the cause of illness is believed to be external such as the sun. Contagion occurs in the older children in this stage: illness is seen to be in objects or people. Colds are caught by someone coming near and transferred by magic. Pre-operational children may see illness or unpleasant procedures as punishment for their naughty behaviour. They are unable to comprehend unpleasant procedures being part of the cure.

In the concrete-operational stage children can apply thinking and reasoning to real objects and events. Contamination children can distinguish from cause and effect, such as bad food will give a tummy ache. However, all illnesses are seen as being caused by contact with the causative agent: if someone has a rash and it is touched then the rash is transmitted. Internalization occurs in the older children in this age group, where illness is seen as internal with an external cause; for example, kissing someone with a cold will cause the germs to go into your mouth and make you ill. Mechanisms of illness remain poorly understood but there is a realization that the body responds to causative agents such as allergens. Children in this age range understand that illnesses are preventable by immunizations and health care (Swanwick 1990).

When caring for children consideration for their conception of illness can ease the path of the child through assessment and treatment to admission or discharge. Be aware of using metaphors when explaining to children as they might confuse or increase fear: for example, white cells 'fighting' infection may give rise to terrifying thoughts of soldiers with guns, missiles and tanks in their blood stream. Despite this acquired understanding, many children regress in behaviour when they become ill, probably as a coping mechanism for the stress associated with hospitalization (Swanwick 1990).

Children aged between 5 and 7 have gained some independence, both socially and intellectually, but their behaviour is unpredictable. They become preoccupied when playing, their perceptions of speed and distance are often wrong and therefore they continue to need supervision, particularly on roads etc.

Much of an early school-goers' time is spent under adult supervision at school or in the home. Increasingly, as they get older, children spend their time away from home in parks and playgrounds unsupervised. Being unsupervised can lead to children using unsuitable areas to play in, such as derelict buildings, water or building sites. They can also indulge in dangerous activities, such as playing with fire, increasing the likelihood of injury. Older children drown in open water, public and private swimming pools; 84% were unsupervised and lacked swimming abilities (Candy et al. 2001).

As children approach adolescence they are more likely to attempt to flaunt their independence, resent rules and authority, and take risks. Peer pressure influences children's behaviour in activities which they know to be dangerous but take part in to avoid losing face in front of their friends. Children will often lie about the mechanisms of injury to prevent detection of a dangerous/banned activity or location.

Hospital attendance is stressful at any age; Wolfer Visintainer (1975) identify five categories which worry a child regarding hospitalization.

1) physical harm
2) fear of the unknown
3) uncertainty
4) separation
5) loss of control.

These five categories were identified following studies on children who were hospitalized; the sudden abrupt attendance in the ED will compound these concerns/fears. Both the child's and the parent's previous experiences of hospital/illness/injury can have a profound effect on the child's attitude and behaviour.

As well as differences in cognition between the ages in this group there are also anatomical and physiological ones (Barnes 2003, Advanced Life Support Group 2001).

ENVIRONMENT AND FAMILY–CENTRED CARE

The Children and Young People's National Service Framework (NSF) (Department for Education and

Skills/Department of Health 2005) and Children's Charter (Department of Health 1995) state that EDs caring for children should provide an environment which, as a minimum, has:

- separate waiting area with play facilities
- separate treatment area suitably decorated and equipped
- private room for distressed parents
- at least one registered sick children's nurse (RSCN) or RN (child)
- liaison health visitor

Many others, such as the Royal College of Nursing (1998), the Audit Commission (1996) and Action for Sick Children (1997), have made similar recommendations regarding the provision of care of children in EDs. While the aim of ED is to provide 24-hour care by paediatric nurses, this is difficult to achieve and must not detract from the skills and experience that general nurses have in caring for children. Paediatric nurses within emergency departments augment the expertise of general nurses; the children's nurse acts as a resource, innovator of practice and educator in all things paediatric.

A sick or injured child is usually accompanied to ED by at least one adult, and sometimes by numerous family members and friends, including other children. Family-centred care should be the aim throughout the child's stay, and both the child and her family should be involved in decisions about care wherever possible (Kennedy 2001, Cudmore & Lakin 1997, Department of Health 1991). Lee (2001) suggests that Casey's model of partnership could be implemented in the ED environment. Casey's model developed from the philosophy stated as: 'The care of children, well or sick, is best carried out by their families with varying degrees of help from suitably qualified members of the health care team whenever necessary'.

The child may require help to meet his needs in order to function, grow and develop. These needs are met by:

- *family care* – the parents carry out family care to help child meet his needs: care given by a nurse if parents absent or unable
- *nursing care* – the nurse gives extra care related to health needs: care given by parents, child or significant others with support and teaching (Casey 1993).

Using Casey's Partnership Model in the emergency department, the nurse determines whether a parent wishes to be involved in their child's care. Some parents may feel unable to be involved, for instance being unable to be present during suturing. Others would expect to be involved, for example, comforting the child during suturing. Parental involvement is not necessarily a time-saving process, as time is required to enable parental participation. Partnership care may result in quicker discharges from ED, for instance for a child with constipation and a reduced re-attendance rate, which is of benefit to the child, family and nurse (Lee 2001).

Children usually benefit from a parent or carer being present during examination/investigation, but pressure should not be placed upon parents/carers if they feel unable to be with their child during specific treatments. It is important for ED nurses to reassure parents that their continuing presence is welcome should hospital admission become necessary.

Should a child need critical intervention, such as resuscitation, many parents would wish to stay with their child. The needs of parents must be considered, with the provision of a nurse to support the parents during this time, keeping them informed, giving explanations of treatments/procedures. Both nurses and medical staff may feel stressed by parental presence in an already tense situation, but in aiming for family-centred care, the parents' and the child's wishes should be respected wherever possible.

The majority of children (60–70%) attend the ED following trauma. Fortunately, most of them will have relatively minor injuries (Morton & Phillips 1996). To the child and parents a minor injury may appear catastrophic. A child-friendly environment, including books, toys, hospital play specialist, will distract and provide a sense of normality for the child, thus helping to reduce the emotional impact of injury. The attitude of multi-professional team, from receptionists to radiologists, towards children and their families plays a large part in reducing the impact of the injury/illness and the ED visit.

Activities and conversation should be related to things included in the child's normal world, such as the current children's films, childhood heroes, pop stars and footballers. Parents and others, especially other children, can be particularly helpful with this. The younger children in this age group appreciate bravery awards and stickers following their treatment.

PAIN ASSESSMENT AND MANAGEMENT

Most children attending ED will require pain relief in some form. Pain assessment can prove difficult, even in older children, and a long-standing problem in paediatric pain management has been the difficulty of objectively assessing pain. An assessment tool such as QUESTT is designed specifically for the assessment of children's pain (Box 17.1).

> **Box 17.1   QUESTT pain assessment tool**
>
> Q – question the child
> U – use pain rating scales
> E – evaluate behaviour and physiological changes
> S – secure parents' involvement
> T – take cause of pain into account
> T – take action and evaluate results
> (Baker and Wong 1998)

The impact of anxiety on a child's pain level should not be underestimated and appropriate measures to reduce anxiety are an important part of pain control. It is imperative that assessment and management of pain are appropriate to the child's understanding and not beyond comprehension. The use of toys and play demonstration can be helpful in reducing anxiety and increasing cooperation in the younger child. This reinforces the need for the nurse to have an awareness of normal childhood development, so communication is effective and pain assessment accurate.

Pain scales, such as numerical continuums, facial expressions and visual analogues, can be a useful aid to pain assessment (British Accident and Emergency Association 1997, Royal College of Nursing 2001) but should not be used in isolation. The use of pain rating scales may be difficult in the ED environment due to anxiety, distress, fear and the unfamiliarity with pain rating scales. Hall (2002) describes a paediatric pain assessment tool designed specifically for ED comprising a mixture of subjective and objective assessments along with examples of injury. The child is asked to choose both a face and a number most appropriate to their degree of pain. The nurse then circles the most fitting behaviour seen in the child. Twycross (1998) suggests that children's perceptions of pain are established prior to a painful episode, thus making the task of pain assessment in ED more difficult.

For many children, immobilization and support of an injured area comprise the first step in pain control, but this should not be used as a substitute for analgesia. ED nurses must not underestimate actual pain, as opposed to the fear of pain and anxiety, as the cause of the child's distress (Morcombe 1998).

For minor injuries, simple analgesia (paracetamol and ibuprofen) can be administered at an early stage, such as at assessment, thus easing the child's passage through ED. Many departments enable the nurse to administer simple analgesia under Patient Group Directives. The start of the pain assessment and management process is at home with the parents administering simple analgesics. Unfortunately it has been found that where parents do not give children analgesia prior to attending ED, they cite not having any suitable analgesics or the accident not occurring at home, and the majority felt that it was the hospital's responsibility (Spedding et al. 1999). Aspirin is not to be used in children under 12 because of the risk of Reye's syndrome (Nunn 1994).

Entonox (50% nitrous oxide, 50% oxygen) is a useful and rapid analgesia for children who are able to hold the mask or mouthpiece (pleasant-smelling masks are available). Its restrictions for use are the same as for adults. A safe dose is one which can be self-administered, and it should not be used for children with chest and moderate to severe head injury. It is useful for dressings, suturing and prior to cannulation (Bruce and Frank 2000).

Children with significant injuries such as displaced fractures, fractured femurs and burns affecting greater than 5% surface area require opiates. These should be given intravenously due to faster action times, ability to titrate dose according to response and reduced risk of tissue storage associated with muscular injections following significant trauma (Advanced Life Support Group 2001). Intravenous cannulation is not easy in an injured/ill or distressed child and repeated attempts should be avoided: seek more experienced help and/or ask for the paediatric team's assistance. Many departments use intranasal diamorphine, thus negating the need for cannulation for opiate administration. Anti-emetics are not routinely used because of a greater risk of extrapyramidal reactions, particularly oculogyric crisis in children under 12 (Hopkins 1992).

Anaesthetic is useful for many procedures. Topical substances containing lignocaine are useful prior to non-urgent cannulation and venepuncture (Smith 1995). Local anaesthetic for suturing and wound cleansing provides pain relief and thus increases the child's cooperation. Unfortunately infiltration with local anaesthetic can be painful; warming the solution, buffering with sodium bicarbonate or applying topical adrenaline cocaine can reduce pain at infiltration. The use of topical adrenaline cocaine especially on facial wounds makes local anaesthetic unnecessary.

In some cases children requiring suturing or other procedure may be unable to cooperate despite all measures of reassurance, hospital play specialist, analgesia etc., or the wound is too large to allow adequate infiltration of local anaesthetic (maximum of 3 mg/kg of 1% lignocaine): these children require general anaesthetic. Some departments advocate the use of sedation for such cases, but this may be problematic in terms of providing adequate staff and resuscitation facilities to ensure the safety of the child, as recommended by the Scottish Inter-Collegiate Guidelines (2002).

Regional nerve blocks are an effective source of pain relief. A femoral block, for example, provides good pain control while X-raying and splinting a fractured femur (Advanced Life Support Group 2001). Children with fractured femurs also require intravenous opiates as the initial pain management.

Where possible all paediatric medications should be prescribed according to the child's weight; where actual weights are not available a child's weight may be calculated using the formula

2 times age + 4

(Advanced Life Support Group 2001).

It is essential for all EDs to keep a guide to paediatric medications such as Medicines for Children (2003) in the children's area and resuscitation room.

MUSCULOSKELETAL INJURIES

As they get older children usually become increasingly competitive, participating in regimented repetitive training, and this creates a potential for serious physical (over-use or acute) and psychological injury (Hawkins et al. 2001). Psychological problems are difficult to measure, whereas acute physical injury can be assessed. Foster and Kay (2003) suggest that the diagnosis of a musculoskeletal problem is essentially clinical and describe comprehensive assessment skills.

There are three main types of musculoskeletal injury associated with children's sport:

- osteochondritis
- specific injury such as fractures
- stress fracture.

Osteochondritis refers to a group of conditions affecting the growth plate. The disorder results from the stresses produced at the bone/ligament junction or articular surfaces during physical activity.

The most commonly affected areas include:

- tibial tuberosity
- metatarsals
- navicular
- lunate
- capitulum
- calcaneum.

Rest is usually sufficient to cure these injuries, but orthopaedic follow-up should be given (Morton & Philips 1996, O'Brennan et al. 2001).

Extensive training without a proper build-up period can lead to stress fractures. Runners and gymnasts are the most likely to incur these injuries. Sports injuries can be prevented with careful supervision, a gradual increase in training activity, and correction of poor technique or inappropriate use of equipment.

FRACTURES

The developmental process of the skeletal system is such that children are prone to incomplete fractures, described as greenstick or torus fractures, with dislocations rare (Davies 2003). These are usually a disruption of the bone cortex on one side as opposed to a complete break. Emergency nurses must be prudent when assessing limb injuries in children as often those with greenstick fractures display no visible signs of bruising, swelling or deformity, leading to these fractures remaining undetected. Most greenstick fractures will heal independently; however, it is common practice to immobilize the fracture with plaster for pain relief.

Mechanism of injury is important, as is exact location of pain and extent of movement and pain association. It is often difficult to make this assessment if the child is very distressed, and simple immobilization and simple analgesia may be useful until after X-ray. Some children sustain fractures which are displaced, and these fractures require reduction to allow healing without deformity to the affected limb. It is preferable to carry out the reduction procedure under general anaesthetic.

Although children most commonly sustain greenstick fractures, they are not exempt from other types of fracture. Fractures through a growth plate (epiphysis) are described as Salter Harris fractures and graded 1–V. They require referral to orthopaedic specialists and may need surgical intervention (Morton & Phillips 1996, Davies 2001).

If a child is discharged with a lower limb cast, her developmental dexterity must be considered. Many 5-to-7-year-olds may be unable to mobilize with crutches partly because of balance and partly because of the weight of the cast. In some cases, a Zimmer frame may be a better aid. Crutches use in the older child may also be difficult due to balance, and schooling needs to be considered, as many schools with a large pupil population or stairs may feel that the child on crutches is at risk of further injury. Parents and children should be made aware of the risks and side-effects of an immobilized limb and be aware of local facilities for review and advice (see also Ch. 5).

LIMPING CHILD

Children with a history of limping frequently attend EDs. Diagnoses include fractures, soft tissue injury, osteomyelitis, septic arthritis, irritable hip, juvenile arthritis, Baker's cyst, Perthes disease and slipped upper femoral epiphysis.

Some children may be systematically unwell; the investigations must exclude infective causes. Investigations may include venepuncture (apply topical anaesthetic cream at triage), X-ray, ultra-sound scan and observation. Management of the child in ED consists of analgesia, support and antipyretics.

Perthes disease is a condition, found in the age range 5–9 years, more commonly in boys, where avascular necrosis of the femoral head occurs. The aetiology is unknown; diagnosis is made by X-ray. Treatment varies from centre to centre and may include immobilization with traction, splints in conjunction with analgesia.

Slipped upper femoral epiphysis, age range 10–15 years, more commonly in boys, confirmed on X-ray, treatment is corrective surgery. The onset can be acute or insidious, with 30% developing the same condition in the opposite limb (Davies 2003, Barnes 2003, O'Brennan et al. 2001, Waterson et al. 1997).

ABDOMINAL PAIN

Children in this age group often attend emergency departments with acute abdominal pain. Assessment and accurate diagnosis can sometimes be made difficult, as discussed previously, by level of cognitive development, pain, effects of hospitalization and level of cooperation by the child.

Children with abdominal pain present with a host of signs and symptoms, including vomiting, altered bowel habits, diarrhoea, constipation, anorexia, not drinking, nausea, frequency of micturition, pain on micturition and pains which maybe colicky, continuous or stabbing in nature.

Urinary tract infection, gastroenteritis, constipation, appendicitis, menarche, period pain, renal stone, obstruction, perforation, inflammatory bowel disease, pneumonia, otitis media, diabetes and psychosomatic pain are all reasons for ED attendance with abdominal pain (Waterson et al. 2000). The history and development of pain provide many clues for diagnosis. Acute pain of sudden onset may indicate obstruction or perforation. A more insidious onset is indicative of appendicitis, and colicky pain is usually associated with intestinal disorders such as gastroenteritis or inflammatory bowel disease.

Assessment of the child with acute abdominal pain as with all ill/injured children begins with a rapid assessment of airway, breathing, circulation and disability and any compromise treated immediately as per resuscitation guidelines.

Further assessment and management includes recording of baseline and subsequent observations,

Box 17.2 Assessment of abdominal pain

The nurse should determine;

The duration of pain
The severity of pain
The exact location and any radiation
Factors which improve or worsen pain
The child's overall posture and level of activity
Associated symptoms, such as, vomiting, nausea, constipation, diarrhoea, dysuria/frequency and vaginal discharge, should be noted
Any obvious social influences, such as problems at school or family stresses, should not be dismissed

urinalysis, pain assessment and analgesics, and may include venepuncture, cannulation, intravenous fluids and specialist opinion if surgical intervention is considered necessary (Box 17.2).

Appendicitis

Appendectomy is the most common operation in childhood apart from ear, nose and throat surgery and is common to all age groups. If appendicitis cannot be ruled out as the cause of abdominal pain, the child is usually admitted to hospital for observation. The pain often subsides and the child is subsequently discharged with a diagnosis of non-specific abdominal pain.

In appendicitis the child usually gives a history of moderate pain, commencing centrally and moving down to the right iliac fossa (RIF). These children are often off their food, but continue to drink. They complain of nausea, and may or may not give a history of vomiting. Altered bowel habits including constipation and diarrhoea may be present.

On assessment, children with appendicitis are moderately unwell, the pulse rate may be raised, and the temperature can be normal or raised and usually ranges from 37.5 to 38.5°C. Abdominal examination will reveal guarding and rebound tenderness in the right iliac fossa area. If appendicitis is suspected, early surgical opinion is indicated. It should be noted, however, that appendicitis can progress to perforation and peritonitis without appropriate treatment.

Constipation

Children with constipation, particularly in the younger part of this age group, often present to ED with acute abdominal pain or rectal bleeding. This may be a result of the commencement of full-time schooling, a hectic morning household and poor condition of school toilets (Barnes 2003).

They may give a history of infrequent bowel activity, associated with small amounts of hard stools. History may consist of colicky abdominal pain, urinary symptoms including retention, anorexia and nausea. Rectal bleeding is not uncommon as a result of anal fissures. Physical assessment usually reveals no abnormality. Examination of the abdomen reveals a loaded descending colon. Abdominal X-ray is not recommended for the diagnosis of constipation (Royal College of Radiologists 1998). Management of constipation may include relief of acute discomfort, either with suppositories or a micro-enema. Many constipated children can be treated at home with oral medications of stool softeners and stimulants (titrated to response), toileting and dietary advice (Dale 2005). The child and parents should be advised that treatment may be necessary for 6–12 months and therefore continued follow-up by their GP, paediatrician (Dale 2005) or nurse led clinic where available (Muir & Burnett 1999) is essential.

Urinary tract infection

Urinary tract infection (UTI) comprises symptoms of infection, together with the presence of pathogenic micro-organisms in the urine, urethra, bladder or kidney. UTI is usually caused by bacteria from the gastrointestinal tract. UTIs are among the most common bacterial childhood infections and in seven-year-olds have an incidence of 2.8% in boys and 8.2% in girls (Coulthard et al. 1997).

A UTI should be considered in all children with undiagnosed malaise or pyrexia of unknown origin. Urinalysis is the most effective way to obtain a definitive diagnosis. It should be performed on any child presenting with dysuria, frequency, haematuria, and sudden onset enuresis, pain in the renal area and suprapubic pain, and any child with pyrexia for which no cause has been established (Morton & Phillips 1996).

Children rarely need admission for UTIs unless they are systemically unwell or unable to tolerate oral antibiotics. Most children can therefore be discharged with oral antibiotics and advice regarding increased fluid intake and supportive care. Paracetamol or ibuprofen relieves pain and high temperature. Parents should also be advised that follow-up from their GP is necessary following a UTI, which may involve radiological imaging and prophylactic antibiotic dependent on the age of the child and local practice (Barnes 2003).

CONSENT

Consent/refusal of treatment is a much-debated topic within the field of adult emergency departments. Consent in paediatrics can also give rise to much discussion and confusion.

Since the Children Act DoH (1989) a child under the age of 16 years of age has been able to consent to treatment if they are deemed Gillick competent or if not Gillick competent a parent can give consent on their behalf (Diamond 2006). Thus some of the children referred to in this chapter may be able to consent to treatment.

In order for a parent or child to give consent they must be given all relevant information and time and opportunity to ask questions; that is, to offer informed consent. A child who fully comprehends what they are consenting to and the consequences of that consent can be said to be Gillick competent (Waterston et al. 1997, Dimond 2001).

In some much-published cases children have refused treatment such as blood transfusions on religious grounds but courts of appeal have overturned the child's refusal and treatment has continued. In an ED where a child refuses consent to treatment an impossible situation arises whereby the nurse must attempt to obtain consent (with parental participation), giving further explanations regarding the necessity of treatment and consequences of refusing treatment. If the child continues to refuse then the best possible alternative treatment is used with comprehensive documentation in the child's notes.

In a life-threatening situation consent is not necessary, if the child is unaccompanied; the welfare of the child is paramount. If parents refuse treatment, e.g. blood transfusion, in a life-threatening situation on the grounds of religious beliefs, professionals who consider the treatment essential acquire consent as for an unaccompanied life-threatening situation.

Many children attend EDs unaccompanied or accompanied by an adult who is not a parent or guardian. Consent can be obtained from those who are:

- Gillick competent
- de facto carers
- from contacting parents to attend ED.

De facto carers include teachers, baby-sitters, step-parents or anyone currently caring for a child; the Children Act DoH (1989) gives such a person the right to make decisions on behalf of the child. Dimond (1996) suggests that ED staff could obtain consent from 'de facto' carers for immediately necessary treatment such as stitches or injections.

HEALTH PROMOTION

Many opportunities exist for health promotion in the ED. The waiting area can be used in a variety of ways to target both parents and children with specific aspects of health promotion and accident prevention. Displays about topical issues such as the prevention of sunburn, safety equipment and meningitis symptoms can provide parents and children with practical commonsense advice. Individual advice supported with written information can help to prevent recurrent accidents, as well as trouble-shooting the specific incident.

Distress is common in children and parents following an accident, even when the physical injury is minor; this is due to the sudden and unexpected nature of the incident, and emotional support may be necessary (Hepinstall 1996). The Child Action Prevention Trust produce a range of age-related leaflets addressing this issue.

Anecdotal evidence suggests an increase in the number of schoolchildren attending ED following incidents of bullying, even during primary school. Bullying involves persistent, deliberate, unprovoked, physical or psychological harm by a more powerful child or young person or group, against a weaker child or group and a proportion of all ages are faced with bullying daily (Smith 1996, Offler 2000).

Children who attend ED frequently with trivial complaints may be being bullied, or the child may disclose bullying at assessment. The nurse must be sensitive/supportive in these cases. Providing information about other agencies such as Kidscape and Childline for ongoing support and management is vital. Bullied children are often reluctant to involve schoolteachers if bullying is occurring in school, but most schools have adopted an anti-bullying policy; gentle persuasion may convince the child that 'telling' will stop the bully and prevent others being bullied. Referral to the school nurse may provide a link within the school environment.

Obese children and young people may be the victims of bullying and as a consequence attend the ED. There is a lack of agreement of the diagnostic criteria for the classification of obesity but studies demonstrate an increased prevalence (Fruhbeck 2000, Ruxton 2004). Childhood obesity may lead to long-term health problems, including hypertension, sleep apnoea, asthma, early puberty, diabetes, back pain and slipped upper femoral epiphysis (Ruxton 2004). Treatment of childhood obesity involves promoting a healthy diet, increased physical activity and a behavioural component (Fruhbeck 2000, Ruxton 2004). In

the ED it involves the treatment of the presenting complaint and promotion of a healthy lifestyle.

Parents attending the ED may be victims of domestic abuse. Domestic violence impacts on the child directly and indirectly and is now a recognized form of child abuse.

Effects of domestic violence on a child include:

- actual physical injury to the child
- emotional effects of witnessing abuse of a parent
- potential difficulties in accessing healthcare. (Spencer 2002, Evans 2001, Evans 2005)

As with bullying, the ED nurse must be sensitive to the needs of the child and abused parent; the ED is for many the first agency the family turns to for help. Physical injuries are cared for and the impact on the child is dealt with as per local child protection policy. The ED nurse should then provide guidance to other agencies such as women's aid groups, the NSPCC, domestic violence units, health visitors and school nurse services.

All children attending the ED are potentially victims of child abuse (Chudleigh 2005, Sanders & Cobley 2005), domestic violence or bullying. The ED nurse must be conversant with trigger factors to these types of incident and be able to provide support and information and refer to the appropriate agency. Although issues of child protection arise across the whole of childhood and beyond, this issue is considered in detail in Chapter 16: Pre-school children.

CONCLUSION

Children attend emergency departments following accidents as a result of the environment in which they live; many attend using the department as a primary health care. Such patients are often labelled as inappropriate attenders; however, Burton (1993) suggests that ED nurses are obliged to meet the needs of all attending children, giving them the best possible service.

The needs of children between the ages of 5 and 13 vary considerably. The ED nurse must have an awareness of the developmental stages of children in order to provide appropriate care. The ED environment is important, as is the attitude of staff to children and their families. Optimum care results from a family-centred approach, with aftercare advice directed at the child and parent in order to achieve concordance.

References

Action for Sick Children (1997) *Emergency Health Services for Children and Young People, A Guide for Commissioners and Providers.* London: Action for Sick Children.

Advanced Life Support Group (2001) *Advanced Paediatric Life Support*, 3rd edn. London: BMJ Books.

Audit Commission (1996) *By Accident or Design: Improving Emergency Care in Acute Hospitals.* London: HMSO.

Barkin RM, Rosen P (1994) *Abuse in Emergency Pediatrics: a Guide to Ambulatory Care*, 4th edn. St Louis: Mosby.

Barnes K (2003) *Paediatrics: A Clinical Guide for Nurse Practitioners.* Edinburgh: Butterworth Heinemann.

British Association for Accident and Emergency Medicine (1997) *Guidelines for Analgesia in Children in A&E.* London: BAEM.

Bruce E, Frank L (2000) Self-administered nitrous oxide (Entonox) for management of procedural pain. *Paediatric Nursing*, **12**(7), 15–19.

Burton R (1993) The child in A&E; a philosophy of care. In: Glasper EA Tucker A (eds) *Advances in Child Health Nursing.* Harrow: Scutari Press.

Candy D, Davies G, Ross E (2001) *Clinical Paediatrics and Child Health.* Edinburgh: WB Saunders.

Casey A (1993) Development and use of the partnership model of nursing care. In: Glasper EA, Tucker A, eds. *Advances in Child Health Nursing.* Harrow: Scutari Press.

Chudleigh J (2005) Safeguarding Children. *Paediatric Nursing*, **17**(1), 37–42.

Coulthard MG, Lambert HJ, Keir MJ (1997) Occurrence of renal scars in children after their first referral urinary tract infection. *British Medical Journal*, **315**, 918–919.

Cudmore J, Lakin K (1997) Child Care in A&E: exploring the issues. *Emergency Nurse*, **5**(5), 10–11.

Dale A (2005) Managing constipation and soiling. *The Practitioner*, **249**, 490–500.

Davies FCW (2003) *Minor Trauma in Children.* London: Arnold.

Department for Education and Skills/Department of Health (2005) *Ill Child Standard, National Service Framework for Children, Young People and Maternity Services.* London: Department of Health.

DoH (1989) *The Children Act.* London: HMSO.

Department of Health (1991) *Welfare of Children and Young People in Hospital.* London: HMSO.

Department of Health (1995) *Children's Charter.* London: HMSO.

Department of Health (2005) *Improving Responses for Children and Young People Requiring Emergency or Urgent Care.* London: Department of Health.

Dimond B (1996) *The Legal Aspects of Health Care.* Mosby: London.

Dimond B (2001) Legal Aspects of Consent 8: children under the age of 16. *British Journal of Nursing*, **10**(12), 797–798.

Evans R (2001) Children living with domestic violence. *Emergency Nurse*, **9**(6), 22–26.

Evans N (2005) Domestic violence: recognising the signs. *Paediatric Nursing*, **17**(1), 14–16.

Foster H, Kay L (2003) Examination skills in the assessment of the musculoskeletal system in children and adolescents. *Current Paediatrics*, **13**, 341–344.

Fruhbeck G (2000) Childhood obesity: time for action, not complacency. *British Medical Journal*, **320**, 328–329.

Hall J (2002) Paediatric pain assessment. *Emergency Nurse*, **10**(6), 31–33.

Hawkins D, Metheny J (2001) Overuse injuries in youth sports: biomechanical considerations. *Medicine & Science in Sports & Exercise*, **33**(10), 1701–1707.

Hepinstall E (1996) *Healing the Hidden Hurt, the Emotional Effects of Children's Accidents.* London: CAPT.

Hopkins SJ (1992) *Drugs and Pharmacology for Nurses*, 11th edn. Edinburgh: Churchill Livingstone.

Kennedy I (2001) *The Report of the Public Health Inquiry into Children's Heart Surgery at the Bristol Royal Infirmary.* London: The Stationery Office.

Lee P (2001) Is partnership in A&E possible? *Journal of Child Health*, **5**(1), 26–29.

Mead D, Sibert J (1991) *The Injured Child – An Action Plan for Nurses.* Harrow: Scutari Press.

Morcombe J (1998) Reducing anxiety in children in A&E. *Emergency Nurse*, **6**(2), 10–13.

Morton RJ, Phillips BM (1996) *Accidents and Emergencies in Children*, 2nd edn. Oxford University Press: Oxford.

Muir J and Burnett C (1999) Setting up a nurse-led clinic for intractable childhood constipation. *British Journal of Community Nursing*, **4**(8), 395–399.

Muller DJ, Harris PJ, Watley L (1986) *Nursing Children: Psychology, Research and Practice.* London: Hodder and Stoughton.

National Institute for Clinical Excellence (NICE) (2005) *Improving Outcomes in Children and Young People with Cancer: The Evidence Review.* London: NICE.

Nunn J (1994) The use of aspirin in children under 12 years old attending a paediatric dentistry department in a dental hospital. *Health Trends*, **26**(1), 31–32.

O'Brennan P, Yassa JG, Ludwig S (2001) *Paediatric Emergency Medicine.* London: Manson Publishing.

Offler E (2000) Bullying: everybody's problem. *Paediatric Nursing*, **12**(9), 22–26.

Piaget J (1983) Piaget's theory. In: P. Mussen (ed). *Handbook of Child Psychology.* 4th edn. Vol. 1. New York: Wiley.

Royal College of Nursing (1998) *Nursing Children in the A&E Department*, 2nd edn. London: RCN.

Royal College of Nursing (2001) *Recognition and Assessment of Acute Pain in Children.* London: RCN.

Royal College of Paediatrics and Child Health (2003) *Medicines for Children.* Southampton: RCPCH Publications.

Ruxton C (2004) Obesity in children. *Nursing Standard*, **18**(20), 47–55.

Sabin MA, Crowne EC, Shield JPH (2004) The prognosis in childhood obesity. *Current Paediatrics*, **14**(2), 110–115.

Sanders T, Cobley C (2005) Identifying non-accidental injury in children presenting to A&E departments: an overview of the literature. *Accident and Emergency Nursing*, **13**, 130–136.

Scottish Intercollegiate Guidelines Network (2002) *Guideline 58: Safe Sedation of Children Undergoing Diagnostic and Therapeutic Procedures.* Edinburgh: SINE.

Smith C (1995) IV cannulation: principles and practice. *Emergency Nurse*, **2**(4), 16–18.

Smith P (1996) *Is Your Child the Playground Bully?* Royal College of Psychiatrists, Child and Adolescent Section, Fact sheet 5. London: Royal College of Psychiatrists.

Spedding RL, Harley D, Dunn FJ McKinnek LA (1999) Who gives pain relief to children? *Journal of Accident and Emergency Medicine*, **16**, 261–264.

Spencer D (2002) Paediatric trauma: when it is not an accident? *Accident and Emergency Nursing*, **10**, 143–148.

Swanwick M (1990) Knowledge and control. *Paediatric Nursing*, **2**(5), 18–20.

Royal College of Radiologists (1998) *Making the Best Use of a Department of Clinical Radiology Guidelines for Doctors*, 4th edn. London: The Royal College of Radiologists.

Twycross A (1998) The management of acute pain in children, *Professional-Nurse*, **14**(2), 95–98.

Visintainer MA, Wolfer JA (1975) Psychological preparation for surgery paediatric patients: the effects on children's and parents stress responses and adjustment, *Paediatrics*, **56**(2), 187–202.

Waterson T, Helms P, Ward-Platt M (2000) *Paediatrics Understanding Child Health*. Oxford: Oxford University Press.

Woodward S (1994) A guide to paediatric resuscitation *Paediatrics Nursing*. **6**(2), 16–18.

Chapter 18

Adolescence

Lynda Holt

INTRODUCTION

Adolescents represent only a small percentage of the total number of patients seen in emergency departments (EDs). Their care, however, needs to be specialized and related to their individual stage of development. This chapter will highlight the common areas of adolescent development, such as risk-taking behaviour, and explore them in relation to ED attendance. Sensation-seeking, leading to potentially deviant behaviour such as violent acts, substance misuse and self-harm, will also be considered, as will the generic effects of illness and injury on adolescents. The impact of caring for adolescents on ED nurses will also be examined. Optimum care environments and appropriate nursing skills will be discussed with regard to the quality of service offered to adolescents attending ED.

ADOLESCENT DEVELOPMENT

The research on adolescent development is vast (Erikson 1965, Leon & Smith 2001, Croghan 2005). An understanding of adolescent development is essential for ED nurses in their daily practice. Adolescence is a period in the life span where the individual, previously dependent on parents and carers for his values and identity, becomes independent and, in this move towards independence, attempts to establish a new and personal identity. The key factors in this process appear to relate to the onset of puberty, i.e. the physical and emotional changes leading to sexual maturity (Bickley & Szilagyi 2003, Tortora & Grabowski 2003), and the need for independence (Erikson 1965).

Cognitively, adolescents are capable of abstract thought and understand many variables within a situation. They should also be able to understand the consequences of their actions (Bernardo & Schenkel 1995). It is a period where group identity is vital, a time of experimentation with self-image, and a time to question fundamental family values. Adolescents are pushing for independence, testing the boundaries of their existing life and, importantly, hoping to find boundaries which will aid the development of their future identity (Croghan 2005).

CARING FOR THE ADOLESCENT IN ED

As a client group, adolescents are considered difficult to care for by the majority of nurses (Holt 1993). In ED, many causes of adolescent attendance can be viewed as self-inflicted, e.g. as a result of alcohol or substance testing, which may render ED nurses less compassionate towards the patient. Caring for adolescents presents a particular challenge, as many nurses are just emerging from adolescence themselves. Kelly (1991) suggested that, to the adolescent, these nurses represent a more realistic role model, enhancing the opportunity for health education. This is particularly pertinent to ED nurses because there is a greater likelihood of interaction with this age group at a time when they are physically and emotionally vulnerable.

Providing ED nurses with a better idea of the process of adolescence may equip them more satisfactorily to meet their patients' needs, which will enable them to recognize normal behaviour instead of reacting to it (Holt 1993).

Nurses are generally less aware of teenagers' needs than those of other age groups. In ED, adult care is the most familiar and, because of the associated anxiety, paediatric care is more often discussed or taught. An understanding of adolescent development could help nurses in ED to provide holistic care. It would also enable nurses to rationalize behaviour such as rebellion, non-conformity, antagonism and paranoia, which is frequently demonstrated in hospital, but is arguably the normal behaviour for an adolescent whose independence has been threatened by illness or injury (Kelly 1991).

Hospital staff, especially in emergency departments, are quick to meet the physical needs of these patients, such as maintaining a safe environment for the drunk teenager or arresting haemorrhage in a patient with slashed wrists, but often with little regard to their emotional needs (Kuykendall 1989). An understanding of these needs, however, could reduce the risk of confrontation and diminish any perceived power struggle. The question for ED nurses is how far these needs can be facilitated within an ED department without compromising the care or well-being of others in the environment. When young

people are asked why they do not use health services they admit to feeling intimidated by both the service and the service providers, they dislike the times and locations, and are concerned about confidentiality and trust (Croghan 2005, Croghan et al. 2004, Leon & Smith 2001).

As with all patients, initial assessment is the key to forming a therapeutic relationship, and the adolescent's response to illness and possible treatment can be quickly gauged, as well as existing coping strategies. Privacy has an important effect on the adolescent because of the significance of self-image; for instance, a wound assessment takes seconds but can cause great embarrassment. Ensuring privacy increases self-esteem and reinforces the adolescent's importance as an individual. Independence is often threatened by hospitalization, even a short period in ED. Including the patient in the care planning and decision-making reduces non-compliance and aggressive behaviour. Separation is greatly underestimated as a stress for adolescents (Blunden 1988). While they demand peer belonging and demonstrate independence, most need and want parental support (Bernardo & Schenkel 1995). Parents themselves often underestimate the support needed and the fears of adolescents. This may be because of swift medical and nursing intervention aimed at promoting physical well-being. While ED nurses are quick to include the parents of a sick child, perhaps, because of the demonstrated independence of adolescents, this inclusion is often overlooked.

The adolescent patient needs to assert his independence, but is not yet ready to cope with the implications of this. In 'crisis' situations, as a visit to ED is often perceived, the ED nurse may be in a position of setting boundaries for the patient. This is not a negative action as it provides the security the adolescent indirectly seeks. All too often, however, on a busy shift, in a packed waiting room, antagonistic behaviour is allowed to escalate into confrontation, often because cues for boundaries have not been recognized by ED nurses inexperienced in adolescent development. Consistency among staff is essential (Gilles 1992). Boundaries for acceptable behaviour should be decided as a matter of policy, and this should be made clear to patients on admission while respecting their independence and individuality. In addition, Knight & Rush (1998) argue that waiting rooms should be made more 'user-friendly' for adolescents, ideally incorporating separate waiting and treatment areas.

Illness or injury often induces developmental regression, forces the adolescent out of his peer group and imposes a fear of rejection. Even in a short admission to ED, nurses need to work towards reducing this anxiety. It is paramount for adolescents to be cared for by staff who are comfortable with them, and can behave as adults, listening to them and respecting their needs. Adolescents are not children and, especially at times of high stress, do not respond well to being railroaded by ED personnel who are threatened or irritated by their behaviour.

PERSONAL FABLE

Despite the upheaval and trauma of adolescence during this life phase, mortality is at its lowest, with the top cause of death being accident-related (Department of Health 2004). An important cause of accident in adolescence is risk-taking behaviour, not just risky sports, but minor law infringement such as failure to wear a safety belt, exceeding speed limits and experimentation with alcohol and illegal substances (Bellis et al. 2005).

A possible explanation of this is the concept of personal fable (Jack 1989) – a belief that despite risk-taking behaviour they will not be affected by life's difficulties. This has both a positive and a negative function, and represents normal cognitive development. Positively, it allows goals to be believed in and attainable, such as dreams of success. Its negative function is that it induces risk-taking behaviour. Normally, consequences of actions are considered, but personal fable gives the security of invulnerability to consequences. This is not unique to adolescents; witness, for example, smoking and lung cancer in older people (Winkenstein 1992).

Personal fable affects not only conformity with perceived authority, but also with chronic illnesses, such as diabetes. It is important for ED nurses to understand this concept in order to intervene in the risk-taking behaviour that can result in an ED attendance. Personal fable is there to protect the self-concept at the vulnerable time of adolescence. It allows conformity with peers despite negative consequences – for instance, the diabetic patient who presents in ED with hypoglycaemia because he has been drinking to conform with peers. The patient can 'blot out' the likely hypoglycaemic attack because being the same is more important. Education and support from ED nurses who understand that this behaviour is not intended to be self-destructive, but is normal adolescent experimentation, can reduce the risk of further occurrence. This perception of invulnerability may contribute to the statistic that the largest cause of adolescent death is from risk-taking – in cars, with fire-arms, in water and with toxic substances (Jack 1989). Sensitive questioning helps adolescents expose their personal myth, recognize their irrationality and induce a change in behaviour.

RISK-TAKING BEHAVIOUR

Most common behaviours evolve from experimentation with alcohol, solvents or drugs, but it can be hard for the busy ED nurse to accept the drunk who is abusive as 'normal' when his behaviour is disruptive and difficult to contain. The majority of adolescents who attend ED with drug- or alcohol-related problems are not abusive, and are there because of an injury or illness related to their risk-taking behaviour. These individuals often present with their peer groups and engage in sensation-seeking behaviour, which can appear threatening to ED nurses. Adequate staffing levels and nurse skill mix, with appropriate back-up such as security officers and an incident alarm, should be available. Sensation-seeking is a normal need for experimentation and new experiences, and adolescents are prepared to take physical and social risks to attain these (Barker 1988). Despite risk-taking and sensation-seeking, most adolescents maintain conventional modes of behaviour and deviants are in the minority. Emergency departments frequently treat adolescents as a result of risk-taking behaviour. A non-judgemental attitude is not always easy to foster, and the ED nurse must be aware of her own vulnerability and biases, as well as understanding adolescent development. This enables the nurse to treat adolescents in an appropriate manner, reduces the risk of confrontation or resentment, and respects the adolescents' rights as individuals.

Not all adolescent risk-taking is because of a low perception of danger. Some revolves around deliberate self-harm. This is usually a cry for help from adolescents who cannot cope with the pressures of growing up. Self-poisoning is the most common reason for hospital treatment (House 1998, Whotton 2002). Only the minority of adolescents take this route, and of these the majority are not clinically depressed. This course of behaviour is not just a result of the strains of adolescence, identity confusion, anger and guilt; it is a way of getting back at those seen as responsible for the torment, such as parents, teachers and peers. A study of 100 children after overdose found that only 6% actually wanted to harm themselves, and over 50% had no idea of the risks associated with the pills taken, reinforcing the need for health education. Those questioned did not consider death a real possibility (Donovan et al. 1985). Adolescent patients often demonstrate this by a blasé attitude towards their actions. Despite low suicide intent, the danger of real harm is great because of low risk awareness. The prevalence of mental health problems among adolescents is estimated at 10–20%, while the incidence of suicide among young men continues to increase and is linked to lifestyle behaviours such as alcohol and drug misuse, and mental health problems (Department of Health 2001a, Marfé 2003). Hawton et al. (1999), following a review based on coroners' and medical records of 174 cases of patients, aged under 25 years, who had committed suicide, found that a previous non-fatal suicide attempt is a predictor for further suicide attempts. Box 18.1 outlines the risk range for suicide among young people.

It is vital that nurses are able to distinguish between normal behaviour and abnormal distress. This can only be achieved by listening to and hearing the adolescent. Nothing should be taken at face value, as the superficial self-confidence and frequent mood changes common to teenagers can mask real and needy patients, as well as making them difficult to nurse. It is recognized that ED is not the ideal place for in-depth discussion, but it may be the only opportunity available to the adolescent. An understanding of why the event occurred is essential before discharging the patient. The adolescent practice of 'dumping distress' on others via self-harm must be controlled and appropriate coping strategies learned in order to prevent further real harm. The ED nurse has a key role to play, by providing constructive advice and follow-up arrangements where appropriate, not by punitive intervention. (See also Chapter 14: Psychiatric Emergencies.)

Box 18.1   Risk categories for adolescent suicide (Marfé 2003)

The young person at extremely high risk:

- has made previous attempts at serious self-harm
- has clear intentions of a wish to die
- has made a deliberate premeditated suicide attempt
- has obtained the agent (tablets etc.) prior to that day
- believes that the agent or his or her actions would cause significant harm
- has specifically arranged a time when he or she reckoned to be alone
- has left a note
- has failed to tell anyone about his or her self-harm attempt
- is still planning serious self-harm
- regrets that he or she was unsuccessful in his or her attempt
- appears to be extremely depressed or despondent

The young person at high risk:

- has tried to seriously self-harm him or herself before
- gives clear reasons for his or her actions, which still pose a risk
- made a suicide attempt that was planned or impulsive
- deliberately bought the agent (tablets etc.) that day, or previously
- was aware that the agent was harmful
- left a note
- was alone when the attempt was made
- is still experiencing suicidal feelings
- is regretful or uncertain about the failed attempt at serious self-harm
- appears extremely depressed

The young person at moderate risk:

- has a history of deliberate self-harm, risk taking or impulsive behaviour
- has a history of poor stress-coping mechanisms
- has no clear intention or a wish to seriously self-harm
- has given clear reasons for actions – but they no longer pose an obvious risk
- has made an attempt to deliberately self-harm, but with no actual suicide intent
- obtained the agent (tablets etc.) impulsively that day
- was not fully aware of the effects of the overdose
- made the attempt at self-harm while others were in the vicinity
- informed others of his or her actions
- is glad he or she did not die
- may still be considering other forms of self-harm (cutting etc.)

The young person at low risk:

- has no history of previous deliberate self-harm or risk-taking behaviour
- has no history of poor stress-coping mechanisms
- has no intentions of, or a wish to, seriously self-harm
- has given clear reasons for his or her actions, which were never intended to pose a risk
- has made his or her self-harm actions known to others appropriately
- accomplished the self-harm when others were in the vicinity
- is not planning self-harm of any kind

SUBSTANCE MISUSE

Within the past 20 years, the worldwide drug culture has evolved dramatically, stemming from two developments. First, the major consumer generation has shifted sharply towards the young, especially adolescent and young adult males; and second, the availability of drugs has become much more widespread (Emmett & Nice 1996). In the UK, around 20–30% of people aged 16–59 years, and about half of those aged 16–29, have taken an illegal substance at some time (Ramsey & Percy 1997). Recent use, which is more likely to reflect regular use, is also highest among people aged 16–29 years, especially if they live in an inner city or are unemployed; up to 18% will have taken one drug, and around 5% will have taken two or more, in the previous month (Ramsey & Percy 1997). In 1994, over 1600 deaths were attributed to misuse of illegal drugs (Home Office 1996). In the UK, it is estimated that 6% of the population, around three million people, take at least one illegal drug in any one year (HMSO 1994). Heroin is the most frequently reported main drug of misuse (64%), followed by methadone (10%), cannabis (9%), cocaine (6%) and amphetamines (4%) (Department of Health 2001b, Rassool 2002). While substance misuse is clearly a problem for young adults as well as adolescents, for convenience the subject will be addressed in this chapter.

In addition, the growth of the rave scene in Britain and designer drugs such as ecstasy, which appear to have become accepted by many as an integral part of relaxation and pleasure, have resulted in a culture in which substance misuse is no longer perceived as an antisocial activity, but where penalties for use and supply are severe (see Box 18.2 and Table 18.1). While the ED nurse will be aware that alcohol is a major causative factor in attendances, there has been a marked increase in attendances as a consequence of other substance misuse.

The mild, moderate and severe effects of drugs of abuse are outlined in Tables 18.2–18.4.

Alcohol

Despite its legal status as a controlled substance, alcohol is the most widely available and commonly used psychoactive substance among adolescents aged 12 to 16 (Rassool & Winnington 2003). Alcohol is a central nervous system depressant. It is absorbed into the bloodstream and starts to have an effect within 5–10 minutes of drinking. The rate of absorption is affected by sex, weight, duration of drinking, nature of drink consumed, food in the stomach, physiological factors, genetic variation and rate of elimination. Paton (1994) suggested that there are 4 million heavy drinkers in the UK, of whom 800 000 are problem drinkers and 400 000 are alcohol-dependent. Boys & Farrell (2001) found that 65% of students were between 13 and 14 years old when they first had their first whole drinking session without their parents knowing. The most popular drinking locations were friends' houses (69%), at home (50%), in parks and on the streets (30%) and in public bars (30%). More than 25% of students aged 15–16 reported three or more binge drinking sessions in the past month (Department of Health 2002). Every year, the adverse effects of alcohol consumption lead to an estimated 1.2 million assaults, result in 150 000 hospital admissions and cost the NHS £1.7 billion (Smith & Allen 2004, Strategy Unit 2003). Concomitant misuse of alcohol is also common among drug misusers. Signs, symptoms and management of alcohol intoxication are addressed in Chapter 14.

Ecstasy

Ecstasy is a synthetic hallucinogenic form of amphetamine. It was first synthesized in Germany in 1910 and patented as an appetite suppressant. It failed commercially and did not reappear until the late 1980s, when it became associated with the 'rave' scene. In its pure form, it is seen as a white powder, but is usually found as tablets or capsules. The colour will depend on any colouring agents that have been added. Ecstasy tablets frequently have images of animals or birds imprinted on them. Ecstasy is generally taken orally and is very rarely injected or smoked (Milroy 1999).

For most users, ecstasy provides a feeling of euphoria, together with an increase in confidence, serenity and empathy towards other people. As an amphetamine derivative, it also provides users with feelings of energy and freedom from hunger. Ecstasy use frequently leads to jaw clenching and teeth grinding (gurning), which causes tooth surface loss (Nixon et al. 2002). While adverse reactions are rare, Cook (1995) and Preston (1992) described the presenting signs of severe reaction as convulsion and collapse, dilated pupils, hypotension, tachycardia, hyperpyrexia and death from disseminated intravascular coagulation. Walsh and Kent (2001) suggest that signs which should alert an ED nurse to an ecstasy-induced collapse include admission from a late night party or rave of a previously fit young person who has collapsed for no apparent reason. Some deaths have been related to cerebral oedema secondary to excess water ingestion, because the drug has an antidiuretic effect on the kidney (Braback & Humble 2001).

Box 18.2 Penalties under Misuse of Drugs Act 1971

Class A, schedule one

- *Simple possession*
  Maximum penalty on indictment is 7 years' imprisonment together with an unlimited fine
- *Possession with intent to supply*
- Possessing a class A, schedule one drug with intent to supply, either by sale or by gift, to another person carries a maximum penalty on indictment of life imprisonment together with an unlimited fine and the seizure of all drug-related assets
- *Supplying to another*
  As for possession with intent to supply
- *Examples of class A, schedule one drugs*
  - LSD
  - magic mushrooms

Class A, schedule two

- *Simple possession*
  Maximum penalty on indictment is 14 years together with an unlimited fine
- *Possession with intent to supply*
  Possessing a class A, schedule two drug with intent to supply, either by sale or by gift, to another person carries a maximum penalty on indictment of life imprisonment together with an unlimited fine
- *Supplying to another*
  As for possession with intent to supply
- *Examples of class A, schedule two drugs*
  - cocaine
  - crack and freebase cocaine
  - heroin
  - methadone
  - ecstasy
  - LSD

Class B, schedule one

- *Simple possession*
  Maximum penalty on indictment is 5 years together with an unlimited fine
- *Possession with intent to supply*
  Possessing a class B, schedule one drug with intent to supply, either by sale or by gift, to another person carries a maximum penalty on indictment of 14 years' imprisonment together with an unlimited fine and the seizure of drug-related assets.
- *Supplying to another*
  As for possession with intent to supply
- *Example of class B, schedule one drug*
  - amphetamine

Class B, schedule two

- *Simple possession*
  Maximum penalty on indictment is 5 years' imprisonment together with an unlimited fine
- *Possession with intent to supply*
  Possessing a class B, schedule two drug with intent to supply, either by sale or by gift, to another person carries a maximum penalty on indictment of 14 years' imprisonment together with an unlimited fine and the seizure of drug-related assets
- *Supplying to another*
  As for possession with intent to supply
- *Examples of class B, schedule two drugs*
  - amphetamines
  - methylamphetamine

Class B, schedule three

- *Simple possession*
  Maximum penalty on indictment is 5 years' imprisonment together with an unlimited fine
- *Possession with intent to supply*
  Possessing a class B, schedule three drug with intent to supply, either by sale or by gift, to another person carries a maximum penalty on indictment of 5 years' imprisonment together with an unlimited fine
- *Supplying to another*
  As for possession with intent to supply
- *Example of class B, schedule three drug*
  Tranquillisers

Class C

- *Simple possession*
  Maximum penalty on indictment is 2 years' imprisonment and/or an unlimited fine
- *Possession with intent to supply*
  Possessing a Class C drug with intent to supply, either by sale or by gift, to another person carries a maximum penalty indictment of 14 years' imprisonment and/or an unlimited fine
- *Supplying to another*
  As for possession with intent to supply
- *Examples of class C drugs*
  - cannabis
  - benzodiazepines
  - temazepam
  - anabolic steroids
  - GHB

Table 18.1   Language of substance misuse (Emmett & Nice 1996)

Word	Meaning
Acid	LSD
Bad trip	A frightening or unpleasant LSD trip
Banging up	To inject drugs
Blow	Herbal cannabis
Buzzing	Feelings after use of ecstasy
Chill out	A period of cooling down to reduce risk of overheating from ecstasy use
Clean	Not using drugs
Coke	Cocaine
Crack	Freebase cocaine
Cut	To mix other substances with a drug to add bulk and weight
Detox	To withdraw from drugs under medical supervision
Dope	Resin and herbal cannabis
Doves	Ecstasy tablets with dove imprint
'E'	Ecstasy
Eggs	Temazepam tablets
Flashback	Tripping out again some time after LSD use. Can be days, months or even years later and is usually a bad trip (q.v.)
GBH	Gamma hydroxybutyrate or sodium oxybate, a liquid hallucinogenic stimulant
Grass	Herbal cannabis
'H'	Heroin
Hash	Cannabis resin
High	The feeling of elation while under the influence of a drug
Hit	To buy or inject drugs
Jack up	To inject drugs
Jellies	Temazepam in capsule form
Joint	A hand-rolled cannabis cigarette
Magic mushrooms	Any of the species of hallucinogenic mushrooms
Main lining	Injecting drugs
Marijuana	Herbal cannabis
Moggies	Mogadon sleeping pills
Poppers	Amyl/alkyl/butyl nitrate
Pot	Cannabis resin
Rock	Freebase cocaine
Score	To purchase drugs
Shoot up	To inject drugs
Smack	Heroin
Snorting	Sniffing cocaine or other drug up the nose
Speed	Amphetamine
Stash	An amount of drugs, usually hidden
Trip	A hallucinogenic experience under LSD
Wacky bacci	Herbal cannabis
Whiz	Amphetamine
Works	Needles and syringes

The control of the patient's temperature is the key to survival, as temperatures of up to 42°C are not uncommon. Cool replacement fluids should be given at as fast a rate as the patient can tolerate and unnecessary clothing should be removed. A brisk fluid-led diuresis should be encouraged; however, if this does not control the rise in temperature then endotracheal intubation, sedation and paralysis will be instituted (Henry et al.

1992). If the temperature continues to rise, dantrolene may be used. This has muscle-relaxant properties and is used in the treatment of malignant hyperthermia following anaesthetic hypersensitivity (Jones 1993).

A central venous catheter should be inserted to measure and guide the rapid dehydration of the patient, and a urinary catheter to monitor renal function. The colour of the urine should be observed for

Table 18.2 Mild clinical effects of drugs of abuse (Schofield et al. 1997)

Clinical effects	MDMA	Amphetamine	Cocaine	Cannabis	LSD
Gastrointestinal effects	✓	✓	✓	✓	✓ (i.v.)
Dilated pupils	✓	✓	✓	✓ (child)	✓
Dry mouth	✓	✓		✓	
Slurred speech			✓	✓ (high dose)	
Salivation					✓
Appetite stimulation				✓	
Chest discomfort		✓	✓		
Agitation	✓	✓	✓	✓ (high dose)	✓
Relaxation				✓	
Tremor	✓	✓	✓	✓ (child)	✓
Ataxia			✓	✓ (child)	✓
Sweating	✓	✓	✓	✓ (child)	
Mild increase in body temperature	✓	✓	✓		
Trismus (jaw clenching)	✓	✓	✓		
Bruxism (teeth grinding)	✓	✓	✓		

Table 18.3 Moderate clinical effects of drugs of abuse (Schofield et al. 1997)

Clinical effects	MDMA	Amphetamine	Cocaine	Cannabis	LSD
Headache	✓	✓	✓	✓	✓ (i.v.)
Hypertonia	✓		✓		✓
Hypotonia				✓	
Hyperreflexia	✓	✓	✓		✓
Hyperventilation	✓	✓	✓		✓ (i.v.)
Incontinence			✓		
Extrapyramidal symptoms	✓		✓		
Tachycardia	✓	✓	✓	✓ (high dose)	✓
Hypertension	✓	✓	✓	✓	
Hallucinations	✓	✓	✓	✓ (high dose)	✓
Paranoia	✓		✓	✓ (high dose)	
Palpitations	✓	✓	✓	✓	
Dehydration	✓	✓			
Hypothermia				✓ (child)	
Drowsiness			✓	✓	

an orange tinge which is suggestive of rhabdomyolysis, the breakdown of skeletal muscle, due to the toxic effects of released globins. Blood tests for creatinine kinase may be ordered to measure this process. Other blood tests may include regular clotting tests, and the patient should be closely observed for clinical signs of coagulation problems. The picture of disseminated intravascular coagulation, falling platelet and fibrinogen count, raised PT and KCCT is an ominous sign (Jones 1993).

Cannabis

Cannabis is the most commonly used illegal drug in the world. It is the collective term for all psychoactive substances derived from the dried leaves and flowers of

Table 18.4 Severe clinical effects of drugs of abuse (Schofield et al. 1997)

Clinical effects	MDMA	Amphetamine	Cocaine	Cannabis	LSD
Pyrexia	✓	✓	✓	✓	✓ (mild)
Delirium	✓	✓	✓		✓
Hypotension	✓	✓	✓	✓ (high dose)	
Convulsions	✓	✓	✓		✓ (i.v.)
Hypoxia	✓		✓		
Coma	✓	✓	✓	✓ (child)	✓
Arrhythmias/ dysrhythmias	✓	✓	✓		
Myocardial infarction			✓		
Rhabdomyolysis	✓	✓	✓		✓ (i.v.)
Renal failure	✓	✓	✓		✓ (i.v.)
Disseminated intravascular coagulation (DIC)	✓	✓	✓		✓ (i.v.)
Pulmonary oedema			✓		✓ (i.v.)
Adult respiratory distress syndrome (ARDS)	✓				
Subarachnoid/intra- cerebral haemorrhage	✓	✓	✓		

the plant *Cannabis sativa* (Schofield et al. 1997). It may be smoked or eaten in food. If smoked, its effects appear within 10–30 minutes and the effects have a duration of 4–8 hours. If eaten, it takes approximately 1 hour to produce its effects. Cannabis comes in three forms:

- herbal – a dried plant material, similar to coarse cut tobacco and sometimes compressed into blocks
- resin – dried and compressed sap, found in blocks of various sizes, shapes and colours
- oil – this is rare; it is extracted from the resin by the use of a chemical solvent and ranges in colour from dark green or dark brown to jet black with a distinctive smell like rotting vegetation.

After use, cannabis has the effect of creating feelings of relaxation, happiness, increased powers of concentration, sexual arousal, loss of inhibitions, increased appetite and talkativeness (Kalant 2004). There is little evidence that smoking cannabis is harmful in the short term, but users will develop a strong psychological habituation with continued use. Furthermore, it seems that adolescents become dependent more readily than adults. For daily or near-daily users, 35% of adolescents became dependent as opposed to 18% of adult users (Chen et al. 1997, Campbell 1999). Withdrawal effects include disturbed sleep patterns, anxiety, panic and restlessness.

It is with these effects that patients may present to the ED department and they should be managed symptomatically.

Amphetamine

Amphetamines are central nervous system stimulants whose action resembles those of adrenaline. They produce a sensation of euphoria and exhilaration as well as increased energy, stamina and strength. They may be injected intravenously, ingested or smoked. Absorbed by the gastrointestinal tract they may have an effect within 20 minutes of ingestion; however, the effects are immediate if injected and last 4–6 hours. They are most commonly seen in the form of a coarse off-white/pink crystalline powder with an average purity of less than 5%.

Signs and symptoms of intoxication include tachypnoea, tachycardia, dilatation of pupils, dry mouth, pyrexia, blurring of vision, dizziness and loss of coordination. The after-effects of lethargy and fatigue can last for several days. Since tolerance develops rapidly, individual response varies greatly, and toxicity correlates poorly with dose. Amphetamines also suppress appetite and, if used regularly, can lead to substantial weight loss (Bellis et al. 2005). Fatalities are rarely reported but predominantly result from convulsions and intracranial haemorrhage. Sedatives, such as chlorpromazine, and antihypertensives may be used for management of the patient.

Cocaine

Cocaine is derived from the leaves of the coca bush, *Erythoxylon coca*, or may be synthesized artificially. It is commonly seen as a white crystalline powder with a sparkling appearance. It is a central nervous system stimulant and is commonly sniffed through the nose or taken by intravenous injection. Effects are felt within a few minutes and last up to half an hour. It may also be neutralized to produce 'crack', which is a potent form of cocaine made by mixing it with baking soda, heating it and then smoking it in cigarettes or a pipe. If smoked or injected, the effects are immediate and last 10–15 minutes. 'Speedballing' or 'snowballing' is a technique particularly prone to fatality and involves mixing cocaine and heroin and injecting the mixture.

The effects of use include feelings of energy, strength, exhilaration, euphoria, confidence and well-being. Users often become very talkative. Adverse effects include agitation, panic and feelings of persecution or threat. Regular use can damage nasal passages and cause exhaustion and weight loss. Tolerance rapidly develops with continued use, and marked physical and psychological addiction occurs.

Snorting cocaine can cause permanent damage inside the nose, and sustained use may lead to frequent nosebleeds and recurrent sinus infections (Villa 1999, Bellis et al. 2005). In extreme cases, use leads to exposure of the septal cartilage and nasal bones, with eventual collapse of the nose (Millard & Mejia 2001). Administering cocaine by rubbing it into the gums or other mouth parts can cause ulcers, lesions and gingival recession (Gandara-Rey et al. 2002). Fatalities may rapidly occur secondary to convulsion, intracranial haemorrhage, intestinal ischaemia, respiratory arrest or cardiac arrhythmias. Sedatives such as haloperidol, diazepam for convulsions and antihypertensives may be required as part of the management regime in ED.

Heroin

Opiates such as heroin are analgesics that depress the central nervous system through suppression of noradrenaline. In its pure pharmaceutical form, heroin is a pure white, fine-grained powder. Medicinally, it is known as diamorphine and is used for severe pain, including chest pain. In its street forms it is coarser and varies in colour from a pinkish cream to dark brown. Heroin can be smoked, sniffed or injected. Intravenous injection (mainlining) results in an almost instantaneous effect ('rush'). It generates feelings of euphoria and inner peace, freedom from fear, worry, pain, hunger and cold, and can last 2–6 hours. As noted previously, it is the most frequently reported main drug of misuse (Department of Health 2001b).

Its adverse effects include depressed breathing, severe constipation, nausea and vomiting. In acute intoxication, symptoms include pinpoint pupils, depression of heart rate and respiration, and suppression of the cough reflex. Severe physical and psychological dependence can occur with continued use. Heroin use carries a high risk of overdose, as the street strength of the drug, which is usually around 20%, can range from 10% to over 60%. In cases of overdose, naloxone is a specific opioid antagonist and is given in a dose of 0.4 mg which can be repeated at intervals of 2–3 minutes up to a maximum of 10 mg.

Methadone

Methadone is a synthetic opiate analgesic which is frequently prescribed by specific medical practitioners, usually GPs or drug clinic physicians. It is used in the treatment of heroin addiction to control withdrawal symptoms. It can be used orally or by injection and generates similar feelings to heroin use, with similar signs, symptoms and management as heroin overdose.

OVERDOSE

The incidence of self-harm, of which 90% of cases involve self-poisoning, now accounts for around 20% of admissions to general medical wards and is the most frequent reason for admission to hospital in young female patients (Merson & Baldwin 1995). Poisonings can be categorized into three groups: accidental, intentional and iatrogenic. Accidental poisoning most commonly occurs among young children, although death is relatively uncommon. Intentional ingestion includes recreational drug use and suicide attempts. Iatrogenic poisoning usually results from unanticipated drug interactions (Zull 1995). In cases of intentional poisoning the ED nurses should ascertain which drugs have been taken by asking the patient or attending friends or relatives (see Box 18.3).

The Children Act gives children under the age of 16 the right to refuse consent to treatment (Department of Health 2001c). Castledine (1994) stressed the importance of establishing a good relationship with the patient, but in all cases a patient must consent if care is to be given or he can sue for assault and battery.

Box 18.3   Information to be determined when interviewing a patient following drug overdose

- What was ingested? Was anyone present at the time to verify the history? Are there any empty or partially filled bottles at home or elsewhere?
- How much was taken? If pill bottles are available, calculate the number of missing tablets from the initial amount prescribed, taking into account the date on the prescription
- What was time of the ingestion? The nurse must take into account the time at which the person was last

seen and when symptoms of intoxication began if the timing is not clear
- What was the route of the poisoning, i.e. oral, intravenous, smoked, inhaled, snorted, subcutaneous?
- Does the patient have a history of substance misuse, depression or schizophrenia?
- What is the patient's medical history, past and present prescription drugs, and allergies?

Castledine suggested that if a patient is mentally confused due to the physical effects of illness or as a consequence of mind-altering drugs, the ED nurse could proceed to treat on the basis of urgency and necessity. Careful recording of the patient's details, and the nursing and medical staffs' actions are important in such cases.

CONCLUSION

Adolescent attendance patterns highlight the need for ED nurses to understand the normal processes through which adolescents pass. Nurses can appear judgemental and less sympathetic towards a patient perceived as being responsible for his own illness (Stockbridge 1993). ED nurses can be affected by the apparent lack of compliance from adolescent patients. This can lead to paternalisms or confrontational

behaviour which destroys the therapeutic relationship and exacerbates conflict. Adolescents cannot be treated wholly as adults as they lack the emotional maturity to cope with independence and still need the emotional support of parents and other carers (Kelly 1991). ED attendance is often a result of normal adolescent behaviour and ED nurses should be equipped with the knowledge necessary to provide appropriate support and education. An environment which provides boundaries, privacy and protected independence, with support, and peer support if appropriate, should be developed.

It is important to remember that psychological distress can be just as great as physical illness or trauma. ED nurses have a responsibility to consider the needs of young people as individuals. Perhaps an alteration of attitude is more important than a vast financial outlay in the improvement of adolescent care.

References

Barker P (1988) *Basic Child Psychiatry*. Oxford: Blackwell.

Bellis MA, Hughes K, McVeigh J, Thomson R, Luke C (2005) Effects of nightlife activity on health. *Nursing Standard*, **19**, 30, 63–71.

Bernardo LM, Schenkel KA (1995) Pediatric medical emergencies. In: Kitt S, Selfridge-Thomas J, Proehl JA, Kaiser J, eds. *Emergency Nursing: A Physiologic and Clinical Perspective*. Philadelphia: WB Saunders.

Bickley LS, Szilagyi PG (2003) *Bates' Guide To Physical Examination And History Taking*, 8th Edn. Philadelphia: Lippincott Williams & Wilkins.

Blunden R (1988) An artificial state. *Paediatric Nursing*, **3**, 12–13.

Boys A, Farrell M (2001) *Survey (2000): a Follow-up Study of Alcohol Use Amongst 15–17-year-olds*. London: National Addiction Centre.

Braback L, Humble M (2001) Young woman dies of water intoxication after taking one tablet of ecstasy. Today's drug panorama calls for increased vigilance in health care. *Lakartidningen*, **98**(8), 817–819.

Campbell J (1999) Cannabis: the evidence. *Nursing Standard*, **13**(44), 45–47.

Castledine G (1994) Ethics and law in ED. *Emergency Nurse*, **2**(1), 25.

Chen K et al. (1997) Relationships between frequency and quantity of marijuana use and last year proxy dependence among adolescents and adults in the United States. *Drug and Alcohol Dependence*, **46**(1–2), 53–67.

Cook A (1995) Ecstasy (MDMA): alerting users to the dangers. *Nursing Times*, **91**(16), 32–33.

Croghan E, Johnson C, Aveyard P (2004) School nurses: policies, working practices, roles and value perceptions. *Journal of Advanced Nursing*, **47**(4), 377–385.

Croghan E (2005) Supporting adolescents through behaviour change. *Nursing Standard*, **19**(34), 50–53.

Department of Health (2001a) *School Nurse Practice Development Resource Pack*. London: The Stationery Office.

Department of Health (2001b) *Statistical Bulletin: Statistics from the British Crime Survey 2001*. London: Department of Health.

Department of Health (2001c) *Reference Guide to Consent for Examination and Treatment.* London: Department of Health.

Department of Health (2002) *Drug Use, Smoking and Drinking Among Young Teenagers in 2001. A Survey Carried out on Behalf of the Department of Health by the National Centre for Social Research and the National Foundation for Educational Research.* London: Department of Health.

Department of Health (2004) *The National Service Framework for Children, Young People and Maternity Services.* London, Department of Health.

Donovan DM, Queiser HR, Salzberg PM et al. (1985) Intoxicated and bad drivers: subgroups within same population of high risk drivers. *Journal of Studies in Alcohol,* **46**(5), 375–382.

Emmett D, Nice G (1996) *Understanding Drugs: A Handbook for Parents, Teachers and other Professionals.* London: Jessica Kingsley.

Erikson E (1965) *Childhood and Society.* Harmondsworth: Penguin.

Gandara-Rey JM, Diniz-Freitas M, Gandara-Vila P, Blanco-Carrion A, Garcia-Garcia A (2002) Lesions of the oral mucosa in cocaine users who apply the drug topically. *Medicina Oral,* **7**(2), 103–107.

Gilles M (1992) Teenage traumas. *Nursing Times,* **88**(27), 58.

Hawton K et al. (1999) Suicide in young people. Study of 174 cases, aged under 25 years, based on coroners' and medical records. *British Journal of Psychiatry,* **175**, 271–276.

Henry J, Jeffreys KJ, Dawling S (1992) Toxicity and deaths from 3,4-methylenedioxymethamphetamine ('ecstasy'). *Lancet,* **340**, 384–387.

HMSO (1994) *Tackling Drugs Together: A Consultation Document on a Strategy for England 1995–1998.* London: HMSO.

Holt L (1993) The adolescent in accident & emergency. *Nursing Standard,* **8**(8), 30–34.

Home Office (1996) *Statistics of Drug Addicts Notified to the Home Office.* Issue 15/96. London: Home Office.

House A (1998) Effective health care. *Deliberate Self-harm,* **4**, 6.

Jack M (1989) Personal fable. *Journal of Pediatric Nursing,* **4**(5), 334–338.

Jones C (1993) MDMA: the doubts surrounding ecstasy and the response of the emergency nurse. *Accident & Emergency Nursing,* **1**, 193–198.

Kalant H (2004) Adverse effects of cannabis on health: an update of the literature since (1996). *Progress in Neuropsychopharmacology and Biological Psychiatry,* **28**(5), 849–863.

Kelly J (1991) Caring for adolescents. *Professional Nurse,* **6**(9), 498–501.

Knight S, Rush H (1998) Providing facilities for adolescents in ED. *Emergency Nurse,* **6**(4), 22–26.

Kuykendall J (1989) Teenage traumas. *Nursing Times,* **85**(27), 26–28.

Leon L, Smith K (2001) Turned upside down: services for young people in crisis. *Young Minds Magazine,* **51**, 22–24.

Lyall J (1990) A time to listen. *Nursing Times,* **86**(14), 16–17.

Marfé E (2003) Assessing risk following deliberate self harm. *Paediatric Nursing,* **15**(8), 32–34.

McCallam I (1990) Growing pains. *Nursing Times,* **86**(34), 62–64.

Merson S, Baldwin D (1995) *Psychiatric Emergencies.* Oxford: Oxford University Press.

Millard DR, Mejia FA (2001) Reconstruction of the nose damaged by cocaine. *Plastic and Reconstructive Surgery,* **107**(2), 419–424.

Milroy CM (1999) Ten years of 'ecstasy'. *Journal of the Royal Society of Medicine,* **92**, 68–72.

Nixon PJ, Youngson CC, Beese A (2002) Tooth surface loss: does recreational drug use contribute? *Clinical Oral Investigations,* **6**(2), 128–130.

Paton A (1994) *ABC of Alcohol* 3rd edn. London: BMA Publishing Group.

Preston A (1992) Pointing out the risk. *Nursing Times,* **88**, 24–26.

Ramsey M, Percy A (1997) A national household survey of drug misuse in Britain: a decade of development. *Addiction,* **92**(8), 931–938.

Rassool G (2002) Substance misuse and mental health: an overview. *Nursing Standard,* **16**(50), 46–52.

Rassool GH, Winnington J (2003) Adolescents and alcohol misuse. *Nursing Standard,* **17**(30), 46–52.

Schofield E, Lawman S, Volans G, Henry J (1997) Drugs of abuse: clinical features and management. *Emergency Nurse,* **5**(6), 17–22.

Smith C, Allen J (2004) *Violent Crime in England and Wales.* Home Office: London.

Stockbridge J (1993) Parasuicide: does discussing it help? *Emergency Nurse,* **1**(2), 19–21.

Strategy Unit (2003) *Interim Analytical Report.* Strategy Unit: London.

Tortora GJ, Grabowski SR (2003) *Principles of Anatomy and Physiology,* 10th Edn. New Jersey: John Wiley & Sons.

Villa P (1999) Midfacial complications of prolonged cocaine snorting. *Journal of the Canadian Dental Association,* **65**(4), 218–223.

Walsh M, Kent A (2001) *Accident & Emergency Nursing: A New Approach,* 4th Edn. London: Butterworth Heinemann Ltd.

Whotton E (2002) What to do when an adolescent self harms. *Emergency Nurse,* **10**(5), 12–16.

Winkenstein M (1992) Adolescent smoking. *Journal of Paediatric Nursing,* **7**(2), 120–127.

Zull DN (1995) Poisoning and drug overdose. In: Kitt S, Selfridge-Thomas J, Proehl JA, Kaiser J. eds. *Emergency Nursing: a Physiologic and Clinical Perspective,* 2nd edn. Philadelphia: WB Saunders.

Chapter **19**

Young adults

Judy Davies

INTRODUCTION

Young adults attending ED are at the peak of life's activity cycle, both physically and sexually. The age group 18–39 years is not, however, homogeneous in its characteristics as it encompasses the period of time in the life cycle from experimentation to full maturity.

As young adults mature from adolescence and settle down, the pattern changes. They have families, face financial burdens, have challenges in or out of work, and may lack traditional family support. Partnership, pregnancy and parenthood may bring a sense of stability and responsibility, although these also carry the risk of stress-related illnesses. For many, the fun of youth is lost too quickly and the responsibilities of adult life come too soon. This chapter considers the range of physical and psychological ailments that affect young adults and bring them to emergency departments.

SPORTING INJURIES

The most popular leisure activity named by young adults is 'going to the pub' (Office of National Statistics 2000). Despite this, many young people's leisure activities involve some kind of sport. Some 53% of 16–24 year old males and 21% of women do physical activity 5 times a week, with 46% of 25–34 year old men and 33% of women doing similarly (Stationery Office, 2000). The most popular sports amongst young adults include walking, gym, cycling and swimming (Office of National Statistics 1997).

It was probably not envisaged that campaigns to encourage people to take more exercise and to be involved in health education programmes, such as 'Look after your Heart' and 'Sport for All', would have the direct consequence of increasing the numbers of personal injuries. The most recent figures available, collected in 18 EDs around the UK, showed that an estimated 912 506 patients sought treatment in emergency departments for sports-related injuries (Department of Trade and Industry (DTI) 2001). They recorded the popularity of two new sporting activities over the previous 5 years which have given rise to associated injuries.

Skateboards remain popular among teenagers and young adults; however, 29% of skateboard injuries involve wrist or ankle fractures (Forsman & Eriksson 2001). Micro-scooter injuries often occur at high speed and involve mainly head, cervical spine and facial bones, because the hands are gripping the steering fork and are unable to protect the face (Exadaktylos et al. 2001). Some DTI groups based in emergency departments are currently making design recommendations to manufacturers.

Although most sports injuries are minor, vigilant triage is essential to identify and prioritize the more serious sports injuries. Ten per cent of all hospital admissions are sports related (Kannus 2000). The most serious are:

- head injuries and airway obstruction
- facial injuries
- spinal injuries
- haemothorax, pneumothorax and tension pneumothorax
- blunt and penetrating abdominal trauma
- pelvic injuries
- muscular skeletal injuries
- compartment injuries.

The most significant non-fatal sporting injuries involve damage to the head or spine. In the UK the greatest number of sporting head injuries arise from golf (28%) and horse riding (16%). Serious spinal injuries are rare, at 17 per week in Great Britain (Eaton 1999), but 20.5% of patients in spinal injury units have sustained their injury as a result of a sporting activity. The most common sports to generate serious spinal injuries are horse riding (6%), diving (6%), rugby (0.5%) and miscellaneous sports, e.g. gymnastics, skiing, motor sports 8% (Grundy & Swain 1996). These injuries have long-term implications for a young person. Paralysis, brain damage or serious reduction in mobility will almost certainly lead to loss of earnings, relationship and sexual problems, depression and a greatly altered lifestyle.

Most deaths from sport arise from professional boxing, followed by horse riding, skating, gymnastics and swimming. Although rare in the young adult, non-accidental sudden death may also occur during sporting activities. The most likely causes are cardiac myopathy, myocarditis, congenital disorders, arrhythmias and conduction disorders. Ruptured aorta and coronary heart disease are more likely to occur in the sports person who is over 39 years (Hillis 2000).

Seventy-five per cent of all sporting injuries are classified as minor and may be seen and treated by sports physiotherapists, GPs, walk-in centres, minor injuries units or in emergency departments. Many are overuse injuries and are usually caused by training errors, excessive load on the body, environmental problems, poor equipment, ineffective rules or violent play (Kannus 2000). Overuse injuries have a better chance of full recovery if treated by a clinician experienced in sports medicine, followed by a correct rehabilitation programme.

In the young adult the muscles are the greatest points of weakness. The knee is the most vulnerable point in children under 15; after this and up to the age of 19 the pelvis is the weakest, with avulsion fractures commonly occurring. From 19 to 30 years of age the hamstring and quadriceps muscles are especially vulnerable. After the age of 30 the tendons start to degenerate and become weaker than the muscles (Noble 1990). A study funded by the Sports Council suggested that annually between 1 and 1.5 million injuries caused by sport resulted in ED attendance and a further 4–5 million injuries resulted in temporary incapacity (Nicholl et al. 1991).

Eighty-two per cent of all patients with sporting injuries are not detained in hospital and are treated in the emergency department, with possible subsequent referral to orthopaedic or physiotherapy clinics. Attendances at these clinics can be greatly reduced by employing a full-time physiotherapist to work in ED (Bakewell 1993). Sporting injuries benefit from quick physiotherapy: haematomas are prevented from fibrosing and long-term injuries avoided (Wardrope & English 1998). The educational value of employing a physiotherapist could be enormous for junior medical staff, for the emergency nurse and, most importantly, for the patient.

The short-term aims of treatment of sporting injuries are pain control, maintenance of range of movements, maintenance of basic strength, and re-establishment of neuromuscular function. After initial first aid, some injuries will require surgery and post-operative rehabilitation (Matthews 2000). Most, however, can be treated conservatively using the following acronym:

P Protection of injured area from further damage
R Rest of part to avoid prolonged irritation
I Ice for control of pain, bleeding, oedema
C Compression for support and control of swelling
E Elevation for decreased bleeding and oedema
S Support for stabilization of injured part

The administration of non-steroidal anti-inflammatory drugs may slightly speed the recovery from injury and also act as an analgesic. Sporting injuries benefit from quick physiotherapy with early controlled mobilization and functional rehabilitation.

ROAD TRAFFIC ACCIDENTS

Despite dramatic falls in child death rates throughout the 20th century, young adults remain the largest accident risk group (Social Trends 2000). In the under-35 age group, injury is the commonest cause of death and has been colourfully described as 'the last great plague of the young' (Skinner et al. 1991).

Many of the more serious injuries of adulthood result from road traffic accidents (RTAs). Road deaths in the UK are now one of the lowest in Europe, with 6 adults per 100 000 and 2 children per 100 000; the highest numbers are in Portugal with 33 adult deaths per 100 000 and 8 children per 100 000 (Office for National Statistics 2000).

While the number of fatal head injuries has begun to decline, a pattern of blunt abdominal trauma has emerged (Cope & Stebbings 1996). The main causes of death from RTAs in young adults are:

- chest, abdominal and pelvic injury
- intracranial injury, excluding skull fracture
- fractures of the skull.

For each fatality on the roads there are 12.6 serious injuries and 50.2 minor injuries: 36% of people with serious spinal injuries receive them as a result of road traffic accidents, 19% from cars or vans, 10% from motorcycles, 4% from pedal cycles and 3% as pedestrians (Grundy & Swain 1996).

The number of pedestrian deaths has remained consistent since 1953. The greatest numbers are among elderly people, with a disproportionately high number also occurring in the age group 1–14 years. The highest number of fatalities for pedal cyclists occur in the 5–14 age group. Those dying in cars, however, are predominantly young adults, but fatalities from motor vehicles, motorcycles and bicycles in this age group have dropped by about one-third. The introduction of the mountain bike has led to a huge surge in the popularity of cycling, with off-road cycling and safety helmets helping to lessen the number of accidents. Legislation limiting the engine capacity of motorcycles that learners can ride and the introduction of a two-part test has led to a 40% reduction in those killed or seriously injured on motorbikes. In the 1980s the imposition of speed restrictions and attention to safer road design by the Ministry of Transport contributed to falling road deaths, as have the recent mandatory use of rear seat belts, crumple zones, anti-brake-lock devices, air bags and seasonal anti drink-drive campaigns. A disproportionately high number of people involved in RTAs have consumed alcohol, and these people are the most likely to sustain serious injuries. Between one in three and one in seven accidental deaths are linked to alcohol and 40% of pedestrians killed in car accidents have blood alcohol levels above the legal driving limit (Keigan and Tunbridge 2003).

Although some accidents involve environmental and vehicular factors, human error is clearly responsible for most accidents. The number of road accidents in the over-25s declines quickly as experience and social maturity develop. Although legislation and attention to environmental issues have reduced the number of road deaths, the problems of inexperience, immaturity, impetuosity and sometimes lack of control are harder to address.

ALCOHOL–RELATED ATTENDANCES

Only 7% of men and 13% of women call themselves non-drinkers. The remaining 80% have widely differing drinking habits, with occupations, genetic and parental influences, life events, race, religion, peer pressure and personality all having an effect on alcohol consumption. The heaviest drinking occurs among young adults in the age range 16–24 years (Royal College of Psychiatrists and Royal College of Physicians 2000). Guidelines recommend that men and women drink no more than four and three units respectively in one day (Department of Health 1995). However, one study of nightclubs found men consuming an average of 15 units and women 10 units during a night out (Deehan & Saville 2003). Young women in particular are drinking more, with the percentage of 16- to 24-year-old women exceeding the recommended weekly drinking limits doubling over the past decade (Rickards et al 2004). The changes in image of pubs to café bars, music pubs, family pubs, nightclubs and rave music venues have all made drinking more accessible to young people. Half of 18–24-year-olds visit pubs at least twice a week and 40% visit nightclubs at least once a fortnight (Mintel 2003).

Every year, the adverse effects of alcohol consumption in England and Wales lead to an estimated 1.2 million assaults, result in 150 000 hospital admissions, and cost the NHS £1.7 billion (Smith & Allen 2004, Strategy Unit 2003). More than 600 000 violent incidents occur in or around pubs every year (Simmons et al. 2002) and at least one in ten nightlife assaults involves the threatened use of glasses or bottles

(Budd 2003), while an estimated 5000 people are injured every year by glass used as a weapon, with many permanently scarred (Deehan 1999).

Alcohol-related attendances in the emergency department may be prompted by injuries, intoxication, medical problems or antisocial behaviour. The former two reasons are most common in the young adult who has had a single episode of heavy drinking, while the latter two are common in the older, habitual heavy drinker. Alcohol acts as a CNS depressant and, although it stimulates conversation and sociability, it also impairs judgement, slows reflexes and can lead to aggressive and violent behaviour. It is tempting when such a patient presents for triage to assess these patients as 'drunk', do an alcometer reading and put them to the back of the queue. However, Moulton and Yates (1999) recommend that, due to the high incidence of trauma in patients with alcohol intoxication, when assessing an intoxicated patient emergency department staff should be aware of the possibility of non-obvious physical injury, including cervical spine and head injury. They advise the following management of the aggressive drunk patient when considering their possible fitness for discharge:

- observe patient carefully, doing head injury observations and blood alcohol readings
- enquire about possible trauma from bystanders
- examine patient, especially head, without personal risk
- undertake blood glucose readings
- get senior medical advice for further management
- observe in hospital, or
- send home with sensible friends with written, explained head injury instructions, or
- send to police custody with written head injury instructions

Ten per cent of adults in the U.K. are classified as 'heavy drinkers', with 1:2000 needing admission to psychiatric hospitals for alcohol-related disease (Goodwin 2000). Unconscious patients brought to the emergency department with acute alcohol intoxication need regular head injury observations, blood sugar readings, fluid replacement of isotonic saline 10 ml/kg in the first hour and airway protection. If there is a possibility of trauma, a cervical spine and CT scan will need to be done. A bottle of spirits may pose no serious problem for the chronic drinker, but for the non-regular drinker with a blood alcohol level of 400 mg/100 ml or over, it can lead to deep coma and death, usually from hypoglycaemia, respiratory depression or aspiration.

Alcoholic coma can be a serious medical emergency requiring admission to hospital. The emergency nurse should be aware that a patient's condition can move from mild to life-threatening as previously ingested alcohol and/or drugs are absorbed (Taylor & Ryrie 1996). Most deaths occur because of respiratory depression or aspiration. Deep alcoholic coma should be treated aggressively with a cuffed endotracheal tube, oxygen and ventilation. If low blood sugar levels necessitate glucose, it should be accompanied by intravenous thiamine. Otherwise, when carbohydrate metabolism begins again, low levels of B1 (thiamine) will precipitate Wernicke's encephalopathy, which consists of ocular muscle palsies, nystagmus, ataxic gait and progressive mental impairment. A patient in alcohol withdrawal is generally dehydrated and orthostatic. Hypoglycaemia, acidosis, hypovolaemia and electrolyte disturbance need treatment with intravenous fluids, CVP line, blood gases, glucose and thiamine.

Zull (1995) noted that, in addition to correction of dehydration and electrolyte abnormalities, the patient may require sedative therapy. Minimal tremulousness in a patient with normal mental status may not require any tranquillizer therapy. However, the patient who is agitated, hallucinating or having seizures, or who has evidence of autonomic hyperactivity, such as fever and tachycardia, should be calmed rapidly. The benzodiazepine sedatives are the preferred agents and diazepam can be given at 15–30-minute intervals, after which the dose and frequency should be decreased or a switch to an oral route made. Drugs such as haloperidol and chlorpromazine are generally avoided because they may increase the risk of seizures. If seizures occur, i.v. diazepam is the treatment of choice.

All emergency departments will have their own regular patients who are heavy drinkers, many of whom will be in their 20s or 30s. Apart from acute intoxication and trauma, they may present with other medical and psychological problems associated with alcoholic liver disease. The most common of these are gastritis, haematemesis, oesophageal varices and pancreatitis. As the disease progresses fits, dementia, cardiomyopathy, strokes and cancers may develop (Edwards et al. 1997). Psychological problems may include parasuicide, depression and acute anxiety attacks. People dependent on alcohol have a mortality rate four times higher than the rest of the population; half of these deaths will be violent and 7% from suicide (Wasserman 2001). After glucose and thiamine for their hypoglycaemia, i.v. diazepam for their fits and cessation of their gastric bleeding, the desire to return to their existing lifestyle will mean that many of these patients will discharge themselves home before they ever reach a ward. Many young adults are ill-informed about safe drinking patterns. Alcohol education continues to receive a low priority in both policy and resources and it is believed that isolated campaigns to educate the public are ineffective (King's Fund 1991).

ACCIDENTS RELATED TO SEXUAL ACTIVITY

The peak of life's sexual activity occurs in young adulthood. Many young men and women come to the emergency department because of their sexually related activities. All of these patients need to be treated with tact and confidentiality by an experienced nurse. It is not the emergency nurse's role to question patients' sexual activities and preferences and it is essential that problems are discussed in a private place, preferably with staff of the same sex. An undisclosed history of rape, buggery, incest, trans-sexualism or transvestism may be reasons for a patient refusing to remove clothing or declining to see a doctor of a particular gender.

Genital trauma may bring an acutely embarrassed patient to the emergency department. Sexual intercourse can cause lacerations to the vagina and penis, which often bleed profusely. Young men may present with pain and bleeding after intercourse because of a torn frenulum, which can normally be treated with a simple frenuloplasty. 'Vacuum cleaner' injuries can be more serious and result in skin loss which may need grafting. Injuries to the penile shaft cause considerable distress to young men and 70% of these arise as a result of sexual practices. The commonest of these injuries is a fracture of the penis. This occurs when the penis is bent acutely during intercourse and the crack of the rupturing tunica albuginea can be heard. The patient suffers pain, deformity and gross swelling, with surgical repair usually needed (Bullock et al. 1995). Human bites to the penis can pose a serious problem and are associated with a 50% infection rate. Suturing, with the additional help of ice packs and pressure, will usually stop the bleeding. Because large numbers of both anaerobic and aerobic organisms are found in human saliva, these bites need to be treated with augmentin (Greaves et al. 1997).

The young, uncircumcised male may present with a paraphimosis after his first sexual encounter. This can normally be reduced using lignocaine and ice packs, followed by manipulation of the retracted foreskin. More rarely a dorsal incision or circumcision may be needed (Burkitt and Quick 2002). Entrapment of the foreskin in a zip can usually be treated conservatively with the aid of mineral oil to the zip and foreskin, by slowly and methodically unzipping the zipper. Tetanus prophylaxis should be considered. Although not common, patients who suffer electric shocks should be questioned about possible burns to the scrotum and penis, since the electrical discharge has a propensity to exit from the genitalia (Bullock et al. 1995).

Both male and female patients may present with foreign bodies in their rectum, vagina or urethra, although they may initially complain of abdominal pain, constipation or rectal bleeding. These are usually inserted for self-exploration, inquisitorial reasons or for sexual pleasure. On other occasions it may be for contraceptive use or as a means of deliberate self-harm (Tanagho & McAninch 2000). These may cause no problems for a long period but can cause patients to present with cystitis, haematuria, discharge, abdominal pain or rectal bleeding. Many of these patients can be treated without admission, but the sexual use of vibrators or other objects may cause serious injury and perforation of the bowel. Fever may also be present if the foreign body has been in situ for a while. Physical examination may reveal the foreign body palpable in, or protruding from, the urethra, vagina and/or anus. Urine and urethral discharge cultures should be obtained and a broad-spectrum antibiotic be prescribed (Kidd 1995).

The most common foreign body is a lost tampon, which can occur because of a broken string, due to the insertion of two tampons for heavy loss or as a result of having sexual intercourse with a tampon in situ. It can easily be removed with the aid of a good light and Cusco's speculum. The prolonged use of large tampons, and also contraceptive diaphragm use, may lead to septic shock (Llewellyn-Jones 2001), a condition caused by a *Staphylococcus aureus* infection. The patient may present with symptoms of a low-grade infection or may be in advanced stages of septic shock. If the latter, their initial treatment will need to encompass a full blood screen, including blood cultures, intravenous fluids and antibiotics, oxygen and regular observations, including capillary refill.

Weekends are a common time for young women to ask for postcoital contraception, when GP surgeries, family planning clinics or pharmacies are closed. Unprotected intercourse, split condoms, or rape may be the reasons for this request. The 'morning-after pill' can be given within 72 hours and is 99% effective. Further details can be found in Chapter 29 (Gynaecological and obstetric emergencies), as can the causes of vaginal bleeding, which brings a considerable number of young women to emergency departments. Miscarriage occurs in 20% of pregnancies and is a source of great distress to many young women and men who come to the emergency department. It is important that these patients are afforded as much privacy and compassion as possible in the emergency environment. The first consideration of the nurse is to establish that the patient is haemodynamically stable, since blood loss can be profuse. After this, pain relief and rapid referral to a gynaecology ward should take place. It is not appropriate for these distressed patients to wait long periods in the department and a nurse-led fast-track system can provide greatly improved care for these young women (Wilson 2000).

In the UK, the occurrence of sexually transmitted infections (STIs) continues to escalate and levels of unwanted pregnancies remain high (Bellis et al. 2004). For various reasons, young men and women may prefer to come to the emergency department with STIs, the principal reason for which may be a desire for anonymity. Patients may be reluctant to go to a general practitioner who is well known to them and their families. They feel, unjustly, that there will be a greater degree of confidentiality in a place where they are not known and to which they will not have to return. Appointments do not have to be made and a decision to seek immediate treatment for an embarrassing problem can be acted upon.

Binge drinking and recreational drug consumption are associated with an increased risk of unprotected sex (Bellis & Hughes 2004). About 10% of young people in some areas have chlamydial infections and levels have more than doubled between 1995 and 2003 (Bellis et al. 2004). Not all STIs require penetrative sex for transmission; for example, syphilis can be spread through oral sex (Cook et al. 2001). Alcohol and some recreational drugs can induce temporary impotence and some clubbers use anti-impotence drugs to enable or enhance sex (Bellish & Hughes 2004). Bellis et al. (2005) also note that women have been reported to use such drugs to improve orgasms. However, such drugs have a range of contraindications, for instance, hypotension and recent stroke and, in combination with alcohol and other drugs, substantially increase the risk of an adverse reaction (Romanelli & Smith 2004).

PSYCHOLOGICAL ILLNESSES IN YOUNG ADULTS

Many find the transition from adolescence to adulthood extremely difficult and stress-related illnesses are common. Those without a strong support network may feel overwhelmed by the problems confronting them. The young adult is at a greater risk of death from suicide than any other age group. The suicide rate rises markedly in the teenage years and it may occur without warning (Lader & Cowen 2001).

Deaths from suicide rose dramatically between 1970 and 1990. Recent analysis, however, shows a decrease in suicides for both men and women between 1960 and 1997 (McClure 2000). Male suicide has continued to rise in areas of high social and economic deprivation, especially among those who experience high levels of unemployment and violence (Office for National Statistics 1998). Three times more men than women successfully commit suicide. In 1998 there was one suicide every 90 minutes in the UK. There is a particularly high rate of suicide amongst young adults and it remains one of the main causes of death for this age group.

Since 1920, the months of April, May and June have consistently been the peak months for suicides. The pattern of suicide and parasuicide (usually known as deliberate self-harm) varies between men and women, with men tending to favour more violent ways of killing themselves, such as hanging, firearms and jumping, while women tend to use self-poisoning (Bird & Faulkner 2000).

Twenty-four per cent of those who successfully committed suicide are recorded as having used the mental health services within the previous week (Bird & Faulkner 2000): 40–50% of those who succeeded in taking their own lives also had a history of self-harm (McClure 2000, Hawton 2004). Deliberate self-harm (DSH) is 3–4 times more common in women than in men. In England and Wales 100 000 patients a year are referred to hospital as a result of DSH. For every suicide there are 30 other cases of self-harm (Evans 1993). Many of these are young adults who take tablets or who inflict wounds on themselves, with 69% of them having been doing so for over 5 years. Those who self-injure tend to do so by cutting, scratching or burning. They may do this for a variety of reasons: physical, emotional or sexual abuse, feelings of low esteem, eating disorders or periods of distress. Sometimes these patients receive poor care in an emergency department from busy nurses who either do not empathize with their problems, do not listen fully or do not give adequate analgesia. Many patients have reported that the way they were received in the emergency department was often crucial, with talking, listening and compassionate care having a very positive effect on their self-esteem (Bird & Faulkner 2000); however, Moore and McLaughlin (2003) argue that when staff are very busy and stressed they can struggle to understand why apparently healthy people have attempted or succeeded in taking their own life. Some will be suicidal while others will not, but those with a past history of DSH are more likely to successfully take their own lives: 20–25% of people who die had come to hospital with self-harm in the previous year (Foster et al. 1997). The difference between the two groups, suicide and self-harm, is not always clear-cut. Those who commit suicide are a small group who tend to plan the act, take precautions against being discovered, use dangerous methods and, in one-sixth of cases, leave a suicide note. The majority of these patients have given a warning of suicidal intent.

Young adulthood is a time when specific mental illnesses can develop. The one which is probably best known as a disorder of the young is schizophrenia, which has a mean age of onset of 31 years in the male and 41 years in the female. Despite the fact that it is believed that this is a disease more prevalent in men, both men and women have a 1% lifetime risk of schizophrenia (Castle et al. 2000). The nurse may first meet the patient with symptoms of disordered thoughts, inappropriate moods, auditory hallucinations or persecutory delusions. These patients can be frightening and difficult to contain if psychiatric referral takes time. Nurses need to understand that the families of these patients bring with them a huge and very varying set of feelings. Some feel total bewilderment, shame, anger, disappointment or grief, while others have still not been able to let go of their hope for a complete cure for the person they love (Jones 2002). The care and nursing management of patients with a psychiatric crisis, including schizophrenia, are considered in detail in Chapter 14 (Psychiatric emergencies).

Several illnesses affect young women in particular. In women under 40, collapse, bradycardia or electrolyte imbalance may arise because of a history of anorexia nervosa or bulimia. Postnatal depression or psychosis may also be seen in the department when young women may present following an overdose, with acute delusions or after being involved in episodes of harm to their children. Certain individuals who are confronted by stress develop anxiety states which vary greatly in severity. These can be a feature of young adult life and symptoms usually persist for an average of 5 years before treatment is sought.

Symptoms include palpitations, tachycardia and chest pain. It is important to get a full history to rule out organic causes such as pneumothorax, infection or myocardial infarct. Individual stress counselling and relaxation groups run by a psychologist or community psychiatric nurse can be very beneficial to help these patients develop coping mechanisms (Hambley & Muire 1997). Life events such as bereavement, divorce, unemployment, marriage, parenthood and physical illness can precipitate these illnesses.

CONCLUSION

Young adults use emergency departments in a different way from children, the middle-aged or the elderly. They may have moved away from the influence and environment of the family and may not be registered with a GP. They rarely have long-term healthcare needs and so tend to use the accident department as a 'drop-in' centre not requiring organized planned appointments.

A survey undertaken in Cambridge calls these young adults 'thresholders'. It finds this generation used to easy solutions and ill-equipped to deal with life's complications (Apter 2002). The commonest reason for attendance is accidental injury. They have a lamentable lack of knowledge of their own bodies and become aggressive or depressed if they have to confront personal injury or disease. They have high levels of anxiety about their body image and a visit to hospital can be an emotionally traumatic time when they become impatient and frightened if they are not treated quickly. This means that the ED nurse needs to be aware that reassurance and explanations are necessary and not be surprised that young people, even in their 20s, want their parents with them. The 18–39 year age range has a diverse group within it and good communication skills are essential to ensure that all patients receive the appropriate treatments for their specific needs. As with every group of patients, the young adult needs tolerance, flexibility and that vital but elusive ingredient, time.

References

Apter T (2002) *The Myth of Maturity: What Teenagers Need from Parents to Become Adults*. London: W.W Norton.

Bakewell P (1993) *A Physiotherapy Research Post in Accident and Emergency*. Norwich: Norfolk and Norwich Hospital.

Bellis MA, Hughes K (2004) Sex potions: relationships between alcohol, drugs and sex. *Adicciones*, 16(4), 251–259.

Bellis MA, Hughes K, Ashton R (2004) The promiscuous ten percent? *Journal of Epidemiology and Community Health* 58(11), 889–890.

Bellis MA, Hughes K, McVeigh J, Thomson R, Luke C (2005) Effects of nightlife activity on health. *Nursing Standard*, 19(30), 63–71.

Bird L, Faulkner A (2000) *Suicide and Self Harm*. London: Mental Health Foundation.

Budd T (2003) *Alcohol Related Assault: Findings From the British Crime Survey*. London: Home Office.

Bullock N, Sibley G, Whittaker R (1995) *Essential Urology*. London: Churchill Livingstone.

Burkitt G, Quick C (2002) *Essential Surgery: Diagnosis, Management.* London: Churchill Livingstone.

Castle D, McGrath J, Kulkarnie J, eds (2000) *Women and Schizophrenia.* Cambridge: Cambridge University Press.

Cook PA, Clark P, Bellis MA et al. (2001) Re-emerging syphilis in the UK: a behavioural analysis of infected individuals. *Communicable Disease and Public Health,* **4**(4), 253–258.

Cope A, Stebbings W (1996) Abdomen. In: Skinner D, Driscoll P and Earlham R, eds. *ABC of Major Trauma.* London: BMJ.

Deehan A (1999) *Alcohol and Crime: Taking Stock.* London: Home Office.

Deehan A, Saville E (2003) *Calculating the risk: Recreational Drug Use among Clubbers in the South East of England.* London: Home Office.

Department of Health (1995) *Sensible Drinking: The Report of an Interdepartmental Working Group.* London: HMSO.

Department of Trade and Industry (2001) *23rd Annual report of Home and Leisure Accident Surveillance System – 1999.* London: HMSO.

Department of Transport (1989) *Road Casualties in Great Britain: 1988.* London: HMSO.

Eaton CJ (1999) *Immediate Medical Care.* Edinburgh: Churchill Livingstone.

Edwards G, Marshall E, Cooke C (1997) *The Treatment of Drinking Problems.* Cambridge: Cambridge University Press.

Evans M (1993) Suicide: a target for health. RCN Nursing Update. *Nursing Standard* **7**(18), 9–14.

Exadaktylos A, Eggli S, Zimmerman H (2001) *British Journal of Sports Medicine.* 35.

Fosman L, Eriksson A (2001) Skateboarding Injuries of Today. *British Journal of Sports Medicine.* **35**: 325–328.

Foster T, Gillespie K, McLelland R (1997) Mental disorders and suicide in Northern Ireland. *British Journal of Psychiatry* **170**: 447–452.

Goodwin D (2000) *Alcoholism: The Facts.* Oxford: Oxford University Press.

Greaves I, Porter K, Burke D (1997) *Key Topics in Trauma.* London: BIOS Scientific Publishers.

Grundy D, Swain A (1996) *ABC of Spinal Cord Injury,* 3rd Edn. London: BMJ.

Hambly K, Murie AJ (1997) *Stress Management in Primary Care.* Oxford: Butterworth/Heinemann.

Harries M et al. (eds) (2000) *ABC of Sports Medicine.* London: BMJ.

Hawton K, Harriss L, Simkin S, Bale E, Bond A (2004) Suicidal behaviour in England and Wales. In: Schmidtke A, Bille-Brahe U, De Leo D, Kerkhof A, eds. *Suicidal Behaviour in Europe: Results from the WHO/EURO Multicentre Study of Suicidal Behaviour.* Hogrefe & Huber: Göttingen.

Hillis WS et al. (2000) *Sudden Death: ABC Sports Medicine.* London: BMJ.

HMSO (1998) *Saving Lives: Our Healthier Nation.* London.

Jones D (2002) *Myths, Madness and the Family.* New York: Palgrave.

Kannus P (2000) *Nature, Prevention and Management of Injury: ABC of Sports Medicine.* London: BMJ.

Kidd PS (1995) Genitourinary emergencies. In: Kitt S, Selfridge-Thomas J, Proehl JA, Kaiser J, eds. *Emergency Nursing: a Physiologic and Clinical Perspective.* Philadelphia: WB Saunders.

King's Fund (1991) *Health of the Nation: Strategy for the 1990s.* London: King Edward Hospital Fund.

Lader M, Cowen P (eds) (2001) *Depression.* Oxford: Oxford University Press.

Llewellyn-Jones D (2001) *Fundamentals of Obstetrics and Gynaecology.* London: Mosby.

Matthews N (2000) *Physiotherapy, Sports Injury and the Reacquisition of Fitness; ABC of Sports Medicine.* London: BMJ.

McClure GM (2000) Changes in suicide in England and Wales 1960–1997. *British Journal of Psychiatry* **176**: 64–67.

Mintel (2003) *Late Licensing UK.* London: Mintel International Group.

Moore K, McLaughlin D (2003) Depression: the challenge for all healthcare professionals. *Nursing Standard,* **17** (26), 45–52.

Moulton C, Yates D (1999) *Emergency Medicine.* Oxford: Blackwell Science.

Nicholl JP, Coleman P, Williams RT (1991) Pilot study of the epidemiology of sports injuries and exercise-related injuries. *British Journal of Sports Medicine* **25**(1), 61–66.

Office for National Statistics (1997) *General Household Survey.* Northern Ireland: Statistics Office.

Office for National Statistics (2000). London: Stationery Office.

Office for National Statistics (1998) *Geographical Variations in Suicide Mortality.* London: Stationery Office.

Parker H, Aldridge J, Measham F (1998) *Illegal Leisure.* London: Routledge.

Rickards L, Fox K, Roberts C, Fletcher L, Goddard E (2004) *Living in Britain: Results from the 2002 General Household Survey.* London: The Stationery Office.

Royal College of Psychiatrists and Royal College of Physicians (2000) *Drugs, Dilemmas and Choices.* Glasgow: Bell and Bain.

Simmonds J, Allen J, Aust R et al. (2002) *Crime in England and Wales 2001/2002.* London: Home Office.

Skinner D, Driscoll P, Earlham R (1991) *ABC of Major Trauma.* London: BMJ.

Smith C, Allen J (2004) *Violent Crime in England and Wales.* London: Home Office.

Social Trends 30 (2000). London: Stationery Office.

Stationery Office (1999) *Mortality Statistics; Injury and Poisoning.* London: Stationery Office.

Strategy Unit (2003) *Interim Analytical Report.* London: Strategy Unit.

Tanagho E, McAnich J (2000) *Smith's General Urology.* New York: McGraw-Hill.

Wasserman D (2001) *An Unnecessary Death.* London: Martin Duntz.

Wilson W (2000) A/E nurses fast-track protocol for miscarriages. *Accident and Emergency Nursing,* **8**(1), 9–12.

Chapter 20

Middle years

Brian Boag

INTRODUCTION

The life continuum represents a sequence of physical, psychological and social attributes that an individual may experience, and will have an influence on how individuals develop within a changing society and cope with the associated demands and crises (Roper et al. 1990). In this chapter the age range of 35–65 will be taken as the nominal age range. This in itself presents the first challenge, as the spectrum of health can often mean a well 35 year-old becoming ill over the 30 years. The opposite can also be observed, as due to the nature of 'health' many people in their forties and fifties become much more aware of their physical being and actively work to ensure they are healthy; therefore one can be a very fit 65-year-old or a 35-year-old whose health status is poor.

This chapter will be an examination of the main concerns faced by those in their middle years and the common presentations to the emergency department. It is worthwhile to note that many illnesses associated with this age group are not physical and a brief examination of the psychological profile of this age group is included. During this age continuum the chances of illness are greatly increased: rates for cancer go up, diabetes rises, joints fail and ischaemic heart disease becomes a more common issue.

CHEST PAIN

Chest pain is a major factor affecting the health of those in the middle years group, with ischaemic heart disease, angina and myocardial infarctions being among the most common. The overall cost of caring for angina has been calculated by Stewart et al. (2003) to be around 1% of the NHS budget, mainly because of hospital bed occupancy and revascularization procedures; however, the burden of chest pain is far greater than the burden of angina. Nilsson et al. (2003) report that 1.5% of primary care consultations are for chest pain, but only 17% of these are associated with definite or possible angina. However, due to health campaigning many present to the emergency department assuming the worst but often have another reason for this.

The patient presenting to the emergency department complaining of chest pain requires careful assessment to determine the symptoms and subtle features which differentiate chest pain that is cardiac in origin from that which is non-cardiac (see Box 20.1). Chest pain can be very frightening for the patient, especially if it is the first episode, and staff need to assess and determine the likely signs of such pain. A number of key characteristics may help the assessing nurse to distinguish cardiac pain from that of other causes:

- *Location.* The location of the pain can give a big clue to the nature of the cause. Cardiac pain is centrally located and chest pain that is peripheral to the sternum is rarely cardiac in nature.

- *Radiation.* Cardiac pain brought on by ischaemia can often radiate to the jaw, neck and arms. Pain

situated over the left anterior chest and radiating laterally may have various causes, such as pleurisy, chest wall injury and anxiety.

- *Provocation.* Anginal pain is precipitated by exertion, rather than occurring after it. It disappears a few minutes after the cessation of activity when blood flow can again match the oxygen requirements of the muscle. In contrast, pain associated with a specific movement, such as bending, stretching or turning, is likely to be musculoskeletal in origin.

- *Character of the pain.* Ischaemic pain is often described as 'dull' or like a heavy object sitting on the chest. Chest pain caused by gastric problems can be described as a bloating or full feeling. Conversely pleural pain may be described as 'sharp' or 'catching' (see Box 20.2).

- *Pattern of onset.* The pain of aortic dissection, massive pulmonary embolism or pneumothorax is usually very sudden in onset (within seconds). Myocardial infarction may build up over several minutes or longer, whereas angina builds in proportion to the intensity of the exertion. Pain which develops over a longer period, such as days or even weeks, is often associated with respiratory illness or muscular damage.

- *Associated features.* The severe pain of a myocardial infarct, massive pulmonary embolus or aortic dissection is often accompanied by autonomic disturbance, including sweating, nausea and vomiting. If the patient is flushed, it may reflect a pyrexia or it may be stress-related. Pallor may be indicative of inadequate cardiac function or shock. Breathlessness is associated with raised pulmonary capillary pressure or pulmonary oedema in myocardial infarction and may accompany any of the respiratory causes of chest pain. Associated gastrointestinal symptoms may provide the clue to non-cardiac chest pain, such as heartburn, peptic ulceration, diarrhoea and vomiting.

On assessment, it is essential to perform a full set of observations. Temperature if high can indicate infection, the rate and depth of the pulse can indicate cardiac damage or arrhythmia, respiration rate can indicate respiratory distress and blood pressure can show cardiac instability. This in conjunction with an ECG can give the assessor a clearer picture as to the nature and cause of the chest pain.

The classic pain of angina pectoris is diffuse and retrosternal and will often diminish after rest. In the case of myocardial infarct, it is localized in the centre

---

Box 20.1   Causes of chest pain

Cardiac
- Angina
- Acute myocardial infarction
- Pericarditis
- Endocarditis
- Genetic abnormality
- Respiratory
- Chest infection
- Embolism
- Pneumothorax
- Asthma
- Chronic conditions

Gastric
- Gastritis
- Ulceration
- Hiatus hernia
- Muscular overuse
- Overuse
- Trauma

Psychosomatic
- Depression
- Bereavement

Box 20.2   Characteristic descriptions of chest pain

Stable angina

Typically constricting, retrosternal pain, radiating to the arms (predominantly to the left), neck or jaw. It often occurs in response to stimuli that increase the oxygen demand of the heart, such as physical exertion or emotion, and is relieved by rest

Unstable angina

As in stable angina, but the periods of pain are prolonged and may occur at rest and have no precipitating factors

Myocardial infarction

Three quarters of patients present with typically severe, crushing, retrosternal pain which may extend to the arms, jaw or back and which often lasts >30 minutes. It is accompanied by nausea, vomiting and sweating. The onset of pain is not always associated with exertion and is not relieved by rest. Some patients have little or no pain, especially the elderly, those from ethnic minority groups (particularly within the Indian subcontinent) and those with diabetes

Pericarditis

The pain is usually sharp and retrosternal and may be more apparent on inspiration. It is often worse when lying flat but is relieved when sitting up or leaning forwards

Pleuritic pain

The pain is usually sharp, localized pain, which is worse on inspiration and coughing

Pulmonary embolism

The pain is pleuritic in nature and may be associated with haemoptysis and breathlessness. Massive PE may produce pain identical in nature to acute myocardial infarction

Oesophageal pain

Oesophageal pain is usually associated with, or eased by, food and is typically worse when lying flat. Oesophageal rupture is usually preceded by vomiting

Aortic dissection

The patient experiences a 'tearing pain', as opposed to the crushing pain of myocardial infarction. This pain is typically felt in the back

Musculoskeletal pain

Pain due to the spinal or muscular disorders can usually be identified by the effect of movement and position. Unlike the other conditions, the chest wall is tender to touch at the specific locations (Adam & Osborne 1997)

Stress–related

The patient will appear flushed and distressed and may be hyperventilating, which will lead to a sensation of central chest pain

---

of the chest, is usually severe in nature, radiating to the left arm and jaw, and is not relieved by rest. Myocardial infarction and its management will be addressed in Chapter 26: Cardiac Care.

It is vitally important to take a careful history from the patient who presents complaining of chest pain. The patient should be encouraged to describe the pain – its intensity, location, duration, what brought it on and whether there is any relevant history (Walsh & Kent 2001). Assessing whether the patient can talk in sentences or whether there is pain on movement can indicate whether the chest pain is respiratory or musculoskeletal in origin. Note also that the fear and anxiety brought on by chest pain can exacerbate symptoms in the patient.

Recording of temperature, pulse and blood pressure and a 12-lead ECG can offer an indication of the likelihood of cardiac-related chest pain. A raised temperature may be a result of the breakdown of cardiac enzymes in response to a myocardial infarct that has happened within the previous few hours or may be a result of underlying infection. Recording of pulse oximetry, which measures arterial oxyhaemoglobin saturation (SpO_2), gives important information about the supply of oxygen to the tissues (Moyle 1994); however, Nicholson (2004) suggests there is no definitive evidence that oxygen has any effect on cardiac ischaemia. Patients whose oxygen saturation levels are under 95% on air are regarded as hypoxic and should be given oxygen via a mask or nasal cannula (Table 20.1). Supplementary oxygen intake to increase oxygen saturation levels helps to relieve tachycardia induced by hypoxia, thereby reducing cardiac workload.

In the absence of pain and with the patient at rest, the 12-lead ECG may be normal; therefore the ECG should also be performed during an episode of chest pain. ST-segment and T-wave changes, which occur during spontaneous chest pain and disappear with relief of the pain, are significant. Even without changes, the ECG should be repeated after 1 hour as the absence of abnormality does not rule out disease. Following myocardial infarction, the levels of some of the myocardial enzymes will rise, and estimation of their serum levels is often of diagnostic importance. In addition, the degree of their elevation may give

Table 20.1 Oxygen masks, flow rates and approximate concentrations of delivered oxygen. (From Jowett & Thompson 1995)

Mask oxygen flow L/min	Edinburgh (%)	MC(%)	Nasal cannulae	Hudson (%)
1	25–30	–	25–30	–
2	30–35	30–50	30–35	25–38
4	35–40	40–70	32–40	35–45
6	–	55–75	–	50–60
8	–	60–75	–	55–65
10	–	65–80	–	60–75

some indication of the size of the infarct (Jowett & Thompson 1995).

Jeremias and Gibson (2005) note that current guidelines for the diagnosis of non-ST-segment elevation myocardial infarction are largely based on an elevated troponin level. While this rapid and sensitive blood test is certainly valuable in the appropriate setting, its widespread use in a variety of clinical scenarios may lead to the detection of troponin elevation in the absence of thrombotic acute coronary syndromes. Many diseases, such as sepsis, hypovolaemia, atrial fibrillation, congestive heart failure, pulmonary embolism, myocarditis, myocardial contusion and renal failure, can also be associated with an increase in troponin level. These elevations may arise from various causes other than thrombotic coronary artery occlusion. Given the lack of any supportive data at present, patients with nonthrombotic troponin elevation should not be treated with antithrombotic and antiplatelet agents. Rather, the underlying cause of the troponin elevation should be targeted. However, troponin elevation in the absence of thrombotic acute coronary syndromes still retains prognostic value. Thus, cardiac troponin elevations are common in numerous disease states and do not necessarily indicate the presence of a thrombotic acute coronary syndrome. While troponin is a sensitive biomarker to 'rule out' non-ST-segment elevation myocardial infarction, it is less useful to 'rule in' this event because it may lack specificity for acute coronary syndromes (Jaffe et al. 2001).

The other measured cardiac enzymes are creatine kinase (CK), lactate dehydrogenase (LDH) and serum glutamic oxaloacetic transaminase (SGOT or AST) and they are released in the first 24 hours after the onset of a myocardial infarct. These enzymes may provide retrospective confirmation of infarction rather than a guide to immediate management (analgesia, aspirin, thrombolysis). If the clinical picture suggests myocardial infarct, the patient should be treated as such; however, these are predominantly undertaken as part of the in-patient workup rather than in the emergency department.

Pain relief may be achieved by administering sublingual GTN tablet or spray, repeated as necessary. Nitrates relax smooth muscle, mainly in the venous system, to increase capacitance and thus reduce cardiac preload. Arteriolar relaxation also occurs, with a fall in peripheral resistance (afterload). The resulting reduction in blood pressure leads to a reduction in chest pain. For patients suspected of having non-cardiac-related chest pain, magnesium trisilicate may relieve symptoms, suggesting an oesophageal or gastric origin of the pain. The use of antacids to differentiate epigastric pain from cardiac pain is common in emergency care; however, consideration must be given to the patient's history, cardiac risk factors and ECG as well as the patient's response to therapy (Novotny-Dinsdale & Andrews 1995). There must always be a high index of suspicion that any chest pain is cardiac in origin until clinical examination and tests prove otherwise (ACEP 2000).

ABDOMINAL PAIN

For many, the onset of abdominal pain occurs for the first time during the middle years and often brings the patient into contact with the emergency department. These abdominal pains range from reflux gastritis through to gastrointestinal haemorrhage; it is therefore that a full and robust history should be taken.

As well as ensuring that the correct cardiovascular observations are taken, it is essential that the assessment nurse gains a full history. This must include:

- *Age.* Some conditions are more likely to occur at different points on the age spectrum.
- *Pain.*
  - Time of onset?
  - Was it a gradual onset or a sudden pain?
  - How does the patient describe the pain, is it stabbing, does it radiate through the back, is it burning?
  - Location of the pain, does it move?
  - Is there any vomiting, what did the vomit look like?
  - Does the pain come, e.g. only after eating, after exercise, at night?
- *Constipation or diarrhoea.* If so when was the last movement, what was the consistency?
- *Temperature.* This can rule out infection or appendicitis.
- *Social history.* Frequent alcohol use, especially binge drinking, can cause ulceration, gastritis, oesophageal varicies or liver disease.

If there is any doubt in the assessing nurse's mind then the patient should be regarded as potentially unwell and regular 15-minute observations commenced. Intravenous access should be established and a full examination of the abdomen undertaken (see Chapter 28: Surgical emergencies).

Obesity has become a major concern for the population of the UK in the past few years and is now a focus of NHS health promotion campaigns. Although not a cause for attendance in the emergency department by itself, morbid obesity can result in many other health presentations (Box 20.3).

It is therefore worthwhile weighing the patient and producing a body mass index (BMI) (Box 20.4) on any patient who is overweight; this can give an indication of potential underlying developing chronic conditions and can also allow the practitioner an opportunity to make a health promotional intervention.

EPIGASTRIC PAIN

Gastritis is a common condition which relates to an inflammation of the stomach lining and involves the symptoms of vomiting. The term gastroenteritis refers to an inflammation of both the gastric and intestinal mucosa. Gastritis is usually associated with dietary indiscretions due to overindulgence of alcohol or food, but it may also be a result of stress, non-steroidal anti-inflammatory drugs (NSAIDs) or uraemia.

The inflammation is usually self-limiting and without sequelae, but patients presenting with gastritis may require antacids to alleviate vomiting and nausea. Advice to patients includes taking clear liquids only until 8–12 hours have passed without vomiting, and then starting with bland foods before gradually resuming a normal diet.

The term 'peptic ulcer' refers to an ulcer in the lower oesophagus, the stomach, the duodenum or the jejunum after surgical anastomosis to the stomach. It is a common condition and has its highest incidence in males aged 40–55 years, with perforation occurring in approximately 5–10% of affected individuals. While epigastric pain resolves with antacids and is self-limiting and short-lived, ulcers are repetitive and are worse after specific foods or drinks. Although peptic ulcer disease is commonly suspected in dyspeptic patients, it is found much less often than suspected when patients undergo endoscopic investigation (Vakil 2005).

Ulceration of the gastric mucosa leads to excoriation and mucous membrane sloughing. An imbalance between pepsin, hydrochloric acid secretion and bicarbonate causes gastric erosion. Bacterial invasion from *Helicobacter pylori* has been implicated as an important aetiological factor in peptic ulcer disease, accounting for 90% of duodenal ulcers and 70% of gastric ulcers (Shearman 1995, Lassen et al. 2004). *H. pylori* causes acute inflammation of the mucosa by causing degeneration, detachment and necrosis of the epithelial cells. Chronic ingestion of medications that irritate the gastric mucosa, such as aspirin or NSAIDs, can also lead to the development of ulcers (Butcher 2004). While duodenal and gastric ulcers are different conditions, they share common symptoms and will be considered together.

The most common presentation is that of recent abdominal pain which has three notable characteristics: localization to the epigastrium, relationship to food and episodic occurrence. The pain is probably caused by acid coming into contact with the ulcer. Occasional vomiting may occur in about 40% of patients with peptic ulcer. In some patients the ulcer is completely 'silent', presenting for the first time with anaemia from chronic undetected blood loss, or as an abrupt haematemesis or acute perforation; in others there is recurrent acute bleeding without ulcer pain between attacks.

Peptic ulceration is an umbrella term used to describe areas in the gastrointestinal tract that have

---

Box 20.3   Health concerns of obesity

- Type II diabetes
- Renal failure
- Cardiovascular disease
- Stroke
- Joint injury, degeneration
- Respiratory problems
- Skin rashes
- Vascular problems
- Ineffective wound healing
- Depression
- Cancer and stomach problems

Box 20.4

Working out a body mass index:
1. Height in meters multiplied by height in meters
2. Weight in kilograms
3. divide 2 by 1.

e.g. a patient weighing 60 kg who is 1.2 meters tall would have a BMI of 41.6
1.2 x 1.2 = 1.44. 60/1.44 = 41.6.

been exposed to, and damaged by, acid and pepsin-containing secretions. The most common sites for peptic ulcers are the stomach (gastric ulcers) and the duodenum (duodenal ulcers) (Elliot 2002). A peptic ulcer may progressively erode the submucosal, muscular and serous layers of the gastrointestinal wall. When perforation occurs, the contents of the stomach escape into the peritoneal cavity; this occurs more commonly in duodenal than in gastric ulcers. The most striking symptom is sudden, severe pain; its distribution follows the spread of gastric contents over the peritoneum. Initially, the pain may be referred to the upper abdomen, but it quickly becomes generalized; shoulder tip pain may occur as a result of irritation of the diaphragm. The pain is accompanied by shallow respirations due to epigastric pain and limitation of diaphragmatic movements. A rapid pulse and reduction in blood pressure indicate shock. Pyrexia may also be present as a result of peritonitis. Pallor, a cold clammy skin, nausea and vomiting may be also evident. The abdomen is held immobile and has 'board-like' rigidity.

Non-operative treatment includes i.v. morphine for pain relief, aspiration of the stomach contents using a nasogastric tube and continuous gastric suctioning, i.v. electrolytes and fluids, and antibiotic therapy. After initial treatment for shock, emergency surgery may be performed to close the perforation or resect the affected area; however, perforation carries a mortality of approximately 10%. The nurse should monitor the patient's vital signs closely for signs of deterioration and offer reassurance to the patient and his family.

Where there is no indication of perforation, the patient is usually managed with a range of anti-ulcer medications such as ranitidine and/or metronidazole, which have antibacterial effects on *H. pylori,* and referred back to his GP.

JOINT INJURY

For some who have had a history of undertaking sport and continue to do so at an aggressive level, there may be injury due to overuse. This will be addressed in further detail in the skeletal injuries chapter (Chapter 5).

DEPRESSION AND LIFE–CHANGING EVENTS

During this phase of life, many people experience life-changing events, including job loss, house moves, children leaving home and bereavement. For many it can be a traumatic time and depression can occur. For some this can manifest itself slowly through a sequence of multiple presentations to the emergency department with psychosomatic presentations of minor illness, and for others it can be manifested as a suicide attempt or through a violent outburst.

For the nurse assessing it is advisable to be aware of the patient with frequent attendance and to ask for a fuller social history. In acute presentations it is essential that a full psychiatric assessment is undertaken by a specialist in mental health as follow-up treatment may be needed. For the partners and relatives of those who have died suddenly, a referral to a chaplain or a bereavement service may help limit the ongoing development of depression and mental illness. These issues are addressed more fully in Chapter 13 and Chapter 14 (Care of the bereaved and Psychiatric emergencies).

HOMELESSNESS

Few would need convincing that the extreme conditions of homelessness, of sleeping rough, are bound to affect health (Joseph Rowntree Foundation 2000, Best 1995). The homeless are disproportionately white, male and middle-aged (Anderson et al. 1993), although there are increasing numbers of young men and women and black and Asian people (Homeless Link 2002, Pleace & Quilgars 1996). In a study of the records of 1873 homeless users of an emergency department compared with 28 420 housed people, a disturbing health profile emerged (North et al. 1996):

- Homeless people's accidents and injuries were four times more likely to be the result of an assault than those of housed people.
- Homeless people had twice the rate of infected wounds compared with housed people. These infections were twice as likely to be severe enough to warrant an admission to hospital for further treatment.
- A substantial proportion (10%) of homeless people attending emergency departments did so for mental health reasons. This was the second largest presenting category for homeless people to emergency departments, but only ranked 10th for housed attenders.
- Homeless people were five times more likely to attend emergency departments due to deliberate self-harm than were housed people. Depression was very common among people of no fixed abode and hostel residents.
- Asthma was twice as common among homeless as among housed attenders.
- Epilepsy was four times as common among homeless as among housed users of the emergency department.

More recent research by Griffiths (2002) has identified that:

- 30–50% of homeless people experience mental health problems
- about 70% of homeless people misuse drugs
- about 50% of homeless people are dependent on alcohol
- rough sleepers are 35 times more likely to kill themselves than the general population and have an average life expectancy of 42 years.

The literature on homelessness reveals the almost universal acceptance that there is a close link between ill health and homelessness (Fisher & Collins 1993, Marren-Bell 1993, Moore et al. 1997). Difficulties in obtaining access to primary health care services have meant that emergency departments have been an important source of health care provision for some homeless men and women. The Scottish Executive Health Department (2001) notes that while emergency departments are often the first point of contact for homeless people, staff may not have received training on homelessness issues and may not be in a position to respond appropriately to homelessness. Minor, acute illnesses pose particular problems for homeless people, who lack the facilities to look after themselves when well, and who are at risk of particular infections and infestations precisely because of their circumstances. Respiratory illness has been found to be a major health problem associated with being homeless (Balazs 1993). Other common conditions are chronic obstructive airways disease, tuberculosis, foot problems, infestations and epilepsy. Homeless people attending emergency departments also exhibit a disproportionate prevalence of infections, scabies and lice (Scott 1993). Emergency admission rates are also higher (Scheur et al. 1991). Low temperature is an important cause of morbidity and mortality among the homeless. In Britain, for each degree Celsius that the winter is colder than average, there are an extra 8000 deaths (Balazs 1993).

Emergency nurses may offer the only social contact for some homeless people. A novel Canadian study found that compassionate care of homeless people who present to emergency departments significantly lowered their repeat visits. The researchers identified 133 consecutive homeless adults visiting one inner-city emergency department who were not acutely psychotic, extremely intoxicated, unable to speak English or medically unstable. Half were randomly assigned to receive compassionate care from trained volunteers. All patients otherwise had usual care and were followed for repeat visits to emergency departments. The researchers found that the attendance by homeless people who received compassionate care was significantly lower. While acknowledging that compassionate care is not necessarily cost-effective if staff costs are taken into account, the authors argued that the basic justification for compassion is decency not economics (Redelmeier et al. 1995).

CONCLUSION

The middle years is a pivotal time frame when things can start to go wrong as the adult moves from being almost always healthy to almost always having a health concern. Through this continuum it is essential that the patient is fully assessed and treated with consideration. It may well be that there is nothing wrong and the concerns are psychological, but now is a good time to begin health promotion, ensuring the middle years adult remains healthy for as long as they can.

References

ACEP (2000) *Clinical Policy: Critical Issues in the Evaluation and Management of Adult Patients Presenting with Suspected Acute Myocardial Infarction or Unstable Angina*. Dallas: ACEP

Adam SK, Osborne S (1997) *Critical Care Nursing: Science & Practice*. Oxford Medical.

Anderson I, Kemp P, Quilgars D (1993) *Single Homeless People*. London: HMSO.

Aro P, Storskrubb T, Ronkainen J, Bolling-Sternevald E, Engstrand L, Vieth M, Stolte M, Talley NJ, Agreus L (2006) Peptic ulcer disease in a general adult population. *American Journal of Epidemiology*. **163**(11), 1025–1034.

Balazs J (1993) Health care for single homeless people. In: Fisher K, Collins J, eds. *Homelessness, Health Care and Welfare Provision*. London: Routledge.

Best R (1995) The housing dimension. In: Benzeval M, Judge K, Whitehead M, eds. *Tackling Inequalities in Health: An Agenda for Action*. London: King's Fund.

Butcher D (2004) Pharmacological techniques for managing acute pain in emergency departments. *Emergency Nurse*, **12**(1), 26–36.

Elliot S (2002) The treatment of peptic ulcers. *Nursing Standard*, **16**(22), 37–42.

Fisher K, Collins J (1993) *Homelessness, Health Care and Welfare Provision*. London: Routledge.

Homeless Link (2002) *An Overview of Homelessness in London.* London: Homeless Link.

Griffith S (2002) *Assessing the Health Needs of Rough Sleepers.* London: Office of the Deputy Prime Minister Homelessness Directorate.

Jaffe AS, The World Health Organisation, The European Society of Cardiology, The American College of Cardiology (2001) New standard for the diagnosis of acute myocardial infarction. *Cardiology in Review*, **9**(6), 318–322.

Jeremias A, Gibson CM (2005) Narrative Review: Alternative causes for elevated cardiac troponin levels when acute coronary syndromes are excluded. *Annals of Internal Medicine*, **142**(9), 786–791.

Joseph Rowntree Foundation (2000) *Research on Single Homelessness in Britain.* London: Joseph Rowntree Foundation

Jowett NI, Thompson D (1995) *Comprehensive Coronary Care*, 2nd edn. London: Scutari.

Lassen AT, Hallas J, Schaffalitzky de Muckadell OB (2004) *Helicobacter pylori* test and eradicate versus prompt endoscopy for management of dyspeptic patients: 6.7 year follow up of a randomised trial. *Gut*, **53**(12), 1758–1763

Marren-Bell U (1993) Homelessness: the A&E response. *Emergency Nurse*, **1**(1), 4–6.

Moore H, North C, Owens C (1997) Health and healthcare for homeless people. *Emergency Nurse*, **5**(1), 25–29.

Moyle JTM (1994) *Pulse Oximetry*. London: BMJ.

Nicholson C (2004) A systematic review of the effectiveness of oxygen in reducing acute myocardial ischaemia. *Journal of Clinical Nursing*, **13**, 996–1007.

Nilsson S, Scheike M, Engblom D, Karlsson LG, Molstand S, Akerlind I, Ortoft K, Nylander E (2003) Chest pain and ischaemic disease in primary care. *British Journal of General Practice*, **53**, 378–382.

North C, Moore H, Owens C (1996) *Go Home and Rest?: The Use of an Accident and Emergency Department by Homeless People.* London: Shelter.

Novotny-Dinsdale V, Andrews LS (1995) Gastrointestinal emergencies. In: Thomas J, Proeh JA, Kaiser, eds. *Emergency Nursing: A Physiologic and Clinical Perspective*, 2nd edn. Philadelphia: Saunders.

Scheur MA, Black M, Victor C, Benzeval M, Gill M, Judge K (1991) *Homelessness and the Utilisation of Acute Hospital Services in London.* London: King's Fund Institute.

Scott J (1993) Homelessness and mental health. *British Journal of Psychiatry*, **162**, 314–324.

Selfridge-Roper N, Logan WW, Tierney AJ (1990) *The Elements of Nursing: A Model for Nursing Based on a Model of Living.* Edinburgh: Churchill Livingstone.

Pleace N, Quilgars D (1996) *Health and Homelessness in London: A Review.* London: King's Fund.

Redelmeier DA, Molin JP, Tibshini RJ (1995) A randomised trial of compassionate care for the homeless in an emergency department. *The Lancet*, **345**, 1131–1134.

Scottish Executive Health Department (2001) *Health and Homelessness Guidance.* Edinburgh: Scottish Executive Health Department.

Shearman DJC (1995) Diseases of the alimentary tract and pancreas. In: Edwards CRW, Bouchier IAD, Haslett C, Chilvers ER, eds. *Davidson's Principles and Practice of Medicine.* 17th Edn. Edinburgh: Churchill Livingstone.

Stewart S, Murphy N, Walker A, McGuire A, McMurray JJV (2003) The current cost of angina pectoris to the National Health Service in the UK. *Heart*, **89**, 848–53.

Vakil N (2005) Commentary: toward a simplified strategy for managing dyspepsia. *Postgraduate Medicine*, **1176**, 13.

Walsh M, Kent A (2001) *Accident & Emergency Nursing: a New Approach.* 4th Edn. Oxford: Butterworth Heinemann.

Chapter 21

Older people

Antonia Lynch

INTRODUCTION

Older people constitute a growing proportion of attendances to the emergency department (ED). This chapter addresses the changing UK demographics, and the physiology of ageing, before considering the assessment of common acute older adult presentations, such as hypothermia, confusion and falls. The effects of polypharmacy and elder abuse will also be described and discussed.

In demographic terms, the UK has an ageing population. From 1971 to 2021 the number of people in the UK aged 65 and over is expected to increase by nearly 70% from 7.3 million to 12.2 million (Office of National Statistics 2006), because average life expectancy in the UK has doubled in the last two hundred years. By 2021, there will be more people over 80 than under the age of 5; over a quarter of the population will be over 60. However, the section of older people which has increased most rapidly, both in actual size and in proportion to the total population, is the 75 years and over group. It is suggested that by 2021 there are expected to be 601 000 people aged 90 and over. These changes are having a major impact on health and social services, and patients over 65 years account for 14–20% (Bridges et al. 1999) of ED attendances. This is likely to rise, considering these demographic changes.

BACKGROUND

There have been concerns about the quality of care delivered to older people for many years. The Health Advisory Service 2000 (1998) identified eight major issues affecting the care of older people (Table 21.1). It was reported that older people waited longer in the ED than any other patient group (Association of

Table 21.1   Concerns about the quality of care for older people

Admission delays
Poor physical environment
Shortage of medical, nursing and therapy staff
Lack of expertise and education in the care of older people
Lack of fundamental care, dignity, respect and assistance with eating and bathing
Low expectations of recovery, lack of awareness of rehabilitation
Poor communication with older people and their families
Poor discharge planning

Health Advisory Service 2000 (1998)

Community Health Councils for England and Wales 2001); however, it was also acknowledged that older people present with more complex needs and take longer to process (Dove and Dale 1986, Clark and Fitzgerald 1999). Meyer and Bridges (1998) found evidence of negative attitudes amongst nurses towards older people in the ED. Spilsbury et al. (1999) interviewed ED patients about their experiences. They reported concerns about lack of assessment, long waiting times, and staff not taking into account their sensory or physical problems while not giving consideration to their privacy, safety and comfort. They also stated that staff did not appear to understand their pre-admission circumstances. Meyer and Bridges (1998) concur with this, stating that ED nurses perceive their role as primarily providing biomedical care rather than nursing care. This prompted the RCN A&E Nursing Association to release a mission statement on the care of older people in the ED, which highlights the need to:

'Provide an environment appropriate to meeting the needs of older people, by creating a culture and supporting practice that is respectful of the complex needs, rights, desires, dignity and life experience' (Sowney 1999)

A report by the UK Standing Nursing Midwifery Advisory Committee (SNMAC 2001) suggested there remained a persistence of negative attitudes about nursing older people and stated that the reasons are complex, including a lack of clinical leadership, management and role modelling. Evers (1984) highlights the role of the sister/charge nurse in determining the style and nature of nursing care and more particularly his or her influence on younger, less experienced nurses.

The National Service Framework for Older People (Department of Health (DoH) 2001a) creates a benchmark to underpin the care of older people. The aim of this document is to address their needs, by promoting knowledge-based practice and partnership working between those who use and those who provide a service (DoH 2001a). This highlights the need for emergency nurses to have expert understanding of the ageing process, specialist assessment whilst also developing practice through leadership, teaching and mentoring (SNMAC 2001).

PHYSIOLOGY OF AGEING

The process of ageing is a continuum progressing throughout the individual's life. It is genetically programmed and influenced by the environment, so the rate of ageing among people varies widely (Cheitlin 2003). Ageing is characterized by a general deterioration of bodily function. Although ageing is considered to be inevitable, the reality is that the rate of deterioration in organ function can be reduced by factors such as regular exercise and accelerated by habits such as cigarette smoking and heavy alcohol consumption. Indeed, there is considerable variability in individuals' susceptibility to ageing. Table 21.2 outlines some of the organ and tissue changes associated with ageing, which will underpin patient assessment.

ASSESSMENT

An older person presenting to the ED requires a thorough physical, psychological and social assessment. Good communication is vital and the emergency nurse must have the ability to listen effectively. As older people's hearing and vision may be impaired and their responses slow, it is therefore important to give the patient time to express themselves freely. It is also important to remember that the history-taking process may take longer than the physical examination, and studies indicate that over 80% of diagnoses are based on the interview alone (Epstein et al. 2003). Patients have previously expressed concerns about lack of assessment and information-giving (Spilsbury et al. 1999). Older people can present with multiple pathologies and the presenting complaint may not be the only condition which needs to be considered.

The emergency nurse needs to elicit why the person has attended the ED. The assessment can begin with a general question that allows full freedom to respond; for example, 'What brings you here?' or 'What can we do for you?' After the patient answers, probe further by asking 'Is there anything else?' It is imperative to remember that patients may also have complex psychological and social causes and may have complicated feelings about themselves, their illnesses or potential treatments. To gain a thorough history, which fulfils

Table 21.2 Physiological changes associated with ageing

System	Pre-existing conditions	Physiological changes	Signs and symptoms	Potential traumatic injuries
Cardiovascular	Coronary artery disease Hypertension Congestive heart failure Myocardial infarction Medications (esp. beta blockers, calcium-channel blockers, anticoagulants)	Fat and fibrous tissue replaces conductive pathways Heart valves thicken reducing compliance Reduced coronary artery flow Lower maximum heart rate Reduced cardiac output	Dysrhythmias Hypertension Inability to meet increased myocardial oxygen demands Heart rate may not rise due to stressors	Aortic arch disruption Myocardial contusion Aneurysm
Respiratory	Chronic obstructive pulmonary disease Asthma Pneumonia Pulmonary oedema Pulmonary embolism Congestive heart failure History of smoking	Non-elastic fibrous tissue Fixed expiratory volume Reduced compliance Reduced vital capacity Reduced alveoli in number and size Reduced peak expiratory flow Increased residual volume Under-ventilation despite normal perfusion Reduced baseline PO_2 Reduced cough reflexes Chest wall stiffness Reduced response to foreign antigen Reduced response to hypoxia or hypercarbia	Increased diaphragmatic breathing Shortness of breath	Increased risk of rib fractures Increased risk of pulmonary contusion Air trapping Atelectasis Increased risk of pneumonia Increased risk of aspiration Increased risk of adult respiratory distress syndrome (ARDS)
Renal	Renal insufficiency	Reduced number of glomeruli Reduced number of nephrons Reduced renal flow Reduced glomerular filtration rate Reduced bladder capacity Reduced drug metabolism	Reduced urinary output	Acute renal failure Increased risk of fluid/electrolyte imbalance and fluid overload

(continued)

Table 21.2   Physiological changes associated with ageing—Cont'd

System	Pre-existing conditions	Physiological changes	Signs and symptoms	Potential traumatic injuries
Central nervous system	Stroke Dementia Alzheimer's Impaired gait		Confusion Altered mental status	Increased risk of subdural haematoma Brain infarct Closed head injury
Gastrointestinal	Reduced calorie intake Reduced glucose tolerance Diabetes	Reduced calorie requirement Reduced body mass Reduced drug metabolism by liver Reduced gastric emptying Reduced gastric motility Reduced oesophageal sphincter	Oesophageal reflux Bowel dysfunction	Increased risk of bowel injuries Mesenteric infarction
Skin and musculoskeletal	Nutritional deficiency Joint disease Arthritis	Loss of skin tone Reduced sensation Loss of resilient connective tissue Reduced mobility Osteoporosis Spondylosis Kyphosis	Bruising Contusions Skin/wound infections	Tetanus Distal radius fractures Fractured hip C1-C2 fractures from falls at ground level Spinal fractures Rib fractures
Immunological	Autoimmune dysfunction	Altered cellular response	Sepsis without pyrexia	
Hepatic	Coagulopathies		Bruising Bleeding	Contusions Bleeding
Endocrine	Diabetes mellitus Diabetes insipidus Thyroid dysfunction			

Adapted from Stevenson (2004).

the patient expectations, the interviewing technique must allow patients time to recount their own stories spontaneously (Bickley 2003). An example of how to structure history taking is provided in Table 21.3.

When first meeting the patient, the nurse should introduce themselves, both as a courtesy and as an opportunity to establish a rapport. If the patient has walked into the department, the nurse should accompany the patient to the cubicle and observe features such as gait, balance and pace.

If the patient needs to get undressed, they should do so themselves, if they are able to. It is important for the patient to feel in control as much as possible. Offering the patient a seat while undressing will allow them to remove their clothes more easily. It also enables the nurse to assess the patient's balance and ability to self-care. It is not essential for patients to remove all their clothing when getting undressed, and undergarments should only be removed if necessary. If the patient is wearing pyjamas or a nightdress on presentation, there is rarely a need to change into a hospital gown; however, the patient will usually require a full examination, and clothing should not inhibit this. The patient may require steps to climb onto the trolley where they are able.

Careful attention should be given to the condition of the patient's skin; inspect the patient for old wounds, unhealed ulcers or bruises. The latter may give an indication of elder abuse (considered later in this chapter). An initial nutritional assessment should be completed.

Not all patients attending the ED require a full set of vital signs and the older person must be assessed individually. For many patients, vital signs will form an integral part of the patient assessment. Older people may have altered vital signs that are normal for them; however, it is imperative to establish their normal baseline. This can be gained from the patient or relative, the computer record system or the patient's Single Assessment Process document (DoH 2001a). For example, the heart rate of an older person is likely to be slower, with arrhythmias being relatively common in otherwise asymptomatic patients. Similarly, the older person's blood pressure is likely to be elevated, usually as a consequence of atherosclerosis. This predisposes the patient to the development of cardiovascular diseases, such as congestive cardiac failure, stroke, transient ischaemic attacks and dementia. If a normally hypertensive patient appears to have a normal blood pressure they may actually be hypotensive. Similarly, if the patient is prescribed and taking beta-blockers they will fail to have a tachycardic response to shock, so the emergency nurse must apply knowledge of pharmacology and altered physiology when analysing vital signs.

A baseline temperature should be recorded. In older people, the temperature is usually recorded as 36.5°C or above, due to the reduction in basal metabolic rate. The patient's respiration rate may be increased due to underlying conditions such as chronic obstructive pulmonary disease or asthma. Poor personal hygiene may reflect difficult socio-economic circumstances of the patient rather than an inability to cope, and the nurse should take this into account when assessing the patient. The patient's pre-existing medical and drug history should be assessed and recorded during the assessment.

As with patients of all ages, the nurse needs to use language the patient will understand and provide frequent orienting information about the time, place and person, including explanations of equipment, procedures and routines. Older people may process information more slowly; the nurse should develop comfortable and natural ways of talking to the patient, bearing in mind normal deterioration in hearing and other special senses that are associated with ageing. Others involved in the care of the patient, such as relatives or ambulance crew, should be consulted about the patient's condition. However, the patient's view should be sought as much as possible, with others used to supplement the information provided by the patient.

ELDER ABUSE

No standard definition of elder abuse applies in the UK; it has no legal status and would not be recognized by many older people (House of Commons Health

Table 21.3	Structured history-taking
Location	Where is the pain/problem?
Timing/onset	When did it start? When did you last feel well? Did it start suddenly or gradually?
Quality	How does the patient describe the pain? Is it constant or intermittent?
Quantity or severity	How does this problem affect their daily living, e.g. SOB, can they walk as far as normal, can they do the stairs?
Aggravating factors	Does anything make it worse?
Relieving factors	Does anything make it better?
Associated manifestations	Are there any other symptoms? E.g. If they are short of breath do they also have a cough?

Committee 2004). The Department of Health (2000) report *No Secrets* notes that their definition is not restricted to older people but refers to a vulnerable person:

> 'A person who is or may be in need of community care service by reason of mental or other disability, age or illness; and who is or may be unable to take care of him or herself, or unable to protect him or herself against significant harm or exploitation.'

This definition has been widely criticized as it assumes a vulnerable person is frail, requiring external support. However, it notes that abuse is a violation of an individual's human and civil rights by a person.

The prevalence of elder abuse in the UK is relatively unknown as there has been little research into this area. It often remains unreported, as older people may be frightened, unable or embarrassed to tell anyone (Neno & Neno 2004). A UK study enquired about abuse caused by family members and close friends; its prevalence was found to be 5% verbal abuse and 2% physical or financial (Ogg & Bennet 1992). However, a survey of community and district nurses indicated that 88% of respondents encountered elder abuse and 12% on a monthly basis (CDNA 2003).

Nurses should have a high index of suspicion when assessing older people, as with non-accidental injury in children. Clinicians must assess whether the mechanism is consistent with the injury or illness presented (Crouch 2003). If emergency nurses know the red flags of abuse (Table 21.4), the right questions to ask (Tables 21.5 and 21.6) and the appropriate action to take in cases of suspected abuse, they can make a critical difference to the welfare of an older person (Gray Vickery 2005). If nurses suspect abuse, attention to detail when documenting is of paramount importance. Document the persons' account in their own words (CDNA 2003) and signs of abuse clearly, and consider the use of illustration through medical photography; this requires specialist consent and adherence to local protocols. Upon detection of abuse local guidelines and policies should be adhered to.

The questions below act as a guide; enquiries must be made sensitively in a private and safe environment, allowing the person time to speak. It is important to find out what the person wants to happen.

Table 21.4   Red flags for identifying elder abuse

For all forms of abuse have a high index of suspicion if the history is inconsistent with the injury or illness

Physical signs of abuse:
- Multiple bruising, e.g. inner thigh or bruising at different stages of healing
- Finger marks
- Burns, especially in unusual places
- An injury similar to the shape of an object
- Unexplained fractures
- Pressure ulcers or untreated wounds
- Attempts to hide part of the body on examination
- Inappropriate use of medications, e.g. overdosing

Signs of sexual abuse:
- Pain, itching or injury to the anal, genital or abdominal area
- Difficulty in walking or sitting because of genital pain
- Bruising and/or bleeding of external genitalia
- Torn, stained or bloody underclothes
- Sexually transmitted disease or recurrent episodes of cystitis
- An uncharacteristic change in the patient's attitude to sex
- Unexplained problems with catheters

Signs of psychological abuse:
- Appears depressed, frightened, withdrawn, apathetic, anxious or aggressive
- Makes a great effort to please
- Appears afraid of being treated by specific staff, carer or relative
- Displays reluctance to be discharged
- Demonstrates sudden mood or behaviour change

Signs of financial abuse: the patient may confide in the emergency nurse
- Unexplained savings account withdrawals
- Inability to explain what is happening to his/her income
- Unpaid bills
- The disappearance of bank statements and valuables, e.g. jewellery, clothes, personal possessions and money

Signs of neglect
- Weight loss
- Unkempt appearance, dirty clothes and poor hygiene
- Pressure ulcers or uncharacteristic problems with continence
- Inadequate nutrition and hydration
- Inadequate or inappropriate medical treatment or withholding treatment
- A patient who is left in a wet or soiled bed

(Adapted from Klein Schmidt 1997, Action on Elder Abuse 2005).

POLYPHARMACY

The use of multiple medications (polypharmacy) is common among older people (DoH 2001a). This is caused by many factors such as coexisting chronic conditions, use of more than one pharmacy, increase in the availability of over-the-counter medicines and multiple prescribing providers. Indeed, interviews carried out with multi-professionals reported that participants admitted that prescribing was sometimes inappropriate and prescribing for chronic diseases was poorly

Table 21.5 Screen for physical abuse with these questions

Has anyone hurt you?
Has anyone touched you without your consent?
Has anyone ever made you do things you didn't want to do?
Has anyone ever threatened you?
Who cares for you at home?
Are you frightened of your care-giver?

Table 21.6 Screen for neglect and financial exploitation with these questions

Are you satisfied with your living situation?
What is a typical day like for you?
Who gives you your medications?
Who helps you with dressing, bathing and/or preparing meals?
Has anyone ever failed to help you when you needed help?

(Adapted from Gray-Vickery 2005).

understood (Spinewine et al. 2005). A US study indicated that 23% of women and 19% of men take at least five prescription drugs (Kaufmann et al. 2002). These figures, however, do not take into account medication that is purchased over the counter.

The effects of polypharmacy may have precipitated the patient's attendance at the ED. Falls and dehydration are common risk factors associated with multiple medications (DoH 2001b). Emergency nurses need to be aware of medicine-related features, which are known to be associated with problems in older people. These are:

- taking four or more medications
- specific medications, e.g. warfarin, non-steroidal anti-inflammatory drugs (NSAIDs), diuretics and digoxin
- recent discharge from hospital.

Social and personal factors associated with medication-related problems are:

- social support – minimal support available
- physical condition – poor hearing, vision and dexterity
- mental state – delirium/dementia
  DoH (2001a).

Patients presenting with polypharmacy should have a detailed drug history recorded; it is good practice to have a pharmacist review medications during the patient's ED episode. However, if this service is unavailable, careful attention should be given to taking and documenting the drug history. In addition to the

drug name, dose and frequency, the source of the history, compliance and concordance should be noted. The key to ensuring safety is appropriate prescribing and monitoring of the patient's condition; 5–17% of preventable admissions are associated with adverse reactions to medications (DoH 2001a). Prescribing should take into account the physiology of ageing, drug interactions, cautions, side-effects and the recommended dose for older people.

Effective communication between the ED and primary care is essential to ensure appropriate and effective monitoring is carried out. General practitioners and patients should be provided with information about medications on discharge; this information must include an explanation of why any changes were made (DoH 2001a).

HYPOTHERMIA

Hypothermia is classified as a core temperature below 35°C; it is associated with a high mortality rate among older people. It is important to ascertain whether hypothermia is caused by environmental exposure or is a consequence of unknown pathology. Common precipitants include immobility (Parkinson's disease, hypothyroidism), reduced cold awareness (dementia), unsatisfactory housing, poverty, drugs, alcohol, acute confusion and infections (Wyatt et al. 2005). Malnutrition may also be a leading factor associated with hypothermia. A well balanced diet is essential to provide the calories needed to generate and maintain adequate heat. A decrease in calorie intake can have a profound effect on the ability to produce heat by shivering (Neno 2005).

Physiology

Body temperature is regulated in the anterior hypothalamus. In cold weather, when the body needs to conserve heat, the hypothalamic heat production centres respond to impulses from the thermoreceptors by causing peripheral vasoconstriction via the sympathetic nervous system. This vasoconstriction enhances the insulating properties of the skin, reducing blood flow to the superficial vessels; the result is less heat being lost from the skin (Pocock & Richards 2004).

The ability of people to respond appropriately to changes in the ambient temperature decreases with age. There is a reduction in the awareness of temperature variances and of thermoregulatory responses. Many older people are unable to discriminate a difference between 2.5 and 5°C (Pocock and Richards 2004). When vasoconstriction fails to raise the body temperature, heat is produced by shivering. However, this response is reduced in older people (Table 21.7).

Table 21.7 Clinical features of hypothermia

Mild hypothermia: 32°C–35°C
Cold skin, pallor
Intensive shivering; loss of shiver response at 34°C
Uncoordinated, slow gait
Confusion, disorientation
Apathy or irritability
Bradypnoea, increased heart rate and blood pressure
May not complain of being cold

Moderate hypothermia: 30°C–32°C
Loss of consciousness
Very cold skin and increased pallor
Shivering stops, muscle rigidity develops
Slowed reflexes
Hypertonic muscles
Bradycardia and hypotension
Atrial and ventricular arrhythmias

Severe hypothermia: below 30°C
Extremely cold skin, extreme pallor, cyanosed
Muscle rigidity may become flaccid below 27°C
Unresponsive
Severe respiratory depression
Atrial and ventricular arrhythmias, ventricular fibrillation and finally asystole

Adapted from Wyatt et al. (2005).

Assessment

Assessment should begin with airway, breathing, circulation and disability; immediate intervention is required if the patient is not breathing or has an absent pulse, when advanced life support should be commenced (Resuscitation Council UK 2005).

Recording of accurate vital signs is essential. The heart rate may be slow or irregular; atrial fibrillation is common due to metabolic disturbances. Similarly the respiration rate may be slower and will be deep or shallow depending on the degree of metabolic acidosis, which is common due to reduced tissue perfusion.

A 12-lead ECG should be recorded and patients with a core temperature <35°C should have continuous cardiac monitoring because of the risk of dysrhythmia or ischaemic changes. The ECG may show a bradycardia or atrial fibrillation: however, in severe hypothermia the ECG may show J waves which occur at the junction of the QRS complex and the ST segment (Haslett et al. 2002). The J wave is a specific finding in hypothermia that disappears when the temperature begins to return to normal (Manning & Stolerman 1993).

Blood screens for FBC, clotting and U&Es should be taken to detect specific metabolic causes, such as hypoglycaemia or hypothyroidism. Arterial blood gas values are useful in determining respiratory status and acid-base balance. Both hyponatraemia and hypokalaemia are frequently found in hypothermia; however, older people who are severely dehydrated or volume-depleted may present with hypernatraemia.

Management

Re-warming may be passive external, active external or active internal (core re-warming). Patients should be re-warmed at a rate that corresponds with the rate of onset of hypothermia (Resuscitation Council UK 2000). In reality this is difficult to gauge. Re-warming should not exceed increases of 0.3–1.2°C per hour in mild hypothermia; however, in severe cases rapid re-warming of 3°C per hour is essential (Carson 1999). Hypothermic patients should be handled carefully; vigorous procedures such as tracheal intubation can precipitate VF (Resuscitation Council 2000).

In mild cases it is sufficient to remove the patient from the cold environment, and prevent further heat loss by wrapping the patient up warmly and providing hot drinks in a warm environment (passive warming). In all cases of hypothermia the removal of wet/soiled clothing should be undertaken as soon as possible, and the patient should be dried and covered with blankets. The patient's head should also be covered, as up to 40% of body heat is lost through the scalp. In moderate cases active external methods should be used which include heated pads, which lie beneath the patient, or warm air-filled blankets (Holtzclaw 2004). In severe cases active external methods may include the use of warm humidified gases, and gastric, peritoneal, pleural and bladder lavage with warm fluids at 40°C (Resuscitation Council 2000).

In hypothermic cardiac arrest the patient requires circulation, oxygenation and ventilation while the core body temperature is gradually raised; this is best achieved by active internal re-warming using cardiopulmonary bypass. Where this facility is unavailable, continuous veno-venous haemofiltration and warming replacement fluids can be used. Death should not be confirmed until the patient has been rewarmed, or until warming attempts have failed to raise the core temperature (Resuscitation Council UK 2000).

During the re-warming phase the emergency nurse must be aware that:

- The patient may become hypotensive as the vascular space expands due to vasodilatation. Patients are therefore likely to require large volumes of fluid. Older people are at greater risk of pulmonary oedema; patients therefore require careful haemodynamic monitoring via arterial blood pressure and central venous pressure and should be transferred to a critical-care environment following the ED episode.

- Peripheral vasodilatation may cause the core body temperature to drop.
- Arrhythmias may occur but tend to revert spontaneously (other than VF) and do not require treatment (Resuscitation Council UK 2000).
- Rapid metabolic changes can occur and should be monitored closely; hyperkalaemia may occur (Resuscitation Council UK 2000).

Following an episode of hypothermia, it will be essential to prevent a recurrence. An in-depth multi-professional assessment, including occupational therapist, nutritionist and social worker, which addresses the predisposing factors that led to the admission is required. Only patients who have had a mild case of hypothermia, i.e. above 34°C, may be discharged following preventive advice. Those with lower core temperatures will require admission. Although increasing severity of hypothermia does worsen prognosis, the major determinant of outcome is the precipitating illness or injury. Reported mortality rates vary from 0% to 85% (Rogers 2004).

CONFUSION

Confusion in older people is a catchall term that covers both dementia and delirium, but may also be a consequence of depression. They are, however, quite different. Dementia is a long-term, non-reversible loss of both short- and long-term memory. Delirium is also known as an acute confusional state, which usually has an organic rather than a psychiatric origin and involves global impairment of mental functions.

The prevalence of older people attending the ED with delirium is 10–12% (Hustey & Meldon 2002).

The ED nurse has an important role in the detection and management of patients with acute delirium. A study by Hustey and Meldon (2002) found that the mental impairment detection rate by emergency doctors was between 28 and 35% and those discharged with delirium had very little discharge advice or follow-up arranged. Information received from the ambulance crew, relatives, home wardens and neighbours can also be crucial in determining the onset and degree of delirium in the patient. This information will be helpful in determining the patient's health and mental status prior to their arrival in the ED.

The aetiology of delirium has to be determined from the history, physical examination and special investigations. This creates a real challenge for emergency nurses, as the history and symptoms can be atypical (Table 21.8); however, linked to knowledge of the altered physiology of ageing, the underlying cause will be found through appropriate investigations.

Assessment

Delirium can result from a pathological lesion within the brain or acting on the brain from a focus elsewhere in the body such as a urine or chest infection. Rapid onset indicates an acute problem. It is therefore important to elicit the time frame for the development of delirium; information can be gleaned unobtrusively from observing and interacting with the patient. The nurse should note the following:

- Is the patient alert?
- Does the patient respond appropriately to questions?
- How is the patient groomed?
- Are the patient's clothes soiled?

Table 21.8 Disorders presenting with atypical features in older people

Disorder	Atypical presentation
Myocardial infarction or pulmonary embolism	Confusion, collapse, breathlessness and palpitations without chest pain
Bronchopneumonia	Confusion, tachypnoea, minimal chest signs, no pyrexia
Appendicitis	Confusion and constipation or diarrhoea, few localizing signs and no pyrexia
Peptic ulcer	Anaemia, haematemesis or malaena without symptoms of dyspepsia
Urinary tract infection	Confusion and urinary incontinence without pyrexia, dysuria or frequency
Dehydration	No thirst, skin changes indistinguishable from those of ageing.
Diabetes mellitus	Asymptomatic until onset of complications, nephropathy, neuropathy or retinopathy
Hypothyroidism	Lethargy and general deterioration with no other characteristic signs and symptoms
Thyrotoxicosis	Apathy, weight loss and cardiac signs without anxiety, excess sweating or heat tolerance
Brain tumour	Confusion, drowsiness and focal neurological signs without headache or papilloedema

Adapted from Edwards et al. (1995).

- Orientation to time, place and person and situation should also be assessed.

Physical examination will provide clues to the cause of the confusional state. Mental function may be impaired in varying degrees; impaired conscious level is a hallmark symptom of delirium. It is important to exclude hypoxia at this point. Observe the patient's work of breathing; checks for cyanosis and vital signs should include a respiratory rate and oxygen saturation monitoring. Temperature, blood pressure, pulse and respirations should be taken to assess for signs of infection, such as urinary tract and chest infections, which are common causes of delirium in older people (Table 21.9). Simple diagnostic tests such as urinalysis will help to identify potential causes. Evidence of dehydration will often be present in the confused, older person. The nurse should observe mucous membranes, skin turgidity and vital signs, as significant dehydration may be the cause of the confusional state. In addition, hypothermia, myocardial infarction, stroke and metabolic disorders such as diabetes mellitus (Table 21.8) may also present as acute confusion; it is therefore necessary to check the patient's blood sugar,

record and analyse a 12-lead ECG and monitor oxygen saturation levels. Blood screening for infections or metabolic causes should also be undertaken. A chest X-ray may confirm a chest infection.

Any of these disorders may lead to delirium and all will require medical management. A history of psychiatric illness should alert the emergency nurse to the possibility of a concurrent mental illness, which could potentiate the confusion. This confusion could be a result of the illness itself or a side-effect of medication the patient is receiving.

Management

There are two key elements to the management of delirium:

- eliminate or correct the underlying aetiological disturbance
- provide symptomatic and supportive care.

Intravenous therapy may be required to correct fluid and electrolyte imbalance. Sedative drugs should not be given unless the patient is at risk of causing harm to themselves. The nurse must ensure environmental risk is assessed; the patient should be nursed in a visible cubicle. Where possible, frequent changes of nurses should be avoided to enable a rapport to be built up with the patient and to facilitate orientation. Effective communication includes ensuring that the patient's hearing aid and spectacles are present and working as necessary.

STROKE

A stroke is defined as a focal neurological deficit due to a vascular lesion which has a rapid onset and lasts longer than 24 hours (Kumar & Clark 2002). Approximately 110 000 people in England have a stroke every year and a further 20 000 people have a transient ischaemic attack (TIA). Stroke is one of the top three causes of death in England, after heart disease and cancer and there are at least 300 000 people living with moderate to severe disabilities as a result of a stroke (NAO 2005, 2007). Although strokes can occur at any age, 70% of strokes occur in those aged over 70 years (Wyatt et al. 2005).

Physiology

Brain tissue is particularly sensitive to the effects of oxygen deprivation, and the effect of occlusion of any part of the vasculature depends on the vessel involved, the collateral blood supply and the duration of occlusion. There are two mechanisms of cerebral injury: cerebral infarction (80%) and intracerebral haemorrhage (20%) (Wyatt et al. 2005). Cerebral infarction is most

---

Table 21.9 Causes of acute confusion

Infection	Hypotension
• Chest	• Acute myocardial infarction
• Urinary	• Hypovolaemia, e.g. gastrointestinal bleed or diarrhoea
	• Sepsis (Gram negative)

Metabolic disturbances	Toxicity
• Uraemia	• Drug, e.g. digoxin or opiates
• Hyponatraemia	• Drug withdrawal
• Hypoglycaemia	• Alcohol withdrawal
• Hypo/hypercalcaemia	• Drug interactions
• Hypo/hyperthyroidism	
• Hepatic failure	
• Hypothermia	
• B12 deficiency	

Hypoxia	Cerebral pathology
• Pneumonia	• Stroke/transient ischaemic attack
• Exacerbation of chronic obstructive pulmonary disease	• Subarachnoid haemorrhage
• Pulmonary oedema	• Subdural haematoma
• Pulmonary embolism	• Tumour
	• Epilepsy – postictal state
	• Encephalitis

Adapted from Haslett et al. (1999).

likely to occur from a thromboembolism secondary to atherosclerosis in the carotid artery and aortic arch (Pocock & Richards 2004). However, this can also be caused by an embolism from atrial fibrillation, valve disease or following a myocardial infarction (Wyatt et al. 2005). Intracerebral haemorrhage is caused by an entry of blood into the brain, which immediately stops function in the area as the neurons are disrupted (Pocock & Richards 2004). This may be caused by hypertension, bleeding disorders and intracranial tumours (Wyatt et al. 2005). Older people who have a stroke are more likely to have other underlying pathology such as COPD, ischaemic heart disease, visual impairments and renal failure; these co-morbidities must be considered at the time of assessment

Assessment

The correct diagnosis must be made through careful history-taking, physical examination and investigations. An acute focal stroke is characterized by a sudden appearance of a focal deficit, most commonly a hemiplegia, with or without aphasia, hemi-sensory loss or visual field defect (Haslett et al. 2004).

Classifications of a focal stroke:
- transient if the deficit disappears in 24 hours; however, 20% of these patients will have a stroke within the first month; they are most at risk within the first 72 hours (Royal College of Physicians 2004)
- completed if the deficit persists but does not worsen
- evolving if the deficit continues to worsen after 6 hours
  Haslett et al. (2002).

The nursing assessment must commence with airway, breathing, circulation and disability. If the patient is unconscious resuscitate as per guidelines, otherwise assess the airway for patency as the patient may have difficulty protecting their own airway (Haslett et al. 2002). Open the patient's airway using manual manoeuvres and inspect for foreign bodies, vomit and suction as necessary. If this is successful insert an oropharangeal or naso-pharangeal adjunct and administer oxygen. If the patient tolerates an airway, the patient will require a definitive airway and the nurse must call for a senior clinician and anaesthetic support.

Assess breathing by observing the rate, rhythm, depth and effort of breathing and monitor oxygen saturation levels; if they are <93% the patient will require an arterial blood gas analysis (Wyatt et al. 2005). Chest auscultation may detect underlying pathology and the patient may require a chest X-ray.

To assess circulation record the patient's temperature, heart rate, blood pressure, blood sugar level and an ECG, particularly looking for atrial fibrillation. Hypertension is commonly noted following a stroke; the only indication for lowering blood pressure in the acute phase is if the patient is at risk of complications of hypertension, e.g. hypertensive encephalopathy, aortic aneurysm and renal involvement (Royal College of Physicians 2004). Blood pressure should return to normal within 24–48 hours spontaneously (Haslett et al. 2002). Intravenous access should be gained and bloods taken for FBC, U&E and a clotting screen if the stroke is suspected to be caused by a bleeding disorder. Patients should have their gag reflex assessed by a trained professional; until this is completed the patient should receive intravenous fluids. Extent of any disability is assessed by recording a full Glasgow Coma Scale.

Management

The patient and their relatives will require an explanation about what is happening and what they can expect to happen during their stay in the ED. It is important to inform family and friends that the patient may be able to understand even if they are unable to communicate verbally; this can be extremely frightening and frustrating for the patient and their family. The emergency nurse needs to be calming and reassuring whilst supporting the patient and their family.

The emergency nurse must possess knowledge of the medical treatment options to influence care and to support the patient and relatives. The nurse must monitor the patient closely to observe for signs of an evolving stroke and this must be communicated to the medical staff. The neurological assessment should include documentation of the localized signs and brain imaging should be carried out as soon as possible or within 24 hours of the onset (Royal College of Physicians 2004). If the pathology or the diagnosis of a stroke is uncertain, an MRI scan should be considered (Royal College of Physicians 2004).

Thrombolysis has the potential to improve the patient's outcome following an ischaemic event; however, there are risks associated with this treatment. This treatment should be given within three hours of onset of an ischaemic stroke, a haemorrhagic stroke must have been excluded, and the patient must not be hypertensive (Haslett et al. 2002, Royal College of Physicians 2005). This procedure must be carried out by specialist staff.

Anti-thrombolytic treatment can be started when a primary haemorrhage has been excluded. Aspirin

300 mg should be given rectally if the patient is dysphagic. Anticoagulation is only necessary if the embolism is from the heart caused by atrial fibrillation; these patients will require oral anti-coagulation with warfarin (Haslett et al. 2004).

The Royal College of Physicians (2004) report that surgical evacuation of a primary intracerebral haemorrhage is not supported by evidence. However, they suggest cases of supratentorial haemorrhage with mass effect should be considered for surgical intervention. They recommend that urgent neurosurgical opinion be sought.

Consideration must be given to pressure area care in the ED, a risk assessment should be performed and this communicated to the ward to ensure the patient has appropriate pressure-relieving aids. The patient's acuity will dictate where they are nursed in the ED; however, as patients can deteriorate rapidly they should be cared for where they can have appropriate monitoring, nursing observation and intervention if required. If the patient is nil by mouth in the ED the patient will require oral care and a nutritional assessment when on the ward.

FALLS

Falls are a major cause of disability and the leading cause of mortality due to injury in the person over 75 years in the UK (DoH 2001a). Traumatic injury caused by falls is the most common surgical reason for presentation to the ED by an older person (Aminzadeh & Dalziel 2002).

Falls can have a profound physical, psychological and social consequence on the patient and their family. Fear of falling or a loss of confidence occurs in approximately half of all older people who fall. This is associated with functional decline, increasing depression, decreased quality of life and further falls (King et al. 1995). Sensitivity is required at this point as it can be embarrassing for an adult who has fallen. If it is not the first time they may feel depressed as they chart their own change in physical state associated with ageing. Sensitive history-taking is more likely to elicit a thorough assessment of both the incident and the patient's ability to cope at home.

Falls can result from the interaction of multiple intrinsic and extrinsic factors. Common intrinsic factors include a history of a previous fall, visual disorders, arthritis, confusion, balance impairment, muscle weakness, sensory impairment and polypharmacy (Sudip et al. 2004, Tideiksaar 2003). Extrinsic factors include environmental hazards such as poor lighting, slippery floors and lack of bathroom rails (Tideiksaar 2003). As a consequence, older people are more likely to sustain falls than younger individuals. Illnesses such as cardiac disease, diabetes and sepsis also contribute to the incidence of falls in older people, as do medications such as diuretics, hypnotics and antihypertensive drugs, due to their hypotensive side-effects (Greaves et al. 1997, DoH 2001a).

The emergency nurse must again assess the older person systematically; airway, breathing, circulation, disability and exposure must be assessed. It is important to ensure that the presentation is caused by a mechanical fall and not by a collapse caused by syncope, postural hypotension, visual problems, polypharmacy or carotid sinus syndrome (British Geriatric Society 2003). Physical examination should include an assessment of standing balance and gait; vital signs should include lying and standing blood pressure, blood sugar monitoring, urinalysis and a 12-lead ECG. Any subsequent investigations may be required dependent on clinical findings.

If a mechanical fall is confirmed it is good practice to have a multi-professional approach to the patient assessment. Occupational therapy (OT) and physiotherapy should be involved in the ED to assess and promote independence. Their assessment may extend to the patient's home if required. As mentioned earlier, the patient may have a loss of confidence and this should form an important part of the discharge decision.

The emergency nurses' role is pivotal to ensuring that the ED assessment is comprehensive and includes a full social history. A study by Bentley et al. (2004) found that the most likely reason for re-attendance at the ED after direct discharge was a fall. In those identified cases, adequate assessment of the patients' social and functional needs was not done and the impact of illness or injury underestimated when considering their ability to cope on discharge.

A risk assessment of the older person prior to discharge should include:

- Medical conditions – a thorough history and examination to exclude underlying pathology and problems associated with polypharmacy which may have caused the fall. If an underlying medical condition is the cause of the fall the patient is likely to require admission to hospital. A full social history must be documented as part of this process.
- Mobility – their ability to walk unaided, with a stick or Zimmer frame, but without carer support, is an important determinant of fitness for discharge. Assessment should be carried out with a multi-professional team.
- Social support – it is important to establish whether the older person lives alone or has formal or

informal support available or whether the ED nurse needs to start coordinating these services in collaboration with primary care.

- Lifestyle – consider whether the injury incurred will enable the older person to function: for example, in a patient who lives alone but has a fractured wrist, an OT assessment should be considered.
- External influences – those living alone in a tower block without working lifts will find it more difficult to mobilize than someone living in sheltered accommodation. The handover ambulance crew can often provide useful information about the environment to which the patient may be returning.

The greatest risk indicator for a future fall is a history of a fall; therefore the assessment and discharge process must be rigorous. There are several tools available; most agree that two predictive risk indicators are a history of falls and polypharmacy (Sudip et al. 2004, Tideiksaar 2003) (Table 21.10). However, remember that seemingly minor infections can cause a fall in older people.

Fractured neck of femur

A frequent and serious consequence of a fall is a fractured neck of femur, with up to 14 000 people a year dying in the UK as a result of an osteoporotic hip fracture (DoH 2001a). Osteoporosis affects 1 in 3 women and 1 in 12 men over the age of 50 years and almost half of all women experience an osteoporotic hip fracture by the age of 70 years (DoH 2001a).

A full assessment of airway, breathing, circulation and disability must be made to ascertain whether the fracture is an isolated injury. This information can be assembled from the history and physical examination. Vital signs need to include a 12-lead ECG to exclude an underlying cardiac cause, which may have precipitated the fall.

Classical features associated with a fractured neck of femur are:

- history of a fall or collapse
- shortened and rotated limb
- groin pain +/− radiating to the knee
- inability to mobilize – some patients can mobilize on a fractured hip; if a patient has difficulty mobilizing associated with hip pain, a fracture needs to be excluded.

Management

Emergency nurses should utilize an integrated care pathway where it exists: this will facilitate a seamless assessment, treatment and referral process for the patient. Ninety per cent of patients should be admitted in two hours and hundred% within four hours (DoH 2006). Patients will require pressure-area care in the ED and consideration should be given to ordering a pressure-relieving mattress.

Analgesia is extremely important in the treatment of hip fractures as pain is likely to be the patients' main problem. Patients with dementia/delirium or cognitive impairment receive less analgesia than those who do not have any cognitive impairment (Heyburn et al. 2000). It is therefore imperative that the emergency nurse is sensitive to subtle non-verbal signs of pain. It must also be remembered that the patient may be pain-free at rest but will have to move for the X-ray and ultimate transfer to a ward or theatre. Analgesia should be administered in accordance with local policy within 20 minutes of arrival; however, greatest efficacy is usually achieved by intravenous opiates titrated to pain; an anti-emetic should also be administered.

The patient will require intravenous access via a cannula; blood should be taken for FBC, U&E along with a group and save as the patient may require blood perioperatively. The patient may need to be nil by mouth immediately and should receive intravenous fluids as per local policy to avoid dehydration.

A fractured neck of femur is associated with significant morbidity and mortality; it is likely to be anxiety-provoking for the patient and their family, and therefore a sensitive explanation of care is required.

CONCLUSION

The care of older people in the ED is an extremely challenging and rewarding element of emergency care. This chapter has covered the physiological affects of ageing, and some of the common presenting complaints associated with older people.

As demographic changes in the population continue to evolve, emergency nurses are required to ensure they have the appropriate knowledge and skills to provide older people with the highest standard of care. The assessment of older people, because

---

Table 21.10 Falls risk assessment tool (Sudip et al. 2004)

Potential risk factors for a fall
History of a fall in the last year
Four or more prescribed medications
Diagnosis of stroke or Parkinson's disease
Reported problems with balance, inability to rise from a chair without using arms

of their social, psychological and physical vulnerability, is a critically important dimension of care in the ED; however, older people should not be seen as a homogeneous group who are all victims or who are automatically infirm because of their age. The ED nurse has an opportunity to challenge stereotypes, provide health promotion and offer guidance on services available to older patients, as well as acting as an advocate for those unable to communicate for themselves. It presents a challenge which ED nurses should embrace as part of their role as health professionals.

References

Action on Elder Abuse (2005) *Indicators of Abuse*. London: Action on Elder Abuse.

Aminzadeh F, Dalziel WB (2002) Older adults in the emergency department: a systematic review of patterns of use, adverse outcomes and effective interventions. *Annals of Emergency Medicine,* **39,** 238–247.

Association of Community Health Councils of England and Wales (2001) *Nationwide Casualty Watch*. London: ACHEW.

Bentley J, Meyer J (2004) Repeat attendance by older people at accident and emergency departments. *Journal of Advanced Nursing,* **48(2),** 149–156.

Bickley LS, Szilagyi PG (2003) *Bates' Guide to Physical Examination and History Taking*. 8th Edn. Philadelphia: JB Lippincott Company.

Bridges J, Spilsbury K, Meyer J, Crouch R (1999) Older people in accident and emergency. Literature review and implications for British policy and practice. *Review in Clinical Gerontology,* **9,** 127–137.

Bridges J, Meyer J, Dethick L, Griffiths P (2005) Older people in accident and emergency: implications for UK policy and practice. *Reviews in Clinical Gerontology,* **14,** 15–24.

British Geriatric Society (2003) *Standards of Medical Care for Older People: Expectations and Recommendations*. London: British Geriatric Society.

Carson B (1999) Successful resuscitation of a 44 year old man with hypothermia. *Journal of Emergency Nursing,* **25(5),** 356–360.

Cheitlin MD (2003) Cardiovascular physiology – changes with ageing. *American Journal of Geriatric Cardiology,* **12**(1), 9–13.

Clarke MJ, Fitzgerald G (1999) Older people's use of the ambulance service, a population based analysis. *Journal of Accident and Emergency Medicine,* **16,** 108–111.

Community and District Nursing Association (2003) *Responding to Elder Abuse*. London: CDNA.

Crouch R (2003) Emergency Care of the Older Person. In: Jones G, Endacott R, Crouch R, eds. *Emergency Nursing Care, Principles and Practice*. London: GMM.

Department of Health (2000) *No Secrets: Guidance on Developing and Implementing Multi-agency Policies and Procedures to Protect Vulnerable Adults from Abuse*. London: Department of Health.

Department of Health (2001a) *National Service Framework for Older People*. London: Department of Health.

Department of Health (2001b) *National Service Framework for Older People. Medicines and Older People, Implementing Medicines-related Aspects of the NSF for Older People*. London: Department of Health.

Department of Health (2006) *Delivering Quality and Value*. London: Department of Health.

Dove A, Dale S (1986) Elderly patients in the accident department and their problems. *British Medical Journal* **292,** 807–808.

Edwards CRW, Bouchier IAD, Haslett C (1995) *Davidson's Principles and Practice of Medicine*. London: Churchill Livingstone.

Epstein O, Perkins DG, Cookson J, De Bono DP (2003) *Clinical Examination*. 3rd edn. London: Mosby.

Evers HK (1984) *Patients experiences and social relations in geriatric wards* (unpublished PhD thesis). Warwick: University of Warwick.

Gray-Vickery P (2005) Elder abuse: are you prepared to intervene? *LPN,* **1**(2), 38–42.

Greaves I, Hodgetts T, Porter K (1997) Care of the elderly. In: Greaves I, Hodgetts T, Porter K, eds. *Emergency Care: A Textbook for Paramedics*. London: Baillière Tindall.

Haslett C, Chilvers ER, Boon NA, Colledge NR (2002) *Davidson's Principles and Practice of Medicine*. 19th edn. London: Churchill Livingstone.

Health Advisory Service (2000) (1998) *Not because they are old: An independent inquiry into the care of older people on acute wards in general hospitals*. London: HAS (2000).

Heyburn G, Jenkinson M, Beringer T, et al. 2000. The efficiency of analgesia in the elderly hip fracture patient. *Age Ageing,* **29** (Suppl 1), 26.

Holtzclaw B (2004) Shivering in acutely ill vulnerable populations. *Advanced Practice in Acute Clinical Care,* **15**(2), 267–279.

House of Commons Health Committee (2004) *Elder abuse: Second report of session 2003–2004*. London: The Stationery Office.

Hustey FM, Meldon SW (2002) The prevalence and documentation of impaired mental status in elderly emergency department patients. *Annals of Emergency Medicine,* **39,** 248–253.

Kaufman DW, Kelly JP, Rosenberg L, Anderson TE, Mitchell AA (2002) Recent patterns of medication use in the ambulatory adult population of the United States. The Slone survey. *Journal of the American Medical Association,* **287**(3), 337–344.

King MB, Tinetti ME (1995) Falls in community-dwelling older persons. *Journal of American Geriatric Society,* **43,** 1146–1154.

Klein Schmidt KC (1997) Elder abuse: a review. *Annals of Emergency Medicine,* **30**(4), 463–472.

Kumar P, Clark M (2002) *Clinical Medicine*. 5th Edn. London: WB Saunders Co.

Manning B, Stolerman DF (1993) Hypothermia in the elderly. *Hospital Practice,* **28**(5), 53–70.

Meyer J, Bridges J (1998) *An action research study into people in the A&E department*. London: City University.

National Audit Office (2007) Joining forces to improve stroke care. London.

National Audit Office (2005) *Reducing Brain Damage: Faster access to better stroke care*. London.

Neno R (2005) Hypothermia: assessment, treatment and prevention. *Nursing Standard*, **19**(20), 47–52.

Neno R, Neno M (2005) Identifying abuse in older people. *Nursing Standard*, **20** (3), 43–47.

Office of National Statistics (2006) *Population Trends*. London: ONS.

Ogg J, Bennet G (1992) Elder abuse in Britain. *British Medical Journal*, **305**, 998–999.

Pocock G, Richards CD (2004) *Human Physiology. The Basis of Medicine*. 2nd Edn. Oxford: Oxford University Press.

Resuscitation Council (UK) (2000) *Advanced Life Support Course. Provider Manual*. 4th edn (Revised). London: Resuscitation Council (UK).

Resuscitation Council (UK) *2005 Resuscitation Guidelines*. London: Resuscitation Council (UK).

Rogers I (2004) Hypothermia. In: P Cameron, G Jelinek, AM Kelly et al. (eds), *Textbook of Adult Emergency Medicine*, 2nd edn. Edinburgh: Churchill Livingstone.

Royal College of Physicians (2004) *National Clinical Guidelines for Stroke*. 2nd edn. Prepared by the Intercollegiate Stroke Working Party. London: Royal College of Physicians.

SNMAC Standing Nursing and Midwifery Advisory Committee (2001) *Caring for Older People: A Nursing Priority. Integrating Knowledge, Practice and Values. Report of the Nursing and Midwifery Advisory Committee*. London: Department of Health.

Sowney R (1999) Older people in Accident and Emergency, a position statement. *Emergency Nurse*, **7**(6), 6–7.

Spilsbury K, Meyer J, Bridges J, Holman C (1999) The little things count. *Emergency Nurse*, **7**(6), 24–31.

Spinewine A, Swine C, Dhillon S, Dean Franklin B, Tulkens PM, Wilmotte L, Lorant V (2005) Appropriateness of use of medications in elderly inpatients: qualitative study. *British Medical Journal*, **331**, 935–940.

Stevenson J (2004) When the trauma patient is elderly. *Journal of Peri Anaesthesia Nursing*, **19**(6), 392–400.

Sudip N, Parsons S, Cryer C et al. (2004) Development and preliminary examination of the predictive validity of the Falls Risk Assessment Tool for use in primary care. *Journal of Public Health*, **26**(2), 138–143.

Tideiksaar R (2003) Best practice approach to fall prevention in community-living elders. *Topics in Geriatric Rehabilitation*, **19**(3), 199–205.

Wyatt JP, Illingworth RN, Clancy MJ, Munro P, Robertson CE (2005) *Oxford Handbook of Accident and Emergency Medicine*. Oxford: Oxford University Press.

PART 5

Physiology for ED practice

PART CONTENTS

Chapter 22

Physiology for ED practice

Marion Richardson

CHAPTER CONTENTS

INTRODUCTION

This chapter explores some of the physiological mechanisms which support normal body function, the failure of which may necessitate nursing intervention in the ED patient. The basic physiological concepts of homeostasis are examined and a number of homeostatic mechanisms described. The importance of temperature regulation is discussed and the homeostatic mechanisms which maintain normal levels of fluids and electrolytes, glucose, blood pressure and haemostasis are outlined. The mechanisms of oxygen and carbon dioxide transport to and from the cells are discussed. Finally, the breakdown of homeostatic mechanisms is considered in a discussion of physiological shock.

HOMEOSTASIS

A single-celled organism, such as an amoeba, requires warmth, oxygen, nutrients and fluids in order to survive and must be able to rid itself of waste products. It interacts directly with the outside world in order to achieve this (see Fig. 22.1). The human body is a highly complex collection of millions of cells, very few of which are in direct contact with the outside world and yet each individual cell has the same survival requirements as the amoeba – a constant supply of fluids, nutrients, oxygen and warmth in order to live and the ability to remove waste products. The external environment (the 'outside world') of the cells in the body is the interstitial fluid that surrounds them (see Fig. 22.2 for body fluid compartments) and this fluid must be kept supplied with all the components which the cells might need. Individual cells need to maintain a constant environment within relatively narrow limits in order to function optimally and this constant state must be maintained whatever

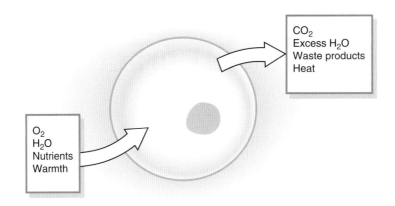

Figure 22.1   Cell homeostasis.

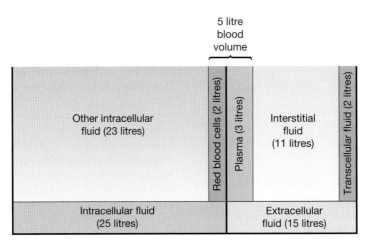

Figure 22.2   Body fluid compartments.

is happening to the body as a whole. The term 'homeostasis', first used by an American physiologist, Walter Cannon, in 1932, refers to the physiological mechanisms which maintain the body in a relatively constant state despite changes in the environment. The word comes from the Greek and means 'standing the same', something of a misnomer since physiological function is never static but constantly fluctuating. Homeostasis is essential if the metabolic activities which occur constantly in all cells are to continue.

Throughout the body there are many self-regulating homeostatic mechanisms which aim to maintain an internal 'steady state'. Most homeostatic mechanisms within the body work by 'negative feedback', where a deviation from normal will cause a response to restore the steady state – thus too little of something will cause more to be produced, too much of something will trigger mechanisms to reduce the amount. Once steady state is reached, the homeostatic mechanisms are switched off. An example of a see-saw is commonly used to illustrate this concept (Fig. 22.3). In order to function, homeostatic mechanisms require specialized receptors to detect deviations from the 'steady state'; they also require a control centre to receive and process the information and the ability to stimulate appropriate body organs and structures to redress the imbalance.

The homeostatic mechanisms involved in temperature regulation, fluid and electrolyte balance, oxygen and carbon dioxide transport and maintenance of blood glucose and blood pressure will be examined in more detail.

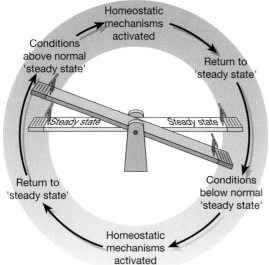

Figure 22.3   Homeostasis: maintaining a steady state.

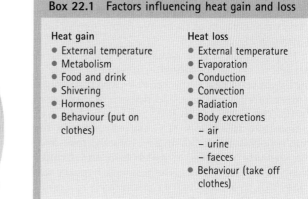

Box 22.1   Factors influencing heat gain and loss

Heat gain
- External temperature
- Metabolism
- Food and drink
- Shivering
- Hormones
- Behaviour (put on clothes)

Heat loss
- External temperature
- Evaporation
- Conduction
- Convection
- Radiation
- Body excretions
  - air
  - urine
  - faeces
- Behaviour (take off clothes)

TEMPERATURE CONTROL

Maintenance of a constant core body temperature, within the internal organs, is essential for optimal functioning of cellular enzymes. Humans are homeothermic and normally maintain a constant core temperature of 37°C regardless of the external temperature. The skin temperature may be several degrees different from the core temperature and varies between areas of the body, as those who always seem to have cold feet and hands will know. Body temperature is usually lower, by about 0.5°C at night and is 0.5–1°C higher in women during the second half of the menstrual cycle as a result of normal circadian rhythms. Children have higher core temperatures than neonates and the elderly, and core temperature can rise by up to 2°C during strenuous exercise. Despite all these normal variations, the body must maintain a careful balance between heat gained and heat lost. A summary of factors influencing heat gain and loss is given in Box 22.1.

Temperature homeostasis

Temperature-sensitive receptors, thermoreceptors, are found peripherally in the skin (sensitive to external temperature changes) and centrally in the hypothalamus in the brain (sensitive to changes in temperature of blood bathing them and thus to core temperature). When stimulated, the thermoreceptors initiate impulses via afferent nerves to the control centre, the temperature-regulating area in the anterior hypothalamus.

When core temperature falls below normal, the hypothalamus acts to conserve heat in the following ways:

- Peripheral vasoconstriction mediated via the sympathetic nervous system closes down the surface blood vessels, ensuring that blood is kept closer to the warm core and heat loss through the skin is minimized.
- Shivering is initiated by the posterior hypothalamus and results in uncoordinated muscle activity which generates heat.
- The thyroid gland is stimulated to produce the hormone thyroxin, which raises the basal metabolic rate of cells, thus increasing heat production.
- Information is relayed to the cerebral cortex and we become conscious of the cold and will take steps to warm ourselves such as putting on extra clothes, turning on the fire, exercising or having a warm drink.

A rise in core temperature above 37°C will stimulate responses aimed at losing heat:

- Peripheral blood vessels are dilated under the influence of the sympathetic nervous system and heat is lost through the skin by radiation, conduction and convection.
- Sweat glands are stimulated, again via the sympathetic nervous system, to increase secretion, and heat is lost by evaporation. Evaporation of sweat is reduced when humidity is high and this is consequently a less effective means of reducing temperature in hot climates.
- Again the cerebral cortex receives information and we take steps to cool down – removing clothes, taking a cold shower, drinking iced drinks.

Once temperature returns to normal levels, the physiological mechanisms are switched off. A diagrammatic representation of thermoregulatory mechanisms is given in Fig. 22.4.

Hypothermia, a core temperature below 35°C, is dangerous and, if not treated, will result in failure of the negative-feedback mechanisms which maintain temperature homeostasis, and damage or death may ensue. The ability to shiver decreases when the core temperature falls below 34°C and consequently the core temperature will fall further. Hypothermia slows the chemical reactions of metabolism and reduces blood flow to all organs. The resultant hypoxia will cause drowsiness and loss of consciousness as a result of cerebral ischaemia. Cardiac arrhythmias will occur at about 25°C and the heart will cease to beat at about 20°C.

The O_2 requirements of the tissues are substantially reduced at low temperatures, and gradual warming of the patient combined with controlled oxygen therapy may result in full recovery provided no physiological damage has occurred. The elderly and neonates are particularly prone to hypothermia because of less efficient thermoregulatory mechanisms, as are those who misuse drugs and alcohol or who live 'rough' and who are not always able to take voluntary measures to regain heat.

Pyrexia or fever occurs when body temperature rises above normal as a result of pyrogens produced by bacteria, viruses or necrotic tissue, which affect the temperature-regulating centre. Head injury and brain damage may have a similar effect. The temperature-regulating centre is 'reset' at a higher level by the pyrogens and the body will continue to produce heat to maintain the higher level until the pyrogens are removed from the body.

Hyperpyrexia, i.e. a core temperature above 40°C, is a dangerous condition. Cellular metabolism is greatly increased and the body is unable to lose the heat produced sufficiently to reduce the temperature. Cells throughout the body are destroyed by literally burning themselves out and irreversible brain damage will occur at about 42°C.

FLUID AND ELECTROLYTE BALANCE

Water is the basis of all body fluids, e.g. plasma, tissue fluids and lymph, and accounts for approximately 60% of total body weight. Body water contains many electrolytes, substances which dissolve and dissociate into ions (develop electrical charges). The main electrolytes in the body are sodium (Na^+), potassium (K^+), calcium (Ca^{2+}) and magnesium (Mg^{2+}), all of which are positively charged *anions*, and the negatively charged *cations* chloride (Cl^-), bicarbonate (HCO_3^-), protein (Pr^-) and phosphate (PO_4^{2-}).

Fluid is either inside the cells (intracellular) or outside the cells (extracellular). Extracellular fluid includes blood plasma, interstitial or tissue fluid which bathes the cells (see above), and small amounts of transcellular fluid, found in body cavities such as intraocular, peritoneal and pleural fluid, cerebrospinal fluid and digestive juices. Figure 22.2 shows how these fluid compartments compare.

Intracellular fluid contains more positively charged potassium and magnesium and negatively charged protein and phosphate than extracellular fluid (which contains more positively charged sodium ions and negatively charged chloride ions) (Fig. 22.5). The ions are prevented from diffusing into other compartments by the selective permeability of the cell membranes and by the presence of a pumping mechanism within cell walls which actively pumps out

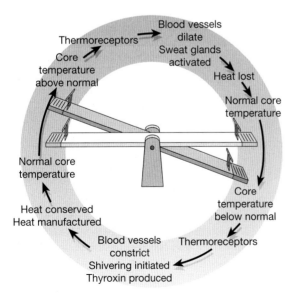

Figure 22.4 Thermoregulation.

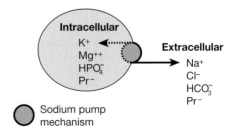

Figure 22.5 Electrolytes in fluid compartments.

sodium and exchanges it for potassium. This difference between intra- and extra-cellular fluid is essential in nerve and muscle cells (excitable tissues), since nerves would be unable to relay messages and muscles unable to contract without it.

The interstitial fluid which bathes cells throughout the body must be maintained in a stable state as it provides the cells with nutrients and maintains the correct temperature for them to function effectively and receives their waste products. Disturbances in the electrolyte content and the concentration, osmolality and osmolarity of the extracellular fluid will affect the intracellular fluid and will impair cell and body function as a result. Normal cell function relies on fluid and electrolyte homeostasis.

Fluids normally enter the body only through the mouth. Thirst is a stimulus triggered when osmoreceptors in the hypothalamus detect a fall in the osmotic pressure of plasma passing over them. Fluid and electrolyte balance by intake alone would be inefficient, since either too much or too little may be ingested for any number of reasons. The body regulates levels of both water and electrolytes at the point of exit, mainly by the action of hormones on the distal tubules of the kidney.

Water balance is coordinated by the thirst centre in the hypothalamus, which controls the release of antidiuretic hormone (ADH). When the concentration of extracellular fluid rises as a result of a fluid intake below body requirements, osmoreceptors in the anterior hypothalamus sense the change and trigger impulses to allow the release of ADH from the posterior pituitary gland. ADH acts on the distal tubules of the kidney so that water is reabsorbed into the circulation. The mechanism is switched off once extracellular osmolarity returns to normal. This is another good example of negative feedback.

The hormone aldosterone, secreted from the adrenal cortex, is responsible for maintaining sodium levels in the body. A fall in blood sodium levels or a rise in serum potassium is detected by specialized cells in the adrenal cortex and increases the release of aldosterone, which acts to reabsorb sodium from the renal tubules and to reduce its excretion in saliva, gastric juices and the skin. Aldosterone production is also stimulated by a fall in the extracellular fluid volume via the renin-angiotensin system activated within the kidney. Potassium balance is closely linked with sodium and when sodium is reabsorbed, potassium is generally excreted. The body is inefficient at conserving potassium and blood levels are not indicative of total body potassium as most of this electrolyte is intracellular.

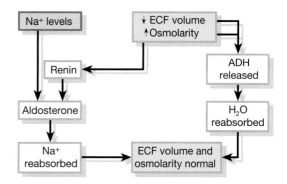

Figure 22.6   Water and sodium balance.

It hardly needs to be said that optimal kidney function is vital for maintaining fluid and electrolyte homeostasis, and damage through whatever cause (trauma, disease, old age etc.) will reduce the efficiency of the homeostatic system.

Fluid and sodium balance are closely linked and hormonal responses are triggered by both changes in extracellular fluid (ECF) volumes and changes in plasma osmolality. A diagrammatic representation is given in Fig. 22.6.

Calcium levels in the body are regulated by the secretion of parathyroid hormone from the four parathyroid glands. The hormone is released directly in response to low extracellular fluid concentrations of calcium and stimulates the release of calcium from bone and its reabsorption from the kidney tubules. In addition, vitamin D is activated and increases the amount of calcium absorbed in the gut from food. When calcium is reabsorbed, phosphate is lost. High calcium levels stimulate the release of calcitonin from the thyroid gland. Calcitonin inhibits the release of calcium from bone and increases its excretion through the kidney until levels return to normal and the mechanism is switched off (see Fig. 22.7).

OXYGEN AND CARBON DIOXIDE HOMEOSTASIS

All cells require oxygen in order to function, and produce carbon dioxide as a result of metabolic activity. These gases are carried to and from the cells in the blood (see below) and their values can be measured as partial pressures (PO_2 and PCO_2). Variations in arterial PO_2 and PCO_2 are sensed by chemoreceptors. Peripheral chemoreceptors in the aortic arch and at the bifurcation of the common carotid artery are particularly sensitive to falls in arterial oxygen levels

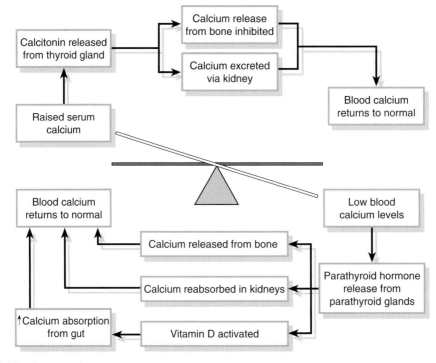

Figure 22.7 Calcium homeostasis.

(P_AO_2), and rises in arterial carbon dioxide (P_ACO_2). Once altered levels are sensed, the respiratory centre in the medulla of the brain is stimulated, via the vagal and glossopharyngeal nerves, and stimulates the phrenic and intercostal nerves to the diaphragm and intercostal muscles. The result is that the rate and depth of respiration are increased and more oxygen is inhaled and delivered to the blood. Once arterial blood oxygen levels are restored to normal, the mechanism is switched off.

Central chemoreceptors on the ventral surface of the medulla monitor the acidity of cerebrospinal fluid and are particularly sensitive to rises in P_ACO_2. Inspiratory neurones in the respiratory centre of the medulla are again stimulated to increase both the rate and depth of respiration until the CO_2 is removed and blown off at the lungs and levels within the blood return to normal. The homeostatic mechanism is switched off once arterial CO_2 levels are normal again.

These homeostatic mechanisms are diagrammatically represented in Fig. 22.8.

In order to understand some common blood gas estimations, the means by which oxygen and carbon dioxide enter and are carried in the blood will be considered.

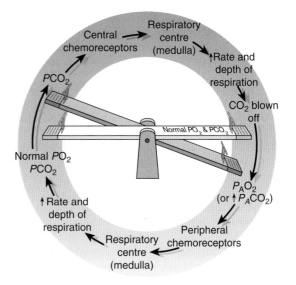

Figure 22.8 Respiratory homeostasis.

Oxygen transport

The atmosphere is composed of a mixture of gases of which the most important physiologically is oxygen. Inspired air consists of approximately 21% oxygen,

79% nitrogen and small amounts of carbon dioxide (0.04%) and other gases, including water vapour. Each gas within this mixture exerts its own pressure, known as the *partial pressure*, and the total pressure of the mixture is equal to the sum of the pressures of all the gases within it (Dalton's law of partial pressures). Atmospheric air pressure at sea level is known to be 101.3 kPa or 760 mmHg, and since oxygen comprises 21% of the mixture, its partial pressure, usually written as PO_2, can be calculated thus:

$$(21/100) \times 101.3 = 21.2 \text{kPa}$$

The PN_2 and PCO_2 can be similarly calculated.

As atmospheric air passes through the respiratory tract, it becomes humidified with more water vapour, which reduces the partial pressure of the other gases as the pressure exerted by the water accounts for a larger proportion of the total pressure. The partial pressures are further modified as the gases combine with the air in the physiological 'dead space' in the respiratory tract before finally meeting and mixing with gases in the alveoli. As a result, the alveolar PO_2 is considerably less than atmospheric PO_2, and alveolar PCO_2 and water vapour pressure are measurably higher, although the total pressure remains the same as atmospheric pressure. Alveolar PO_2 is 13.3 kPa and alveolar PCO_2 is 5.3 kPa, and it is these amounts of gas that are available at the alveolar capillary membrane in the lungs where gaseous exchange takes place. Blood within the alveolar capillaries contains less oxygen and more carbon dioxide than alveolar air as a result of cellular metabolism which removes oxygen from arterial blood and replaces it with carbon dioxide produced as a result of metabolic activity. Blood arriving at the lungs has a PO_2 of 5.3 kPa and a PCO_2 of 6.1 kPa.

In the alveoli, gaseous exchange is possible because of the very thin pulmonary membrane between the alveoli and capillaries and the vast network of capillaries surrounding them (Fig. 22.9). The existence of a pressure gradient, i.e. different pressures on either side of the membrane, results in movement of oxygen into the blood and carbon dioxide out of the blood and into the alveoli ready to be expired. Blood leaving the lungs for the heart contains oxygen and carbon dioxide at virtually the same partial pressures as those contained within the alveoli, so that the normal pulmonary vein and systemic arterial partial pressure of oxygen (P_AO_2) is 13.3 kPa and P_ACO_2 is 5.3 kPa (Fig. 22.10); these quantities of gas are carried within the blood to the tissues.

At the tissues, gases diffuse in the opposite direction across pressure gradients and thin membranes. Oxygen is given up to the tissues and replaced with

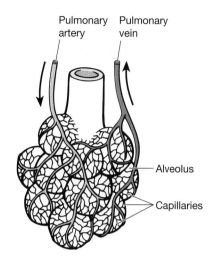

Figure 22.9   Capillary network surrounding the alveolus.

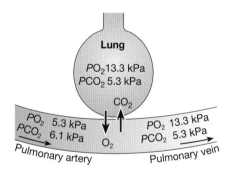

Figure 22.10   Gaseous exchange across the alveolar-capillary membrane.

carbon dioxide produced by the tissues. Partial pressures of oxygen and carbon dioxide within the cells are the same as those in blood arriving at the lungs (Fig. 22.11), since the gases cannot cross the thicker membranes of blood vessels in the rest of the circulation.

Oxygen is not simply carried around the circulation dissolved in blood, as a blood volume in excess of 80 litres would be required to supply the 250 ml of oxygen required every minute when the body is at rest. Oxygen carried by this means accounts for only 1% of the total oxygen transported in the blood, but it is an important 1% as this is the only oxygen that exerts a pressure: not only does it maintain the pressure gradients necessary for diffusion, but it is this that is recorded when arterial blood gases are measured. Normal P_AO_2 and P_ACO_2 are the same as

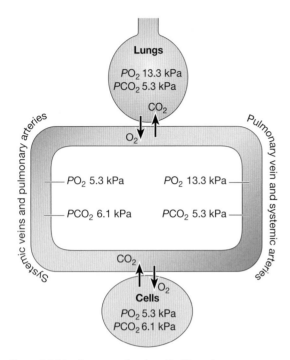

Figure 22.11   Oxygen and carbon dioxide exchange throughout the body.

the pressures within alveolar air, i.e. 13.3 and 5.3 kPa, respectively. This PO_2 governs the far greater amount of oxygen that can be transported in the blood bound to haemoglobin. Normally, 99% of oxygen is carried bound to haemoglobin (Hb) and, once bound, is no longer free to exert a pressure or to be measured in blood analysis. As the O_2 in solution is used, some of the bound O_2 will be released so that the ratio of 1% in solution: 99% bound to Hb is always maintained.

Haemoglobin is a conjugated protein found in red blood cells and consists of four haem groups containing iron and four polypeptide chains. Each of these haem groups can combine with one molecule of oxygen to form oxyhaemoglobin, which is bright red and gives arterial blood its distinctive colour. This process is known as oxygenation. Normal Hb is approximately 15 g/dl and each gram of Hb can carry 1.34 ml O_2, so that the total oxygen capacity of the blood, i.e. the total amount that could be carried, is $15 \times 1.34 = 20.1$ ml/dl. This equation is simpler if SI units are used – normal Hb is 2.2 mmol/L blood and each molecule of Hb can combine with four molecules of O_2, so the oxygen capacity is 8.8 mmol/L (1 mmol $O_2 = 22.4$ ml). Amounts of oxygen carried bound to Hb can thus be far in excess of the normal

requirements of the body. A simple sum will allow us to see that the body, which needs 250 ml of O_2 each minute at rest, actually has theoretically available 8.8×22.4 (= 197.12 ml per litre) $\times$ 5 litres pumped out of the heart each minute, i.e. 986 ml per minute.

In normal physiological circumstances, not quite all the available haemoglobin binding sites become bound with oxygen but about 97–98% do – this is the 'oxygen saturation' that is recorded by pulse oximetry. There are many reasons why pulse oximetry may give misleading information but an important physiological reason is that while Hb may be fully bound with O_2, Hb levels may be very low – pulse oximetry readings will be within normal limits but the blood is unable to carry sufficient oxygen to supply the needs of the cells throughout the body – examples are in severe anaemia or in hypovolaemia (see section on shock below).

Oxygen does not bind to each haem molecule with the same ease, and a graph plotting Hb saturation against PO_2 is not linear. The rate at which they bind is dependent on the PO_2. The first haem group combines with O_2 with relative difficulty, the second and third groups combine more readily and the fourth combines with the greatest difficulty of all. It will be seen from Fig. 22.11 that at a PO_2 of 5.3 kPa, as in blood arriving at the lungs, almost 70% of the Hb sites are bound with oxygen and exposure to a PO_2 of 13.3 kPa at the alveoli will allow up to 98% of the Hb to become saturated with O_2. At the tissues, O_2 is unloaded from the haem molecules in response to the fall in PO_2, so that a tissue PO_2 of 5.3 kPa will mean that oxygen from the 70–97% range can be removed for use.

The 's' shape of the oxygen–haemoglobin dissociation curve is important physiologically for a number of reasons. Normal physiological function occurs over only a small part of this curve (Fig. 22.12) and a large reserve is available in the event of a fall in arterial PO_2, such as in lung disease, during exercise or at altitude. Even at a PO_2 of only 8 kPa, 90% saturation of Hb with oxygen will be achieved in blood leaving the lungs (point I in Fig. 22.12). During strenuous exercise, it is possible to achieve a PO_2 at the tissues of as little as 2 kPa and this will allow 80% of the bound oxygen to be released (point II in Fig. 22.12), thus supplying the increased amount of oxygen required by the tissues.

Several factors affect the ease with which O_2 binds with Hb and will influence the position of the oxygen–haemoglobin dissociation curve. The factors influencing 'shifts' in the curve are summarized in Fig. 22.13. The result of a shift to the left is that

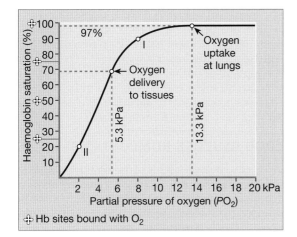

Figure 22.12 The oxygen dissociation curve.

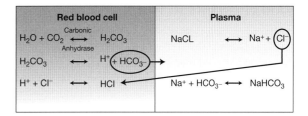

Figure 22.14 Respiratory homeostasis.

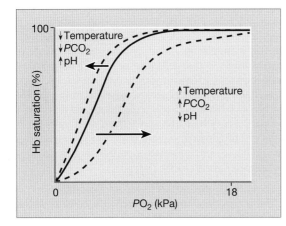

Figure 22.13 Factors influencing a shift in the dissociation curve.

loading of Hb with O_2 occurs more readily, i.e. at a lower PO_2, while a shift to the right facilitates release of the O_2 at the tissues.

Carbon dioxide transport

Carbon dioxide is transported around the body in three ways:

- 7% in simple solution
- 23% bound to the globin portion of haemoglobin and influenced by PCO_2
- 70% as bicarbonate (hydrogen carbonate) ions.

Tissue cells constantly produce CO_2 and this diffuses across a pressure gradient into the capillaries supplying the tissue. Some remains dissolved in the plasma or binds to Hb but most crosses into the red blood cells (erythrocytes), where the presence of an enzyme, carbonic anhydrase, promotes the conversion of CO_2 and water within the cells to carbonic acid. The carbonic acid then dissociates into hydrogen and bicarbonate according to the equation

$$H_2O + CO_2 \leftrightarrow H_2CO_3 \leftrightarrow H^+ + HCO_3^-$$

HCO_3^- is then removed to the plasma where it is transported combined with sodium found in the plasma as sodium bicarbonate $NaHCO_3$.

CO_2 carried in this way does not exert a pressure within the blood and the equation reverses readily when blood arrives at the lungs so that CO_2 is readily released to be blown off. Fig. 22.14 shows this process diagrammatically.

OXYGEN THERAPY

The aim of oxygen therapy is to raise the PO_2 in the lungs, thus increasing the pressure gradient across the alveolar capillary membrane and allowing more oxygen to enter the blood for transport to the tissues. There are, however, potential hazards which should be considered when oxygen therapy is indicated.

Patients with long-term respiratory disease may rely on low PO_2 levels to stimulate the respiratory centre (hypoxic drive) rather than rises in PCO_2 levels. High levels of oxygen administered to these patients will cause respiratory depression and possibly apnoea.

High concentrations of O_2 over prolonged periods may cause lung damage with oedema. Concentrations of administered O_2 should be kept as low as possible whilst maintaining adequate blood gas levels.

Compressed O_2 is very drying and should be humidified prior to administration. Patients receiving O_2 will require regular mouth rinses.

In neonates, particularly premature infants, blindness caused by retrolental fibroplasia, i.e. fibrosis behind the lens of the eye, may develop as a result of high-level O_2 administration.

VARIATIONS AT ALTITUDE AND DEPTH

As altitude increases, for example during flight or when ascending mountains, barometric pressure falls. At 10 000 feet (300 metres) total atmospheric pressure is 70 kPa or 523 mmHg and the PO_2 will be 21% of this, i.e. 15 kPa. Alveolar PO_2 at this height will be reduced to approximately 9 kPa, causing a marked reduction in the pressure gradient across the alveolar capillary membrane. Hypoxic hypoxia (a deficiency of O_2 at the tissues caused by low P_AO_2 levels) may become apparent in anyone above 10 000 feet unless supplementary oxygen is administered. Normal blood oxygen saturation of 98% at sea level will be reduced to 87% at 10 000 feet and to only 60% at 20000 feet. In pressurized aircraft cabins, pressure is usually maintained at about 8000 feet and the fit adult can readily adjust to cope with the resultant physiological alterations.

The symptoms of hypoxia include increases in heart and respiratory rate, headache, fatigue, nausea and dizziness. Perhaps the most threatening factor is that the onset is insidious and may occur in the carer as well as the patient. Prevention of hypoxia should always be the primary concern.

Pressures within body cavities alter with changes in barometric pressure. At altitude, gases within the cavities expand and then contract again during descent. These effects are particularly noticeable in the smaller body cavities, such as the middle ear and sinuses. Normally expanding and contracting gases will pass through the eustachian tubes or the sinus cavities so that the pressure changes are equalized. In individuals with allergies, a cold or sinus infection, this movement of gases is limited or obstructed and painful otitis media or sinusitis may result. Those patients in whom respiration is compromised require careful monitoring and any pneumothorax must be treated prior to air transport as it will be likely to collapse further at altitude. Endotracheal tube balloons, intravenous fluid bags, antishock trousers and pneumatic splints are also subject to pressure changes and need close observation to ensure accurate functioning.

Gas pressures increase below sea level and at as little as 10 metres deep in sea water (10.4 metres in fresh water) atmospheric pressure is doubled (i.e. 202.6 kPa) and consequently all the partial pressures of the constituent gases are doubled. Divers and underwater tunnel workers breathe air at high pressure to equalize the pressures on the chest wall and abdomen. Nitrogen dissolves in plasma and interstitial fluid at these pressures but as long as ascent to the surface is slow and controlled, the dissolved N_2 will diffuse at the lungs and be breathed off. If ascent is too rapid, however, the N_2 forms bubbles in the tissues and decompression sickness results. With the current popularity of scuba diving, it is important to be aware of the symptoms of this sickness (joint pain, especially in the limbs, dizziness and fatigue, shortness of breath) as patients may present in departments a day or more after their dive and far from the coast.

BLOOD GLUCOSE HOMEOSTASIS

Cells need a constant supply of nutrients from which to extract energy for cell work and glucose plays an important role in this as it is a major substrate for the manufacture of adenosine triphosphate (ATP) within the cells. This is particularly true in the brain, where 90% of the cellular energy required for metabolism is derived from glucose. Glucose is obtained from food and food substrates and the body has efficient glucose storage mechanisms for use in times of plentiful supply (for example, following a meal) and equally efficient means of releasing the stores during fasting states. Two hormones – insulin and glucagon – are responsible for maintaining blood glucose within relatively narrow limits so that cells throughout the body receive a constant and adequate supply (see Fig. 22.15).

Following a meal, glucose crosses from the gut into the blood stream and the high levels are detected in the pancreas where the specialized beta cells in the islets of Langerhans are stimulated to secrete insulin. Insulin has a number of ways of reducing blood sugar (by negative feedback):

- encourages the entry of glucose into cells throughout the body, especially the cells of skeletal muscle, to be used to manufacture ATP
- turns glucose into the storage form glycogen (this process is known as glycogenesis) for storage in cells and in the liver
- slows down the processes which turn fats and proteins into glucose.

If blood sugar is low, the alpha cells of the islets of Langerhans are stimulated and secrete the hormone glucagon. This leads to a number of physiological alterations aimed at raising the blood glucose levels:

- acts on liver cells to convert stored glycogen back to glucose (glycogenolysis) and release it back into the blood
- encourages the liver to manufacture glucose from lactic acid and from some amino acids (gluconeogenesis) and release it into the blood

When blood levels have returned to normal, the mechanism is switched off.

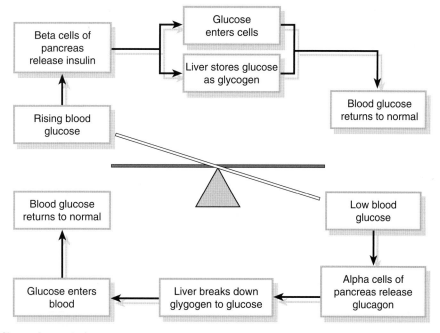

Figure 22.15 Glucose homeostasis.

BLOOD PRESSURE HOMEOSTASIS – A MORE COMPLEX MECHANISM

The maintenance of blood pressure is essential to life and the body initiates a number of mechanisms to restore pressure to normal resting state. A fall in blood pressure is detected by baroreceptors (pressure receptors) in the aortic arch and carotid arteries and information is relayed to the cardiovascular control centre in the medulla. The sympathetic nervous system is stimulated here and acts to bring about peripheral vasoconstriction so that blood pressure is increased in vessels supplying the vital organs.

The fall in blood pressure is also detected in the kidney where the juxtaglomerular cells release the enzyme renin. Renin converts a plasma protein, angiotensinogen, into angiotensin I and this, in turn, is converted into angiotensin II when it meets angiotensin-converting enzyme (ACE) in the blood vessels. Angiotensin II stimulates the release from the adrenal glands of aldosterone, which increases the amount of sodium and water reabsorbed into the blood as it passes through the kidneys. Angiotensin II also stimulates the release of adrenaline from the adrenal glands and this enhances and maintains the vasoconstrictor effect of sympathetic nervous stimulation described above. Two distinct negative-feedback mechanisms – vasoconstriction and fluid retention –

can be seen acting together to increase venous return to the heart and maintain normal blood pressure.

A number of homeostatic mechanisms using negative feedback to maintain a relatively constant internal environment within which cells can function optimally have been examined. There are examples of physiological positive-feedback mechanisms, where too much produces more and too little produces even less, in the body and two of these will now be explored. In the first, the positive-feedback loop is broken once the desired effect has been achieved. In the second, the desired effect is unachievable and the positive feedback continues until the patient's death unless appropriate interventions are made to break the loop.

HAEMOSTASIS – AN EXAMPLE OF POSITIVE FEEDBACK WITH A CUT-OFF MECHANISM

Haemostasis, the arrest of bleeding, is a homeostatic process designed to maintain the body's blood volume. Haemostasis takes place only where blood vessels are damaged as it is essential that blood in the rest of the circulation remains fluid. Normally the haemostatic process will control bleeding in all but large arteries and veins; intervention will be needed if bleeding is to be arrested in these large vessels.

The process of haemostasis can be divided into stages, although physiologically it occurs as a continuous process:

1. Myogenic reflex. Damaged vessels will normally dilate immediately after injury under the influence of histamine released by mast cells in response to the trauma. Within seconds the vessels constrict and the cut ends retract as platelets within the vessels begin to clump together and release powerful vasoconstrictors, serotonin (also called 5-hydroxytryptamine or 5HT) and thromboxane A. This so-called 'myogenic reflex' occurs even in large vessels and lasts for approximately 20 minutes, enough time for stages two and three to commence.

2. Platelet plug formation. When blood vessels are cut, filaments of collagen and elastin are exposed and attract passing platelets which adhere to them. This adherence causes the release of adenosine diphosphate (ADP) from the platelets, red blood cells and vessel walls. ADP triggers a change in the shape of the platelets which encourages them to clump together. Other substances, including serotonin, also encourage platelet clumping until a plug of platelets is formed which is large enough to close the wounded vessel. A platelet plug is formed within a few seconds of injury and is sufficiently strong to stop bleeding in smaller vessels. The plug must then be stabilized by fibrin fibres or it will break down after about 20 minutes and bleeding will start again.

3. Fibrin clot. Fibrin is an insoluble protein that is laid down as a mesh of fine threads which adhere to one another and to blood cells and platelets. They become entangled in the platelet plug, attract more cells to plug the damaged area and gradually make the clot firmer and more stable. Fibrin is formed by a complex process initiated when tissues are damaged. The complexity of the process is important since clotting within undamaged vessels would be highly undesirable. The early stages of fibrin formation also trigger the complicated clotting cascade involving 13 different factors, mostly blood constituents, which ultimately results in a blood clot. Blood is prevented from clotting, or the process is prolonged, if any of the factors is absent (as in haemophilia) or by the use of anticoagulants (such as heparin or aspirin), which prevent their production. The positive feedback of this clotting mechanism stops once the cascade is complete.

4. Fibrinolysis. During this stage fibrin is broken down and removed by phagocytes. The enzyme plasmin, which is responsible for this process, may be activated by streptokinase and other fibrinolytic agents.

SHOCK – WHERE HOMEOSTASIS FAILS AND UNCONTROLLED POSITIVE FEEDBACK ENSUES

Shock is a complex clinical syndrome characterized by a lack of adequate tissue and organ perfusion to such an extent that the oxygen and nutritional needs of the cells cannot be met. Cells and organs throughout the body are unable to function adequately and will fail and die unless both the cause and the symptoms of shock are treated.

Shock is commonly classified according to its pathophysiological cause, but any condition, physical or psychological, which reduces the blood supply to the tissues is a potential cause of shock.

Classification of shock

There are three distinct mechanisms which may lead to hypoperfusion of the tissues:

- Hypovolaemia – there is insufficient blood to carry the oxygen and nutrients needed
- Pump failure (cardiogenic) – the heart is unable to pump the blood around the body effectively
- Distribution problems – blood volume and cardiac output are essentially adequate but widespread vasoconstriction leads to pooling of blood and reduces venous return to the heart. Neurogenic, septic and anaphylactic shock all fall into this category.

Hypovolaemic shock. The causes of hypovolaemia are:

- loss of blood through haemorrhage
- loss of plasma as in severe burns and peritonitis
- loss of body fluids through diarrhoea, vomiting or sweating
- failure to drink sufficient fluids.

Fifteen per cent or more of total blood volume may be lost before signs of hypovolaemic shock are noted in an adult.

Cardiogenic shock ('pump failure'). Events which reduce the ability of the heart to pump efficiently result in cardiogenic shock. These include:

- myocardial infarction
- cardiac arrhythmias
- cardiac tamponade.
- disorders in the lungs, e.g. tension pneumothorax or pulmonary embolus.

Neurogenic shock. In neurogenic shock, sympathetic and parasympathetic nervous control is lost. The venous 'tone' essential to the maintenance of normal blood pressure and venous return is lost and blood pools in the venules and capillaries. Common causes include:

- severe head injury
- spinal injury
- drug reaction and anaesthetics
- neurological illness, e.g. Guillain-Barré syndrome.

Intense pain and severe fright may also result in neurogenic shock.

Septic shock. Damage is caused by overwhelming bacterial infection, usually by Gram-negative bacilli such as *Escherichia coli, Peseudomonas* and *Klebsiella*. The bacteria cause damage by releasing endotoxins which cause vasodilatation and increased capillary permeability. Fluid leaks out of the capillaries, causing hypotension and ultimately hypovolaemia. Septic shock often has an insidious rather than a sudden onset and is sometimes referred to as 'hot shock' because sufferers are pyrexial as a result of the precipitating infection. 'Toxic shock' is a type of septic shock and is generally associated with menstruation and prolonged use of tampons. The causative organism in this instance is *Staphylococcus aureus*.

Anaphylactic shock. Anaphylaxis occurs as the result of an antigen:antibody response in sensitive individuals. Antigens combine with immunoglobulin E (IgE) antibodies on the surface of mast cells throughout the body and these cells degranulate and release histamine and prostaglandins into the circulation. Under their influence, capillaries become more permeable, and widespread oedema results, including laryngeal oedema, which can rapidly cause death if not treated with adrenaline. Antigens may be introduced by the following routes:

- by injection, e.g. animal or insect bites and stings, drug therapy and mismatched blood transfusion
- by ingestion – food (shellfish, cheese, egg, nuts are some common causes of allergic reaction) or orally administered drugs
- by inhalation, e.g. dust and chemicals.

It will be noted that, whatever the initial cause of shock, venous return will be increasingly reduced and the cardiac output will continue to fall – a clear example of positive feedback at work.

Physiology of shock

Whatever the initial cause of shock, the pathophysiological response is the same (Fig. 22.16). Cells throughout the body are deprived of oxygen, resulting in cell membrane damage. Histamines and kinins are

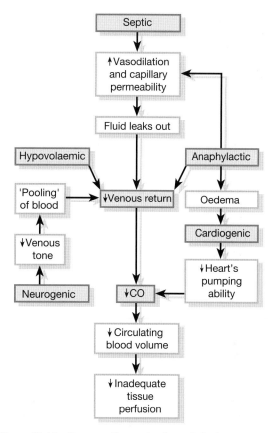

Figure 22.16   The causative mechanisms of shock.

released in response to the damage and cause vasodilation and increased capillary permeability. White blood cells leak out of the capillaries and proteins pass into the extracellular fluid. Oedema occurs within the cells and the interstitial fluid volume increases as the fluid compartments break down. The result is a decrease in the circulating blood volume and a consequent reduction in venous return, in the amount of blood available for oxygenation and in cardiac output (CO). Metabolism continues within the cells despite the lack of oxygen, and lactic acid, produced as a result of cellular metabolism, builds up causing metabolic acidosis.

Compensatory mechanisms – the early stage
In the initial stages of shock, the body's homeostatic mechanisms are triggered and attempt to return the body to 'steady state'.

Sympathetic nerves are stimulated by the fall in arterial blood pressure and a fall in PO_2. They act to preserve blood supply to the vital organs, i.e. the heart and the brain, by vasoconstriction and by increasing heart rate, although stroke volume, the volume pumped by each contraction, diminishes. This may be felt as a rapid, weak pulse.

The skin becomes cold as blood is diverted to the vital organs and patients may become confused and disoriented as blood supply to the brain is reduced.

The fall in PO_2 levels triggers deep and rapid breathing ('air hunger') but this will only rectify the situation if sufficient blood is passing through the system for adequate oxygenation to occur.

The fall in PO_2 at the tissues means that more O_2 can be released from Hb, but demand will exceed supply unless intervention occurs. Administered O_2 will only partially rectify the situation.

In the early stages of shock, interstitial fluid is returned to the circulation through the capillary walls in an attempt to raise the circulating blood volume, but once cell damage begins this mechanism also fails. Sodium and water are preserved in the body by the production of ADH and aldosterone and this further helps to raise blood volume. Urine output falls as a result.

Progressive shock – when compensatory mechanisms are not enough

Without intervention, these compensatory mechanisms ultimately fail and cells throughout the body begin to malfunction. Some of the resulting effects are:

- Metabolic acidosis causes hyperventilation and this causes respiratory acidosis in addition as too much CO_2 is blown off.
- PCO_2 falls, causing a reduction in blood flow to the brain and a reduced level of consciousness.
- Adrenaline and noradrenaline are produced in response to sympathetic nervous stimulation and cause vasoconstriction, which causes further hypoxia by decreasing blood flow through the lungs. Surfactant production in the lungs starts to fail and the lungs begin to collapse, making breathing more difficult. Fluid leaks from the pulmonary capillaries and pulmonary oedema results.
- Reduced blood volume and flow result in poor renal perfusion with resultant oliguria.
- In the liver, cells can eventually no longer conjugate bilirubin; it is returned to the circulation and jaundice becomes apparent.
- Poor blood flow through the gut leads to breakdown of the gut lumen. Gut contents cross

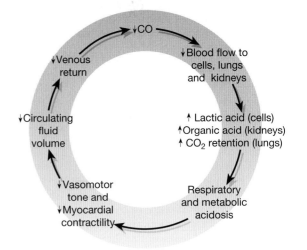

Figure 22.17   The vicious circle of irreversible shock.

into the circulation and blood passes into the gut – haematemesis and melaena are indications that this is happening.
- Disseminated intravascular coagulation occurs when the clotting system is activated by enzymes released from the breakdown of cells and this further reduces blood flow.
- The heart's pumping ability is so reduced that it is unable to supply even the needs of the cardiac muscle and it becomes weaker and weaker.

Irreversible shock – the final stage

The vicious circle described above, with its many positive-feedback mechanisms, is illustrated in Fig. 22.17. Early intervention may mean that homeostasis can be restored but once cell breakdown and acidosis reach a critical level, the damage is irreversible and death will ensue despite all intervention.

CONCLUSION

A basic understanding of physiological mechanisms employed to maintain homeostasis is vital if the ED nurse is competently to manage the complex assaults on normal body systems that are regularly witnessed in patients attending ED.

Further Reading

Edwards S (2001) Shock: types, classifications and explorations of their physiological effect. *Emergency Nurse*, **9**(2), 29–38.

Godfrey H (2004) *Understanding the Human Body: Biological Perspectives for Healthcare*. Edinburgh: Churchill Livingstone.

Gosling P, Alpar E (1999) The metabolic and circulatory response to trauma. In: Alpar E, Gosling P (eds). *Trauma: A Scientific Basis for Care*. London: Edward Arnold.

Hartshorn JC, Sole ML, Lamborn ML (1997) *Introduction to Critical Care Nursing*. Philadelphia: WB Saunders.

Jones G (2002) Anaphylactic shock. *Emergency Nurse*, **9**(10), 29–35.

Montague SE, Watson R, Herbert RA (2005) *Physiology for Nursing Practice*, 3rd edn. London: Baillière Tindall.

Silverthorn DU (2001) *Human Physiology: An Integrated Approach*, 2nd edn. New Jersey: Prentice Hall.

Thibodeau GA, Paton KT (2005) *The Human Body in Health and Disease*. Missouri: Elsevier Mosby.

Chapter 23

Wound care

Elaine Cole, Antonia Lynch & Tanya Reynolds

CHAPTER CONTENTS

INTRODUCTION

Wound management forms a large percentage of the Emergency Department (ED) nurse's workload, and with changes in working patterns, the ED nurse may be the only health professional involved in a patient's care. It is important that traumatic wound care in ED is seen as more than the best way to achieve technical closure. Wound care is about an extensive knowledge of skin anatomy, the physiological processes of healing, the causes and impact of wound infection and empowerment of patients to manage their own wounds. This chapter aims to provide the knowledge base needed for safe and effective wound management.

ANATOMY OF THE SKIN

The skin covers the whole of the body (Baggaley 2001), representing up to 15% of body weight (Flanagan & Fletcher 1997). Its thickness varies around the body, with areas of greatest friction, such as the soles of the feet, being thickest and areas of low friction, like eyelids, being the thinnest. The skin has five primary functions (Box 23.1):

- protection
- sensation
- thermoregulation
- vitamin D synthesis
- excretion and reserve.

The skin is made up of two main parts, the epidermis and the dermis, which cover the subcutaneous fat layer and deep structures (see Fig. 23.1).

Epidermis

This is subdivided into five distinct layers. Working from the surface these are as follows:

Box 23.1 Functions of the skin

- Protection from:
  - bacteria and viruses
  - heat and cold
  - dehydration
  - some chemical substances
  - mechanical damage

- Sensation
  - largest sensory organ
  - contains nerve endings – most concentrated in fingertips and lips
  - sensitive to touch, pain, heat, cold, vibration and pressure
  - skin hairs are also sensitive to touch, reducing risk of injury to the skin

- Thermoregulation
  The skin is responsible for maintaining the body's core temperature. It is controlled by the hypothalamus. The skin stabilizes heat generated by metabolism. This is done by heat conduction, convection and radiation from the skin surface. Heat loss is also influenced by vasodilation and constriction, varying the amount of blood flowing beneath the skin surface. This mechanism also prevents excessive heat loss in cold weather. Sweat production and evaporation have a cooling effect. The body is insulated from the environment by a layer of subcutaneous fatty adipose tissue

- Vitamin D synthesis
  Vitamin D is synthesized from ultraviolet light falling on the skin. Vitamin D is necessary for calcium absorption. Vitamin D can also be synthesized from dietary intake

- Excretion and reserve
  Some gaseous exchange takes place through skin. Sodium and urea are excreted via sweat. The skin provides a water reserve which is drawn into the circulating blood volume in cases of sudden fluid loss, such as haemorrhage or chronic dehydration. The fat layer can also be converted into energy

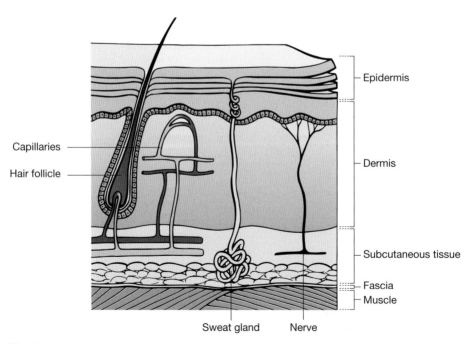

Figure 23.1 Skin structure.

Stratum corneum. This outer layer consists of dead cells. They contain keratin, which absorbs water, making the skin susceptible to maceration if constantly exposed to water. These cells shed continuously at a rate of 1 500 000 per hour. The whole layer is replaced every 24 hours (Collier 1996). The primary function of this layer is to act as a barrier.

Stratum lucidum. This layer of dead cells is found in areas needing extra protection, such as the soles of the feet and the palms of the hands.

Stratum granulosum. These cells are dead granular cells, not yet flattened, and contain cytoplasmic granules which are the precursor to keratin.

Stratum spinosum. These form a layer of living cells which act as intracellular bridges preventing cell separation.

Stratum basale. This layer lies next to the dermis. These cells are responsible for germination of new epithelial cells and are reliant on the dermis for nutrients from the blood supply.

Dermis. This is made up of two primary layers of connective tissue, ground substance and cells. The ground substance supports fibres and cells of the dermis. It forms a jelly-like matrix which is susceptible to some microorganisms, e.g. *Clostridium* and *Streptococcus pyogenes*. These dissolve the matrix, creating a tract for deep infection. The fibres contained include collagen. This gives strength to the jelly-like matrix tissue and the water-holding element of the skin, with reticular formation surrounding the collagen bundles and elastin. Cells in the dermis include:

- Fibroblasts – used in wound healing. These lie between bundles of collagen and act to synthesize elastin and collagen.
- Tissue macrophages – these phagocytic cells engulf debris and matter during healing.
- Tissue mast cells – found near hair follicles and blood vessels, these cells produce histamine and heparin.
- Transient cells – these move between dermis and blood vessels. They include neutrophils, lymphocytes and monocytes. Quantities vary at different stages of healing.

The dermis is formed of two distinct layers. The papillary layer lies next to the basal layer of the epidermis. It is composed of connective tissue, and houses capillary vessels, nerve endings, temperature and touch sensors, and lymph vessels. The roots of sebaceous glands, sweat glands and hair follicles are also found in the dermis. This layer is largely responsible for the tensile strength of skin. The reticular layer is at the base of the dermis; blood vessels and collagen fibres increase in size in this layer. There is no real physiological separation between the papillary and reticular layers, more a gradual change from one to the other.

WOUND HEALING

Terminology and the number of stages in the healing process vary between texts (Collier 1996, Desai 1997). The general consensus is that four phases of healing occur. They usually follow a set pattern (Clark 2002), but can occur concurrently, and different parts of the same wound can heal at different rates (see Table 23.1). Wound healing can be complex and is affected by the mechanism of injury and the general health of the patient.

Four phases of wound healing

Haemostasis
The body's initial response to a cut in the skin is bleeding. This extravasation initiates platelet activity and coagulation of blood. It also results in vasoconstriction and release of histamines and ATP, which also attract leucocytes. Platelets begin to aggregate and the coagulation cascade results in the development of a fibrin mesh, or beginnings of a scab, which temporarily seals the wound (Baggaley 2001).

Inflammatory
As well as a haemostatic response, the body also responds to tissue trauma by releasing prostaglandins and activated proteins which initiate vasodilation in the area. This has two main functions:

1. It increases blood supply to the area
2. It increases capillary permeability.

This is to enable plasma to leak into tissues around the area of injury. This creates wound exudate.

Table 23.1 Phases of wound healing

Duration	Phase	Signs
First hour	Haemostasis	Initial vasoconstriction Coagulation of wound
10 minutes–5 days	Inflammatory	Vasodilation, pain, heat, swelling
3 days–1 month	Proliferation	Wound size diminishing Surrounding skin of normal colour Less pain
3 weeks–1 year	Maturation	Wound healed Scarring fades

Neutrophils leak into the area of the wound and offer initial protection from infection by engulfing and digesting bacteria. Neutrophils have a short life span, and so are replaced by monocytes which are capable of phagocytosis. These promote new tissue formation and angiogenesis, and continue to engulf and destroy bacteria and debris from the wound, including old neutrophils (Whitby 1995).

The signs of an inflammatory response are often confused with infection, so it is important to establish a clear history of the duration since injury. Inflammatory responses usually occur before infection has had time to develop. The signs of the inflammatory response include:

- redness – because of local vasodilatation
- heat – because of increased blood supply and metabolic activity
- oedema – because increased capillary permeability allows fluid to leak into the extracellular space
- pain – due to pressure of fluid in tissues and chemical irritation from enzymes such as prostaglandin.

This inflammation is vital to the natural healing. If it is suppressed by drugs or illness healing will be delayed. For this reason non-steroidal anti-inflammatory drugs (NSAIDs) are not recommended in the initial management of wounds. Macrophages are essential for transition into the proliferation stage of healing, as they begin to produce transforming growth factor (TGF), which promotes angiogenesis and the formation of new tissues. Macrophages also produce fibroblast growth factor (FGF), which stimulates fibroblast production.

Proliferation

This starts 3–5 days post-injury. As its name suggests, this part of the healing process is about growth and reproduction of tissue to replace that lost in injury. By day five the wound surface will only be 7% of its pre-injury tensile strength (Waller 2004). In order to produce new tissue, the wound needs a good oxygen supply and essential nutrients such as vitamin C. As angiogenesis occurs in response to wound hypoxia and TGF, new capillary loops develop and the wound is oxygenated. Three distinct processes occur during the proliferation phase.

1. **Granulation.** This is the formation of new tissue up from the base, and in from the sides of a wound. It is dependent on the division of endothelial cells forming new capillary loops, until eventually they meet up with existing undamaged blood vessels. At the same time, fibroblasts begin to produce a network of collagen and ground substance which fills

tissue spaces and begins to bind fibres together. Collagen synthesis depends on adequate nutrients, i.e. vitamin C, copper and iron (Flanagan 1997). These can usually be obtained from a healthy diet. Collagen forms in a haphazard and jelly-like structure, and with adequate vitamin C matures into a strong cross-linked structure which gives the tissue its tensile strength.

2. **Contraction.** This occurs at the same time as epithelialization. In wounds where tissue loss has occurred, once the wound bed has filled with healthy granulation tissue, myofibroblasts develop which contract and pull the wound edges together, therefore decreasing the overall size of the wound.

3. **Epithelialization.** This is the resurfacing of the wound by regeneration of epithelial cells. This will only occur where basal cells are in contact with the dermal layer, and therefore in deep wounds regeneration will only occur around wound margins until granulation has taken place. In wounds of varying depth, small islands of epithelialization will occur in superficial parts of the wound. This gradually migrates across wound surfaces until epithelialization is complete. The attachment of this layer to dermal connective tissue is fragile and easily displaced. Regeneration therefore continues until the epidermis has regained its usual thickness. Epithelial regeneration requires a warm, moist environment. If a wound surface has dry scabs or necrotic areas, these will form a barrier to migration of new cells. Cells eventually burrow under scabs.

As the wound cavity is filled with granulation tissue and the surface is regenerated with epithelial cells, the proliferation stops. If this does not happen, e.g. if overgranulation occurs due to continued hypoxic stimulation, perhaps as a result of local ischaemia, then excessive scar tissue is formed (Flanagan & Fletcher 1997).

Maturation

This begins around 3 weeks after injury, and is a process of returning the area to its usual functional structure. The process is twofold.

1. Collagen is remodelled, sometimes over a period of years. The aim of this is to gradually replace newly formed type III collagen, laid down in the proliferation phase, with stronger more organized collagen fibres. The amount of collagen does not change; its bundles become thicker and shorter and hold the wound together more tightly. Although the skin and wound scar become stronger, the area only usually regains about 80% of the pre-injury tensile strength (Brown 1988). This takes a long time; at 3 months post-injury 50% of tensile strength is considered good healing (Morrison 1992).

2. The second part of the process is the rationalization of blood vessels bringing extra nutrients to the area. This process occurs gradually, and its progression can be monitored by the gradual fading of the scar. It will become paler and flatter as blood vessels diminish. Once maturation is achieved the scar will appear white; it is avascular, has no sebaceous glands and no hairs (Flanagan 1997) (Table 23.1).

Scarring

Dermal damage results in an abnormal formation of connective tissue. This is permanent and manifests as a scar on the skin surface. Scarring follows three phases, although the time span increases with age, skin pigmentation and as a result of poor general health (Table 23.2). Certain areas of the body are notorious for poor scarring – the shoulder, knee, and sternal areas, which are areas under a lot of tension and motion (Bayat et al. 2003, Capellan & Hollander 2003).

Keloid scarring results from the formation of large amounts of scar tissue in the proliferation phase of healing. It results from an increase in collagen synthesis and lysis to an extent where tissue formation exceeds cell breakdown (Bryant 1992). Keloid scarring is also considered to be related to the melanocyte-stimulating hormone as it is much more common in people with heavily pigmented skin, predominantly those aged 10–30 years (Bayat et al. 2003, Mustoe 2004). Tissue growth is persistent, with scarring often being much larger than the original wound. Early effective wound management can reduce the risk of keloid scarring.

Hypertrophic scarring forms in a similar fashion to tissue growth, but follows the line of incision. This type of scarring is more common in the young and in fair-skinned people and typically occurs after burn injury on the trunk and extremities. In these scars, there is an imbalance in collagen synthesis versus collagen degradation. The resulting wounds are red and raised and can be itchy. In the majority of cases, this is temporary and resolves without treatment although it may take a year or more.

Tattoo scarring results from gravel or foreign bodies being left in a wound. It forms unsightly purple or blue blotches in the scar and is difficult to remedy after initial wound healing. Generally, scars that lie parallel to the body's natural tension lines have a better cosmetic prognosis.

Factors affecting wound healing

Although patients with sudden traumatic wounds do not have the same physiological and educational preparation as patients undergoing surgery, many of the influences on wound healing can be optimized by effective education and empowerment during their initial visit for wound management. Clinical factors affecting healing potential can also be identified at this early stage, and the patient's care can be designed to accommodate them. The main influences on wound healing are listed in Box 23.2.

Nutrition

Nutrition deserves more elaborate exploration, as it is fundamental to adequate healing and is often overlooked both in discharge information and in promoting well-being in hospital in-patients. Malnutrition affects healing in several ways:

- poor healing with reduced tensile strength and an increased risk of wound dehiscence (McLaren 1992)
- an increased likelihood of infection (Lansdown 2004, Dickson 1995)
- poor quality scarring.

Protein and calorie intake need to be above normal recommended levels to support additional collagen synthesis and metabolic activity (Table 23.3).

Vitamin deficiency

Vitamin C is essential for the synthesis of collagen; a deficiency reduces wound tensile strength, increases the fragility of capillaries and impairs angiogenesis. Vitamin A supplement improves healing in patients on corticosteroids (Pinchofsky-Devin 1994). It can help to restore inflammatory response and reduces the risk of wound infection. Similarly, a vitamin A deficiency increases infection risk. Vitamin B complex is necessary for wound strength as it contributes to cross-linking of collagen fibres. Vitamin K is essential for the clotting process in early wound healing (Lansdown 2004).

Table 23.2	Scar formation
No. of weeks post–injury	Scar characteristics
0–4 weeks	Soft, weak scarline
4–12 weeks	Scar contracts, becomes harder and stronger
12–52 weeks	Scarline flattens and becomes soft and supple, moving easily with surrounding skin. Gradually, whitens as vascularity decreases. Skin does not regain pre-injury elasticity

Box 23.2   Factors affecting wound healing

- **Age**
  With age, all metabolic processes slow down and collagen production is lower; therefore wounds heal more slowly and have less tensile strength
- **Tissue perfusion**
  Many diseases cause hypoxia and reduced tissue perfusion. Those with a significant effect on wound healing include:
    - anaemia
    - peripheral vascular disease
    - respiratory disease
    - arteriosclerosis
    - dehydration.
    The result of this is reduced fibroblast activity and collagen synthesis, reduced epithelial regeneration and greater susceptibility to infection because of decreased leucocyte activity
- **Other diseases**
  These include diabetes, immune disorders and cancer, because of dampened inflammatory response and susceptibility to infection. Also, inflammatory conditions, liver failure and uraemia
- **Psychological factors and body image**
  Stress and anxiety supress the immune system and are linked with sleep disturbance. This has been shown to delay healing (Pediani 1992). Anabolic healing is enhanced by sleep. Altered body image can occur from seemingly minor wounds and this can adversely affect healing in terms of stress and compliance with wound care strategies

- **Poor wound care**
  Inadequate wound cleansing or inappropriate wound dressing is an avoidable factor in healing
- **Nutrition**
  Protein, vitamins and trace elements are vital for prompt, adequate wound healing. These include:
    - iron
    - copper
    - zinc
    - vitamin A
    - vitamin C
    Vitamins B, E and K also influence healing, and adequate protein and calorie intake is also necessary
- **Hydration**
  To maintain metabolism, between 2 and 2.5 L of fluid in 24 hours is needed. Less than this will result in fluid being drawn from interstitial spaces. Patients who are already clinically dehydrated will have delayed healing
- **Smoking**
  Both carbon monoxide and nicotine, as end-products of smoking, have an adverse effect on peripheral tissue perfusion, therefore increasing hypoxia risk. There is also an increased risk of thrombus formation in smokers (Sianna et al. 1992)
- **Drug therapy**
  Anti-inflammatory agents, immunosuppressive drugs, cytotoxics and corticosteroids all impinge on the healing process

Trace element deficiency

Iron deficiency has two significant impacts on wound healing: first, in patients with anaemia, oxygen transportation is reduced and therefore tissue perfusion is inhibited; and second, iron is a necessary co-factor in collagen synthesis. Copper deficiency is rare but where it occurs, enzyme activity is restricted and collagen cross-linkage is impaired. Zinc deficiency delays wound healing because it slows collagen synthesis, reduces wound strength and decreases speed of epithelialization.

Table 23.3   Calorie and protein intake in wound healing

	Energy (kcal)	Protein (g)
Men	2150–2510	54–63
Women	1680–2150	42–45

WOUND ASSESSMENT

It is essential that an accurate history is elicited from the patient to ensure systematic assessment and appropriate management of the wound. As with all patients attending the ED, the immediate history of events leading up to ED attendance is imperative. Assessment should consider when, where and how the injury occurred. The mechanism of injury gives important clues to the type of wound being dealt with. Table 23.4 relates the mechanism of injury to wound type. The type of skin damage of injury is usually related to mechanism of injury (Fig. 23.2).

The size, shape, wound depth and anatomical site of the wound should be assessed and documented. Diagrams in the patient's notes, or a photograph with a measurement scale, are useful if the wound is likely to need follow-on care.

Table 23.5 demonstrates the essential principles of wound assessment.

Table 23.4   Mechanism of injury: wound classifications

Mechanism of injury	Type of wound	Appearance	Special considerations
Blunt force such as a direct blow to the skin causing tearing or splitting of the skin (Cole 2003)	Laceration	Irregular break of the skin	
Caused by a sharp cutting implement such as a knife, broken glass or a metal edge (Milroy & Rutty 1997)	Incision	Straight, clean cut	
Caused by an object penetrating the skin and possible underlying structures	Penetrating	Appearance may be deceptive; this type of wound needs careful exploration	There may be underlying injury or a foreign body present
Tissue is crushed by the force of the injury, causing skin and underlying structures to split open (Walsh & Kent 2001)	Crush	Jagged with skin loss	This type of wound may be unsuitable for suturing and may need closure using adhesive tissue strips
Skin is forced against a resistant surface in a rubbing or scraping fashion (Trott, 1997)	Abrasion	Superficial skin loss, friction burn	
Blunt trauma	Contusion	Damage to vessels beneath surface with or without lacerations	
Trapped between shearing forces	De-gloving injury	Full thickness skin loss	There may be damage to underlying structures (Dandy & Edwards 2003)
Thermal sources Caused by intense heat or cold or substances, steam, flame, sun exposure, friction, radiation	Burn	Classified as superficial, partial thickness and full thickness. See wound assessment	
Chemical sources Acids or alkalis. Specialist advice should be sought for chemical burns, an antidote may be needed			There is a risk of underlying tissue damage
Electrical currents			

Wound examination

Effective wound examination should reveal the extent of tissue damage, the degree of contamination and specifically the integrity of the nerves, tendons and vascular supply (Autio & Olson, 2002; Clark, 2004). It should also exclude the presence of foreign bodies (FBs). All findings should be documented, including the normal ones.

Most traumatic wounds occur in unsterile conditions, and therefore all carry a risk of infection. A number of factors affect infection potential, such as mechanism of injury, degree of tissue loss, age of the wound prior to cleansing and anatomical location. All traumatic wounds should be considered contaminated; some of these will appear clean on initial examination, while others will be obviously contaminated. It is important to assess the degree of contamination carefully before a management plan is decided upon, as a

direct correlation exists between the degree of contamination and the incidence of infection (Edlich et al. 1988). The distinction between 'clean' and 'dirty' wounds lies with how contaminants are removed. In clean wounds, simple wound cleansing is adequate, whereas dirty wounds require surgical cleaning, removal of contaminants or excision of devitalized tissue (Dimick 1988).

Excessive bleeding and macerated or badly damaged tissue can detract from a thorough examination. Bleeding should be controlled to allow an accurate examination to be carried out (Clark 2004). Assessment of vascular integrity should include the patient's estimation of blood loss, together with objective evidence of haemorrhage. The wound should be carefully inspected for continuous oozing of blood (suggestive of venous bleeding), spurting of bright-red blood (indicative of arterial injury) and haematoma formation, which could

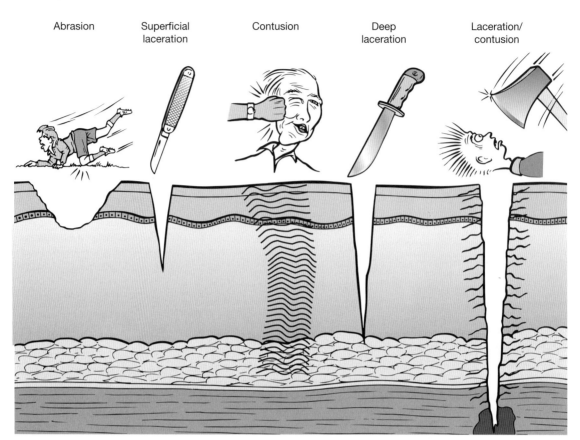

Figure 23.2 Mechanism of injury and skin damage.

Table 23.5 Wound assessment

Assessment question	Rationale
How did the wound occur?	–To establish mechanism of injury and classification of wound –To exclude serious or other injuries –To assess potential contamination risk (Clark 2004)
When did the injury occur?	–To ensure it is appropriate for primary closure –To assess for infection risk (wounds >6 hours old are more prone to infection; Moulton & Yates 1999)
Site and depth of wound	–To ascertain the most appropriate method of wound closure (e.g. wounds over joints or requiring high tensile strength usually require sutures; Autio & Olson 2002) –To ensure base of wound can be visualized
Past medical history	–To detect pathology that may delay or influence healing
Medication history	–To detect medication that may delay or influence healing –To avoid prescribing contraindicated medications as part of wound management
Allergies	–To avoid allergic reactions during the wound management process and during subsequent treatment
Tetanus status	–To ensure the patient has tetanus immunity
Occupation and dominant hand	–To assess the effect of the injury on the patient's lifestyle –To ensure treatment is appropriate for the patient's lifestyle

pose a risk to healing in the form of potential infection. Haemostasis is usually achieved through direct pressure and elevation of the injured area. Where bleeding cannot be controlled specialist input should be sought. Vascular integrity distal to the wound can be assessed by observing skin colour distally to the wound, feeling skin temperature, and checking distal pulses and the speed of capillary refill (ASSH 1990).

Nerves have both a sensory and a motor function and therefore both can be checked to eliminate injury. Sensory function distal to the wound should be assessed either by use of a cotton wool wisp, to detect the absence or presence of sensation, or by gentle pin-prick tests to assess sharp and dull sensation. Motor function should be assessed, particularly in hand or wrist injuries, and this can be done by assessing a variety of movements of the patient's hand and wrist (Trott 1997).

Tendon injury should also be identified and eliminated as part of the examination stage of wound management. Tendons can often be partially severed and still retain their function, so elimination of this type of injury should be done in two ways. An initial systematic examination of the patient's function in the affected limb may demonstrate reduced power or function. This should be followed by direct visualization of the wound to discover any structural damage (Trott 1997). This is particularly important in hand injuries where extensor tendon injuries are common, e.g. mallet finger. Flexor tendon injuries following injury to the palmar aspect of the hand are less common, but have a high incidence of disability when missed, as they leave the patient unable to bend the injured digit. Flexor tendon injury is difficult to detect as tendons contract when cut and are therefore not always visible at the wound edges. If the mechanism of injury and initial examination suggest tendon injury, the wound should be explored until tendon edges or an intact tendon are visualized. Specialist referral is necessary for wounds such as flexor tendon injuries or wounds involving cosmetic challenges such as the vermillion border or the cartilage of the ear (Reynolds 2004).

During examination and cleansing, FBs should be excluded. Likely FBs include glass, metal, plastic or grit, all of which could lead to infection or tattooing if left in situ. If the history suggests that glass or any other radio-opaque FB may be present in the wound, an X-ray is a useful way of locating or excluding this (Miller 1995).

WOUND PAIN

Wound pain is initiated by the inflammatory response and is a normal part of the healing process. It is

Box 23.3 Pain triggers

- Inflammatory response
- Atmospheric exposure – drying to wound
- Tissue tension – due to oedema and angiogenesis
- Irritation from cleaning solutions
- Dressings too tight
- Wound complications, such as infection

caused by a combination of noxious stimuli, including histamine and peptides, such as substance P (a pain transmitter) and prostaglandin (a chemical stimulus for pain). Box 23.3 highlights some of the pain triggers. Part of the pain response is to protect the wound from further injury. The impact of wound pain should not be underestimated and analgesia suitable for the stage of wound healing should be used.

There is conflicting evidence about the use of NSAIDs and wounds (Hawkey 1999, Patterson et al. 1997). NSAIDs are thought to have the potential to affect platelet activity by inhibiting clumping and coagulation, as well as the potential interference with the inflammatory phase of healing, where mediators and white cell activity are so important. While analgesia for burns (and wounds) should be a top priority, the potential inhibition of inflammation tends to indicate that other analgesia, such as paracetamol and codeine-based drugs, may be preferable. Opiates should be avoided for ED patients who will invariably be discharged.

Non-pharmacological methods of pain relief should also be considered. If ongoing wound care will be needed, e.g. in management of burns, patients should be prescribed analgesia to take prior to dressing changes. Appropriate explanations of interventions and psychological support will help to alleviate pain (see also Ch. 24).

WOUND CLEANSING

There are two important considerations in wound cleansing.

- The way it is carried out
- The solution used.

Wound cleansing is essential for the prevention of infection, tattoo scarring and exclusion of foreign bodies. The practitioner carrying out this cleansing prior to wound closure has a responsibility to ensure that the wound is decontaminated and if any doubt exists the wound should not be closed.

Cleansing solutions

Wound cleansing solutions have been the subject of much debate over recent years. In many emergency departments, normal saline is the cleanser of choice because of its safety and cost-effectiveness (Dulecki & Pieper 2005). Like tap water, it is most effective when warmed to body temperature. Studies have demonstrated that both normal saline and tap water are comparable for wound irrigation in terms of infection rates and healing (Bansal et al. 2002, Valente et al. 2003). Riyat & Quinton (1997) cultured tap water from various outlets in an emergency department and grew no bacteria. A systematic review by the Cochrane Group (Fernandez et al. 2003) suggests that clean, drinkable water is a safe, cheaper alternative to normal saline. Nevertheless water quality may influence outcomes (Betts 2003) and therefore it should be drawn from a tap that is frequently used, from a direct water supply with a nozzle that is regularly swabbed for contamination. Both water and normal saline are less likely to impede the natural healing process compared with other commercial irrigants or detergents such as povidone iodine (Dulecki & Pieper 2005).

Antiseptic solutions include cetrimide and chlorhexidine. They generally claim to destroy bacteria and have a detergent component for wound cleansing. Most, however, need to be in contact with bacteria for 20 minutes to have any effect (Russell et al. 1992) and are not recommended for routine wound closure (Holt 2000).

Povidone-iodine is a broad-spectrum antiseptic agent and is the cleansing agent of choice for contaminated wounds. Iodine is more effective than other antibacterial agents, particularly against Gram-negative bacteria (Trott 1991). It has a slow release capacity where povidone acts as a carrier gradually releasing iodine into the tissues. It has been suggested that this reduces tissue toxicity and irritation but preserves antibacterial properties (Trott 1991). There is continued concern over the use of povidone-iodine (Cole 2003) partly because the concentration of iodine in commercial preparations remains cytotoxic to the fibroblasts needed for wound healing and therefore reduces the tensile strength of the wound and slows the epithelialization process. Rabenberg et al. (2002) in a study using human skin samples found that diluting povidone-iodine solution 1 part solution to 9 parts water provides a safe antibacterial yet non-toxic compromise.

Desloughing solutions such as hydrogen peroxide are not effective as a routine treatment. Their ability to destroy bacteria is considerably reduced once in contact with blood or pus. While the oxidizing activity does remove slough, it also breaks down granulating wound tissue. If diluted to a strength which is non-toxic to tissues, the hydrogen peroxide is no longer effective on bacteria. Hydrogen peroxide should only be used as a one-off treatment for extremely sloughy wounds and the area should be irrigated with saline afterwards. This makes its use in traumatic wound management very limited. There is some evidence that using hydrogen peroxide to irrigate cavity wounds can cause emboli (Haller et al. 2002, Henley et al. 2004) so care should be taken when doing this. The National Institute for Health and Clinical Excellence (NIHCE) recommends considering other agents, and suggests that using hydrocolloids or hydrogels, among others, would be more acceptable to patients in terms of comfort and acceptability (NICE 2005).

Eusol (Edinburgh University Solution Of Lime) type preparations are rarely used and there is no clinical indication for their use in any circumstances. Considerable evidence exists to highlight the limited antibacterial effects of sodium hypochlorite and their devastating degree of tissue damage is well documented (Brennan & Leger 1985, Dealey 1994). Table 23.6 lists cleaning solutions and their properties.

Cleansing methods

It is now accepted practice that swabbing a wound with cotton wool or gauze is not the most effective method of cleaning a wound. Fibres can be left in situ and bacteria can be distributed around the wound (Cole 2003). Acute, traumatic wounds should be irrigated with a degree of pressure (using a steripod©; a pressurized canister of solution or a syringe and needle) to clean the wound and remove debris (Towler 2001). To be effective, the mechanical force used must exceed that of the adhesive forces of the contaminant (Dulecki & Pieper 2005). The amount of pressure needed for adequate irrigation with minimal damage to tissue is approximately 5 to 8 psi. Studies have demonstrated that this pressure can be achieved using a 19 g needle (Stevenson et al. 1976, Singer et al. 1994). Wound irrigation should continue until all obvious contamination has been removed.

In some cases, such as dirty abrasions and gritty wounds of varying depths, surgical scrubbing of the wound is indicated. The procedure should be carried out in a gentle manner so that further tissue damage is avoided; small circular movements are more effective than scrubbing across the wound (Trott 1991). If this is necessary adequate anaesthesia or analgesia will be required.

Table 23.6 Properties of cleaning solutions

Solution	Antibacterial activity	Tissue toxicity	Advantages	Disadvantages
Tap water	None	None	Cheap Easily accessible Large volumes	Potential for environmental contamination
Normal saline	None	None	Isotonic Gentle	Cost (compared with tap water)
Povidone iodine	Gram −ve Gram +ve	Toxic at >5% (sold in 7.5 and 10% solutions only)	Highly antibacterial	Potentially delays healing at strengths commonly used
Chlorhexidine	Strong Gram-positive, slight Gram-negative	Low toxicity	No clinical advantages	Antibacterial action reduced when in contact with blood or pus
Cetrimide	Low activity	Irritant	Good detergent	Antibacterial properties inactivated by blood and pus. Easily contaminated by infection
Hydrogen peroxide	Weak action on anaerobic surface	Very toxic to cells	No clinical advantages	Inactivated by pus

Chronic wounds

Chronic wounds are different so the practitioner should consider whether the wound needs cleansing. Unless there is obvious contaminant such as pus, most chronic wounds do not require cleaning. Small amounts of crust and serous fluid should be left in situ as these are natural by-products of the wound healing process.

LOCAL ANAESTHESIA

Local anaesthesia (LA) is used to ensure that wound cleansing or closure using sutures or staples is a painless procedure. Local infiltration of lignocaine or topical application of gel is usually adequate. Some patients find the administration of LA uncomfortable; therefore, careful explanation, expectations of procedure, encouragement and reassurance are helpful in reducing the anxiety and pain of LA administration (Quaba et al. 2005). For further information see Chapter 25: Local and regional anaesthesia.

WOUND CLOSURE

The closure of traumatic wounds in the ED can be categorized into two types:

- Primary wound closure – where edges of wounds are brought together preferably within the first 12 hours after injury
- Secondary closure – where the wound heals by granulation and epithelialization. Purposeful delay allows an intervention, such as the use of antibiotics, before the wound is closed. This may

happen following debridement of the wound edges.

Primary wound closure

Primary closure should only be carried out once the wound is thoroughly cleaned, foreign bodies have been eliminated and there is minimal or no tissue loss. While it is not suitable for all wound types, primary closure does improve healing and cosmetic appearance. Primary closure occurs when the wound has been brought together by sutures, staples, tissue adhesive, adhesive tissue strips and hair ties (Fig. 23.3). Primary closure entails aligning skin layers and underlying structures, eliminating any dead space and so reducing the risk of haematoma and infection (Castille 1998, Clark 2004).

The time elapsed since initial injury must be considered when undertaking primary closure. Wounds are normally closed up to 6 to 12 hours post injury, but this may differ according to the site of the wound. A face, for example, should be considered for primary closure up to 24 hours post-injury (Holt 2000). Similarly, if a wound is heavily contaminated or in an anatomical site prone to infection, such as the hand, safe primary closure times are considerably shorter.

Suturing

Sutures are appropriate for the management of specific wounds, such as deep, large or jagged wounds, those under tension, mobile areas or wounds in awkward places (Autio & Olson 2002). Wound closure using sutures can be more painful than other

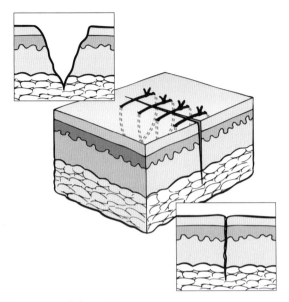

Figure 23.3   Primary closure.

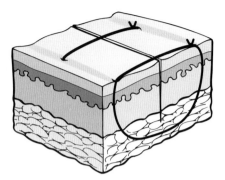

Figure 23.4   Everting wound edges with square sutures.

techniques, usually due to the need to infiltrate the area with local anaesthesia prior to suture insertion.

The wound depth is partial or full dermal depth, and neurovascular damage should be excluded before wound closure. Healing occurs across wound layers, so it is important to accurately match each skin layer. It is important to eliminate the dead space below the superficial layer of the wound (Atiyeh et al. 2002) as this provides an ideal location for bacterial colonization (Richardson 2004a). In addition, because scars contract during the maturation phase of healing, everted wound lines will flatten to the normal plane of the skin. Achieving proper wound edge eversion lies with suturing technique.

The most commonly used technique in ED is an interrupted suture (Jay 1999). This is basically a square suture, with width and depth of suture equal. This helps to evert wound edges. If suture width is greater than its depth then the wound edges will roll or invert (see Fig. 23.4). After thorough wound cleansing the initial suture should be placed centrally, to divide the lesion into two smaller wounds. Further sutures should then be placed strategically along the wound so that the tension remains constant throughout (Cole 2003). This can be achieved by having all of the knots on the same side.

Suture types   Suture products vary greatly, but general principles for use can be adapted. Sutures are designed to be absorbed or removed (see Table 23.7).

Sutures are either absorbable or non-absorbable, with the latter being commonly used for wounds where only the skin requires closure. Where there are deeper structures exposed, such as subcutaneous fat and muscle, then absorbable sutures may be used. These will dissolve over a longer period.

Non-absorbable sutures are used for dermis and epidermal skin closure. They are either monofilament or multifilament. Monofilament nylons and polypropylene are the most commonly used because they carry a low infection risk and are of a high tensile strength as they are made from single strands and not braided. Because they are synthetic, they are far less likely to cause an inflammatory response, which is common with silk and other organic sutures (Cole 2003). These sutures need removing.

Absorbable sutures, such as catgut or synthetic polymers, are used for deeper tissue structures as well as the inside of the mouth and perineum. They are broken down by protein synthesis over about 3–4 weeks and therefore do not need removal. Monofilament synthetic polymers are most commonly used as they have a lower infection and inflammation risk than catgut, but they do take longer to reabsorb.

Sutures are measured by gauge, and choice of suture size will be influenced by the extent and site of the wound. The common range of suture sizes found in an ED will be from 3/0 to 6/0, with the lower number indicating the thicker gauge and the higher indicating the finer. A general guide for sutures sizes and wounds can be seen in Table 23.8.

It is usual to utilize a reverse cutting needle for suturing (Clark 2004). This type of needle is manufactured to facilitate ease of use on tissue such as skin. The type and size of needle is depicted on the suture packet. Suture packs usually contain forceps, suture holder and scissors. Forceps may be toothed or non-toothed but regardless of the type used care should be taken not to crush the wound edges (Richardson 2004b).

Table 23.7 Suture material

Type	Description	Ease of use	Tensile strength	Inflammatory reaction risk	Infection risk
Silk	Organic, non-absorbable	Easy	Low	High	High
Nylon	Synthetic, non-absorbable monofilament	Moderate	High	Low	High
Polypropylene	Synthetic, non-absorbable monofilament	Difficult	High	Low	High
Catgut (plain or chrome)	Organic from sheep, absorbable	Moderate	Moderate	High	High
Polyglycolic acid	Synthetic braided, absorbable	Moderate	High	Low	Medium
Polydioxanone	Synthetic monofilament, absorbable	Easy	High	Low	Low

Table 23.8 A guide to suture size

Area	Size of suture	Suggested removal
Face	6/0 nylon	5 days (in some circumstances removal after 3 days may be appropriate)
Scalp	3/0 nylon	7 days
Arms, upper legs, torso	4/0–5/0 nylon	5–7 days
Hands, lower legs, extensors	3/0–4/0 nylon	7–10 days

Complications of suturing Sutured wounds do not need a dressing unless there is associated skin loss or the sutures are in need of protection, e.g. where the patient is a young child or a person working in a dirty environment. Dressings should provide a warm environment and be permeable to allow the wound to breathe. Some patients prefer sutured wounds to be dressed, however, and this should also be taken into consideration. See Table 23.9.

Staples

Staples are usually associated with surgical wounds, but they also have a place in the closure of acute traumatic wounds, particularly those in the scalp. Staples have the same tensile strength as sutures and can be used for linear wounds of moderate tension. Evidence suggests that overall, staples are quicker and cheaper than sutures for closing scalp wounds (Hogg & Carley 2002) and are associated with good cosmesis (Autio & Olson, 2002). Staples offer a low level of tissue reactivity and better resistance to infection than sutures (Edlich & Reddy 2001). Skill is required to insert staples, and failure to align tissue edges correctly can cause scar deformity (Richardson 2004b). In common with sutures, local anaesthesia should be used prior to insertion of staples. Staples require special equipment for removal and they should be removed in 5–7 days.

Tissue adhesive

Tissue adhesives (TA) are a useful method of closing simple traumatic wounds. TA is usually supplied in sterile units, which can be disposed after single use. It is easy and quick to use, and less painful than other methods (Mattick 2002). Wound contamination rates are lower than that of sutures (Quinn et al. 1997) and it achieves good cosmetic results (Farion et al. 2003). Risk of needlestick injuries is eliminated as no sharps are used (Richardson 2004b). TA is particularly useful in the management of acute wounds in children due to its ease and rapidity of use (Barnett et al. 1998).

When applying TA, it is essential that bleeding has been stopped, or the adhesive will not work. Application of TA is normally a two-person technique, and should not be attempted by a lone practitioner, unless the wound is very small and the edges well apposed and the practitioner is skilled in its application.

The wound edges should be apposed as closely as possible, while the adhesive is applied either in a continuous line or dotted along the wound edges (Cole 2003). The wound edges should be held together for at least 30 seconds to allow polymerization to occur (Richardson, 2004b), although individual manufacturers' instructions should be followed. TA should *never* be instilled into the wound and then the wound edges pushed together, as this will cause pain and excessive scarring. It will also increase the risk of infection.

Table 23.9   Complications of suturing

Complication	Comment	Solution
Patient fainting	Patient inadequately prepared	Lie patients down while suturing
Sutures too tight	Can result in split sutures and/or devitalized tissue. Can also increase scarring	Tie sutures tight enough to ensure edges are everted. If suture appears too tight remove and replace it
Sutures too loose	Will not hold tissue in apposition and may delay healing or cause a scar	Tie sutures tight enough to ensure edges are everted. If suture appears too loose remove and replace it
Wound edges overlapping	Will not heal optimally and will leave a poor cosmetic finish	Ensure wound edges are apposed and everted
Wound edges inverted	Can result in a depressed scar and delay healing	Ensure wound edges are apposed and everted
Sutures too near to wound edge	May tear skin	Ensure sutures are 4–5 mm from wound edge. Do not suture thin, friable skin: consider other wound closure methods
Sutures too far from wound edge	May cause increased tension and 'cross hatch' scarring	Ensure sutures are 4–5 mm from wound edge
Infection	May cause delayed wound healing, scarring and systemic illness	Scrupulous cleansing and aseptic technique

(Adapted from Clark, 2004 & Richardson, 2004b)

Care should be taken when using adhesive on the face to avoid it running into the eyes. This can be avoided by always having the patient lying down and covering the eyes with a damp gauze pad during application.

Following application the patient should be instructed to start washing the affected area with soap and water after five days and the adhesive will start to gently dissolve.

Adhesive tissue strips

Adhesive strips are available in different widths, can be elasticized to allow ease of movement (Richardson 2004b) and have several advantages over suturing. They are usually less traumatic and painful for the patient, tissue trauma is decreased and there is little risk of reaction to the material being used. There is a lower risk of induced wound infection (Edlich & Reddy 2001).

Adhesive tissue strips are useful for wounds that are superficial, straight and where skin edges can be aligned and there is minimal wound tension (Autio & Olson 2002). They are also useful for flap wounds and patients with frail skin, such as the elderly or patients on steroid therapy, where a suture might tear the skin, e.g. a pre-tibial laceration. They are unsuitable for wounds where bleeding cannot be stopped and for hirsute areas such as the scalp (Cole 2003). Care should be taken when using them on confused or non-compliant patients, as they can be easily removed (Fig. 23.5).

When applying adhesive tissue strips, ensure that the surrounding skin is clean and dry to allow adequate adhesion (Richardson 2004b). Following the same principles as suturing, and after the wound edges have been apposed, either with forceps or gloved fingers, the first closure should be made in the centre of the wound. Subsequent strips should be placed to bisect the resulting smaller wounds until closure is complete (Richardson 2004b). Tension should be even across the wound and small gaps should be left between the strips to allow exudate to escape (Cole 2003). Adhesive tissue strips can be used in conjunction with other wound-closure techniques for support.

Adhesive tissue strips require minimal follow-up after application (Autio & Olson 2002), allowing the patient to care for the wound themselves, if they have been given appropriate advice.

A dressing is not strictly necessary over these wounds, but may be used if the wound needs extra protection. Adhesive strips should be removed after 3–4 days from the face, and 5–7 days in most other areas. Patients with friable skin or pre-tibial lacerations should have adhesive strips in place for at least 10 days.

Patients can remove adhesive strips themselves without the need to return to a healthcare professional. Specifying to the patient how long, removal should take place after 5–7 days by gently peeling back both ends of the strip, while supporting the skin, towards the centre of the wound.

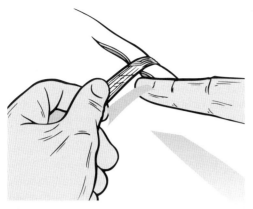

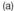
(a)

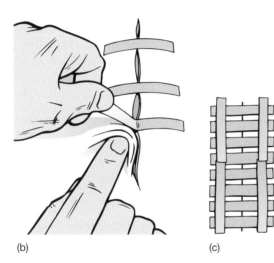

(b)   (c)

Figure 23.5   Application of adhesive tapes.

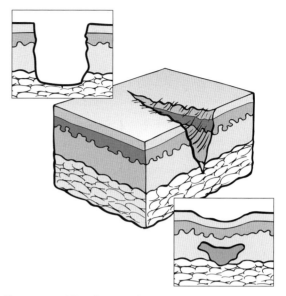

Figure 23.6   Wound granulation.

Hair apposition technique (hat)

This is an underused technique, which can be used for superficial wounds on the scalp that are not actively bleeding (Cole 2003). Ong et al. (2002) suggest that this should be the first choice for scalp wounds; however, the patient's hair needs to be long enough to tie. It may be used in situations when other more conventional methods of wound closure may be inappropriate, such as with children or adults who refuse sutures due to needle phobia. However, this method is only suitable for superficial scalp wounds (Richardson 2004b).

HAT is a quick and relatively painless method of wound closure which compares with suturing for wound healing, risk of infection and wound breakdown, but is superior in terms of scarring, overall complications and procedure-related pain (Ong et al. 2002).

The wound edges are pulled together by the hair on either side, which is then tied in a knot. Alternatively, the hair can be twisted rather than tied, and secured with a drop of tissue adhesive (Hock et al. 2002). The patient needs to be advised not to pull on the hair tie with a brush or a comb. After five days the patient should treat the wound as for tissue adhesive.

Secondary closure

This occurs by granulation when primary closure is contraindicated (see Fig. 23.6). Wounds healing by secondary closure usually require a dressing. The purpose of a wound dressing is to create the optimal healing environment for that particular wound (Box 23.4).

See Table 23.10 for an overview of common types of dressings.

Wound humidity

Epithelialization of a wound is 40% faster when the wound surface is covered with a film dressing (Collier 1996). This is because the moist wound surface allows epithelial cells to slide across it as they regenerate. Wound pain is also reduced in a moist healing environment (Eaglestein 1985).

Gaseous exchange

The benefit of wound oxygenation depends on the depth and stage of healing.

> **Box 23.4 The optimum wound dressing. (After Dealey 1994)**
>
> - High humidity between wound surface and dressing
> - Allows gaseous exchange
> - Provides thermal insulation
> - Impermeable to bacteria
> - Removes excess exudate
> - Free of particles and toxic wound contaminants
> - Can be removed without causing further tissue trauma

For superficial regenerating wounds involving the epidermis, semi-permeable film dressings are advantageous (Dealey 1994). However, gaseous exchange from the wound surface is inhibited by exudate, making atmospheric oxygen through permeable dressings an unreliable source of oxygenation.

For wounds which heal by granulation, some degree of tissue hypoxia is necessary to stimulate angiogenesis and fibroblastic activity (Knighton et al. 1981). Where healing is by granulation, hydrocolloid dressings are effective. Cherry & Ryan (1985) suggested that the low PO_2 produced under the dressing stimulates the formation of vascular tissue and therefore speeds up wound healing.

Thermal insulation

A constant wound temperature of 37°C promotes mitotic and macrophage activity (Collier 1996). If the thermal environment is kept stable under a dressing, this cellular activity is further enhanced. If that wound becomes exposed, perhaps for a dressing change, its surface temperature drops and cellular activity is inhibited. It can take up to 3 hours for this activity to return to normal (Myers 1982). Dressings should therefore only be removed when clinically indicated, as removing dressings has the potential to delay healing.

Permeability to bacteria

Dressings should provide the wound with protection from microorganisms. They should also contain any existing bacteria within the dressing. Any dressing which becomes wet, or where wound exudate soaks through, becomes a passage for infection both into the wound and out from it, and should be changed. Certain types of dressing, such as gauze and some tulle dressings, allow tracts to be created, therefore increasing the infection rate.

Removal of excess exudate

Although the wound surface should be moist, excessive exudate causes skin maceration around the wound. For this reason, the dressing chosen should be of an absorbency level suitable for the amount of exudate. Many commercial dressings are made in a variety of absorbencies. Absorbent pads may be necessary but should only be used over a primary dressing (Holt 2000).

Removal without causing tissue trauma

Dressings which stick to the wound surface should be avoided, particularly dry dressings on open wounds. Exudate can also cause a dressing to stick if it dries, which is why dressings with adequate absorbency are essential. Newly granulating tissue is fragile and easily destroyed in dressing removal. Dressings should be removed slowly while supporting the wound surface in order to reduce the risk of tissue trauma.

Types of dressing

Many wound dressing products are available for hospital use, either for general use or by medical prescription. These can be broadly grouped into seven categories (Table 23.10).

Wound dressings most commonly used in ED warrant further consideration.

Dressings which promote regeneration

These are used for grazes, abrasions, minor burns and other superficial wounds involving the epidermis. The most effective dressings for this are semi-permeable films or membranes. They provide the moist environments needed and some thermal protection; however, membranes have limited absorbency for light exudate. Neither should be used on infected wounds.

Non-adherent dressings also tend to be used for superficial wounds; however, not only do they have little absorbency, but they cannot provide a moist environment for regeneration and are therefore not recommended.

Dressings which promote granulation

These are used for wounds involving the dermal layer where tissue loss has occurred. Occlusive hydrocolloid dressings provide a warm, moist environment and promote granulation. They are designed to absorb moderate amounts of exudate and can be left in place for several days. As exudate is absorbed into the dressing, a distinctive odour is produced, which although it is not offensive can cause some concern

Table 23.10 Wound dressings

Wound	Dressing classification	Product example	Indications	Contraindications	Application
Abrasion	Non-stick silicone dressing	Mepitel	Anticipated adherence trauma, superficial wounds, granulating wounds, minor burns	Infected, heavily exudating wounds	Can be left in situ for 7 days. Initial wound may be reviewed after 2–3 days to check for possible infection
Epithelializing wounds	Semi-permeable film	Opsite	Superficial regenerating wounds, sites of primary closure	Infected wounds, exudating wounds	Apply to dry skin if it becomes loose or exudate builds up
Infected	Povodine iodine impregnated tulle gras	Inadine	Infected or potentially infected wounds	Non-infected wounds	Apply directly onto wound. 48 hours maximum between changes
Sloughy	Hydrogel	Intrasyte gel, granugel	Slough, small areas of necrosis	Non-sloughy wounds	Gel should be covered with a semi-permeable film. May need a secondary dressing. Review depends on wound size and amount of exudate
Exudating	Hydrophilic/hydrophobic foam	Lyofoam	Heavily exuding wounds	Dry wounds	Apply shiny side of dressing to wound. May require a secondary dressing. Review depends on wound size and amount of exudate
Granulating	Hydrocolloid	Granuflex, Duoderm	Granulating wounds and burns. Can also be used to deslough wounds	Infected wounds	Apply gel side directly onto wound. Does not need a secondary dressing. Can be left in situ for up to one week, depending on wound size. Waterproof
Bleeding	Haemostatic	Kaltostat	Bleeding wounds	Dry or infected wounds	Initial review after 24–48 hours for an infection check. Dressing may stick to the wound. Needs to be soaked for removal

for patients if it is not expected. Hydrocolloid dressings should not be used on infected wounds.

Impregnated tulle

Tulle dressings such as Inadine are useful for treating superficial wounds with moderate infection.

WOUND INFECTION

Most traumatic wounds occur in unsterile conditions, and therefore all carry a risk of infection. But just because contaminants can get in does not mean that all wounds become infected. A number of factors affect infection potential such as mechanism of injury, degree of tissue loss, age of the wound prior to cleansing and anatomical location.

It is important to recognize infection and differentiate from the normal inflammatory response. Accurate history-taking and the duration of the injury are important factors in differentiation. Signs of infection include:

- redness
- swelling
- increased pain
- skin warm to touch
- purulent discharge
- odour
- breakdown of the wound
- systemic symptoms
- pyrexia
- tachycardia
- tachypnoea.

Patients with a suspected wound infection should have a wound swab taken for culture and sensitivity prior to considering antibiotic therapy. Patients who suffer unexpected traumatic wounds are at greater risk of infection if they are malnourished, immunosuppressed or taking steroids.

WOUNDS THAT REQUIRE SPECIAL CONSIDERATION

Bite wounds

Bite wounds make up a small but significant proportion of injuries seen in the ED and warrant special consideration because of their potential for infection. About 1 in 5 people bitten by a dog seek medical attention and 1% of those seeking attention require admission to hospital (Dire 1992). It has been estimated that dog bites account for 60–90% of bites; cat bites for 5–18%, and human bites for 4–23% (Smith et al. 2000, Dire 1992, Richardson 2006). Between a third and half of all mammalian bites occur in children (often bitten by a household pet).

Bite wounds most commonly occur on the hands and are potentially at high risk for infection. The reasons for this are twofold; first, because of the number of pathogens found in the perpetrator's mouth, both human and animal; second, because of the way the pathogens are transferred – usually by deep, penetrating puncture wounds, which means that bite wounds, especially those from animals, tend to be heavily contaminated. All these factors mean that a bite wound can lead to complications such as local wound infection, lymphangitis, abscess formation, septic arthritis and potentially rarer complications such as meningitis (Brook 2003, 2005).

Human bite wounds to the hand, particularly from clenched-fist injuries, may not present initially as a bite-injury, and may accompany other co-existing injuries, such as fractures to metacarpals. Nonetheless, these should be treated as bite injuries (Cole 2003). Where a human bite is sustained, consideration should be given to the possibility of transmission of other diseases, such as hepatitis B (HBV) and HIV. The greater risk is with potential HBV transmission and so the opinion of a virologist should be sought, with a view to the patient commencing an accelerated course of HBV vaccine. HIV levels are low in saliva and so the risk of transmission via human bites is thought to be negligible (Eckerline et al. 1999). Rigorous wound management can go some way to reducing the infection risk (Kizer & Callahan 1984, Bower 2002).

The closure of bite wounds is a subject of ongoing debate, with some authors advocating delaying closure of hand wounds (Dearden et al. 2001, Bower 2002) for 24–48 hours. Suturing may be appropriate where cosmetic appearance is of a primary concern, such as on the face (Chen et al. 2000, Correira 2003).

The use of prophylactic antibiotics can be controversial, but they should always be considered (Stefanopoulos et al. 2004). There is general agreement that prophylactic antibiotics should be given when the bite is sustained on the hand, head, neck or groin (Taplitz 2004) or if the wound is considered to be high-risk, such as very deep wounds (Taplitz 2004, Brook 2005).

Insect bites and stings

Insect bites and stings are seen commonly in this country throughout the summer and early autumn months although they can occur at other times. Commonly, people attend the ED following a sting from an insect of the classification Hymenoptera such as a wasp or bee, which has not resolved or from which they are suffering ill-effects.

Reactions to an insect sting range from local to systemic (Brinker et al. 2003). The majority will be local and will consist of symptoms such as localized pain, redness and itching. For these reactions, the treatment is symptomatic and the use of antihistamines and simple analgesics will usually result in a resolution of symptoms. Where cellulitis has developed, the patient should be treated with antibiotics and reviewed within 24 hours to ensure the infection is resolving. It is helpful to mark the outer border of the erythema with a marker pen so that the patient, and also the practitioner who reviews the patient, can see if there is an improvement of symptoms.

Where patients have a systemic reaction due to anaphylaxis, treatment must be prompt and should follow the UK Resuscitation Council Guidelines (Resuscitation Council 2004).

Abrasions

Abrasions are caused by shearing trauma to the epidermis and dermis, resulting in the variable loss of these two layers of skin and potentially deeper layers of tissue such as fat and muscle (Trott 1997). These injuries can be small or can potentially cover a large surface area of the body, such as in the case of the cyclist who comes off a bike at speed and slides along a road.

Due to the nature of these injuries, they are often contaminated with dirt, debris and sometimes tar from road surfaces. This debris, if not removed at initial presentation, can become trapped under the skin and lead to unsightly tattooing, which is very difficult to remove later (Trott 1997, Richardson 2004b).

Analgesia should be given some time prior to cleansing to make the patient more comfortable. Large pieces of grit or dirt can be removed using forceps or by gentle scrubbing with a surgical sponge (Trott 1997). The patient may require additional pain relief such as inhaled nitrous oxide, local anaesthetic infiltration or even intravenous opiates, if the area is particularly large or painful. A non-adherent dressing can be applied (see Table 23.10).

Minor burns

Most minor burns are dealt with in EDs and in the community (McKirdy 2001). Minor burns are usually considered to be where the surface area of the burn is less than 5% (Harulow & Holt 2000) with only superficial or partial thickness involvement. Minor burn injuries will heal in the same manner as a minor wound, with epithelialization complete within 7–14 days.

Initial treatment should start with cooling the burned area in water and giving the patient analgesia. Intact reddened skin can be treated with non-perfumed emollients such as Vaseline or E45 cream. The patient should be encouraged to keep flexion surfaces (McKirdy 2001) such as the hands and fingers, for example, mobile.

Partial-thickness burns need to be protected against infection and encouraged to heal. Individual gauze and pad dressings for hand and finger burns should be avoided as the mobility of the hand will be impeded (Cole 2003). A burn bag or glove filled with silicone or paraffin is an effective alternative as a method of allowing movement, moisture and collection of exudate. Non-flexure surfaces may be dressed with a semi-permeable film dressing (DuKamp 2000); however, there may be leakage in cases of large amounts of exudate. Multiple layers of sterile paraffin tulle dressing (*at least* 4) or a non-stick silicone dressing (e.g. Mepitel©) may be useful alternatives.

The management of partial-thickness burn blisters is contentious. It is suggested that a blister should be deroofed as not doing so could increase the size of the lesion (Collier 2000); however, this is contradicted by Flanagan and Graham (2001), who describe the detrimental and deepening effects of exposing a burn injury to air. Furthermore, calmodulin, a protein found in burn blisters, has been shown to have a positive effect on healing (DuKamp 2000, Flanagan Graham 2001), indicating the need to leave the blister intact during the inflammatory phase. Many patients find it very painful to have a blister deroofed in the first day or two following a burn injury; therefore the blister may be left intact and covered with a protective dressing. When the devitalized tissue has become loose and grey it is ready for debridement (Cole 2003).

TETANUS PROPHYLAXIS

Clostridium tetanii are anaerobic bacteria found in the soil and animal faeces which cause tetanus. They enter the circulatory system through a wound and, while the effects of tetanus in the UK are generally controlled by an immunization programme, if acquired the disease can prove fatal (Cassell 2002). It is essential to establish the tetanus status of a patient with an acute wound.

The Health Protection Agency (2003) states that lifelong immunity to tetanus is achieved after 5 doses of a vaccine such as Revaxis© (Adsorbed Diphtheria, Tetanus and inactivated Poliomyelitis vaccine 0.5 ml), delivered in 3 doses as a primary course, followed by a booster 10 years later and a final booster again 10

Table 23.11 Anti-tetanus prophylaxis

Immunization status	Clean wound	Tetanus–prone wound	
	Vaccine	Vaccine	Human tetanus immunoglobulin
Fully immunized, has received a total of five doses of vaccine at appropriate intervals	None required	None required	Only if high risk, e.g. contamination with manure
Primary immunization complete, boosters incomplete but up to date	None required (unless next dose due soon and convenient to give now)	None required (unless next dose due soon and convenient to give now)	Only if high risk, e.g. contamination with manure
Primary immunization incomplete or boosters not up to date	A reinforcing dose of vaccine and further doses as required to complete the schedule	A reinforcing dose of vaccine and further doses as required to complete the schedule	Yes: one dose of human tetanus immunoglobulin to be given in a different site
Not immunized or immunization status unknown or uncertain	Immediate dose of vaccine followed, if indicated, by completion of the full five dose course	Immediate dose of vaccine followed, if indicated, by completion of the full five-dose course	Yes: one dose of human tetanus immunoglobulin to be given in a different site

Adapted from Department of Health (2005)

years later (Reynolds & Cole 2006). Lifelong immunity may not protect against tetanus-prone wounds. These may include wounds that have been crushed, devitalized or contaminated by dirt (Rhee et al. 2005), wounds that are more than six hours old or wounds that have been in contact with soil or manure. Patients with tetanus-prone wounds may need human tetanus immunoglobulin 250 IU intramuscular injection for further protection. See Table 23.11 for Department of Health recommendations.

WOUND CARE AND NURSING DOCUMENTATION

The NMC (2005) has guidelines on record-keeping and state that it is an integral part of nursing practice which should be factual, consistent and accurate. Dimond (2002) suggests that failure to maintain a reasonable standard of record-keeping could be evidence of professional misconduct. Documentation must be clear, legible, timed and dated, signed for, unambiguous and fully completed.

When assessing and describing a wound it is essential that the correct terminology is used. This is important for two reasons. First, from a medico-legal perspective, patient's notes are sometimes called in evidence during a coroner's or criminal investigation. Therefore an accurate record of how the wound occurred and the subsequent treatment undertaken is mandatory.

Second, poor descriptions of injuries are common (Milroy & Rutty 1997) and therefore, if in doubt about the causation of the wound, it is preferable to describe it as a wound. Photography can be used to record the initial wound and its subsequent progress during treatment and provides a useful objective record of the injury (Bianco & Williams 2002).

DISCHARGING PATIENTS

It is important that patients fully understand what has happened to them during their time in the ED and what to expect in terms of wound healing and wound management. Patient education will ensure compliance with treatment regimes. Flanagan (1997) highlighted the importance of a number of factors influencing a patient's ability to manage an injury at home (see Box 23.5). Patients should have access to wound-care materials if appropriate, and access to advice and support from the ED staff.

If the patient has a co-existing illness or condition which may influence their wound healing status, they should be given the appropriate advice related to their condition. For example, patients taking anti-coagulants may need sutures or tissue strips left in situ for longer periods. All information should be

Box 23.5 Personal influences on wound healing

- **Knowledge and understanding** – the patient's and carer's level of knowledge will affect their ability to promote wound healing. The nurse needs to ensure the patient understands wound care guidance and any dieting changes necessary
- **Compliance** – this is complex and is influenced by the success of treatment so far, the duration of injury, previous experience and the degree of trust in the health care professional
- **Motivation** – this may be influenced by the carer's fear, guilt and how the patient sees the injury in relation to the rest of her life
- **Attitude** – a positive attitude to recovery will enhance motivation and compliance, particularly if supported with appropriate education
- **Body image** – this may impact on how the patient cares for the wound
- **Financial status** – this affects the patient's ability to comply with healthcare advice

given in both written and verbal format (using health advocates as required).

If you are referring the patient to another health-care provider for follow-up, it is good practice to give the patient a discharge letter summarizing care to date and the materials for the next dressing. If ongoing wound care will be needed, e.g. in management of burns, patients should be prescribed analgesia to take prior to dressing changes.

CONCLUSION

Wound care is an important part of the ED nurse's work and is an area of practice where nurses have a great deal of experience and influence. It is imperative that, in addition to good wound-management skills, the nurse also has an in-depth knowledge of wound healing, the threats to healing and the range of wound care methods available.

References

ASSH (American Society for Surgery of the Hand) (1990) *The Hand: Examination and Diagnosis*. Philadelphia: Churchill Livingstone.

Atiyeh BS, Ioannovich J, Al-Amm CA et al. (2002) Management of acute and chronic open wounds: the importance of moist environment: I optimal wound healing. *Current Pharmacological Biotechnology*, **3**, 179–195.

Autio L, Olson KK (2002) The four S's of wound management: staples, sutures, steri-strips and sticky stuff. *Holistic Nursing Practice*, **16**(2), 80–88.

Baggaley A (ed.) (2001) *Human Body*. London: Dorling Kindersley Limited.

Bales S, Jones V (1997) *Wound Care Nursing: a Patient Centred Approach*. London: Baillière Tindall.

Bansal BC, Wiebe RA, Perkins SD et al. (2002) Tap water for irrigation of lacerations. *American Journal of Emergency Medicine*, **20**, 469–472.

Barnett P, Jarman FC, Goodge J et al. (1998) Randomised trial of histoacryl blue tissue adhesive glue versus suturing in the repair of paediatric lacerations. *Journal of Paediatrics and Child Health*, **34**(6), 548–550.

Bayat A, McGrouther DA, Ferguson MWJ (2003) Skin scarring. *British Medical Journal*, **326**, 88–92.

Betts J (2003) Wound cleansing with water does not differ from no cleansing or cleansing with other solutions for rates of wound infection or healing. *Evidence Based Nursing*, **6**(3), 81.

Bianco M, Williams C (2002) Using photography in wound assessment. *Practice Nursing*, **13**(11), 505–508.

Bower M (2002) Evaluating and managing bite wounds. *Advances in Skin and Wound Care*, **15**(2), 88–90.

Bray JJ, Cragg PA, Macknight ADC et al. (1999) *Lecture Notes on Human Physiology*, 4th edn. Oxford: Blackwell Science.

Brennan SS, Leger DJ (1985) The effect of antiseptics on healing wounds: a study using the rabbit ear chamber. *British Journal of Surgery*, **72**(10), 780–782.

Brinker D, Hancox JD, Bernardon SO (2003) Assessment and initial treatment of lacerations, mammalian bites and insect stings. *American Association of Critical-care: Nurses Clinical Issues*, **14**(4), 401–410.

Brook I (2003) Microbiology and management of human and animal bite wound infections. *Primary Care Clinics in Office Practice*, **30**(1), 25–39.

Brook I (2005) Management of human and animal bite wounds: an overview. *Advances in Skin & Wound Care*, **18**(4), 197–203.

Brown G (1988) Acceleration of tensile strength of incisions treated with EGF and TGF. *Annals of Surgery*, **208**, 788–794.

Bryant RA (ed.) (1992) *Acute and Chronic Wounds*. St Louis: Mosby Year Book.

Capellan O, Hollander JE (2003) Management of lacerations in the emergency department. *Emergency Medicine Clinics of North America*, **21**(1), 205–231.

Cassell OCS (2002) Death from tetanus after pre-tibial laceration. *British Medical Journal*, **324**, 1442–1443.

Castille K (1998) Suturing. *Nursing Standard*, **12**(41), 41–48.

Chen E, Hornig S, Shepherd SM et al. (2000) Primary closure of mammalian bites. *Academic Emergency Medicine*, **7**(2), 157–161.

Cherry G, Ryan T (1985) Enhanced wound angiogenesis with a new hydrocolloid dressing. In: Ryan T, ed. *An Environment for Healing: the Role of Occlusion*. London: Royal Society of Medicine.

Clark A (2004) Understanding the principles of suturing minor skin lesions. *Nursing Times*, **100**(29), 32–34.

Clark JJ (2002) Wound repair and factors influencing healing. *Critical Care Nursing Quarterly*, **25**(1), 1–12.

Cole E (2003) Wound management in the A&E department. *Nursing Standard*, **17**(46), 45–52.

Collier M (1996) The principles of optimum wound management. *Nursing Standard*, **10**(43), 47–53.

Collier M (2000) Expert comment on managing burn blisters. *NT Plus*, **96**(4), 20.

Correira K (2003) Managing dog, cat and human bite wounds. *Journal of American Academy of Physicians Assistants*, **16**(4), 28–37.

Dandy DJ, Edwards DJ (2003) *Essential Orthopaedics and Trauma*. 4th edn. London: Churchill Livingstone.

Dealey C (1994) *The Care of Wounds*. Oxford: Blackwell Scientific.

Dearden C, Donnelly J, Dunlop M et al. (2001) Traumatic wounds: local wound management. *NT Plus*, **97**(35), 55–57.

Department of Health (2005) Tetanus.

Desai H (1997) Aging and wounds. *Journal of Wound Care*, **6**(4), 192–196.

Dickson J (1995) The problem of hospital induced malnutrition. *Nursing Times*, **92**(4), 44–45.

Dimick A (1998) Delayed wound closure: indications and techniques. *Annals of Emergency Medicine*, **17**(12), 1303–1304.

Dimond B (2002) *Legal Aspects of Nursing*. Harlow: Pearson Longman.

Dire DJ (1992) Emergency management of dog and cat bite wounds. *Emergency Medicine Clinics of North America*, **10**(4), 719–736.

DuKamp A (2000) Managing burn blisters. *NT Plus*, **96**(4), 19–20.

Dulecki M, Pieper B (2005) Irrigating simple acute traumatic wounds: a review of the current literature. *Journal of Emergency Nursing*, **31**(2), 156–160.

Eaglestein W (1985) Experiences with biosynthetic dressings. *Journal of the American Academy of Dermatology*, **12,** 434–440.

Eckerline C, Blake J, Koury R (1999) Puncture wounds and bites. In: *Topics in Emergency Medicine: A Comprehensive Study Guide*. 5th edn. New York: McGraw-Hill.

Edlich RF, Reddy VR (2001) Revolutionary advances in wound repair in emergency medicine during the last three decades: a view towards the new millennium. 5th Annual David Boyd Lecture. *Journal of Emergency Medicine*, **20**(2), 167–193.

Edlich R, Rodeheaver G, Morgan R (1988) Principles of emergency wound management. *Annals of Emergency Medicine*, **17**(12), 1284–1302.

Farion KJ, Osmond MH, Hartling L et al. (2003) Tissue adhesive for traumatic lacerations: a systematic review of randomised controlled trials. *Academic Emergency Medicine*, **10**(2), 110–400.

Fernandez R, Griffiths R, Ussia C (2003) *Water for Wound Cleansing (Cochrane Review). The Cochrane Library. Issue 4.* Chichester: John Wiley & Sons.

Flanagan M (1997) *Wound Healing*. Edinburgh: Churchill Livingstone.

Flanagan M, Graham J (2001) Should burn blisters be left intact or debrided? *Journal of Wound Care*, **10**(1), 41–45.

Flanagan M, Fletcher J (1997) Wound care: the healing process. *RCN Nursing Update (Nursing Standard, suppl.)*, **11**(40), 5–17.

Haller G, Faltin-Traub E, Kern C (2002) Oxygen emobolism after hydrogen peroxide irrigation of a vulval abscess. *British Journal of Anaesthesia*, **88**(4), 597–599.

Harulow S, Holt L (2000) Burns. In: Dolan B, Holt L, eds. *Accident and Emergency: Theory into Practice*. London: Baillière Tindall.

Hawkey CJ (1999) Cox-2 inhibitors. *Lancet*, **353**(9162), 1439–1440.

Health Protection Agency (2003) *Tetanus: Information for Health Professionals*. London: HPA.

Henley N, Carlson DA, Kaehr DM, Clements B (2004) Air embolism associated with irrigation of external fixator pin sites with hydrogen peroxide. A report of two cases. *Journal of Bone Joint Surgery: American volume*, **86**(4), 821–822.

Hock M, Ong E, Ooi SBS et al. (2002) A randomized controlled trial comparing the hair appositionapposition technique with tissue glue to standard suturing in scalp lacerations. *Annals of Emergency Medicine*, **40**(1), 19–26.

Hogg K, Carley S (2002) Staples or sutures for repair of scalp laceration in adults. *Emergency Medicine Journal*, **19**(4), 327–328.

Holt L (2000) Wound care. In Dolan B, Holt L, eds. *Accident and Emergency: Theory into Practice*. Edinburgh: Baillière Tindall.

Jay R (1999) Suturing in A&E. *Professional Nurse*, **14**(6), 412–415.

Kane D (2001) Chronic wound healing and chronic wound management. In: *Chronic Wound care: A Clinical Source Book for Health Care Professionals*, 3rd edn. Pennsylvania: Health Management Publications.

Kizer K, Callahan M (1984) A new look at managing mammalian bites. *Emergency Medicine Reports*, **5**(8), 53–58.

Knighton D, Silver I, Hunt T (1981) Regulation of wound healing angiogenesis: effect of oxygen gradients and inspired O_2 concentration. *Surgery*, **90**, 262–270.

Lansdown ABG (2004) Nutrition 2: A vital consideration in the management of wounds. *British Journal of Nursing*, **13**(20), 1199–1208.

McKirdy L (2001) Management of minor burns. *Journal of Community Nursing*, **15**(10), 28–33.

McLaren SMG (1992) Nutrition and wound healing. *Journal of Wound Care*, **1**(3), 45–55.

Mattick A (2002) Use of tissue adhesives in the management of paediatric lacerations. *Emergency Medicine Journal*, **19**, 382–385.

Miller M (1995) Principles of wound assessment. *Emergency Nurse*, 3(1), 16–18.

Milroy CM, Rutty GN (1997) If a wound is 'neatly incised' it is not a laceration. *British Medical Journal*, **314**, 1702.

Morrison MJ (1992) *A Colour Guide to the Nursing Management of Wounds*. London: Mosby.

Moulton, C, Yates D (1999) *Lecture Notes on Emergency Medicine*. Oxford: Blackwell Science.

Mustoe TA (2004) Scars and keloids. *British Medical Journal*, 1329–1330.

Myers J (1982) Modern plastic surgical dressing. *Health and Social Services Journal*, **92**, 336–337.

National Institute for Health and Clinical Excellence (NIHCE) (2005) *Skin Disorders and Wounds*. London: NIHCE.

Nursing & Midwifery Council (2005) *Guidelines for Records and Record Keeping*. London: NMC.

Ong MEH, Hock M, Ooi SM et al. (2002) A randomized controlled trial comparing the hair apposition technique with tissue glue to standard suturing in scalp lacerations (HAT study). *Annals of Emergency Medicine*, **40**, 19–26.

Patterson DR, Ptacek JT, Carrougher GJ, Sharar S (1997) Lorzepam as an adjunct to opioid analgesics in the treatment of burn pain. *Pain*, **72**, 367–374.

Pinchofsky-Devin G (1994) Nutritional wound healing. *Journal of Wound Care*, 3(5), 231–234.

Quaba O, Huntley JS, Bahia H et al. (2005) A users guide for reducing the pain of local anaesthetic administration. *Emergency Medicine Journal*, **22**, 188–189.

Quinn J, Maw J, Ramotar K et al. (1997) Octylcyanoacrylate tissue adhesive versus suture wound repair in a contaminated wound model. *Surgery*, **122**(1), 69–72.

Rabenberg VS, Ingersoll CD, Sandrey MA et al. (2002) The bacterial and cytotoxic effects of antimicrobial wound cleansers. *Journal of Athletic Training*, **37**(1), 51–54.

Resuscitation Council (UK) (2004) *ALS Course Provider Manual*. 4th edn (revised). London: UKRC.

Reynolds T (2004) Ear, nose and throat problems in accident and emergency. *Nursing Standard*, **18**(26), 47–55.

Reynolds T, Cole E (2006) Techniques for acute wound closure. *Nursing Standard*, **20**(21), 55–64.

Rhee P, Nunley MK, Demetriades D et al. (2005) Tetanus and trauma: a review and recommendations. *Journal of Trauma, Injury, Infection and Critical Care*, **58**(5), 1082–1088.

Richardson M (2004a) Acute wounds: an overview of the physiological healing process. *Nursing Times*, **100**(4), 50–53.

Richardson M (2004b) Wound care: procedures for cleansing, closing and covering acute wounds. *Nursing Times*, **100**(4), 54–58.

Richardson M (2006) The management of animal and human bite wounds. *Nursing Times*, **102**(3), 34–36.

Riyat MS, Quinton DN (1997) Tap water as a wound cleansing agent in A&E. *Journal of Accident and Emergency Medicine*, **14**, 165–166.

Russell A, Hugo W, Ayliffe G (1992) *Principles and Practice of Disinfection, Preservation and Sterilisation*. Oxford: Blackwell Scientific.

Sianna J, Franklin B, Grottup F (1992) The effect of smoking on tissue function. *Journal of Wound Care* 1(2), 37–41.

Singer AJ, Hollander JE, Subramanian S et al. (1994) Pressure dynamics of various irrigation techniques commonly used in the emergency department. *Annals of Emergency Medicine*, **24**, 36–40.

Smith PF, Meadowcroft AM, May DB (2000) Treating mammalian bite wounds. *Journal of Clinical Pharmacy & Therapeutics*, **25**(2), 85–99.

Stefanopoulos P, Karabouta Z, Bisbinis I et al. (2004) Animal and human bites: evaluation and management. *Acta Orthopaedica Belgica*, **70**(1), 1–10.

Stevenson TR, Thacker JG, Rodeheaver GT et al. (1976) Cleansing the traumatic wound by high pressure syringe irrigation. *Journal of American College of Emergency Physicians*, **5**, 17–21.

Taplitz RA (2004) Managing bite wounds. *Postgraduate Medicine*, **116**(2), 49.

Towler J (2001) Cleansing traumatic wounds with swabs, water or saline. *Journal of Wound Care*, **10**(6), 231–234.

Trott A (1997) *Wounds and Lacerations: Emergency Care & Closure*. St Louis: Mosby.

Trott A (1991) *Wounds and Lacerations: Emergency Care and Closure*. St Louis: Mosby Year Book.

Walsh M, Kent A (2001) Soft tissue injury. In: Walsh M, Kent A, eds. *Accident & Emergency Nursing*. 4th edition. Oxford: Butterworth Heinemann, pp. 97–11.

Waller R (2004) Wound care and repair. In: Cameron P, Jelinek G, Kelly AM, Murray L, Brown AFT, Heyworth J, eds. *Textbook of Adult Emergency Medicine*, 2nd edn. Edinburgh: Churchill Livingstone.

Walsh M, Kent A (eds) (2001) Soft tissue injury. In: *Accident & Emergency Nursing*, 4th edition. Oxford: Butterworth Heinemann.

Whitby (1995) The biology of wound healing. *Surgery*, **13**(2), 25–28.

Chapter 24

Pain and pain management

Marion Richardson

CHAPTER CONTENTS

INTRODUCTION

Pain is a primitive, multi-dimensional experience with physiological, psychological, social and emotional components. The International Association for the Study of Pain Subcommittee on Taxonomy (1979) describe pain as 'an unpleasant sensory and emotional experience associated with actual or potential tissue damage or described in terms of such damage'. Pain is also a valuable and necessary part of the body's defence mechanism and usually indicates that something is wrong, for example, physical damage or disease (O'Hara 1996).

This chapter will consider the physiological and psychological elements of pain and will identify assessment tools that may be used in the emergency department. Pharmacological and non-pharmacological methods of pain management will be considered and the nurse's role in relieving pain and suffering will be explored.

FEELING PAIN

Pain is felt when sensory nerve endings are stimulated and neurones relay information to the brain. Specialized pain receptors, known as nociceptors, are found in free nerve endings close to mast cells and small blood vessels which all work together to respond to pain (McHugh & McHugh 2000). Nociceptors are found in large numbers in the skin, arterial walls, periosteum and joint surfaces and in smaller numbers in all of the deep tissues of the body (Marieb 2004).

There appear to be two distinct types of nociceptor – high-threshold mechanoreceptors which respond to strong mechanical stimulation and polymodal nociceptors which respond to mechanical, thermal and chemical stimuli (McHugh & McHugh 2000). Mechanical stimuli include compressing or stretching tissues and thermal stimuli can be produced by excess heat or cold, though it appears that both of these types of stimuli may actually act through chemical mediators to stimulate the nociceptors (Allan 2005). Chemical stimulus occurs as a result of the substances which are released from damaged tissues, e.g. prostaglandins, serotonin, bradykinin and histamine (Cross 1994). Examples of tissue damage when such chemicals are released are infection, ischaemia, inflammation, ulceration and nerve damage (Godfrey 2005).

Once nociceptors are stimulated, the sensory, or afferent, nerve fibres of which they form part carry impulses to the spinal column. Two types of fibre are involved in this transmission:

A-delta fibres respond to stimulation of the high-threshold mechanoreceptors. The fibres are small in diameter and are myelinated; they transmit pain impulses rapidly (about 12–30 metres a second) and

are known as 'first' or 'fast' fibres. Pain sensation is usually sharp or pricking.

C fibres connect to the polymodal receptors. They are smaller, unmyelinated fibres which conduct at 0.5–2 metres a second and are known as 'second' or 'slow' pain fibres. Pain sensation is burning, dull and poorly localized (McHugh & McHugh, 2000).

In the spinal cord

Information carried by the neurones is relayed to the substantia gelatinosa in the dorsal horn of the spine where the A-delta and C nerves terminate and synapse with T (transmitter) neurones (see Fig. 24.1). The T neurones cross the spinal cord and ascend on the opposite side, carrying pain information to the brain. The neurochemical transmitters which are released to allow this transfer of information to occur are substance P and glutamate. The T neurone ascends via the spinothalamic tract to the thalamus

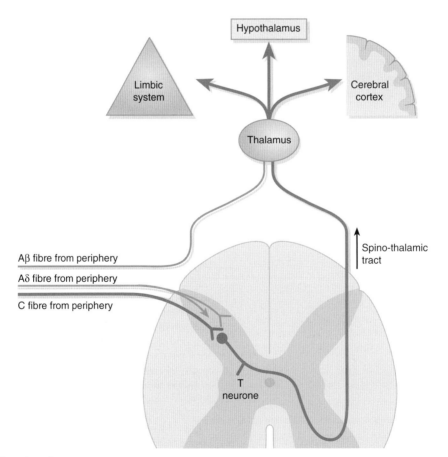

Figure 24.1 The pain pathway.

in the brain and connects there with a third neurone which relays the information to the cerebral cortex; this allows us to localize pain and interpret the stimuli. This perception of pain in the brain is vital as it allows us to do something to relieve or alleviate the situation. Fibres from the thalamus also connect with the hypothalamus, accounting for the changes in the autonomic nervous system outlined below, and to the limbic system where emotional responses are generated (Godfrey 2005).

A–beta nerve fibres

Other sensory (afferent) nerve fibres are not involved in carrying pain information, including A-beta fibres, which attach to low threshold mechanoreceptors. These fibres are thicker and heavily myelinated and conduct information such as touch, pressure and temperature (but not pain) very rapidly (30–100 metres per second). They account for 60–70% of all sensory fibres (Bentley 1998). These fibres also enter the spine at the dorsal horn but do not synapse with other neurones or cross the spine; instead they ascend to the brain in the ipsilateral column of nerve fibres and relay information to the lower medulla where they synapse with connecting neurones to the thalamus and cerebral cortex.

Opioids and opioid receptors

While substance P and glutamate have been implicated in the transmission of pain, other neurochemicals appear to possess analgesic properties. These include endorphins and enkephalins, which are produced by the body and have an analgesic action similar to that of morphine. These chemicals were only isolated in the body as recently as 1975 and have been the subject of much research since that time. There are receptors for endorphins and enkephalins throughout the brain and spinal cord. Further research is required, but the existence and action of these chemicals help to explain phenomena such as the placebo response, where an individual perceives pain relief even though no analgesic agent has been given. It appears to be that, in such cases, the mere expectation of pain relief is sufficient to release psychogenically the endogenous opiates, which would then cause a genuine analgesia even without the administration of an analgesic drug (Allan 2005).

EFFECTS OF PAIN

Physiological effects

The physiological responses that occur when the nociceptors are stimulated are similar to those of the stress ('fight or flight') response. The sympathetic nervous system is activated and this results in tachycardia, tachypnoea, hypertension, sweating and pallor. The sympathetic system causes general vasoconstriction, but dilates the arteries supplying vital organs such as the muscles (O'Hara 1996). Tidal volume and alveolar ventilation may be reduced, as is gastric motility. Skeletal muscle spasm may occur and hormonal changes may cause electrolyte imbalances and hyperglycaemia (Sutcliffe 1993).

Non–physiological effects

There is evidence that everyone has the same pain threshold – that is, they perceive pain at the same stimulus intensity. Sternback & Tursky (1965) found that there was no difference among four different ethnic groups in the level of electric shock that was first reported as producing a detectable sensation. Heat, for example, is perceived as painful by everyone at the 44–46°C range when it begins to damage tissues (Marieb 2004). The sensory conducting apparatus, in other words, appears to be essentially similar in all people so that a given level of input always elicits a sensation. However, an individual's tolerance of and response to pain will be affected by a number of factors other than those described above. The different thresholds associated with pain are identified in Box 24.1.

Although there is evidence that everyone, regardless of cultural background, has a uniform threshold, cultural background does have a powerful effect on the pain tolerance levels. Sternback & Tursky (1965) reported that the levels at which subjects refused to tolerate electric shocks, even when they were encouraged by experimenters, depended in part on the ethnic origin of the subject. For the emergency nurse,

---

Box 24.1   Pain thresholds

- **Sensation threshold** – the lowest stimulus value at which a sensation, such as tingling or warmth, is first reported
- **Pain perception threshold** – the lowest stimulus value at which the person reports that the stimulation feels painful
- **Pain tolerance (or upper threshold)** – the lowest stimulus level at which the subject withdraws or asks to have the stimulation stopped
- **Encouraged threshold** – the highest stimulus level the subject will tolerate after being encouraged to tolerate higher levels than identified in the pain tolerance threshold

this may explain the differing reactions to pain of individuals from different cultural backgrounds.

Anxiety and the experience of pain have also been linked (Cave 1994, Hayward 1975). As long ago as 1975, Hayward's work demonstrated that if patients were given information regarding their post-operative pain, they experienced less pain and required less analgesia. Walsh (1993), in a study of patients with relatively minor problems, found that 90% had pain and many were also anxious. He suggested that this may be due to a variety of reasons, such as:

- the sudden and unexpected disruption of the illness or injury
- fear of treatment
- fear of the possible long-term effects of the illness or injury
- fear of the unknown hospital treatment.

Because pain is not simply a physiological phenomenon, the experience of pain is unique for each person (Sofaer 1992). As McCaffery (1983) noted, 'pain is always a subjective experience and pain is what the patient says it is and exists when the patient says it does'.

PAIN THEORIES

Pain was originally thought to be due to the activities of demons and evil spirits or to be the penalty for wrongdoings. A number of theories have been proposed and developed in order to understand and explain the process of pain. Two will be considered here: the specificity theory and the gate control theory.

Specificity theory

The traditional specificity theory was developed by Descartes in 1644 (Godfrey 2005). Descartes thought that there was a direct link from the point of pain to the brain; it suggests that pain is a specific sensation and that the intensity of pain is proportional to the extent of the tissue damage (Watt-Watson & Ivers Donovan 1992). According to this theory, pain associated with a minor cut gives minimal discomfort, whereas pain associated with major trauma hurts far more. It is now known that pain is not simply a function of the amount of bodily damage, but is influenced by attention, anxiety, suggestion, experience and other psychological variables (Melzack & Wall 1982). However, while current research indicates that conduction of pain impulses is more complex than was originally proposed, the recognition of the specific pain pathways inherent in the specificity theory certainly made the idea of pain pathways credible and provides the basis for surgery in intractable pain. The procedure interrupts the pain pathway and impulses do not reach conscious level (Hallet 1992).

Gate control theory

The gate control theory of pain proposed by Melzack & Wall (1965) revolutionized the understanding of pain. They proposed the idea of a 'gate' in the substantia gelatinosa of the dorsal (or posterior) horn of the spinal cord through which pain information must pass on its way to the brain. The substantia gelatinosa is an area of special neurones located close to each posterior column of grey matter and extending the length of the spinal cord. A number of factors can block or close the 'gate' to pain messages, but equally other factors will open the gate and allow pain to be experienced by the individual. When nerve impulses from the nociceptors are brought to the dorsal horn by A-delta and C fibres and relayed to the T neurones, the gate is opened.

The T neurones can, however, be inhibited by other neurochemical transmitters released by tiny interneurones in the substantia gelatinosa. The large-diameter A-beta fibres (see above) synapse with these interneurones and thus inhibit transmission of information to the T neurone (see Fig. 24.2). Inhibition of the T neurone reduces the flow of pain information to the brain, effectively 'closing' the pain gate. As activity in the A-beta fibres (touch, pressure, temperature) increases, less pain is felt, while an increase in activity in the small diameter A-delta and C fibres means that more pain is perceived (Barasi 1991). This is the basis for many of the non-pharmacological pain-relieving measures, including 'rubbing it better', the application of heat or cold, electrical stimulation and counter-current irritation, all of which stimulate the A-beta fibres and so reduce the pain messages being relayed to the brain.

The gating mechanism is also affected by information flowing from the brain down descending inhibitory pathways. These fibres originate in a number of areas of the brain (reticular formation, periaqueductal grey matter, raphe nuclei) and synapse with the inhibitory neurones in the substantia gelatinosa of the spine, releasing the neurotransmitters serotonin and noradrenaline (Barasi 1991). The inhibitory interneurones in the dorsal horn of the spine are excited and this suppresses pain transmission to the brain via the T neurone. Allowing the brain to release these endogenous opiates is a key factor in pain relief and

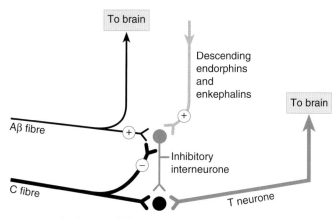

Figure 24.2 Inhibitory interneurone and pain transmission.

several methods can be employed in emergency settings to try to achieve this:

- use of sensory input, such as distraction, guided imagery and hypnotism
- reducing fear and lowering the level of anxiety
- patient education about the cause and relief of pain.

The neurochemical transmitters secreted by the inhibitory interneurones are natural opioids (endorphins, enkephalins and dynorphins) and these inhibit the T neurone. They also block the release of substance P from the A-delta and C fibres and block the receptors for substance P on the T neurones (Godfrey 2005).

If the inhibitory interneurones are stimulated, either by the A-beta fibres or by input from descending brain pathways, fewer pain impulses will be relayed to the T fibres and so less pain information will be carried to the brain.

Melzack & Wall (1965) felt that this theory explains why the relationship between pain and injury is so variable and why the location of pain can differ from the site of injury. It also explains how pain can persist in the absence of injury or after healing and why the nature and location of pain can change over time. Hallet (1992) suggested that the gate control theory expands the role of the spinal cord; it is not just a relay station, but a centre for filtering and integrating incoming sensory information.

ASSESSING PAIN

Individuals not only feel and react differently to pain, but describe it differently as well (Sofaer 1998). It is difficult to measure pain as it is a subjective phenomenon, and this is further complicated where patients are unable to describe their pain because of the location or severity of their injury or because they are

unconscious or intubated. The aim of pain assessment is to take the patient's subjective experience and transform it into objective data which health professionals can understand and use to plan relevant pain-relieving measures and measure their effect.

In some situations it will be immediately obvious that the patient is profoundly distressed and requires urgent intervention, e.g. the patient suddenly presenting to the emergency department with severe crushing chest pain. Intervention in these circumstances should be immediate and only a brief assessment of the situation is required. In other circumstances, however, a more thorough assessment is required and should be ongoing in the light of the patient's clinical condition. Hallet (1992) identified the range of information that should be included when making pain assessments (see Box 24.2).

Pain assessment tools

A number of pain assessment tools are used in ED (Longstaff 1997, O'Hara 1996). Visual analogue scales (VAS) can be used to measure pain and treatment effectiveness and satisfaction. The VAS consists of a line that ranges from 'no pain' to 'worst possible pain'. A numerical interpretation may be attached by the nurse in order to facilitate documentation. The advantages of a VAS are as follows:

- it is sensitive to small changes
- it can be used to measure pain intensity
- it can be used to measure pain relief
- it is easy for the patient to use.

The disadvantages of VAS are that:

- pain is scored on a single dimension only
- some patient groups, such as the visually impaired or the elderly, may find it difficult to use.

Box 24.2   Detailed pain assessment. (After Hallet 1992)

Location
The location should be identified as specifically as possible. For instance, abdominal pain may be localized to the lower or upper left or right quadrant, epigastrium or mid-abdomen. The site may be well defined or diffuse or the pain may radiate, involving a wide area. Observing the pain's location(s) on the patient's body can help to localize the sites of pain, as well as identifying physical changes at the site, such as swelling or discoloration.

Intensity
The intensity or severity of pain experienced should be translated into words or numbers that can provide objective data for ongoing assessment. Visual analogue scales and numerical scales, with or without written descriptions, are often used.

Quality
A description of pain, using the patient's own words, is helpful in determining the origin of pain, its cause and possible pain relief measures. For instance, patients with cardiac-related chest pain may describe it as 'crushing', whereas patients with non-cardiac-related chest pain may describe a 'sharp' pain, usually related to inspiration. Other words used to describe pain are throbbing, stabbing, cramping, hot-burning and aching.

Onset and duration
When the pain first began and how the pain has changed over time should be determined. If the pain varies over the course of a day, this variation and the circumstances surrounding the variation should be noted. The pattern may be constant, intermittent, variable etc.

Relief measures
The efficacy of measures used by the patient to relieve pain should be identified. Any medications, including analgesia, taken by the patient prior to attendance at ED should be recorded.

Exacerbating factors
Often patients may be comfortable at rest, but have difficulty moving due to pain. For instance, patients with abdominal pain may be more comfortable sitting upright than lying flat on the ED trolley. In most instances, the ED nurse should support patients by making them as comfortable as possible, except where this may compromise their safety such as lying over the end of the trolley.

Associated symptoms
Associated symptoms can include nausea and vomiting, profuse perspiration, fainting, inability to perform usual functions, dulling of senses, apathy, clouding of consciousness, disorientation and inability to rest and sleep.

For children over the age of 3 years and those unable to grasp the concept of linear scales, pain rating scales using pictures of faces have become popular. The faces, which are in increasing degrees of distress, are shown to patients, who are then asked to point to the one which depicts the amount of pain they are feeling. However, concern about pain scales has been expressed by Mather & Mackie (1983), who noted that children played down their pain because they did not want to be given an injection. In this instance, the children were capable of evaluating their pain and using the visual analogue scale available to do this. However, the consequences of pain reporting were unpleasant, e.g. administration of an injection, and so the pain report was inaccurate.

Similarly, adult patients, particularly those who are elderly, may minimize their pain reports and will suffer in silence because they do not want to be seen as a 'nuisance' to nursing staff or to their families. The emergency nurse should therefore reassure patients that their needs are being taken seriously and evaluate pain requirements and relief at regular intervals. As none of these assessment tools is of use in the semi-conscious patient or in infants, the nurse must use her observational skills and knowledge of physiological responses to pain to estimate its severity. The most important observations include facial expression, grimacing, movement, posture and interaction with others. In severe pain, the patient's blood pressure and pulse rate may rise, and respirations may increase and therefore should be recorded.

PHARMACOLOGICAL PAIN MANAGEMENT

Most acute pain is managed solely with drugs. In the three months from October to December 2004, approximately 1.7 million items of opioid analgesic items were prescribed in the UK along with 8.4 million non-opioid analgesic items, mostly NSAIDs and paracetamol and its combinations (Prescription Pricing Authority 2006).

Drugs that are used to relieve pain work in several ways: by altering the pain sensation, depressing pain perception or modifying the patient's response to pain. As a general principle, drugs are used most effectively if their selection is based on the cause and intensity of pain. They can be delivered in a variety of ways, including:

- orally
- rectally
- intramuscularly
- epidurally
- intravenously
- topically
- subcutaneously
- by inhalation

Analgesics act in the brain, spinal cord, nerve endings and at the site of tissue damage to reduce the amount of pain being felt. They are selective as they are able to diminish pain without affecting other sensations (O'Hara 1996). Analgesics can be divided into two groups: opiates and non-opiates.

Opiates

Opiates are used in the treatment of moderate to severe pain and work by binding to the opiate receptors in the CNS and thus modulate the transmission of pain (nociceptive) messages via the 'gate' in the spinal cord. Opiate analgesics may also initially produce sedation, reduce fear and anxiety and promote sleep. Opiates stimulate the chemoreceptor trigger zone (CTZ) in the brain stem, causing nausea and vomiting in about 30% of patients. They can also produce respiratory depression by acting on respiratory centres in the brain. The antidote naloxone can reverse this effect.

Morphine
Morphine is a derivative of the opium poppy and is an extremely effective analgesic agent. In the emergency department, it is usually administered intravenously. It alleviates pain and anxiety; however, the nurse should note the following (Greenstein & Gould 2004):

- the pupils of the eye are constricted due to an effect on the nucleus of the third facial nerve
- morphine stimulates the vagus nerve, which may present difficulties when morphine is used for the pain of coronary thrombosis as it may further reduce the pulse rate and blood pressure
- morphine causes spasm of the sphincters, including the sphincter of Oddi, and therefore should not be used in pancreatitis.

In trauma cases, oral or intramuscular morphine should not be given as the shocked patient will have poor perfusion. This leads to limited absorption of the drug initially and bolus absorption following resuscitation (Driscoll et al. 1994).

Diamorphine
The actions of diamorphine are similar to those of morphine, but it is 2.5 times more potent as an analgesic agent (Thompson & Webster 1992) and is the drug of choice in the management of severe central chest pain. Intravenous administration should be accompanied with anti-emetics, and the depressant effects on the respiratory centre need to be borne in mind, particularly in patients with chronic chest disease. Diamorphine is usually administered in dose of 2.5–5 mg i.v., repeated as necessary. Diamorphine, a class A controlled drug, is also known as heroin and the antidote naloxone 0.4 mg i.v. should always be available.

Pethidine
Pethidine is a synthetically derived analgesic which has similar actions to diamorphine and is chemically related to atropine. It is less powerful than morphine but has a lower risk of respiratory depression and does not cause constriction of the pupils; it is therefore used in head injuries where observation of the pupil size may be important (Goldstein & Gould 2004). Unlike morphine, it does not cause spasms of the sphincters and is the analgesic of choice in pancreatitis. It is worthy of note that pethidine can react with monoamine oxidase inhibitor (MAOI) drugs and cause severe hypertension (Carr & Mann 2000).

Non-opiates

Effective relief can be achieved with oral non-opioids and NSAIDs. These drugs are appropriate for treating much pain after minor surgery, such as incision and drainage, or on discharge home, for instance, following musculoskeletal injury. Two examples of non-opiates are entonox and NSAIDs.

Entonox
This gaseous mixture of 50% oxygen and 50% nitrous oxide can be effective as a short-term analgesic agent. Its primary use is to provide pain relief to conscious patients who are able to use the demand valve system of delivery for analgesia during unpleasant procedures, e.g. during splinting (Adam & Osborne 1997). It is contraindicated when there is a pneumothorax or a fracture to the base of the skull (Driscoll et al. 1994).

Non-steroidal anti-inflammatory agents (NSAIDs)
These are the most widely used analgesics. Commonly used NSAIDs include aspirin, indomethacin and ibuprofen. They are effective particularly in relieving pain associated with inflammation, such as musculoskeletal disorders, trauma to peripheral tissues and headache. Some studies have shown that NSAIDs provided pain relief equal to or better than

10 mg intramuscular morphine (McQuay and Moore 1998). NSAIDs also act on the hypothalamus to reset the body's thermostat during febrile episodes, reducing the temperature.

NSAIDs inhibit the enzyme cyclo-oxygenase and thus affect the body's production of prostaglandins (Carr & Mann 2000), which cause pain and inflammation. However, prostaglandins are also responsible for maintaining the mucous lining of the gastric mucosa. As a consequence, the use of NSAIDs can lead to gastric damage, which may range from nausea or 'heartburn' to gastrointestinal bleeding. This can be ameliorated by recommending the patient to take the NSAIDs with meals and/or milk. NSAIDs can also trigger asthmatic reactions, and patients should be asked if they suffer from asthma before NSAIDs are prescribed or dispensed. In the past 5 years, selective cyclo-oxygenase II specific inhibitors (COX-II) have been developed which produce analgesia with fewer side effects.

NON-PHARMACOLOGICAL PAIN MANAGEMENT

In addition to pharmacological interventions, there is a wide range of pain-relieving strategies that can be employed by the nurse to relieve patient pain and suffering. McCaffery (1990) has suggested that a combination of pharmacological and non-pharmacological methods probably yields the most effective relief for the patient.

Information

Attention to factors identified by the patient and, for example, to his level of anxiety regarding pain is essential. Hayward's (1975) classic study showed that patients who were kept informed about the level of discomfort and pain they could expect reported lower levels of pain. It is both unwise and unethical for the nurse to state that a patient will not feel pain before a painful procedure. This is especially true for children, who may subsequently lose trust in their health carers. Honesty with reassurance can do much to alleviate the mental suffering associated with current or impending pain from nursing and medical procedures.

Immobilization and elevation

These simple but effective measures can do much to alleviate pain and suffering and are particularly useful for patients who have sustained musculoskeletal injuries. The nurse can use slings, splints, pillows or blankets to place the injured limb in a comfortable position and should advise the patient to move it as little as possible. Swelling and pain, particularly when associated with soft tissue injury, can also be reduced by elevation of an injured limb (Walsh 1996).

Warm and/or cold compresses

For patients who have sustained musculoskeletal injuries, superficial burns or other injuries, the use of cold compresses can reduce swelling and alleviate pain. They act by reducing the release of pain-causing chemicals, such as lactic acid, potassium ions, serotonin and histamine (Lee & Warren 1978). The nurse should ensure that the cold compress does not cause further injury, such as frostbite, and therefore ice should be placed in a plastic bag and covered with a paper or cloth towel. The use of gel packs which can be kept cool in the fridge or warmed in hot water can reduce this risk.

Warm compresses may also be used to reduce pain by triggering pain-inhibiting reflexes through temperature receptors. They are particularly effective for muscle and joint pain. However, because warmth increases swelling and the tendency to bleed, it is contraindicated after trauma. Because heat can burn, it should be used with particular caution over areas with impaired sensation or in patients with limited or no ability to communicate.

Distraction

McCaffery (1990) defined distraction as simply focusing attention on stimuli other than the pain sensation. One of the most frequently used distraction techniques in ED involves breathing exercises. Patients are directed to focus their breathing by concentrating on inhalations and exhalations. Appropriate use of humour is also a successful distraction strategy that has been shown to improve the release of the body's natural endorphins (Watt-Watson & Ivers Donovan 1992).

CONCLUSION

The emergency nurse has a key role in the assessment and management of pain. This chapter has outlined the physiological and psychological effects of pain as well as a number of assessment tools the nurse may employ in the emergency department. Pharmacological and non-pharmacological means of delivering pain relief have also been considered. Non-pharmacological methods in particular are usually effective, simple to apply and easy to learn.

The emergency nurse has a responsibility to obtain a working knowledge of the range of strategies available to decrease pain and to use them to alleviate patient suffering and improve the quality of care.

References

Adam SK, Osborne S (1997) *Critical Care Nursing: Science and Practice*. Oxford: Oxford Medical.

Allan D (2005) Sensory Receptors and Sense Organs. In: Montague SE, Watson R, Herbert RA, eds. *Physiology for Nursing Practice*, 3rd edn. London: Elsevier.

Barasi S (1991) The physiology of pain. *Surgical Nurse*, **4**(5), 14–20.

Bentley J (1998) The science of pain: an update. In: Sofaer B, ed. *Pain – Principles, Practice and Patients*. Cheltenham: Stanley Thorne.

Carr ECJ, Mann EM (2000) *Pain: Creative Approaches to Effective Management*. Basingstoke: Macmillan Press.

Cave I (1994) Pain in A&E: the patient's view. *Emergency Nurse*, **2**(2), 19–20.

Cross SA (1994) Pathophysiology of pain. *Mayo Clinic Proceedings* **69**, 375–383.

Davis P (1993) Opening up the gate control theory. *Nursing Standard*, **7**, 25–26.

Driscoll P, Gwinnutt C, Brook S (1994) Extremity trauma. In: Driscoll PA, Gwinnutt CL, LeDuc Jimmerson C, Goodall A, eds. *Trauma Resuscitation: The Team Approach*. Basingstoke: Macmillan.

Godfrey H (2005) *Understanding the Human Body: Biological Perspectives for Healthcare*. Edinburgh: Churchill Livingstone.

Greenstein B, Gould D (2004) *Trounce's Clinical Pharmacology for Nurses*, 17th edn. Edinburgh: Elsevier.

Hallet N (1992) Pain: prevention and cure. In: Royle JA, Walsh M, eds. *Watson's Medical-Surgical Nursing and Related Physiology*. London: Baillière Tindall.

Halliday T, Robinson D, Stirling V et al. (1992) Book 3, the senses and communication. In: *Biology, Brain and Behaviour*. Milton Keynes: Open University.

Hardy JD, Wolff HG, Goodell H (1952) *Pain Sensations and Reactions*. Baltimore: Williams and Wilkins.

Hayward J (1975) *Information: A Prescription Against Pain*. London: RCN.

IASP subcommittee on taxonomy (1979) Pain terms: a list with definitions and notes on usage. *Pain* **6**, 247–252.

Lee JM, Warren MP (1978) Clinical applications of cold for the musculoskeletal system. *Cold Therapy in Rehabilitation*. London: Bell & Hyman.

Longstaff M (1997) Methods: pain measurement in A&E. *Emergency Nurse* **4**(4), 20–22.

Marieb EN (2004) *Human Anatomy and Physiology*, 6th edn. San Francisco: Pearson Benjamin Cummings.

Mather L, Mackie J (1983) The incidence of post-operative pain in children. *Pain* **15**, 271–282.

McCaffrey M (1983) *Nursing the Patient in Pain*. London: Chapman & Hall.

McCaffrey M (1990) Nursing approaches to non-pharmacological pain control. *International Journal of Nursing Studies* **27**, 1–5.

McHugh JM, McHugh WB (2000) Pain: neuroanatomy, chemical mediators and clinical applications. *AACN Clinical Issues*, **11**(2), 168–178

McQuay M, Moore A, Justins D (1997) Treating acute pain in hospital. *British Medical Journal* **314**, 1315–1331.

McQuay H, Moore A (1998) *An Evidence-Based Resource for Pain Relief*. Oxford: Oxford University Press.

Melzack R, Wall PD (1965) Pain mechanisms: a new theory. *Science* **150**, 971–979.

Melzack R, Wall PD (1982) *The Challenge of Pain*. New York: Basic Books.

O'Hara P (1996) *Pain Management for Health Professionals*. Chapman and Hall: London.

Prescription Pricing Authority (2006) *Analgesics and NSAIDs Prescribing*. London: PPA

Sofaer B (1992) *Pain – A Handbook for Nurses*, 2nd edn. London: Chapman & Hall.

Sofaer B (1998) *Pain – Principles, Practice and Patients*. Cheltenham: Stanley Thorne.

Sternback RA, Tursky B (1965) Ethnic differences among housewives in psychophysical and skin potential responses to electrical shock. *Psychophysiology* **1**, 241–246.

Sutcliffe AJ (1993) Pain relief for acutely ill and injured patients. *Care of the Critically Ill* **9**(6), 266–269.

Thompson DR, Webster R (1992) *Caring for the Coronary Patient*. Oxford: Butterworth Heinemann.

Walsh M (1993) Pain and anxiety in A&E attenders. *Nursing Standard* **17**(7), 40–42.

Walsh M (1996) *Accident and Emergency Nursing: A New Approach*, 3rd edn. Oxford: Butterworth Heinemann.

Watt-Watson JH, Ivers Donovan M (1992) *Pain Management: Nursing Perspectives*. St Louis: Mosby Year Book.

Chapter 25

Local and regional anaesthesia

Paula (Polly) Grainger*

CHAPTER CONTENTS

INTRODUCTION

Local anaesthesia is a method of rendering surgical interventions painless to a conscious patient while also being spontaneously reversible, enabling the complete recovery of function following the treatment.

The first recorded use of a local anaesthetic was the application of cocaine to the cornea by Freud and Koller in 1884 (Gajraj 2003); since then the field of local and regional anaesthesia has developed hugely. The development of other agents, notably procaine in 1904 and lignocaine in 1947, along with the pioneering of increasingly sophisticated techniques, has led to a growth in the use of local anaesthetics to achieve pain-free procedures.

Local and regional anaesthetics are suitable for the management of the pain that many patients present to the emergency department (ED) with, and they can be used either as an adjunct to treatment or as definitive treatment in itself. This chapter will describe the pharmacology of local anaesthetics and applicable aspects of the physiology of the conduction of the pain signal, discuss the advantages and disadvantages associated with their use, review the various methods of use and outline the principles of managing patients undergoing these procedures in the ED. Chapter 24 discusses other aspects of pain and pain management in the ED situation.

* The author would like to thank Roxanne McKerras for her support and advice in writing this chapter.

PHARMACOLOGY OF LOCAL ANAESTHETICS AND APPLICABLE ASPECTS OF THE PATHOPHYSIOLOGY OF THE CONDUCTION OF THE PAIN SIGNAL

Pain that is classified as nociceptive is caused by tissue damage in which inflammatory mediators are released from tissues and bathe and sensitize the nociceptors (Butcher 2004). Local anaesthetics address this type of pain. They act by blocking the conduction of the nerve impulses when it is applied either locally to the nerve fibre endings or regionally to the nerve trunks which convey the impulses from the affected area.

The sensation of pain is created through four stages, the first of which is transduction. This is the passage of an impulse along a nerve axon triggered by a noxious stimulus which releases sensitizing substances causing an action potential (McCaffery & Passero 1999). This action potential is dependent upon the interchange of sodium ions and to a lesser extent potassium ions across the nerve cell membrane. During the resting phase the cell membrane is largely impermeable to sodium ions. This, in combination with the sodium pump, raises the concentration of sodium in the extracellular fluid to 10 times that inside the cell. This contrasts with that of potassium ions, the concentration of which is 30 times greater inside the nerve cell compared with the outside. This ratio of sodium to potassium gives rise to a possible electrical potential across the cell membrane of -90 millivolts (mV), the inside being negatively charged compared to the outside; however, the resting cell membrane electrical potential is -70 mV to enable the passage of other ions across the membrane (Tortora & Grabowski 2003). When stimulus energy is applied to the cell membrane it becomes permeable to sodium ions, leading to an influx into the cell where there is an exchange with potassium ions. This interchange of ions reverses the electrical potential difference, the inside of the cell transiently becoming positive with respect to the outside to about $+40$ mV. The depolarization travels the length of the nociception fibres in milliseconds, causing the impulse to be experienced as a conscious sensation in the brain (McCaffery & Passero 1999), in this case pain. For this to occur, a critical level of depolarization of the cell membrane must be reached, known as the threshold potential.

Local anaesthetics work by binding to the sodium channels in the membrane, thereby preventing changes to membrane permeability. They can be considered as having a membrane-stabilizing effect by blocking the depolarization of the membrane

(Fatovich & Brown 2004). The smaller the diameter of nerve fibre, the more sensitive it is to the effects of local anaesthetic. The clinical sequelae following injection are initial loss of autonomic function, followed by loss of pain sensation, then touch and pressure sensation and finally motor function: recovery proceeds in the reverse order (Rosenbery 2000). The interference with autonomic function means that all local anaesthetics, with the exception of cocaine, cause local or regional vasodilatation depending on the technique used. This vasodilatation can lead to rapid dispersal, thereby minimizing the duration of the local anaesthetic. To address this effect a vasoconstrictor such as adrenaline can be added, which can delay absorption, prolonging anaesthesia and preventing flooding of the circulation (Fatovich & Brown 2004). The normal duration of action for lignocaine of 15–45 minutes when infiltrated subcutaneously can be increased by 50% by the addition of adrenaline (De Jong 2001). If adrenaline is used, the total dose should not exceed 0.5 mg/ml or the concentration 1:200 000 (BNF 2006).

The duration of action is dependent upon:

- the drug used
- the concentration and dose of local anaesthetic
- the mode of drug administration
- the rate of diffusion from the injection site to the axon.

This latter point is important as it emphasizes the need to allow sufficient time for the local anaesthetics to work before commencing the procedure.

CLASSIFICATION OF LOCAL ANAESTHETICS

The ideal local anaesthetic should possess the following characteristics:

- non-irritant
- rapid onset of effect
- non-toxic
- have a duration of action appropriate to the procedure
- leave no local after-effects.

Local anaesthetics can be divided into two chemical groupings: amides and esters. The amino-amides are slowly metabolized by the liver and can therefore only be used in those patients whose liver function is uncompromised. This group includes the drugs lignocaine, bupivacaine, etidocaine and ropivicaine. Amino-esters are broken down more readily in the plasma by pseudocholinesterase, and then by the liver to para-aminobenzoic acid, and include cocaine, procaine, amethocaine (tetracaine) and chloroprocaine (Chan et al. 2002). The properties of four commonly used local anaesthetics are outlined in Table 25.1.

BENEFITS OF LOCAL ANAESTHETICS

In the ED setting local and regional anaesthesia either enables otherwise painful procedures to occur, leading to the patient's discharge from ED rather than admission to an inpatient bed; or it can ensure a patient's comfort while waiting for surgical intervention after their transfer from the ED.

The principal benefit of local anaesthesia is the absence of those complications which may arise from the use of general anaesthetics and intubation. These include: the laryngeal and cough reflexes remain unimpaired, reducing the risk of respiratory obstruction and respiratory function is not automatically depressed, making them ideal for patients with poor lung function. Also the patient does not experience the discomforts associated with general anaesthesia, such as nausea, vomiting, dizziness and/or a sore throat. The associated shorter recovery time also facilitates an earlier discharge. In addition, many, though not all, minor procedures can still be performed even if the patient has eaten.

The numbing effect of local anaesthetics on the surgical site usually lasts beyond the operative period, providing highly specific, temporary postoperative pain relief. Also, because the patient remains conscious, they are able to cooperate if required, and report any abnormalities, making the early detection of complications more likely (Rivellini 1993).

DISADVANTAGES AND LIMITATIONS OF LOCAL ANAESTHESIA

The first major disadvantage with local anaesthesia is that, while patients may not feel pain, they will often experience other sensations associated with the procedure, such as pressure and movement. Because they are conscious they will also be able to see, hear and smell all that is going on. There will be many patients who simply do not wish to be awake because they would rather not know anything; they may find the feelings of numbness, paraesthesia, paralysis and the sense of being detached from the affected part of the body disconcerting (Rivellini 1993). For this reason many, although not all, children and adults with learning difficulties are not be suitable candidates for treatment under local or regional anaesthesia. The use of local anaesthetic requires the active cooperation of the patient and so may not suitable for confused, aggressive and agitated people. Children and patients with learning difficulties may pose a challenge for the nurse but they should by no means automatically be excluded from the use of local anaesthesia.

A second disadvantage is that the use of local anaesthetic may be limited by the suitability of the surgical site. In addition, some of the procedures involved for regional anaesthesia may be perceived as technically difficult and require a high level of expertise beyond that of the majority of ED medical and nursing staff. However, standardized training in the use of each technique could and should be available and local anaesthesia has been recommended as a practical alternative to general anaesthesia (Graham et al. 1997).

Table 25.1 The pharmacology of common anaesthetics used for infiltration, field blocks or regional blocks (BNF 2006, Rayner-Klein & Rowe 2005, Fatovich & Brown 2004, Chan et al. 2002)

Agent	Group	Concentration	Max. single dose without adrenaline	Onset of action for infiltration	Duration of action for infiltration (minutes)	Onset of action for nerve block	Duration of action for nerve block
Lignocaine (Lidocaine)	Amide	1–4%	4.5 mg/kg, max 200 mg	Fast	60–120	4–10 minutes	60–120 minutes
Prilocaine (Citanest)	Amide	1%	6 mg/kg, max 400 mg	Slow	60–120	Fast	30–90 minutes
Bupivicaine (Marcain)	Amide	0.25–0.5%	2–2.5 mg/kg max 150 mg	Moderate	240–480	8–12 minutes – up 30 for full effect	240–480 minutes
Ropivicaine (Naropin)	Amide	7.5–10 mg/ml	30–40 ml of 7.5 mg/ml max 300 mg	Not indicated	N/A	8–12 minutes	Long

It is important to remember that while the term 'local' is used, local anaesthetics are only minimally metabolized at the site of injection; most pass ultimately into the bloodstream and, potentially, may produce systemic toxic effects. These result from the membrane-stabilizing effects on other cells, notably those of the cardiovascular and central nervous systems.

Allergic reactions to local anaesthetic drugs are uncommon; those seen are generally caused by the preservative added (e.g. methylparaben) rather than by the anaesthetic drug (Chan et al. 2002). Also allergic reactions have been confused with systemic toxicity; however, the amino-ester drugs have a higher frequency of allergic reactions than the amino-amide group (Fatovich & Brown 2004) and adverse side-effects have been reported (BNF 2006). The potential effects of toxicity are listed in Box 25.1.

Other potential toxic effects include hypotension due to loss of vascular tone, respiratory depression and allergic reactions (BNF 2006), although the latter two are uncommon.

TYPES AND USES OF LOCAL ANAESTHESIA

The types of local anaesthesia are categorized according to the method of administration or site of injection

---

Box 25.1 Potential toxic effect of local anaesthetics (in order of increasing plasma levels)

Central nervous system
- Paraesthesia of mouth and tongue
- Dizziness and light-headedness
- Tinnitus
- Visual disturbance
- Talkativeness
- Feelings of disorientation
- Confusion
- Agitation or tremor
- Drowsiness
- Convulsion
- Coma

Cardiovascular system
- Myocardial conduction
- Sinus bradycardia
- AV block
- Reduced cardiac output
- Hypotension
- Resistant ventricular arrhythmias
- Apnoea
- Cardiac arrest (highest plasma levels)

---

and are broadly divided into local or regional (Rivellini 1993):

- Local
  - topical
  - infiltration
- Regional
  - peripheral nerve block
  - haematoma block
  - intravenous regional (Bier's) block
  - epidural (extradural) block
  - spinal (subarachnoid) block.

Local anaesthesia is used for relatively minor procedures, whereas regional anaesthesia is reserved for those that are more complex or requiring a longer duration of action. The intravenous regional block is a useful option in the ED although in some departments it is underutilized; however, the last two techniques are not usually seen in ED and are therefore beyond the scope of this chapter.

Surface or topical application

This involves direct application of the local anaesthetic to mucous membranes, intact skin or open wounds, such as grazes. Suitable sites for topical anaesthesia include the cornea, conjunctiva, upper airway, epidermal and dermal layers of the skin, and urethra. Local anaesthetics for this purpose come in various forms, including aerosol sprays, liquid solutions, creams, jellies, balms and ointments as seen in Table 25.2. One local anaesthetic used as a topical agent is cocaine. The initial formulation of tetracaine (amethocaine) 4%, epinephrine (adrenaline) 1:2000–1:4000 and cocaine 4% (TAC) gained widespread acceptance in North America and largely supplanted infiltration anaesthesia (Grant & Hoffman 1992). Unlike other local anaesthetics, cocaine potentiates the action of the sympathetic nervous system thus causing local vasoconstriction and it is highly effective on very vascular areas, such as the nasal membranes. It also causes dilatation of the pupil when used on the cornea. Cocaine, however, has powerful central effects, making it too dangerous to inject: it also has complex administrative and financial issues resulting from its being a drug of addiction, which has led to the development of cocaine-free alternatives in the last decade (Eidelman et al. 2005).

These alternatives include creams and jellies containing a combination of lignocaine and prilocaine which can be used prior to venepuncture or cannulation in children. One example of such a topical anaesthetic is the Eutectic Mixture of Local Anaesthetics (EMLA®) cream. The 'eutectic' property refers to the

Table 25.2 Topical anaesthetics (McCaffery & Passero 1999, Lander & Weltman 2002, Butcher 1994, Dunn et al. 1997)

Type	Agent	Onset	Duration (minutes)	Skin condition
TAC	Tetracaine (amethocaine) 4%, epinephrine (adrenaline) 1:2000–1:4000 and cocaine 4%	20 minutes	30-45 – after removal of solution/gel	Intact skin only
EMLA cream	Prilocaine 2.5% and lignocaine 2.5%	60 minutes for venepuncture to 120 minutes for cannulation (maximum effect 2–3 hours post application)	60-120 – after removal of cream	Intact skin only
Ametop gel	Tetracaine (amethocaine) 4%	30 minutes for venepuncture to 45 minutes for cannulation for maximum effect	120-180 – after removal of cream	Intact skin only
ALA, LET, LAT or XAP	Tetracaine (amethocaine) 0.5%, lignocaine (lidocaine) 4% and adrenaline (epinephrine) 0.05%	10 minutes (up to a maximum of 30 minutes)	15-60 – after removal of solution/gel	Intact skin or into/onto wounds
Refrigerant spray	ethylchloride, fluroethyl or Frigiderm	Cools <10°C within 10–15 seconds		Intact skin only
Ophthalmic use	Tetracaine hydrochloride 0.5–1%	<1 minute	20-40	N/A

liquefaction of the constituents, prilocaine and lignocaine (McCaffery & Passero 1999). EMLA cream is applied only to intact skin (BNF 2006) for cutaneous anaesthesia. To do this a thick layer is applied under an occlusive dressing and left for 60–120 minutes, dependent on the indication for its use. Numbing of the skin should occur one hour after application, reaching a maximum at two to three hours (one hour for children less than three months old). The effect lasts for one to two hours after removal of the cream (Lander & Weltman 2002). However, this time lag sometimes makes it impractical for use in ED especially when a painful activity needs to be performed before that time. An alternative option is 4% amethocaine gel (Ametop®), which is similarly indicated for local topical anaesthesia prior to venepuncture or venous cannulation. As with EMLA, this gel is applied to the site required and sealed with an occlusive dressing; however, it is ready for the procedure to occur after 30 minutes for venepuncture and after 45 minutes for venous cannulation as it is has a faster action. Like EMLA, it should only be applied to intact skin as it is rapidly absorbed and it should not be applied to inflamed, traumatized, highly vascular surfaces or mucous membranes (BNF 2006).

A further option is a solution or gel containing, amethocaine (tetracaine / pontacaine), lignocaine (lidocaine/xylocaine) and adrenaline (epinephrine), known as ALA, LET, LAT or XAP (according to country of use), which can be made by the hospital pharmacy (McCaffery & Passero 1999). It is a faster-acting option and can be applied directly into or onto a wound in conjunction with the application of a piece of gauze soaked in the solution and left on the wound with a clear non-absorbent dressing used to hold it in place for 10 minutes (up to a maximum of 30 minutes). This can provide sufficient anaesthesia lasting up to 15 minutes to enable wound cleansing and closure with sutures if required (McCaffery & Passero 1999). Care should be taken to avoid the mucous membranes to avoid systemic absorption and possible toxicity, and the eyes should be avoided also due to the risk of causing corneal abrasions (McCaffery & Passero 1999). The benefit of these topical treatments is that they are painless to use.

Other uses of anaesthesia include those for ophthalmic procedures in ED such as irrigation or examination, in which case tetracaine® (amethocaine) 0.5–1% is the drug of choice because of its profound effect. Lignocaine can also be used alone in a 4% solution or a 1–2% jelly form for relief from the discomfort of procedures such as urinary catheterization. Chronic long-term use of topical preparations can lead to sensitization and local allergic reactions.

An alternative to EMLA and amethocaine topical agents is the use of cryoanaesthesia via a refrigerant spray, with which the rapid cooling of the skin causes superficial anaesthesia suitable for immediate pinpoint pain relief (Brown 2004). Examples of these sprays are ethylchloride, fluroethyl and dichlorotetrafluoroethane (Frigiderm)®. Refrigerant sprays work by extremely rapid cooling of the skin (<10°C within 10–15 seconds of application); however, their duration of action is briefer than that provided by EMLA, Amethocaine gel or ALA and this sudden cooling can be distressing and children particularly may object to it (McCaffery & Passero 1999). Refrigerant sprays should be used with caution as prolonged application can cause frostbite. Table 25.2 summarizes the various drugs available for topically applied local anaesthesia.

Local infiltration and field block

The difference between these two methods of drug administration is that local infiltration involves the injection of the anaesthetic drug directly into the subcutaneous tissue involved, while a field block involves injecting the chosen drug into the surrounding area for treatment (Chan et al. 2002). The latter has the advantage of avoiding distortion of the wound edges. Care needs to be exercised to avoid injection of large volumes of local anaesthetic as this can lead to localized oedema, causing distortion of wound edges and tissue hypoxia, which makes the apposition and healing of the wound edges difficult. It is imperative to avoid introducing lignocaine directly into a vein due to its cardiac arrhythmia properties.

Local infiltration and field block are ideal methods of anaesthesia for the suturing and extensive cleansing of minor wounds and the drainage of superficial wound abscesses. Note that the local anaesthetic may be less effective when used for infiltrating an abscess due to the altered pH of the infected tissue/fluid, and it is recommended that infiltration is not used for inflamed or infected tissues (BNF 2006). While these methods provide excellent levels of pain relief the act of infiltration or injection can be painful. Warming the vial between the hands prior to drawing up and use can relieve this discomfort to some extent. Buffering the lignocaine with sodium bicarbonate 8.4% has been seen to significantly decrease the pain perceived by the patient on infiltration by raising the pH of the solution (Achar & Kundu 2002, Chan et al. 2002). However, this latter option significantly decreases the solution's shelf-life, limiting the anaesthetic's efficacy to one week post combination with the sodium bicarbonate, and it is recommended to only mix the two drugs together immediately prior to the procedure. Lignocaine 1 or 2% with or without adrenaline (dependent on the wound location) is the drug of choice for these methods of administration due to its rapid onset. Toxicity can be avoided if the dose of lignocaine does not exceed 3 mg/kg body weight (Chan et al. 2002), which is approximately 20 ml of a 1% solution in an adult, increased to a maximum of 500 mg if the lignocaine solution contains adrenaline (BNF 2006).

Haematoma blocks and peripheral nerve blocks

Haematoma blocks are principally used for the reduction of wrist fractures. They involve injecting the anaesthetic drug directly into the haematoma surrounding the fracture (Chan et al. 2002). The benefit of this type of block is that it is easy and quick to give and is sufficiently effective to enable the reduction and immobilization of the fracture; however, a peripheral nerve block is more selective in that the local anaesthetic drug is injected around nerve trunks supplying the injury/operation site.

Peripheral nerve blocks are occasionally mistakenly referred to as haematoma blocks; however, a peripheral nerve block affects a larger area and in a dermatonal pattern (McCaffery & Passero 1999). Various peripheral nerve blocks using local anaesthetic agents have been described in order to reduce pain and facilitate treatments; these nerve blocks are used to administer an anaesthetic agent locally to nerves serving particular parts of the body. The techniques for administering peripheral nerve blocks are also more difficult than that of haematoma blocks; however, they provide excellent analgesia over limited fields with minimal systemic effects, and are generally easy to perform, inexpensive and safe. They also act as muscle relaxants as the motor fibres are also blocked. Care should be taken not to exceed maximum local anaesthetic doses (shown in Table 25.1).

The most frequent uses of regional nerve blocks in the ED setting are ring blocks to achieve anaesthesia of a digit and femoral blocks for pain relieve of a hip or femur fracture. A ring block involves injection into the base of the finger via the interdigital web; bilateral infiltration is required to ensure blockage of all four digital nerves. Brachial plexus or axillary blocks can be used to achieve anaesthesia of the forearm and hand, for which the local anaesthetic is injected into the neurovascular sheath surrounding the axillary artery and the median, radial and ulnar nerves. A number of options are available for femoral blocks, which differ according to the experience and skill of the practitioner and include the lateral cutaneous nerve of thigh, subcostal nerve, femoral nerve, sciatic nerve, triple nerve block (femoral, obturator and sciatic nerves), psoas (lumbar plexus) block or continuos epidural block (Parker et al. 2002). The triple nerve femoral block using a three-in-one injection method has been found to effectively reduce pain and the need for opiates and can be given by all grades of medical staff trained in the procedure (Fletcher et al. 2003). The main advantage of the triple nerve block is it requires fewer injections and avoids the pain involved in injection directly into already sensitive tissue.

Potential complications, as with all nerve blocks, relate to the possibility of damage to surrounding structures (Rivellini 1993). It is imperative that adrenaline is not added to the local anaesthetic solution for any procedure where it may compromise the flow of blood to an area which has an end-arteriole blood supply, as the adrenaline leads to vasoconstriction and can cause the occlusion of the supplying arteries: these include fingers or toes, skin flaps with marginal viability, penis and tips of the ears or the nose-tip (Achar & Kundu 2002, McCaffery & Passero 1999). It should also be noted that the onset and duration of action of the various drugs differ according to the site of injection: for example, there has been seen a difference of up to 25 minutes for onset time and 6 hours difference of duration time of bupivacaine when comparing an intercostal nerve block with a brachial plexus block (Chan et al. 2002).

Intravenous regional anaesthesia (Bier's block)

The technique of intravenous regional anaesthesia (IVRA) was first described by Karl Bier in 1908 and the technique later became known as a Bier's Block (Brill et al. 2004). It is used primarily to achieve anaesthesia below the elbow, although it can also be used for procedures below the knee and in ED the main uses of this technique are for the manipulation of Colles' and Smith fractures. Contraindications for the use of IVRA are outlined in Box 25.2. The use of IVRA has been found to provide better relief from pain and it facilitates better limb reduction with a reduced risk of re-dislocation or the need for re-plastering in comparison to the use of haematoma blocks (Handoll 2005).

Two points of intravenous access are required, one for access to enable the administration of other drugs as required and the other for administration of the regional anaesthesia. This second line should preferably be placed distally to the injury (Dunn et al. 2003) or at the antecubital fossa (Blyth et al. 1995). The injured limb is then elevated for between 30

> **Box 25.2   Contraindications for the use of intravenous regional anaesthesia:**
>
> - Patient refusal
> - Peripheral vascular disease including
>   - Sickle cell disease
>   - Raynaud's disease
> - Severe atheroma
> - Unstable epilepsy
> - Heart failure
> - Systolic blood pressure >200 mmHg
> - Severe liver disease
> - Anticoagulant therapy
> - Confusion/uncooperative patient
> - Compromised limb circulation
> - Compartment syndrome in the injured limb
> - Injuries at the tourniquet site (humerus) including fractures or soft tissue injuries
> - Local infection, e.g. cellulitis

seconds and 2 minutes following insertion of the intravenous cannula to drain some of the blood from the veins in order to reduce the dilatation of the local anaesthetic (Dunn et al. 2003). A cuffed tourniquet, underlaid by wool, is placed around the upper arm and inflated to a pressure at least 100 mmHg above the patient's systolic blood pressure.

The local anaesthetic, e.g. 40 ml prilocaine 0.5%, is injected into the collapsed veins of the limb, which will cause the limb to develop a blue, mottled appearance. The maximum length of time for which the cuff can remain inflated is 1.5 hours; however, pain from the direct compression of nerve and muscle tissue will be evident after 30 minutes and may be unbearable after an hour. This discomfort may be eased by the use of a double-cuff. When this is used, the proximal cuff is inflated prior to infiltration. Following infiltration the distal cuff is inflated and the proximal cuff let down. Thus, the tourniquet effect is maintained by the distal cuff, which is located over an area of the limb that has been anaesthetized (Rivellini 1993).

It is imperative that the pressure in the cuff is maintained constantly for at least 30 minutes to permit fixation of the local anaesthetic to the tissues of the limb (Rivellini 1993). Release or leakage of the anaesthetic into the systemic circulation prior to this time can lead to cardiovascular and CNS depression and therefore the presence of resuscitation facilities and circulatory access are mandatory for this procedure.

NURSING IMPLICATIONS OF PROCEDURES INVOLVING LOCAL ANAESTHETICS

Preoperatively

The patient's past and current medical history should be assessed and factors that might contraindicate the use of local anaesthetics should be noted, in particular previous allergic reactions. A baseline of the current neurovascular status of the proposed surgical site should be established. When intravenous regional anaesthesia is proposed the patient's baseline cardiovascular status in the form of their haemodynamic observations and their weight is necessary. The nurse needs to be familiar with the technique to be used, the length of time the block will last and whether any vasoconstrictive agent has been added (Rivellini 1993).

Thorough preparation of the patient includes the provision of information about both the nature of the procedure and the feelings the patient may experience during it. Explanation of sights and sensations which may result from the procedure needs to be given before they occur, e.g. that local anaesthesia will remove the sensation of pain but not the sensation of pressure or that during intravenous regional anaesthesia a change of limb colour associated with the infiltration of local anaesthetic is expected.

Informed consent will need to be obtained. For minor procedures such as suturing this can be obtained verbally, but for techniques involving intravenous regional anaesthesia formal written consent will be required.

Intraoperatively

Special consideration should be given to the fact that patients are awake. Careless remarks should be avoided and technical terms, when used, even between staff, need to be explained. The focus of conversation should be the patient rather than the procedure. Where conscious awareness of the procedure causes distress, social conversation can be used to distract the patient (Edwards 1994).

Constant vigilance is required to assess for signs of toxicity and allergic reaction. The neurovascular function of the affected area should be continuously observed and compared with that of equivalent unaffected areas. This is particularly pertinent with procedures involving manipulation of a limb or the application of a plaster cast, as the complications of either are mimicked by the action of local anaesthetic. The tourniquet time, where appropriate, should be noted. The patient should be encouraged to report any discomfort experienced.

Postoperatively and advice for discharge

Pain provides a protective function both as an initiator of reflex mechanisms and by alerting the person when a body part has sustained trauma. In eliminating pain, local anaesthetics eliminate these protective mechanisms. Nurses will need to consider measures to ensure the safety of the patient and the body part involved; for example, the patient's limb should not be allowed to rest on or become trapped in cot sides. The transient loss of motor function necessitates that affected extremities will need to be supported in anatomically neutral positions. A sling will serve both to protect and to support the weight of an arm. Any attempt at using the affected area until full sensation has returned should be discouraged. The post-anaesthesia levels of sensory and motor function should be continually assessed and delays in expected dissipation times reported. It is vital that care is taken to differentiate between paraesthesiae related to dissipation of the block and those of neurovascular compromise (Jasinski & Snyder 1996). These observations should be documented at least once prior to discharge.

The residual effect of the local anaesthetic will provide immediate pain relief. However, as this is only temporary, postoperative analgesia will need to be prescribed and administered before the effect dissipates. As far as possible, it is helpful to give some indication as to the possible levels of discomfort the patient may experience once the local anaesthetic has worn off. This will help the patient to determine whether this is normal or an indicator of residual or developing complications.

CONCLUSION

This chapter has highlighted both the rationale for the use of local anaesthetics and the nursing implications. Local anaesthetics are a valuable tool in the options available in ED care. Used with vigilance they can provide an alternative to the torture of the 'one quick pull' or the fear of 'being put to sleep', and improve the experiences of the patients and their supporters while in ED.

References

Achar S, Kundu S (2002) Principles of Office Anesthesia: Part 1. Infiltrative Anesthesia. *American Family Physician,* **66**(1), 91–95.

Blyth MJG, Kinninmonth AWG, Asante DK (1995) Biers Block: a change of injection site. *Journal of Trauma-Injury & Critical Care,* **39**(4), 726–728.

Brill S, Middleton W, Brill G, Fisher A (2004) Bier's Block; 100 years old and still going strong! *Acta Anaethesiologica Scandinavia,* **48**(1), 117.

British National Formulary [BNF] (2006) *British National Formulary No. 51.* London: British Medical Association and the Royal Pharmaceutical Society of Great Britain.

Brown A (2004) Pain relief. In: Cameron P, Jelinick G, Kelly A-M, Murray L, Brown A, Heyworth J, eds. *Textbook of Adult Emergency Medicine,* 2nd edn. Edinburgh: Churchill Livingstone.

Butcher D (2004) Pharmacological techniques in managing acute pain in emergency departments. *Emergency Nurse,* **12**(1), 26–36.

Chan SK, Karmakar MK, Chui PT (2002) Local anaesthesia outside the operating room. *Hong Kong Medical Journal,* **8**(2), 106–113.

De Jong RH (2001) Local anaesthetics in clinical practice. In Waldman SD, ed. *Interventional Pain Management,* 2nd edn. Philadelphia: WB Saunders Company.

Dunn R, Dilley S, Brookes J, Leach D, Maclean A, Rogers I (2003) *The Emergency Medicine Manual,* 3rd edn. Adelaide: Venom Publishing.

Edwards B (1994) Local and regional anaesthesia. *Emergency Nurse,* **2**(2), 10–15.

Eidelman A, Weiss JM, Enu IK, McNicol E, Lau J, Carr DB (2005) Topical anaesthetics for repair of dermal lacerations (Protocol). *The Cochrane Database of Systematic Reviews,* Issue 3. London: John Wiley & Sons.

Fatovich DM, Brown AFT (2004) Pain relief in emergency medicine. In: Cameron P, Jelinick G, Kelly A-M, Murray L, Brown A, Heyworth J, eds. *Textbook of Adult Emergency Medicine.* 2nd edn. Edinburgh: Churchill Livingstone.

Fletcher AK, Rigby AS, Heyes FL (2003) Three-in-one femoral nerve block as analgesia for fractured neck of femur in the emergency department: a randomized control trial. *Annals of Emergency Medicine,* **42**(4), 596–597.

Gajraj N (2003) Round the block one more time. *The Lancet,* **361**(9375), 2165.

Graham CA, Gibson AJ, Goutcher CM, Scollon D (1997) Anaesthesia for the management of distal radius fracture in adults in Scottish hospitals. *European Journal of Emergency Medicine,* **4**(4), 210–212.

Grant S, Hoffman R (1992) Use of tetracaine, epinephrine, and cocaine as a topical anesthetic in the emergency department. *Annals of Emergency Medicine,* **21**, 987–997.

Handoll HHG (2005) Anaesthesia for treating distal radial fracture in adults. *Cochrane Review, Cochrane Collaboration.* London: John Wiley & Sons.

Jasinski D, Snyder C (1996) Invasive interventions. In: Sallerno E, Williams J, eds. *Pain Management Handbook: An Interdisciplinary Approach.* St Louis: Mosby.

Lander JA, Weltman BJ (2002) Topical anaesthetics (EMLA and AMETOP creams) for reduction of pain during needle insertion in children (Protocol). *The Cochrane Database of Systematic Reviews,* Issue 4. London: John Wiley & Sons.

McCaffery M, Passero C (1999) *Pain: Clinical Manual,* 2nd edn. St Louis: Mosby.

Parker MJ, Griffths R, Appadu BN (2002) Nerve blocks (subcostal, lateral cutaneous, femoral, triple, psoas) for hip fractures. *The Cochrane Database of Systematic Reviews,* Issue 1. London: John Wiley & Sons.

Rayner-Klein J, Rowe CA (2005) Analgesia and anaesthesia. In: O'Shea RA, ed. *Principles and Practice of Trauma Nursing,* Edinburgh: Elsevier Churchill Livingstone.

Rivellini D (1993) Local and regional anaesthesia. *Nursing Clinics of North America,* **28**(3), 547–572.

Rosenbery PH (2000) *Local and Regional Anaesthesia.* Oxford: Blackwell Publishing.

Tortora GJ, Grabowski SR (2003) *Principles of Anatomy and Physiology.* 10th edn. New Jersey: John Wiley & Sons.

PART **6**

Emergency care

PART CONTENTS

Chapter **26**

Cardiac emergencies

Jamie Walthall

CHAPTER CONTENTS

INTRODUCTION

Cardiovascular disease accounts for approximately 40% of all deaths under the age of 75 years in Europe (Resuscitation Council (UK) 2005). One-third of all people suffering from myocardial infarction will die prior to reaching hospital, with a high proportion of these dying within one hour from the onset of symptoms (Resuscitation Council (UK) 2000). In the UK, coronary heart disease is among the biggest killers. More than 1.4 million people suffer from angina and 300 000 have myocardial infarctions (MI) every year (Department of Health 2000). Thus, EDs will see a high proportion of patients suffering from a cardiovascular disorder.

The aim of this chapter is to give a systematic approach to the multiple problems that may be encountered by cardiac patients. A general overview of anatomy and physiology has been included to enable the disease process to be more accurately defined. The management of the particular cardiac problems described in this chapter is set out as a suggested guideline and is not a definitive directive for all cardiac patients, as each problem should be judged on an individual basis.

RELATED ANATOMY AND PHYSIOLOGY

The heart can be described as a muscular pump containing four chambers, situated at an oblique angle in the mediastinal cavity (Tortora & Grabowski 2000) (Figs 26.1 and 26.2).

As the heart beats it expels blood into two closed circuits. The first circuit is fed from the left side of the heart. This supplies oxygenated blood from the lungs to the systemic circulation. The second circuit is the pulmonary circuit. This enables the right side

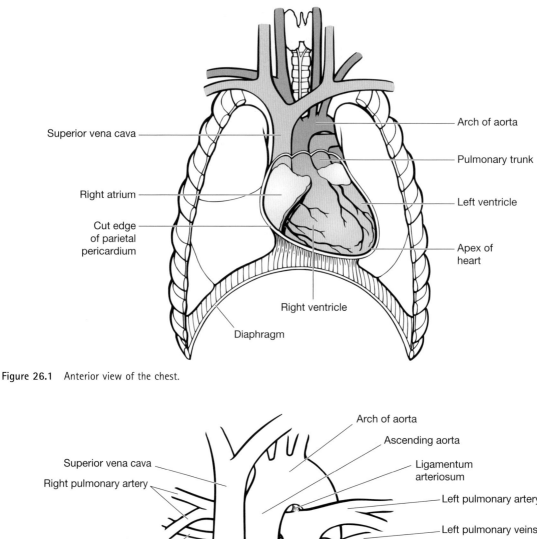

Figure 26.1 Anterior view of the chest.

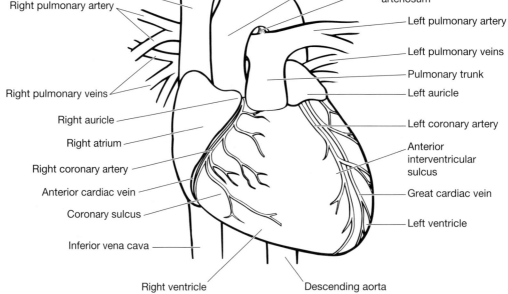

Figure 26.2 Anterior external view of the heart.

of the heart to receive deoxygenated blood which is then pumped back to the lungs via the pulmonary artery (Marieb 2000).

The heart is composed of a triple layer, which enables the protection of the inner components (Tortora & Grabowski 2000):

- The pericardium – the outer layer is composed of thick fibrous tissue that surrounds and protects the heart.
- The myocardium – this is the muscular layer that forms the basis of the pumping action of the heart. It is present within both the atria and the ventricles, with the ventricles having the greater ratio of muscle.
- The endocardium – this is composed of a thin layer of endothelial and connective tissue covering the inside of the heart, including the valves, which enables a smooth flow of blood through the heart, with little resistance.

Cardiac valves (Fig. 26.3)

The atrioventricular (AV) valves refer to the mitral and tricuspid valves, which lie between the atria and the ventricles, the mitral on the left and the tricuspid on the right. The valves are supported by a network of strands called chordae tendineae. The passive movement of blood from the atria to the ventricles, across the AV valves, occurs in the cardiac cycle in the phase known as ventricular filling. As the pressure in the ventricles increases, the valves are forced to close, preventing a back-flow of blood.

At the origin of the aorta and the pulmonary artery sit the semilunar valves. These consist of three cusps, and prevent the back-flow of blood into the heart. During ventricular diastole (relaxation), these valves are closed, but as ventricular systole (contraction) occurs the valves are forced to open and blood is ejected out into either the aorta or the pulmonary artery. Should these valves be diseased or damaged, stenosis or regurgitation may occur. More often than not this precludes the need for the surgical intervention.

Coronary circulation

To maintain oxygenation and the supply of nutrients, the heart derives its own blood supply via the coronary arteries (see Fig. 26.4). The left and right coronary arteries originate from the aorta. As suggested, they branch into a network of arteries supplying both the right and left sides of the heart.

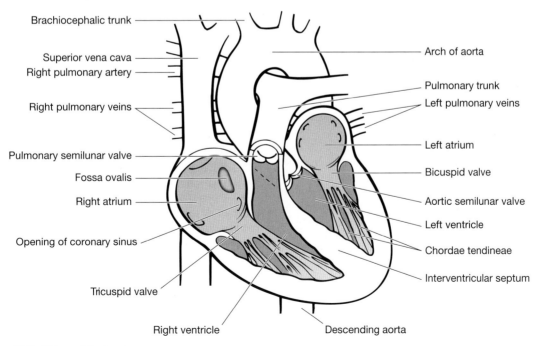

Figure 26.3   Valves of the heart.

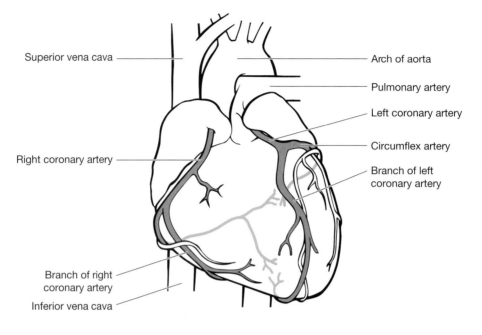

Figure 26.4 Coronary circulation.

THE CARDIAC CYCLE

The cardiac cycle is divided into three main phases (Tortora & Grabowski 2000):

- ventricular relaxation (diastole)
- ventricular filling
- ventricular contraction (systole).

For simplification only the left side of the heart will be explained.

Ventricular relaxation. This follows ventricular contraction (systole). The ventricles relax, resulting in pressure within the left ventricle falling below that of the aorta, and thus the aortic valve closes. As Tortora & Grabowski (2000) indicate, all valves within the heart are now closed. At the same time, blood is passively flowing into the left atrium via the pulmonary system. As pressure and volume within the left atrium increases, the mitral valve opens and the second phase of the cardiac cycle is now entered.

Ventricular filling. Tortora & Grabowski (2000) identified that the ventricular filling phase of the cardiac cycle is divided into three stages. The first stage is referred to as rapid ventricular filling and involves passive filling of the left ventricle from the left atrium. The second stage of ventricular filling is known as diastasis and refers to slow ventricular filling. At the end of diastasis, the pressures in the left atrium and the left ventricle are now equal. The third stage of

ventricular filling is due to the contraction of the atrium, with blood being forced into the left ventricle.

Ventricular contraction. As the left ventricle starts to contract the mitral valve closes. The left ventricle is now a closed chamber. The muscles within the left ventricle start to contract and there is a resultant increase in pressure. Once the pressure in the left ventricle is greater than that of the aorta, the aortic valve opens and blood is ejected out (the stroke volume). As the pressure in the left ventricle drops with the expulsion of blood, the aortic valve closes and the cardiac cycle starts again.

ASSESSMENT

The presenting history when a patient attends the ED with a cardiac event remains one of the most crucial aspects in aiding diagnosis The history provides subjective information about the presenting complaint, symptoms, past medical history and any other relevant information (Alexander et al. 2000). During initial assessment, the patient's need for immediate care must be paramount. Hence, the use of the ABC principle should be initiated automatically (Box 26.1).

The remainder of the assessment should include:

- Assessment of patient's appearance – this should include pallor, posture and any non-verbal signs.

Box 26.1   ABCs

A   Check the patency of the **airway**
B   Check the adequacy of the **breathing**
C   **Circulation:** signs of shock, pallor etc.

- Pain assessment – location, type, site and severity of pain, including any measures taken to relieve the pain.
- Baseline observations – these should include blood pressure, pulse, temperature, respiration and oxygen saturation. Often temperature is forgotten, but the incidence of a mild pyrexia is a common response to muscle damage (Alexander et al. 2000).
- Electrocardiograph (ECG) – note any arrhythmia and use of cardiac monitor.

Clinical investigations

Clinical investigations to support assessment should include blood analysis (see Box 26.2) and chest X-ray to determine heart size and detect oedema (Jowett & Thompson 2002).

Box 26.2   Blood analysis in cardiac patients

- **Cardiac enzymes** – these indicate muscular damage which may suggest cardiac ischaemia (Julian 1988)

- **White cell count** – a raised white cell count in the cardiac patient is usually indicative of myocardial damage

- **Erythrocyte sedimentation rate (ESR)** – a raised ESR may indicate an increase in fibrinogen due to myocardial necrosis

- **Urea and electrolytes (U&E)** – any change in the sodium or potassium should be noted as these ions are related to cardiac cells and their function

- **Glucose** – the appearance of hyperglycaemia can be stress-related and linked to any acute changes in the myocardium, e.g. myocardial infarction (Woods et al. 2000)

- **Lipids** – these will give an indication as to the risk factors incorporated with ischaemic heart disease; they include cholesterol and triglycerides

- **Clotting screen** – this is useful when the patient may be anticoagulated

BASIC ECG INTERPRETATION

It is important for ED nurses to accurately record and interpret an ECG of a patient presenting with a cardiac condition. An inherent and rhythmical electrical activity is the reason for the heart's continuous beating (Tortora & Grabowski 2000). The cardiac cells (myocardial cells) located within the myocardium undergo chemical changes, which in turn trigger electrical impulses (action potentials) and result in myocardial contraction.

The normal heartbeat is known as sinus rhythm. In essence, this means that the impulses have been generated by the normal heart conductive system (Fig. 26.5). These electrical impulses can be recorded via an ECG. To obtain a 12-lead ECG, electrodes are placed across the chest and each limb (see Fig. 26.6).

Having positioned the ECG electrodes, it is important to understand the representation being made by each electrode. The heart's electrical impulses start at the SA node and depolarize down the conductive system as far as the apex of the heart. This directional flow is known as the cardiac vector. The four limb leads attached as shown in Fig. 26.7 form what is known as the Einthoven triangle. The fourth lead not shown within the triangle acts as an earth and helps to standardize recordings. Leads I, II and III are known as bipolar leads, because each lead represents the electrical activity between two poles:

- Lead I represents electrical activity from the right arm to the left arm.
- Lead II represents electrical activity from the right arm to the left leg.
- Lead III represents electrical activity from the left arm to the left leg.

Leads AVR, AVL and AVF are known as unipolar leads. They read electrical impulses from one electrode, with the ECG machine calculating the effect of the other limb leads to give an average reading between the points of the triangle formed by the bipolar leads.

The abbreviations for the unipolar leads are as follows:

- A – augmented (amplified)
- V – vector (force of direction of impulse)
- R, L, F – the direction being viewed, i.e., right, left or foot.

Thus, AVR looks at the right atrium (although in practice this is of little consequence), AVL looks at the lateral aspect of the heart, and AVF looks at the inferior aspect (see also Box 26.3). The chest leads are a much more simplified version for looking at

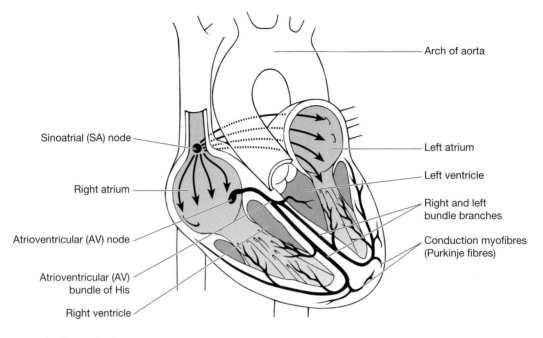

Figure 26.5   Cardiac conduction.

the frontal plane of the heart. These are unipolar leads which pick up electrical activity from the point at which they are placed (Box 26.3):

- V1 is placed over the 4th intercostal space to the right of the sternum.
- V2 is placed over the 4th intercostal space to the left of the sternum.
- V1 and V2 thus view the anterior surfaces of the right and part of the left ventricles.
- V3 is placed on the chest midway between V2 and V4; hence it is useful to apply V4 before V3. V3 looks at the septum.
- V4 is placed on the 5th intercostal space, midway along the clavicular line, and views the septum and the anterior wall of the left ventricle.
- V5 is placed along the same line as V4, but anteriorly to the midaxillary line.
- V6 is again placed along the same line as V4 and V5, but rests on the midaxillary line.
- V5 and V6 view predominately the lateral wall of the left ventricles.

Components of a normal ECG

The ECG complex is made up of a sequence of electrical events occurring in the heart. The activity starts with impulses being transmitted from the sinoatrial node across the atria. As the atria depolarize, the P wave is created. The AV node filters and holds atrial impulses to allow significant ventricular filling time prior to contraction. This is represented as a straight line (isoelectric line) on the ECG and is called the P-R interval. As depolarization occurs through the bundle branches, and a wave of depolarization spreads across, the QRS complex is created on the ECG. This is followed by a short resting period, depicted again as an isoelectric line called the ST segment, before the T wave is created by ventricular repolarization (Fig. 26.8).

When this is all put together, a single heartbeat is represented in the ECG trace as shown in Fig. 26.9.

Basic rhythm recognition

To make an accurate analysis of cardiac activity it is necessary to obtain a 12-lead ECG trace as opposed to a rhythm strip. The rhythm strip only shows one view of the heart which is dependent on the electrode positioning. As a result, myocardial damage or stress can easily be missed.

Once the 12-lead ECG has been obtained (see Fig. 26.10), it is necessary to work through each lead methodically, looking at each waveform to ensure that any changes/abnormalities are recognized. To interpret an ECG, the ED nurse should start by looking at the rhythm strip to determine whether a

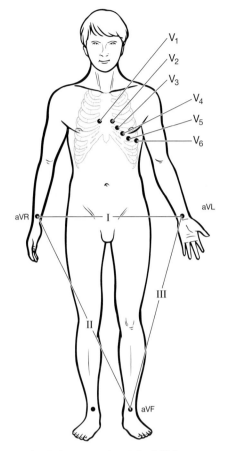

Figure 26.6 Lead placements for 12-lead ECGs.

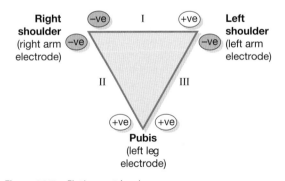

Figure 26.7 Einthoven triangle.

Box 26.3 Areas of heart shown in specific leads

I	Left lateral surface
II	Left lateral and inferior surface
III	Inferior surface
AVR	Right atrium
AVL	Left lateral surface
AVF	Inferior surface
V_1	Right anterior
V_2	Right anterior surface and some of left anterior surface
V_3	Septal area
V_4	Anterior surface of left ventricle
V_5	Left anterior/lateral surfaces
V_6	Lateral aspect of left ventricle

ECG tracings are standardized so that heart rate can be calculated from the tracing. Most ECG machines are set to pass paper through at 25 mm/s. As graph paper is standardized, one small square represents 0.04 s (1 mm of paper), one large square represents 0.2 s (5 mm of paper) and five large squares represent 1 s (25 mm of paper). Therefore, if there is one QRS complex per five large squares, the heart rate would be approximately 60 beats/min. Once an approximate rate is established, the nurse should look at the make-up of the repetitive complexes, checking whether the P waves are followed by the right length of interval and the QRS complex is followed by a T wave (see Box 26.4).

Once a basic rhythm has been established from the rhythm strip, attention should be focused on the various leads to determine whether any area of the heart is damaged or ischaemic. It is important that ECG interpretation does not take precedence over the patient's clinical condition. The clinical picture and condition of the patient are by far the best indicators of overall well-being. For this reason there is no substitute for the ED nurse's fundamental assessment skills.

CARDIAC ARREST

Cardiorespiratory arrest is defined as the sudden cessation of spontaneous respiration and circulation (Jowett & Thompson 2002). The main causes of cardiac arrest are:

- ventricular fibrillation (VF)/pulseless ventricular tachycardia (VT)
- asystole
- pulseless electrical activity (PEA)

basic rhythm is present. If a rhythm exists, complexes will be repetitive and components of those complexes will form the same pattern. It is also necessary to determine whether this pattern is occurring at regular intervals or not. Once an underlying rhythm is established, the rate of the rhythm should be determined.

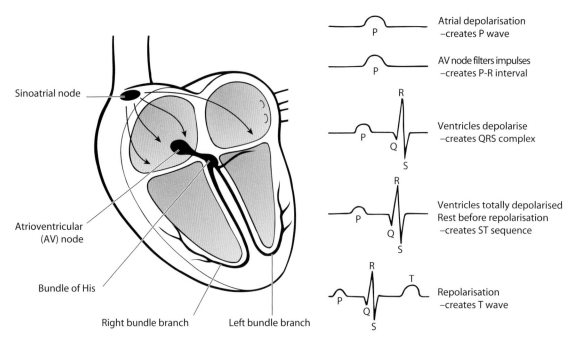

Sinoatrial node

Atrioventricular
(AV) node

Bundle of His

Right bundle branch   Left bundle branch

P — Atrial depolarisation
–creates P wave

P — AV node filters impulses
–creates P-R interval

P, Q, R, S — Ventricles depolarise
–creates QRS complex

P, Q, R, S — Ventricles totally depolarised
Rest before repolarisation
–creates ST sequence

P, Q, R, S, T — Repolarisation
–creates T wave

Figure 26.8   Electrical activity of the heart in relation to the ECG recording.

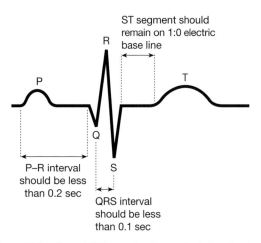

ST segment should
remain on 1:0 electric
base line

P–R interval
should be less
than 0.2 sec

QRS interval
should be less
than 0.1 sec

Figure 26.9   Normal ECG complex from a single heartbeat.

It is identified by:

- sudden loss of consciousness
- absence of a central pulse (carotid/femoral)
- absence of respiration.

Systemic management

In EDs, cardiac arrests in most instances are anticipated. Therefore, the ED nurse is responsible for (Alexander et al. 2000):

- recognizing cardiac arrest
- correct procedure for summoning help
- commencing basic life support (Fig. 26.11).

Ventricular fibrillation (VF)

The most common cause of cardiac arrest is usually VF or pulseless ventricular tachycardia (VT), which has an 80–90% mortality rate for patients outside the hospital environment (Colquhoun et al. 1999). In VF, the cardiac cycle is disrupted and the cardiac cells behave chaotically, depolarizing in a disoriented and disorderly fashion or fibrillation (Fig. 26.12). As a result, cardiac output is compromised to the extent that blood circulation stops. This results in hypoxia, loss of consciousness within 10–20 seconds and absence of respiration. The physiology of VT is discussed later in this chapter. Simply put, the ventricular contractions occur at such a rate that ventricular filling time is inadequate and cardiac output is compromised. In severe cases, circulation ceases as in VF.

Immediate management

Cardiac arrest management has been standardized by the development of advanced life support (ALS) protocols (ILCOR 2005a, Resuscitation Council (UK) 2005). If the VF arrest is witnessed and monitored, a precordial thump may be of benefit in an attempt to

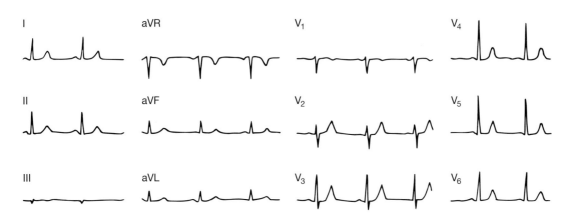

I   aVR   V₁   V₄

II   aVF   V₂   V₅

III   aVL   V₃   V₆

Figure 26.10   A normal 12-lead ECG trace.

Box 26.4   ECG analysis

- **Rhythm.** Is it regular? Are the R–R intervals equal? To check this, place a piece of paper on the trace and mark off three R waves, moving the paper alone to see if other R waves match this pattern.

- **Rate.** Sinus, tachycardic or bradycardic?

- **P waves.** Are P waves present? Are they of a uniform shape? Do they precede the QRS complex? These represent atrial activity or abnormality

- **QRS complex.** Normal width/shape? These represent ventricular activity or abnormality

- **T waves.** Are the ST segments above or below the isoelectric line? Uniform shape and size?

- **Intervals.** Are all the intervals normal?
  P–R 0.12–0.2 s
  QRS 0.07–0.1 s
  Q–T 0.33–0.43 s
  P–R and Q–T intervals vary with heart rate

Unresponsive ?

↓

Shout for help

↓

Open airway

↓

Not breathing normally?

↓

Call 999

↓

30 chest compressions

↓

2 rescue breaths
30 compressions

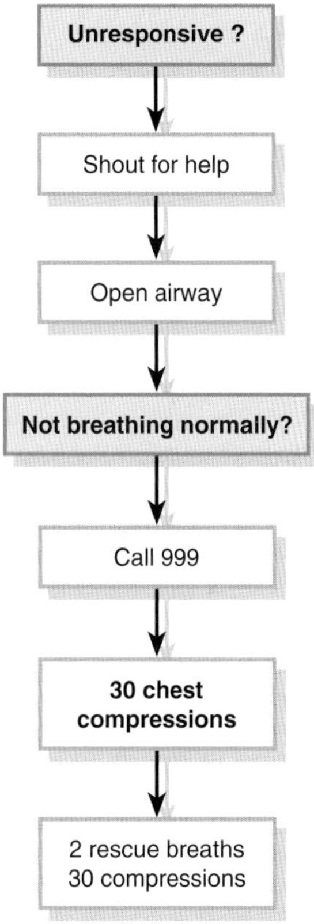

Figure 26.11   Adult basic life support (Resuscitation Council 2005).

'shock' the heart and restore normal electrical activity (Caldwell et al. 1985). Potential complications of the precordial thump include rhythm deteriorations, such as rate acceleration of VT and asystole (Krijne 1984, Sclarovsky 1981). A precordial thump is most likely to be successful in converting VT into sinus rhythm. Successful treatment of VT by precordial thump is much less likely (Resuscitation Council 2005). Having reviewed the evidence, the International Liaison Committee on Resuscitation [ILCOR] (2005b) recommends one immediate thump may be considered after a monitored cardiac arrest if an electrical defibrillator is not immediately available.

The optimum first-line treatment for VF and pulseless VT is early defibrillation. The aim of defibrillation is to depolarize the myocardium simultaneously, to allow normal cardiac cell function to resume (Colquhoun et al. 1999). A key factor in reducing mortality lies with the speed of defibrillation, which should be given without delay (ILCOR 2005b). For

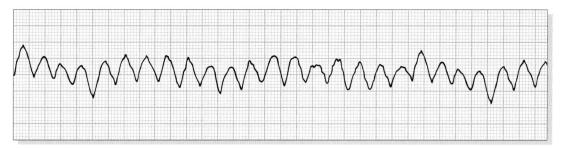

Figure 26.12 Ventricular fibrillation.

this reason, ED nurses should be appropriately skilled in performing defibrillation as they are likely to be the first personnel in attendance.

Defibrillation

The paddles of the defibrillator are positioned to enclose as much myocardium as possible (Skinner & Vincent 1997) (see Fig. 26.13). A conductive medium, such as jelly pads, should always be used, both to enhance contact and to reduce skin damage. Good contact with the chest is vital to maximize conduction and prevent 'arcing' of electrical current. The paddles should be placed firmly over jelly pads and perpendicular pressure should be applied (approximately 8 kg). One paddle should be placed to the right of the sternum, below the right clavicle in the midclavicular line, and the other vertically in the mid-axillary line, approximately level with the V6 electrode position or the female breast. This position should be clear of any breast tissue (Resuscitation Council (UK) 2000).

Prior to defibrillation, GTN patches and external pacing generators should be removed. Internal pacers or defibrillating systems do not preclude the need for external DC shock in the case of VF or pulseless VT; however, the electrode should be placed away from the device. The defibrillation regime should follow the algorithm shown in Fig. 26.14.

As even short interruptions to perform rhythm analysis causes significant interruptions in CPR and thus survival, the Resuscitation Council (UK) (2005) now recommends a single-shock strategy. The rationale is that with the first wave of biphasic waveforms exceeding 90%, failure to terminate VF/VT successfully implies the need for a period of CPR, to improve myocardial oxygenation, rather than a further shock. The Resuscitation Council (UK) (2005) notes that even if defibrillation is successful in restoring a perfusing rhythm, it is very rare for a pulse to be palpable immediately afterwards, and the delay in trying to palpate a pulse will further compromise the myocardium if a perfusing rhythm has not been restored (van Alem 2003). The SOS-Kanto study group (2007) found in witnessed out of hospital

cardiac arrest, cardiac–only resuscitation improved survival rate.

The safety of the resuscitation team is paramount and it is the responsibility of the person administering DC shocks to ensure that other team members are clear of the patient. This should be ascertained verbally and visually before proceeding with defibrillation. ALS courses provide a standardized approach to training for all team members and should be a priority for ED nurses.

Asystole

This is total cessation of circulation, brought about by the lack of cardiac pacemaker activity, either natural or artificial (Colquhoun et al. 1999) (Fig. 26.15). Asystole accounts for 25% of all cardiac arrests within the hospital environment (Jowett & Thompson 2002). The treatment is continued cardiac compression with ventilation. Adrenaline and atropine are used to stimulate cardiac activity, but the prognosis for a successful resuscitation remains poor, with the overall survival rate being about 17% of the survival rate with VF/VT rhythms.

Pulseless electrical activity (PEA)

This presents as a full QRS complex on the heart trace, but with the absence of any palpable pulse, hence the lack of systemic circulation. The causes are divided into the categories primary and secondary (see Box 26.5).

For the resuscitation attempt to be of any success, the cause must be isolated and the appropriate treatment initiated, namely the Non VF/VT side of the algorithm shown in Fig. 26.14.

Drug therapy

Pharmacological intervention may be used during cardiac arrest to (Jowett & Thompson 2002):

- correct hypoxia and acidosis
- accelerate or reduce the heart rate
- suppress ectopic activity
- stimulate the strength of myocardial contraction.

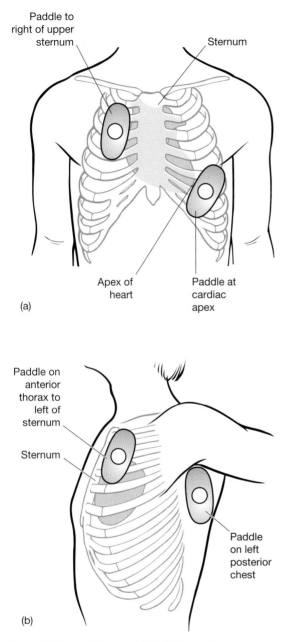

Figure 26.13   Positioning of defibrillator paddles.

Adrenaline   Adrenaline (adrenaline) is the first drug used in cardiac arrest. Its therapeutic action is to improve coronary and cerebral perfusion. To date, clinical evidence that adrenaline improves survival or neurological recovery in humans is absent (ILOCR 2005a). Adrenaline is an alpha- and beta-agonist and acts upon receptor sites to increase circulation to vital sites (Opie 2000). Its action in cardiac arrest is to cause vasoconstriction, increasing cerebral and coronary perfusion.

Atropine   Atropine is used to block the action of the vagus nerve, thereby increasing sinoatrial node activity. However, the efficacy of this drug has been questioned, as repeated doses reduce electrical stability of the heart, increasing the risk of VF (Opie 2000). The dose in asystole is 3 mg once only.

Amiodarone   Amiodarone is used to increase the duration of the action potential in both the atrial and ventricular myocardium, thus prolonging the QT interval. Amiodarone 300 mg is considered for use in treating shock-refractory cardiac arrest due to VF or pulseless VT after the third shock. Lidocaine may be given as an alternative if amiodarone is not available; however, both should not be given.

Calcium salts   In cardiac cell activity, calcium ions play a vital role in contraction, as well as during the cell's action potential. Calcium is indicated during resuscitation from PEA when the cause is

● hypocalcaemia
● hyperkalaemia
● overdose of calcium-channel-blocking drugs
● overdose of magnesium (e.g. during treatment of pre-eclampsia (Resuscitation Council (UK) 2005).

Sodium bicarbonate   Controversy continues as to the efficacy of this drug and its routine use is not recommended. It may be considered for the reversal of life-threatening hyperkalaemia, pre-existing metabolic acidosis or tricyclic antidepressant overdose (ILCOR 2000a).

Whether the resuscitation is successful or not, thought and consideration for family or relatives must be a priority. Clear lines of communication must exist between medical and nursing staff and any family/friends. If the need to break bad news arises, ideally the doctor and the ED nurse should perform this, with one or the other actually breaking the news. More often than not these simple communication skills are forgotten (see Box 26.6). A detailed discussion of this subject is given in Chapter 13 (Care of the Bereaved).

Ethical considerations

Occasionally the subject of 'do not attempt resuscitation' orders (DNAR) will present itself. In a joint statement from the British Medical Association and Royal College of Nursing (Resuscitation Council 2001), it was determined that the overall responsibility for decisions about CPR and DNAR rests with the consultant in charge of the patient's care. This decision should

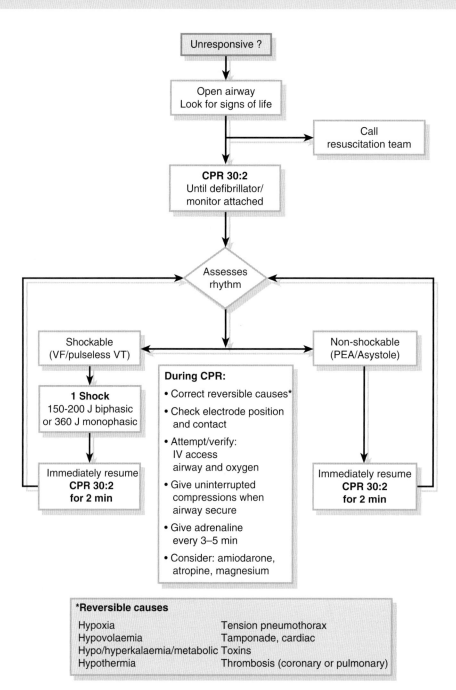

Figure 26.14 Universal algorithm (Resuscitation Council 2005).

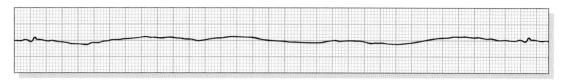

Figure 26.15   Asystole.

Box 26.5   Causes of electromechanical disassociation

Primary causes
- Myocardial infarction (particularly inferior wall)
- Drugs (beta-blockers or calcium antagonists) or toxins
- Electrolyte abnormalities (such as hypocalcaemia, hyperkalaemia)
- Atrial thrombus or tumour (myxoma)

Secondary causes
- Tension pneumothorax
- Pericardial tamponade
- Cardiac rupture
- Pulmonary embolism
- Prosthetic heart valve occlusion
- Hypovolaemia

Box 26.6   Communicating with relatives/friends

- Prepare yourself. Compose your thoughts
- Enter the room/area with another person, e.g., a doctor or nurse
- Confirm that you are talking to the correct relatives/friends
- Spend time with the relatives. Avoid appearing harassed or impatient
- Maintain eye contact when talking
- Be prepared to emphasise and repeat any information
- Avoid using the wrong terms, i.e. 'slipped away' or 'passed on'. Be honest, say the person has died
- Don't be afraid of silences
- Be prepared for wide variety of reactions

---

involve the medical and nursing staff, the patient (if possible) and the family and must be clearly documented, including the date, decision and the reasons for it (Resuscitation Council 2001, Alexander et al. 2000). It is also discussed in Chapter 13 (Care of the bereaved).

RHYTHM DISTURBANCES

It is important when caring for a patient with a presenting cardiac condition that the recognition of any abnormalities is accurate and prompt. Reference to the UK treatments algorithms for tachycardias and bradycardias may prove useful to the ED nurse when considering the management of arrythmias (Resuscitation Council (UK) 2005). Rhythm disturbances can be divided into two groups: ventricular and atrial arrhythmias. Those commonly treated in ED are discussed below.

Ventricular Ectopics (VEs)

This is due to premature discharge of an ectopic ventricular focus (Schamroth 2001) (Fig. 26.16). The impulse avoids travelling through conducting tissue, but travels through ordinary muscle structure. Causes of VEs include:

- hypoxia
- myocardial ischaemia
- hypokalaemia
- hypercalcaemia
- acidosis
- caffeine
- digoxin toxicity.

Assessment
The aim of assessment is to determine both causative factors and level of systemic compromise. This should include pulse speed, regularity and pressure, respiration and blood pressure. Repeated VEs reduce ventricular filling time and can result in a reduction of circulatory volume. A 12-lead ECG should be obtained to confirm diagnosis. ECG characteristics are shown in Table 26.1.

Management
The patient may present with palpitations or shortness of breath. Immediate treatment of ventricular ectopics can include the use of anti-arrhythmic drugs, such as intravenous amiodarone. For long-term control, oral preparations such as beta-blockers, calcium-channel blockers or amiodarone can be used. Correction of the urea and electrolyte imbalance can lead to the resolution of VEs.

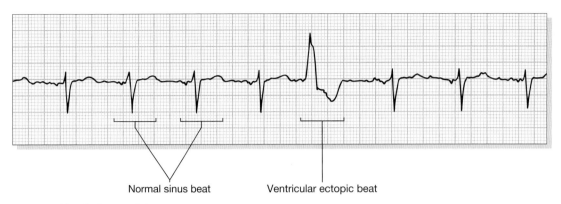

Normal sinus beat   Ventricular ectopic beat

Figure 26.16   Ventricular ectopic beat.

Table 26.1	ECG characteristics of ventricular ectopics
Component	**Finding**
Rhythm	Irregular, due to premature beats
Rate	60–100 beats/min
P wave	Not related to QRS complex of the VE
QRS	Wide and bizarre complex of a VE

Ventricular tachycardia (VT)

Ventricular contraction is stimulated from within as ventricular myocardium and does not follow normal electrical conductivity (see Fig. 26.17). The causes of VT are the same as those of VEs, but it is considered more dangerous due to its capacity to significantly decrease cardiac output. The cardiac output is compromised due to the shortening of the cardiac cycle, and thus there is a reduced amount of blood available for ejection (Woods et al. 2000). The ventricular myocardium is not able to sustain rapid contraction over prolonged periods and there is therefore a tendency for VF to follow untreated VT.

Assessment
This is the same as assessing a patient with multiple VE's. The important factor is determining the degree of systemic compromise through levels of consciousness, pulse, respirations and blood pressure. ECG characteristics are shown Table 26.2.

Management
Presenting symptoms may include shortness of breath, palpitations, dizziness and diaphoresis. Treatment may incorporate the use of 300 mg amiodarone

Table 26.2	ECG characteristics of ventricular tachycardia
Component	**Finding**
Rhythm	Either regular or slightly irregular
Rate	Faster than 100 beats/min
P waves	Dissociated from QRS complexes
QRS	Wide and bizarre

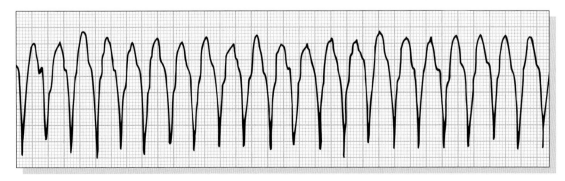

Figure 26.17   Ventricular tachycardia.

i.v. over 20–60 minutes, followed by an infusion of 900 mg over 24 hours (Resuscitation Council (UK) 2005). If initial drug therapy is not successful and the patient is showing signs of cardiovascular compromise, cardioversion with synchronized DC shock should be carried out. The patient should be sedated for this procedure, unless his clinical condition is deteriorating too rapidly to facilitate this. If VT becomes pulseless at any time, emergency defibrillation should be carried out, and the algorithm in Fig. 26.14 followed.

Supraventricular tachycardia (SVT)

This does not always stem from atrial activity, but it does originate from above the ventricles and it is difficult to pinpoint the exact causative factor from the ECG (Fig. 26.18). The atria can depolarize in a retrograde fashion or a circular fashion depending on the causative factors.

Causes include:

- atrial tachycardia
- atrial flutter/fibrillation
- stimulants, e.g. caffeine or nicotine
- idiopathic.

Assessment
This should concentrate on determining the patient's capacity to compensate for the rapid heart rate. Pulse, respirations and blood pressure are vital indicators. The patient will probably be aware of palpitations or 'pounding' in his chest and may complain of pain, dizziness and shortness of breath. The ECG characteristics are shown in Table 26.3.

Management
Depending on the patient's tolerance of the SVT, vagal stimulation can be attempted to slow down the heart rate. This can be achieved by carotid sinus massage and is sufficient to control SVT in about 20% of cases (ILCOR 2005a); however, overzealous treatment can result in profound bradycardia or VF

Table 26.3 ECG characteristics of supraventricular tachycardia

Component	Finding
Rhythm	Regular
Rate	>100 and up to 280 beats/min
P wave	Not usually visible
QRS	Usually narrow

(Skinner & Vincent 1997). Drug therapy of choice is adenosine, with the initial dose of 6 mg given by rapid bolus injection. If required, two further doses of 12 mg can be administered. Adenosine works by depressing AV node conduction and therefore prevents re-entry rhythms from sustaining SVT, allowing sinus rhythm to return. Side-effects of adenosine are common, and the nurse should expect the patient to be flushed, nauseous and have some chest discomfort. These effects are short-lived and should have passed in a matter of minutes (Opie 2000). If the patient's condition continues to deteriorate, a synchronized DC shock is indicated.

Atrial ectopics

This is a premature discharge of an ectopic atrial focus from a point other than the sinoatrial node (Julian 1998) (Fig. 26.19). Causes include:

- alcohol
- mitral valve disease
- coronary artery disease
- hyperthyroidism
- heart failure
- viral infections.

It can also occur in healthy individuals.

Assessment
Diagnosis is made on ECG tracing as the patient is usually unaware of the occurrence of atrial ectopics. Pulse rate should be checked for irregularity and

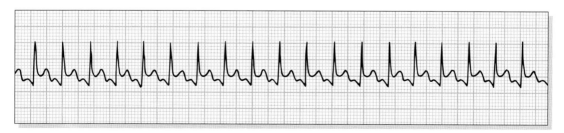

Figure 26.18 Supraventricular tachycardia.

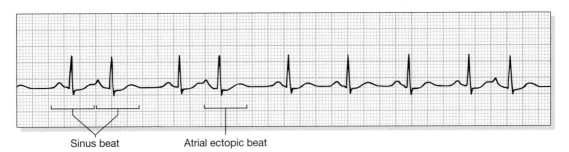

Sinus beat   Atrial ectopic beat

Figure 26.19 Atrial ectopic beats.

respiration may be slightly increased. ECG findings are shown in Table 26.4.

Management
The patient is usually unaware, but can present with shortness of breath. The treatment of atrial ectopics is not usually required unless the patient shows signs of compromise. Drugs used include disopyramide.

Atrial fibrillation

Atrial fibrillation (AF), which affects 5–10% of older people (Houghton & Gray 1997), is a rapid and disorganized depolarization occurring throughout the atrial myocardium, replacing normal rhythmic activity by the SA node (Hand 2002). Every minute 400–600 impulses reach the AV node from different atrial foci rather than the SA node but only 120–180 of these reach the ventricles to produce QRS complexes (Fig. 26.20). Causes include:

- hypertension
- ischaemic heart disease
- binge alcohol drinking
- atrial septal defect
- pulmonary embolus
- pneumonia
- cardiomyopathy
- idiopathic
- rheumatic heart disease
- myocardial infarction
- mitral valve disease.

Assessment

The fast pace at which the atria depolarize leads to failure of the atria to contract effectively, causing them to quiver. This means that the ventricles do not fill adequately, which can lead to a 10–15% fall in cardiac output (Houghton and Gray 1997). Patients with AF often present with palpitations or symptoms of an underlying cause. Respirations, pulse and blood pressure should be ascertained. The patient may complain of weakness, dizziness or shortness of breath. ECG changes are listed in Table 26.5.

Table 26.4 ECG characteristics of atrial ectopic beats

Component	Finding
Rhythm	Slightly irregular
Rate	Usually within normal limits
P wave	Precede every QRS
QRS	Normally no change is seen

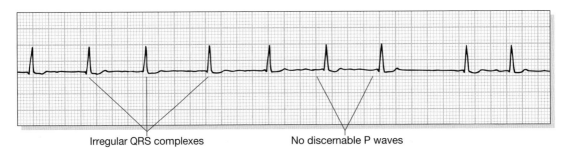

Irregular QRS complexes   No discernable P waves

Figure 26.20 Atrial fibrillation.

Table 26.5	ECG characteristics of atrial fibrillation
Component	Finding
Rhythm	Irregular
Rate	Variable, but usually >100 beats/min
P waves	Not present
QRS	Normal

Management

The aim of treatment of AF is usually to eliminate the cause in order to control the ventricular rate, thereby optimizing cardiac function, reducing the risk of embolism and restoring sinus rhythm (Hand 2002). If the duration is less than 48 hours, and rhythm control is considered appropriate, this may be attempted using amiodarone 300 mg i.v. over 20–60 min followed by 900 mg over 24 hours (Resuscitation Council (UK) 2005). If the patient is severely compromised, cardioversion may be necessary. Other symptoms can include an increased risk of thrombus formation, and hence the need for anticoagulants.

Atrial flutter

Atrial flutter occurs when there is rapid atrial excitement and is much less common than atrial fibrillation. The term flutter is used as the P waves appear 'sawtoothed' (O'Connor 1995) (Fig. 26.21). It is almost always associated with significant cardiac abnormalities (Hand 2002). The atrial rate can be anything between 250 and 350 beats/min, but the ventricular rate is much lower because of AV filtering which acts as a 'gatekeeper'. In contrast to atrial fibrillation, the rate is regular.

The causes include:

- ischaemic heart disease with left ventricular dysfunction
- mitral valve disease
- acute MI
- hypertension

Assessment

Assessment is the same as for AF (see Table 26.6).

Management

Hudak et al. (1998) suggest that slowing down the rhythm using adenosine or vagal manoeuvres should increase the degree of AV block and make the rhythm more apparent. Although drugs can be used to control the ventricular rate, the aim should be to restore sinus rhythm. If the patient is compromised, oxygen will be required (Hand 2002). Treatment comprises digoxin or verapamil, or in severe cases cardioversion may be required. Other drugs which may aid treatment include amiodarone, beta-blockers or disopyramide.

HEART BLOCK

Heart block occurs when the impulses from the atria to the ventricles are delayed at the AV node (Hampton 2003). There are, for the purpose of this chapter, three types of heart block:

- first-degree heart block
- second-degree heart block
- third-degree (complete) heart block

These can be a complication of a myocardial infarction.

First–degree heart block (Fig. 26.22)

As can be seen from the rhythm strip, the P-R interval is prolonged. This is due to the delay at the AV node,

Table 26.6	ECG characteristics of atrial flutter
Component	Finding
Rhythm	Usually regular
Rate	Variable, but usually >100 beats/min
P Waves	Usually obscured by flutter waves
QRS	Normal, may be widened by bundle branch block

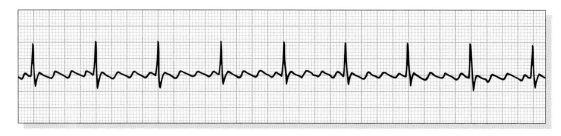

Figure 26.21 Atrial flutter.

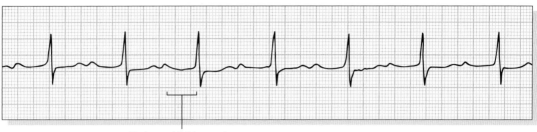

Prolonged P-R interval

Figure 26.22   First-degree heart block.

where impulses conduct to the ventricles but with delayed conduction times (Jacobson 2000, Jowett & Thompson 2002). The ECG characteristics are given in Table 26.7.

Management
In most instances the patient remains asymptomatic and does not require any further treatment, but for the reasons of safety should be re-evaluated at regular intervals.

Second-degree heart block (Fig. 26.23)

There are two types of second-degree block: type I (Wenckebach) and type II (see Table 26.8 for ECG

Table 26.7   ECG characteristics of first degree heart block

Component	Finding
Rhythm	Regular
Rate	Sinus, between 60 and 100 beats/min
P wave	Normal
P–R interval	Prolonged, i.e. >0.20 s
QRS	Normal

Table 26.8   ECG characteristics of second degree heart block

Component	Finding
Rhythm	Regular
Rate	Sinus or atrial beats
P waves	Normal
P–R interval	Can lengthen or can be normal
QRS	Normal

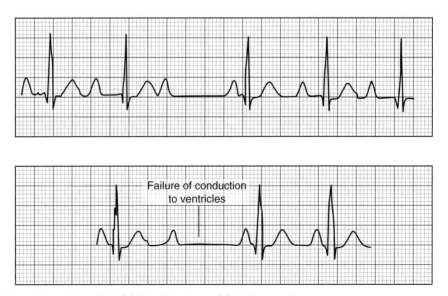

Failure of conduction to ventricles

Figure 26.23   Second degree heart block (a) Wenckebach type. (b) Mobitz type II.

characteristics). In type I, second-degree AV block a gradual lengthening of the P-R interval occurs because of lengthening AV conduction time, until an atrial pulse is non-conducted, so a P wave is not followed by a QRS. Then the sequence begins again. The blocked P wave may occur occasionally or frequently, regularly or irregularly. Of the second-degree heart blocks, type I is the most common, is usually transitory and rarely progresses to complete heart block. It produces few or no clinical symptoms although a 2:1 type block may develop with haemodynamic instability. In type II second-degree AV heart block, a P wave is blocked without progressive antecedent P-R elongation and occurs almost always in a setting of bundle branch block. Type II second-degree block is often caused by irreversible damage and frequently progresses to complete heart block. Clinical symptoms such as dizziness or faintness may occur with frequent non-conducted P waves (Erickson 1996, Wyatt et al. 1999).

Management

Depending on the patient's tolerance to the rhythm, there may or may not be a need for treatment. If the patient is compromised, i.v. atropine is the first-line drug for bradycardias. Then consider adrenaline and seek expert help. The patient may need temporary pacing to avert the need for pacemaker insertion in a compromised patient if sudden complete heart block develops (Hand 2002).

Third-degree (complete) heart block (Fig. 26.24)

This type of heart block is characterized by the unrelated impulses sent between the atria and the ventricles. When this occurs there is no correlation of the electrical activity and a disassociation develops between the atria and ventricles. This in turn means that the cardiac output is reduced to the point where the patient usually becomes symptomatic.

Assessment

A nodal rhythm gives a rate of around 40–60 beats, while a ventricular rhythm gives a rate of 30–40 beats/min. If this so-called 'escape' rhythm does not develop, ventricular standstill will occur and this is fatal if not treated (Hand 2002). It is important to assess the level of circulatory compromise as a treatment guideline. Some patients will present profoundly, with a history of collapse. This is due to severe circulatory collapse as a result of poor cardiac output due to decreased atrial and ventricular synchronicity. The ECG characteristics are given in Table 26.9.

Management

Treatment ultimately depends on the symptoms encountered. If the cause is acute inferior MI, drug toxicity, acute pericarditis or myocarditis, total AV block is usually a passing phenomenon. Drug therapy includes atropine and isoprenaline, but in most instances requires the insertion of either a temporary or a permanent pacing system to maintain the patient's cardiac equilibrium. In cases of profound collapse, external pacing is necessary to maintain circulatory volume. Nolan et al. (1998) estimate that up

Table 26.9 ECG characteristics of third degree heart block

Component	Finding
Rhythm	Regular
Rate	Normal atrial rate, but the ventricular rate can be less than 45 beats/min
P wave	Normal, but shows no relation to the QRS complexes
P-R interval	No consistent P-R interval exists
QRS	Normal, although sometimes wide

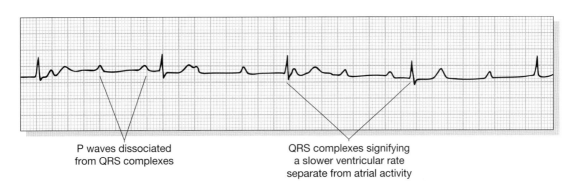

P waves dissociated from QRS complexes

QRS complexes signifying a slower ventricular rate separate from atrial activity

Figure 26.24 Complete (third degree) heart block.

to 89% of patients who develop complete heart block following anterior MI die, often from pump failure due to ventricular damage.

PACING

It is sometimes necessary to support a patient's conductive system by means of a pacing system. The purpose of pacemakers is to control the electrical activity of the heart (Julian 1998). Both temporary and permanent pacing systems contain two components:

- pulse generator (pacing box) – this forms the electrical supply source for pacing; the box usually contains batteries as its power source
- pacing catheter – this conductive wire has either one or two electrodes to provide an electrical stimulus to the heart, once the pacing catheter electrodes are in direct contact with the myocardium.

There are currently three types of pacemaker available:

- non-invasive temporary pacing
- temporary (transvenous) pacing
- permanent pacing

Non-invasive temporary pacing (NTP)

This system of pacing is used predominately by EDs to treat symptomatic bradycardias and ventricular asystole. Most EDs in the UK have access to a defibrillator with pacing facilities, e.g. the Physio Control Lifepak 20. The advantages of NTP include its ability to be initiated rapidly, its ease of use and the fact that CPR can be continued without risk to the user. To use NTP, two large electrodes are placed on the chest as shown in Fig. 26.25.

Once NTP has been commenced it is important to look for signs of electrical and mechanical capture. When looking for signs of electrical capture, a heart trace can provide the evidence required. A pacing spike should be followed by a wide QRS and a tall broad T wave (Fig. 26.26). Mechanical capture is seen by the improvements in the patient's condition.

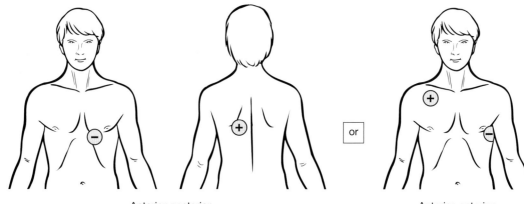

Anterior-posterior

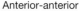

Anterior-anterior

Figure 26.25   Positioning of pacing pads for non-invasive temporary pacing.

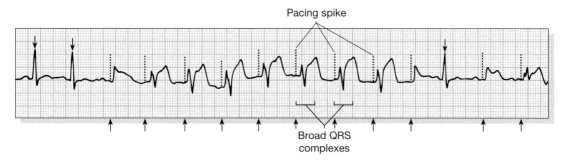

Figure 26.26   Non-invasive temporary pacing.

Compared with other forms of pacing, NTP is, on the surface, a more favourable approach to emergency pacing.

Temporary pacing (transvenous)

The indications for the insertion of a temporary transvenous pacing wire include (Timmis & Nathan 1997):

- extreme bradycardia
- complete heart block
- asystole
- very occasionally for tachycardias.

A bipolar pacing catheter is inserted through a central or peripheral vein (subclavian, external jugular or antecubital fossa) under sterile conditions, using ECG monitoring and fluoroscopy equipment. A local anaesthetic is used prior to insertion. Once the pacing catheter has been sited, the electrodes are then connected to the external pulse generator (pacing box). Complications include:

- pneumothorax
- infection
- cardiac perforation
- arrhythmias

Permanent pacing

The decision to use an implantable pacing system remains dependent on the patient's symptoms. Symptomatic patients are fitted with a permanent pacemaker by inserting the power source (lithium-driven) with a subcutaneous pocket under the clavicle or axilla. The procedure is performed under a local anaesthetic. The majority of permanent pacemakers fitted today have an approximate life span of 15 years.

ACUTE CHEST PAIN

Acute coronary syndromes

These consist of:

1. Non-Q wave myocardial infarction, now better known as non-ST elevation MI or non-STEMI (subendocardial or intramural wall damage)
2. Q wave myocardial infarction (full thickness myocardial necrosis) known as ST segment elevation MI (STEMI)
3. Unstable angina (myocardial ischaemia without necrosis).

Non-ST segment elevation myocardial infarction can occur with partial or transient blocking of the coronary artery. This can produce less extensive damage to the surrounding muscle. However, testing serum troponin levels will show that necrosis has occurred. With Q wave myocardial infarction, sometimes the typical ST changes are not seen; however, if ischaemia persists, typical Q waves will appear on the ECG.

Unstable angina is a symptom, not a disease, brought on by inadequate coronary blood flow to the myocardium (Jowett & Thompson 2002, Woods et al. 2000). Castle (2003) notes that while the myocardium has no 'pain fibres', ischaemic hearts do produce lactic acid, bradykinin, adenosine, prostaglandins, potassium and carbon dioxide. Each of these has been linked with the stimulation of pain fibres in coronary arteries or the transmission of pain as a noxious stimulus (Jowett & Thompson 2002). It usually presents as central chest pain with either a rapid or gradual onset over several minutes, with possible radiation to the jaw, back and arms. It can occur at rest or on exertion. When chest pain has been unremitting for 20 minutes at rest, myocardial infarction should be considered (Braunwald et al. 2000). Other associated symptoms include breathlessness, dizziness, belching and epigastric discomfort after eating.

Assessment

When a patient presents to the ED with chest pain secondary to unstable angina it is usually because previous attempts to relieve the pain have failed. On average patients delay seeking medical care for acute MI symptoms for two or more hours (Zerwic 1999); however, prompt assessment of the patient with acute coronary syndromes is critical as the incidence of ventricular fibrillation is greater during the first hour after the onset of acute MI symptoms (Barnason 2003).

It is very often difficult to distinguish between unstable angina and acute MI during the initial assessment of the patient, thus the management in the first few hours will often be similar to that for an MI. When assessing the patient it is important to gain a detailed history. This should include: the type (e.g., crushing, burning, sharp), severity and duration of the pain, what the patient was doing when the pain started, and whether anything has been taken to relieve it. Any radiation of pain should be noted because it helps to confirm a clinical picture of cardiac pain. Any symptoms associated with the onset of pain or still present are also important as they act as an indication of the level of systemic compromise resulting from myocardial hypoxia. The patient's medical and drug history should also be noted.

Physical assessment should include baseline observations of pulse rate, regularity and pressure, respirations and blood pressure. These should enable the ED nurse to determine the impact of the angina on the patient's overall condition. Temperature should also be checked, as a rise in temperature can be indicative of tissue breakdown, consistent with a myocardial infarction. Cardiac monitoring, 12-lead ECG recording and X-ray help complete the clinical picture. The ECG may show any associated rhythm disturbance and most importantly any ischaemic changes to the myocardium as a result of hypoxia. ECG changes may show as ST-segment depression in the area affected by hypoxia (see Fig. 26.27, Table 26.10).

Clinical investigations include blood analysis to detect electrolyte imbalance, cardiac enzymes or cardiac troponins consistent with myocardial infarction. Blood should be taken for full blood count, urea and electrolyte levels, glucose (which can rise after acute infection) and cardiac enzymes and troponins. Detection of raised troponin levels indicates a diagnosis of non-ST-elevated MI, and absence of detectable troponin is indicative of unstable angina (Fox 2004). Troponin reaches detectably raised levels hours after a cardiac event, and so may not be abnormal at initial presentation. Raised levels can be detected three to four hours after the event and remain elevated for up to two weeks. Coady (2006) argues this is important if the patient re-presents within this timeframe.

Table 26.10	Classification of angina
Classification	**Characteristics**
Stable angina	Condition in which the frequency and severity of angina remain well controlled and unchanged over months
Angina decubitus	Pain occurring when lying down
Unstable angina	Condition in which the pain is increasing in frequency, severity and duration. Occurs with less activity or at rest
Printzmetal's angina	Unusual form where pain occurs at rest or long after activity has ceased. Accompanied by transient ST-segment elevation. Coronary artery spasm without underlying disease is often the cause
Crescendo angina	Form of angina where chance of an MI occurring within a few days is high
Intractable angina	Continued pain with increasing frequency, despite treatment

French & White (2004) recommend that troponin levels should be measured at presentation, at 6 to 9 hours and at 12 hours to ensure correct diagnosis. It is important to note that troponins are specific to myocardial injury rather than to myocardial infarction so other causes of cardiac damage should be excluded through the patient history and clinical examination. In addition, elevated troponin levels may be present in other conditions, such as renal failure, sepsis and heart failure, so it is important this test is used as part of an overall clinical assessment (Fox 2004, Coady 2006). A chest X-ray is useful to detect any cardiac failure or enlargement. Isoenzymes may also be useful if other trauma, such as cardiac massage, has taken place.

Management

It is useful to obtain i.v. access early in the patient's management in order to administer pain relief or supportive drugs if necessary. The aim is to restore a normal blood flow through the coronary arteries, so that myocardial oxygen supply and demand is met. It is important that oxygen therapy is commenced at the earliest opportunity. This both acts as a pain-relieving agent and reduces the likelihood of tissue damage. It is necessary to reduce the workload of the heart, which relieves the symptoms experienced by the patient. Sublingual glyceryl trinitrate (GTN) is an effective first-line treatment. It works by causing

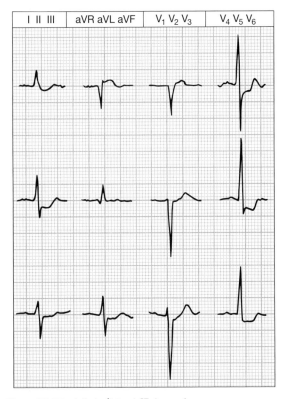

Figure 26.27   Inferior/lateral ST depression.

venous and coronary artery dilatation. This in turn causes a reduction in preload and consequently a reduction in afterload (Khan 2000), therefore allowing blood to flow with less effort from the myocardium, increasing the amount of oxygen to the heart and subsequently decreasing chest pain. Diamorphine is the preferred agent for the treatment of patients with ongoing chest pain. It relieves chest pain and anxiety, which decreases myocardial oxygen consumption. Opiate and GTN substances should also be given as an i.v. infusion titrated to the patient's pain blood pressure, to ensure that vasodilatation is not excessive. Aspirin should as be given as a general measure.

Other drugs that can be used include:

- beta-blockers
- calcium antagonists.

Other aspects in the management of unstable angina include a reduction in activity and adjustments in lifestyle, if risks to the patient's health have been noted. If symptoms do not settle with analgesia, or if ECG changes persist after pain subsides, the patient should be admitted for observation and specialist management.

Myocardial infarction

Myocardial infarction (MI) is defined as the death or necrosis of part of the myocardium due to the reduction or cessation of blood flow (Alexander et al. 2000). The treatment of acute MI remains a major medical challenge, with over 300 000 patients presenting annually in the UK (Department of Health 2000). The major cause of the final event leading to acute MI is thrombosis formation in a narrowed coronary artery from ruptured or fissured atherosclerotic plaque. Subsequent vessel occlusion and thrombosis cause myocardial hypoxia and necrosis. Myocardial hypoxia may also be caused by coronary artery spasm and dissecting aortic aneurysm. Complete necrosis occurs in 4 to 6 hours and the area surrounding the zone of necrosis is ischaemic. Damage of the myocardium predisposes the patient to pump failure and various dysrhythmias secondary to conduction defects and irritability of myocardial tissue. The location and size of the infarct depend on the coronary artery affected and where the occlusion occurs. Most acute MIs are caused by a blockage of the left anterior descending coronary artery, which causes involvement of the anterior wall of the myocardium (Barnason 2003, Doering 1999) (Fig. 26.28).

The crucial aspect in the management of MIs is rapid commencement of treatment as soon as possible after the onset of symptoms. In ED, rapid treatment relies on accurate and thorough assessment by ED nurses.

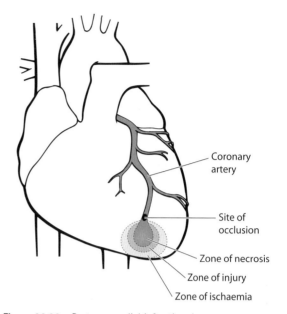

Figure 26.28 Post-myocardial infarction damage.

Assessment

Assessment of patients having an MI should follow the same structure as a patient with acute coronary syndrome. In addition, the patient is likely to appear:

- pale
- sweating or clammy
- short of breath
- possibly cyanosed
- nauseous and vomiting
- anxious.

The 12-lead ECG is an important tool in the diagnosis of an MI, but should be taken in context with the overall clinical picture. The ECG usually demonstrates specific changes in the areas of myocardial damage. These are linked to the time span of injury and duration of pain. During the first hour of pain there is little change to the ECG; however, T waves may flatten. After this, the ST segment may elevate and during the next 12–24 hours Q waves begin to develop as myocardium becomes necrotic and electrical conduction ceases. In general, ST segment elevation myocardial infarctions are associated with a larger region of myocardial necrosis, higher enzyme levels, fresh coronary thrombosis, frequent vomiting, congestive heart failure, conduction defects, dysrhythmias and less collateral circulation (Barnason 2003). T waves become inverted because repolarization changes. In some instances, the ECG trace will remain with Q waves and inverted T waves in damaged areas. In other instances, T waves will turn upright after a period of time (see Fig. 26.29).

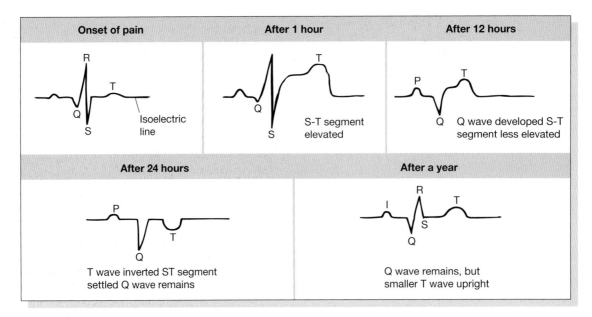

Onset of pain	After 1 hour	After 12 hours
Isoelectric line	S-T segment elevated	Q wave developed S-T segment less elevated

After 24 hours	After a year
T wave inverted ST segment settled Q wave remains	Q wave remains, but smaller T wave upright

Figure 26.29   ECG changes following myocardial infarction.

In addition to the progress of the MI, the ECG will also depict the areas of the myocardium affected by the infarct (see Box 26.3).

Blood pressure   In the majority of cases the blood pressure appears low. This is due to poor ventricular function and a reduced cardiac output. The frequency of BP recordings should be of an optimum level to detect any further changes in the patient's condition.

Pulse   Predominately the patient will be tachycardic as a response to the decreased cardiac output, but the anxiety levels should also be taken into account as these can also induce a tachycardia due to the sympathetic response. Specific side-effects of infarction should also be considered. Bradycardia is frequently associated with inferior infarction.

Respiration   Tachypnoea or dyspnoea will usually be evident. These can indicate levels of hypoxia and the onset of pulmonary oedema. Oxygen therapy is vital in MIs to ensure that the myocardium is receiving as much oxygen as possible.

Temperature   is sometimes forgotten, but in the instance of an MI a mild pyrexia can be indicative of muscle damage due to an inflammatory response (Woods et al. 2000).

Blood analysis   Similar to chest pain from unstable angina, blood analysis should include cardiac enzymes and cardiac troponins (troponin I and troponin T). Following an MI there is a rise in the levels of myocardial enzymes present. Assessment of troponins, which are highly sensitive and more specific than creatinine kinase, can now identify smaller areas of myocardial necrosis than previously (Coady 2006). It is these enzymes that aid in the diagnosis of an MI (Jowett & Thompson 2002) and they include (see also Table 26.11):

- creatinine kinase (CK)
- lactic dehydrogenase (LDH)
- aspartate aminotransferase (AST)

Table 26.11   Cardiac enzyme changes following a myocardial infarction

Enzyme	Released into circulation		
	Initially	Peaks	Range (normal)
Creatinine phosphokinase (CPK)	6 h	18–36 h	200–1000 u/ml (100 u/ml)
Serum aspartate transferase (formerly glutamic oxalo-acetic transaminase, SGOT)	12–24 h	36–48 h	>100 u/ml (50 u/ml)
Lactic dehydrogenase (LDH)	2–3 days	7 days	
Troponin	4–6 h	10–24 h	<0.5 ng/ml

- cardiac troponins (troponin I and troponin T).

CK, LDH and AST are released in the first 24 hours after the onset of a myocardial infarct. These enzymes may provide retrospective confirmation of infarction rather than a guide to immediate management (analgesia, aspirin, thrombolysis). While troponin is a sensitive biomarker to 'rule out' non-ST-segment elevation myocardial infarction, it is less useful to 'rule in' this event because it may lack specificity for acute coronary syndromes (Jaffe et al. 2001).

Changes to other levels are as follows:

- *Full blood count*. A rise in both the white blood count and ESR is indicative of muscle necrosis.
- *Urea and electrolytes*. Sodium and potassium ions are important in cardiac function due to their involvement within the action potential. This analysis is also important as it helps to determine if there is any renal function impairment present.
- *Glucose*. As previously stated, a rise in the blood glucose can be indicative of stress-related hyperglycaemia. However, 5% of cardiac patients admitted to hospital have previously undiagnosed diabetes (Alexander et al. 2000).
- *Lipids*. Raised cholesterol and triglycerides are common in ischaemic heart disease.

Chest X-ray may show fluid levels associated with oedema or an enlarged heart.

Management
The aim of care is to (Alexander et al. 2000):

- limit the infarction size
- re-establish an optimal cardiac output
- relieve pain
- detect and prevent any life-threatening complications.

Oxygen therapy should be commenced as early as possible in an attempt to limit myocardial damage and relieve pain. Pain control in patients with an MI should be achieved by using i.v. opiates, such as diamorphine or cyclomorph. These provide pain relief but also have a mild diuretic effect, hence enabling a better ventricular function (Opie 2000). An anti-emetic, such as cyclizine or metoclopramide, is also indicated as it reduces any previous nausea and counteracts the nauseated feelings associated with opiates.

Thrombolytic therapy
Thrombolytic therapy is vital if the integrity of the myocardium is to be preserved. Rapid administration of thrombolytic therapy reverses the effects of ischaemia and injury before necrosis can occur, therefore dramatically changing the outcome for the patient (Quinn & Thompson 1995).

Thrombolytic therapy is well established as a treatment that reduces mortality (Fibrinolytic Therapy Trialists' Collaborative Group 1994) after STEMI. The amount of time that passes from onset of symptoms to myocardial salvage relates directly to patient mortality. There is a decrease in lives saved from 65 per 1000 patients treated with thrombolytic therapy within an hour of onset of symptoms to 29 per 1000 patients treated at between three and six hours (Boersma 1996, Castle 2006). Thrombolytic therapy retains a clinical benefit for up to 12 hours after onset of symptoms and, under specific conditions, benefit may be evident for up to 24 hours (Late Assessment of Thrombolytic Efficacy Steering Committee 1993). Currently 61% of suitable patients receive thrombolytic therapy within three hours of onset of symptoms, with 40% receiving treatment in less than two hours (Birkhead et al. 2004).

The Department of Health (2000) recommends thrombolytic drug therapy within 20 minutes of the patient's arrival at hospital. The National Service Framework for Coronary Heart Disease (Department of Health 2000) has stimulated a major reorganization of how thrombolysis is delivered through the measurement of treatment times and has seen a move a way from coronary care unit led thrombolysis services to services being led in ED (Castle 2006). It is essential that predetermined protocols exist for the treatment of these patients and that criteria are set down to facilitate the administration of thrombolytic drugs as early as possible (ILCOR 2005c).

Thrombolytic therapy dissolves the thrombus/clot occluding a coronary artery and restores blood flow to the myocardium, therefore limiting damage. Therapy is administered via an intravenous route, usually prepared as an infusion.

There are four thrombolytic agents available for use in the management of STEMI; streptokinase, and three fibrin-specific agents, alteplase, reteplase and tenecteplase. Streptokinase is a bacterial protein that reduces circulatory fibrinogen and clotting factors V and VIII (Alexander et al. 2000); however, it is also associated with significant incidence of hypotension, bradycardia and allergic reaction when compared with third-generation thrombolytic agents such as alteplase, reteplase and tenecteplase (Castle 2006). Recombinant tissue-type plasminogen activator (tPA) (alteplase) is a single bolus, fibrin-specific and works mainly on dispersement of the clot, therefore reducing the risk of systemic effects (see Box 26.7).

During therapy, the ED nurse should be vigilant for signs of reperfusion (see Box 26.8) and complications. Blood pressure and ECG monitoring should be frequent, and the patient should not be left unattended. Complications include reperfusion arrhythmias, including VF, allergic reactions and hypotension. The patient may feel flushed, generally unwell and have a headache. Bleeding episodes can also occur.

Other drugs of benefit include aspirin, which inhibits platelet aggregation and reduces blood viscosity, therefore reducing the risks of further thrombus activity. For the appropriate management of patients suffering from an MI, ED staff must be aware of current trends and treatments in cardiac care in order to understand more fully, and care more competently for, this group of patients. For optimal care, patients with an acute MI should be 'fast-tracked' to coronary care units at the earliest opportunity.

ACUTE CARDIAC FAILURE

In 1995 the New York Heart Association renamed and reclassified all types of heart failure under the heading of 'heart failure'. There are now four classifications of heart failure, but for the purposes of this chapter the term is used to depict the clinical manifestations that relate to this condition. Heart failure is characterized as the heart's inability to provide an adequate cardiac output for the body's metabolic requirements (Alexander et al. 2000).

Acute left ventricular failure (LVF)

Left ventricular failure often presents suddenly and is usually associated with pulmonary oedema. LVF is also a frequent complication of MI. Common causes include:

- myocardial infarction
- coronary artery disease
- diabetes mellitus
- cardiac drugs – beta-blockers, or calcium antagonists
- alcohol
- hypertension
- cardiomyopathy
- valvular disease
- arrhythmias
- hypertension
- pericarditis
- pericardial effusion
- pregnancy
- severe anaemia
- ventricular or atrial septal defect

The mechanics of LVF mean that the heart is regarded as a failing pump, with more blood remaining in the ventricle at the end of each cardiac cycle (Tortora & Grabowski 2000). Often, this build-up of pressure results in blood being forced to seep back into the lungs, causing an increase in pressure and resulting in pulmonary oedema. In response to the pump mechanism failing, blood can also back up from the right ventricle into the systemic circulation, causing peripheral oedema due to the increase in capillary pressure causing fluid to seep into the tissues. This is most noticeable in the ankles and feet.

Assessment

Typically, LVF and pulmonary oedema occur in the night or early hours of the morning due to an increase in venous return when lying down. The usual presentation in ED includes:

- cold/clammy appearance
- severe dyspnoea
- cyanotic appearance
- tachycardia
- raised jugular venous pressure (JVP)

The assessment findings are summarized in Box 26.9.

Immediate priorities for care
- Airway assessment
- Oxygen therapy
- Baseline observations
- Cardiac monitoring
- Intravenous or central line access
- Diuretics
- Catheterization for urine output measurement.

Box 26.9   Assessment findings in left ventricular failure

- **Respirations.** Airway is of paramount importance, as the presence of pulmonary oedema exacerbates any shortness of breath and causes hypoxia. Depending on the severity of the hypoxia, airway adjuncts such as oropharyngeal or nasopharyngeal airways may be required. Extreme cases may require intubation and ventilation.

- **Pulse.** Tachycardias are prominent in LVF with the heart beating faster in an attempt to compensate for the reduced cardiac output

- **Blood pressure.** Hypotension is usually present due to the failure of the pumping mechanism and hence a reduced cardiac output

- **Temperature.** Possible occurrence of pyrexias

- **Urine output.** With the use of diuretics, it is vital to keep an accurate hourly record of the output to monitor the effectiveness of the diuretics

- **Cardiac monitoring.** This should be maintained throughout the stay in the emergency department and on transfer. Rhythm changes, such as increasing ventricular ectopics, or left bundle branch block should be considered. Profuse sweating may make electrode placement difficult to achieve

- **Central venous pressure monitoring.** This measurement is important in monitoring and maintaining the haemodynamic status of the patient

---

Clinical investigations should include:

- Blood chemistry analysis – both to monitor renal function and to maintain adequate potassium levels if loop diuretics, such as frusemide, are being administered
- Cardiac enzymes/cardiac troponins – to check for muscular damage
- Full blood count – a low haemoglobin would show any evidence of anaemia
- Arterial blood gases – monitor frequently to assess respiratory function
- Chest X-ray – useful in determining the degree of pulmonary oedema and any evidence of heart enlargement.

Management
The aims of first-line management are:

1. to relieve symptoms
2. to treat the underlying cause.

Oxygen therapy is vital to counteract the effects of hypoxia. Positioning is also important in LVF, as sitting patients in an upright position reduces venous return. LVF is highly treatable and good nursing and medical care should provide symptomatic relief very quickly for the patient. Symptomatic relief comes in the form of i.v. diuretics, namely frusemide, due to its rapid onset of action. This type of diuretic is a potent 'loop diuretic' causing almost immediate diuresis. In severe cases, inotropic drugs may be required, such as dobutamine, dopamine or adrenaline to increase the contractility of the myocardium and thus to assist the left ventricular function. Other drugs of note include vasodilatation agents such as ACE inhibitors, nitrates and calcium-channel blockers. These reduce preload and thus enable an increase in the cardiac output (Nicholas 2004).

Cardiogenic shock

Shock is defined as impaired organ perfusion, which if left uncorrected will lead to irreversible cell damage and multiple organ failure and death (Timmis & Nathan 1997). In the case of cardiogenic shock, the degree of heart failure is so severe that the extreme reduction in cardiac output leads to inadequate organ perfusion. It can occur because of one significant or multiple smaller infarcts in which over 40% of the myocardium becomes necrotic, a ruptured ventricle, significant valvular dysfunction or at the end stage of heart failure. It can also result from cardiac tamponade, cardiomyopathy, pulmonary embolism or dysrhythmias (Smeltzer & Bare 2000). Kinney and Packa (1996) suggest a mortality rate of at least 80% during the course of MI, with the incidence of cardiogenic shock among survivors of MI likely to be 6–20%, indicating the seriousness of the condition (Hand 2002).

Assessment

Patients presenting with cardiogenic shock require urgent attention as they are acutely ill. The patient will appear clinically shocked and hence consideration must be given to the following symptoms:

- acute dyspnoea
- profound hypotension
- pale/cyanotic
- cold/clammy
- arrhythmias

The assessment findings are summarized in Box 26.10.

Priorities for care

Ideally the patients should be cared for in the resuscitation environment with:

- cardiac monitoring
- i.v. access and CVP access
- oxygen therapy
- baseline observations
- catheterization.

Clinical investigations include:

- *Renal care* – urine measurement is vital to measure the effectiveness of drug therapy and U&Es to monitor potassium levels
- *Blood analysis* – for routine FBC and cardiac enzymes/cardiac troponins
- *ECG* – may show multifocal ventricular ectopics

Box 26.10 Assessment findings in cardiogenic shock

- **Blood pressure.** Severe hypotension, due to a radically reduced cardiac output

- **Pulse.** Tachycardia; the heart rate increases to compensate for the reduced cardiac output, but in profound stages the rate may become weaker and arrhythmias may occur

- **Respirations.** Oxygen therapy is vital if hypoxia is to be restricted. An upright posture will help to reduce venous return. Again, in extreme cases intubation and ventilation may be required. Arterial blood gases must be performed on a regular basis to monitor levels of hypoxaemia and any rise in the carbon dioxide levels.

---

indicative of an irritable ventricle, or ischaemic changes suggestive of an acute MI
- *Chest X-ray* – evidence of pulmonary oedema and cardiac enlargement may be present.

Management

Close, frequent observations and cardiac monitoring are vital if life-threatening abnormalities are to be detected. Adequate i.v. access is essential if the haemodynamic status of the patient is to be stabilized. Aggressive i.v. diuretic therapy should be administered to this end and its effectiveness monitored. Volume replacement is sometimes necessary, but should be titrated to CVP and pump functioning. Vasodilators (i.v. nitrates) and inotropic agents (dobutamine, dopamine or adrenaline) may be used to support the cardiovascular system. Rapid administration of alteplase to dissolve thrombi has been shown to increase aortic pressure and survival significantly (Hand 2002). On occasions an intra-aortic balloon pump may be required to support the left ventricle. Thought and consideration must be given to the family and/or friends as this undoubtedly will be a very stressful experience for them.

VIRAL/INFLAMMATORY CONDITIONS

Pericarditis

Acute pericarditis is an acute inflammation of the pericardial sac. The presence of a respiratory tract infection may indicate a viral infection. Causes of pericarditis include:

- idiopathic (non-specific)
- bacterial infection
- viral infection
- pregnancy
- uraemia
- connective tissue disease, e.g. systemic lupus erythematosus (SLE), arthritis
- following an acute MI
- hypothyroidism
- neoplasm, e.g. breast, lung, etc.
- radiation.

Assessment

The patient with pericarditis presents in ED with sharp chest pain localized to the retrosternal area and left precordium. It is typically pleuritic and positional, worsening on deep inspiration, coughing or movement. Other symptoms include:

- dyspnoea
- fever
- production of sputum

- weight loss
- on auscultation of the chest, the sound of a friction rub confirms the diagnosis of pericarditis.

Immediate priorities for care

- baseline observations
- cardiac monitor
- intravenous access
- oxygen therapy.

Specific investigations should include:

- *ECG* – the classical sign seen on the ECG, of which 90% are abnormal in patients with acute pericarditis, is the presence of widespread concave ST elevation, often referred to as saddleback. Late presentations of pericarditis can include generalized T wave inversion on most leads (Humphreys 2006)
- *Blood analysis* – U&Es due to the possibility of uraemically induced pericarditis as a result of decreased renal function
- *FBC* – a raised white cell count would be indicative of bacterial infections
- *Blood culture* – to investigate for infections
- *Chest X-ray* – this is usually normal, unless the presence of a pericardial effusion shows cardiac enlargement.

Management

The immediate management is pain relief. In the initial stages the use of opiates may be required, e.g. diamorphine, or if the pain is less acute, NSAIDs are given, particularly ibuprofen due to its rare side-effects, favourable impact on coronary flow and large dose range (300–800 mg every 6–8 hours).

With viral pericarditis no further treatment is required. For bacterial pericarditis, antibiotic therapy should be initiated. If pericarditis is left uncorrected, it can become potentially life-threatening, leading to pericardial effusion and cardiac tamponade.

Endocarditis

Endocarditis is caused by either bacterial or fungal infiltration of the heart valves or endocardium and should be considered a multisystem disease (Lee 2004). It is prevalent in a heart already damaged by congenital or acquired heart abnormalities. The main characteristic of endocarditis is a vegetative growth on the leaflets of the valves, causing dysfunctional or incompetent valvular action.

Assessment

The symptoms of endocarditis include:

- anaemia
- rigors

- heart murmur
- night sweats
- fever (present in 80–85% of cases Karchmer 1997)
- haematuria
- chills.

Immediate priorities for care

A major complication of endocarditis is heart failure. Hence, on presentation in the ED, the patient, along with the symptoms listed above, may be acutely short of breath, dyspnoeic and pale. Thus, immediate priorities are:

- oxygen therapy where required
- baseline observations – check temperature for recurrent pyrexias
- i.v. access.

Specific investigations include:

- ECG – to detect damage or stress to the heart
- blood analysis – FBC for possible raised white cell count in response to an infection
- U&E – imbalance may occur if heart failure is present
- blood cultures – these are performed to enable isolation of the causative pathogen, so that the correct antibiotics are used to target the source of the infection.

Management

This is dependent upon the causative factor for endocarditis; there are three approaches:

- bacterial endocarditis – suggested antibiotics include benzylpenicillin and gentamicin
- fungal endocarditis – amphotericin is the drug of choice
- surgical intervention – to replace the diseased valve
- antibiotic prophylaxis is required when undertaking any dental work. This is necessary to reduce the risk of reinfection.

The overall mortality for endocarditis is 20–25%. Primary treatment failure can occur even with combined medical and surgical treatment if the organism is *Staph. aureus*, enterobacteriacae or fungi (Lee 2004).

Cardiomyopathy

Cardiomyopathy is a broad term that includes sub-acute or chronic disorders of the myocardium. Heart failure often results from cardiomyopathy and not from coronary artery disease as previously thought (Laurent-Bopp 2000). The definition and diagnosis of cardiomyopathy are ambiguous due to the fact that it is a disease of the heart muscle of an unknown cause.

There are four classifications of cardiomyopathy:

- dilated cardiomyopathy (DCM)
- hypertrophic cardiomyopathy
- arhythmogenic right ventricular cardiomyopathy
- restrictive cardiomyopathy.

Assessment

The majority of patients in the acute phase will be suffering from heart failure due to their cardiomyopathy. Other symptoms include:

- dyspnoea, because of heart failure
- fatigue, because of hypoxia due to inadequate cardiac output
- chest pain related to a decreased cardiac output (mainly with hypertrophic cardiomyopathy)
- syncope
- palpitations
- anxiety
- depression.

Immediate priorities for care

In the presence of heart failure or an acute episode, the priorities should be:

- cardiac monitoring for ventricular arrhythmias, suggestive of a stressed heart
- oxygen therapy
- i.v. access
- baseline observations
- ECG
- routine FBC and U&Es

- chest X-ray – this will show cardiac hypertrophy and may show pulmonary oedema.

During non-acute phases, patients with cardiomyopathy are usually asymptomatic.

Management

A fundamental goal of treatment in cardiomyopathy is the alleviation of symptoms and the prevention of sudden cardiac death (Cruickshank 2004). The only true treatment to offer a cure is heart transplantation. During the interim period, the use of ACE inhibitors such as captopril may be of benefit. Other drugs used in the treatment of cardiomyopathy include:

- diuretics
- amiodarone to control ventricular arrhythmias
- prophylactic anticoagulants, e.g. warfarin – these are indicated as the risk of thrombus formation and subsequent pulmonary embolus is great.

CONCLUSION

The diversity of cardiac conditions presenting in ED is vast. It is therefore essential for ED nurses to understand the principles of a systematic approach to the elements of cardiac care. This chapter has explored one of the most exciting aspects of ED nursing by identifying distinct aspects of patient care and subsequent management.

References

Alexander MF, Fawcett JN, Runciman PJ (2000) *Nursing Practice: Hospital and Home – The Adult*, 2nd edition. Edinburgh: Churchill Livingstone.

Barnason S (2003) Cardiovascular emergencies. In: Newberry L, ed. *Sheehy's Emergency Nursing: Principles and Practice*, 5th edn. St Louis: Mosby.

Birkhead JS, Walker L, Pearson M, Weston C, Cunningham AD, Rickards AF (2004) Improving care for patients with acute coronary syndromes: initial results from the National Audit of Myocardial Infarction Project. *Heart*, 90(9), 1004–1009.

Boersma E, Maas A, Deckers J, Simoons M (1996) Early thrombolytic treatment in acute myocardial infarction: reappraisal of the golden hour. *The Lancet*, 348(9030), 771–775.

Braunwald E, Antman EM, Beasley JW et al. (2000) ACC/ AHA guidelines for the management of patients with unstable angina and non-ST-segment elevation myocardial infarction: executive summary and recommendations. A report of the American College of Cardiology/American Heart Association task force on practice guidelines (committee on the management of patients with unstable angina). *Circulation*, 102(10), 1193–1209.

Caldwell G, Millar G, Quinn E (1985) Simple mechanical methods for cardioversion: defence of the precordial thump and cough version. *British Medical Journal*, 291, 627–630.

Castle N (2003) Effective relief of acute coronary syndrome. *Emergency Nurse*, 10(9), 15–19.

Castle N (2006) Reperfusion therapy. *Emergency Nurse*, 13(9), 25–35.

Coady E (2006) Managing patients with non-ST-segment elevation in acute coronary syndrome. *Nursing Standard*, 20(37), 49–56.

Colquhoun MC, Handley AJ, Evans TR (1999) *ABC of Resuscitation*, 4th edn. London: BMJ.

Cruickshank S (2004) Cardiomyopathy. *Nursing Standard*, 18(23), 46–52.

Department of Health (2000) *National Service Framework for Coronary Heart Disease*. London: HMSO.

Doering LV (1999) Pathophysiology of acute coronary syndromes leading to acute myocardial infarction. *Journal of Cardiovascular Nursing*, 13(2), 1–20

Erickson BA (1996) Dysrhythmias. In: Kinney MR, Packa DR, Andreoli KE, Zipes DG, eds. *Comprehensive Cardiac Care*, 8th edn. St Louis: Mosby.

Fibrinolytic Therapy Trialists' Collaborative Group (1994) Indications for fibrinolytic therapy in suspected acute myocardial infarction: collaborative overview of early mortality and major morbidity results from all randomized trials of more than 1,000 patients. *The Lancet*, **343**(8893), 311–322.

Fox KA (2004) Management of acute coronary syndromes: an update. *Heart*, **90**(6), 698–706.

French JK, White HD (2004) Clinical implications of the new definition of myocardial infarction. *Heart*, **90**(1), 99–106.

Jaffe AS, The World Health Organisation, The European Society of Cardiology, The American College of Cardiology (2001) New standard for the diagnosis of acute myocardial infarction. *Cardiology in Review*, **9**(6), 318–322.

Hampton J (2003) *The ECG Made Easy*, 6th edn. Edinburgh: Churchill Livingstone.

Hand H (2002) Common cardiac arrhythmias. *Emergency Nurse*, **10**(3), 29–38.

Houghton A, Gray D (1997) *Making Sense of the ECG: A Hands-on Guide*. London: Arnold.

Hudack C et al. (1998) *Critical Care Nursing: A Holistic Approach*. Philadelphia: Lippincott.

Humphreys M (2006) Pericardial conditions: signs, symptoms and electrocardiogram changes. *Emergency Nurse*, **14**(1), 30–36.

International Liaison Committee on Resuscitation [ILCOR] (2005a) Part 4: Advanced life support. *Resuscitation*, **67**, 213–217.

International Liaison Committee on Resuscitation [ILCOR] (2005b) Part 3: Defibrillation. *Resuscitation*, **67**, 203–211.

International Liaison Committee on Resuscitation [ILCOR] (2005b) Part 5: Acute coronary syndromes. *Resuscitation*, **67**, 249–269.

Jacobson C (2000) Arrhythmias and conduction defects. In: Woods SL, Froelicher ESS, Motzer SU (eds) *Cardiac Nursing*, 4th edn. Philadelphia: Lippincott, Williams and Wilkins.

Jowett NI, Thompson DR (2002) *Comprehensive Coronary Care*, 3rd edn. London: Baillière Tindall.

Julian P (1998) *Cardiology*, 7th edn. London: Baillière Tindall.

Karchmar AW (1997) Infective endocarditis. In: Braunwald E (ed.) *Heart Disease: A Textbook of Cardiovascular Medicine*, 5th edn. Philadelphia: WB Saunders.

Kern KB, Hilwig RW, Berg RA, Sanders AB, Ewy GA (2002) Importance of continuous chest compressions during cardiopulmonary resuscitation: improved outcome during a simulated single lay-rescuer scenario. *Circulation*, **105**, 645–649.

Khan MG (2000) *Manual of Cardiac Drug Therapy*, 6th edn. London: WB Saunders.

Kinney MR, Packa DR (1996) *Comprehensive Cardiac Care*. St Louis: Mosby.

Krijne R (1984) Rate acceleration of ventricular tachycardia after a precordial chest thump. *American Journal of Cardiology*, **53**, 964–965.

Lange C (1994) *A Guide to ECG Patterns* (2nd issue). London: Blue Sensor Medicotest.

Laurent-Bopp D (2000) Cardiomyopathies and myocarditis. In: Woods SL, Froelicher ESS, Motzer SU, eds. *Cardiac Nursing*, 4th edn. Philadelphia: Lippincott, Williams and Wilkins.

Late Assessment of Thrombolytic Efficacy Steering Committee (1993) Late assessment of thrombolytic efficacy (LATE) study with alteplase 6–24 hours after onset of acute myocardial infarction. *The Lancet*, **342**(8874), 759–766.

Lee M (2004) Heart valve emergencies. In: (Cameron P, Jelinek G, Kelly AM, Murray L, Brown AFT, Heyworth J, eds), *Textbook of Emergency Medicine*, 2nd edn. Edinburgh: Churchill Livingstone.

Marieb E (2000) *Human Anatomy and Physiology*, 5th edn. California: Benjamin Cummings.

Nicholas M (2004) Heart failure: pathophysiology, treatment and nursing care. *Nursing Standard*, **19**(11), 46–51.

Nolan I et al. (1998) *Cardiac Emergencies: A Pocket Guide*. Oxford: Butterworth Heinemann.

O'Connor S (1995) *The Cardiac Patient. Nursing Interventions*. London: Mosby.

Opie L (2000) *Drugs and the Heart*, 5th edn. London: WB Saunders.

Quinn T, Thompson DR (1995) Administration of thrombolytic therapy to patients with acute myocardial infarction. *Accident and Emergency Nursing*, **3**, 208–214.

Resuscitation Council (UK) (2001) *Decisions Relating to Cardiopulmonary Resuscitation: A Joint Statement from the British Medical Association and the Royal College of Nursing*. London: Resuscitation Council.

Resuscitation Council (UK) (2005) *Advanced Life Support Course Provider Manual*, 5th edn. London: Resuscitation Council.

Schamroth L (2001) *An Introduction to Electrocardiography*, 8th edn. Oxford: Blackwell Scientific.

Sclarovsky S, Kracoff OH, Agmon J (1981) Acceleration of ventricular tachycardia induced by a chest thump. *Chest*, **80**, 596–599.

Skinner D, Vincent V (1997) *Cardiopulmonary Resuscitation*, 2nd edn. Oxford: Oxford University Press.

Smeltzer S, Bare B (2000) *Brunner and Suddarth's Textbook of Medical and Surgical Nursing*. Philadelphia: Lippincott.

SOS–Kanto study group (2007) Cardiopulmonary resuscitation by bystanders with chest compression only (SOS–Kanto): an observational study. *Lancet*, **369**, 920–926.

Timmis AD, Nathan AW (1997) *Essentials of Cardiology*, 3rd edn. Oxford: Blackwell Scientific.

Tortora GJ, Grabowski S (2000) *Principles of Anatomy and Physiology*, 9th edn. New York: Harper Collins.

van Alem AP, Sanou BT, Koster RW (2003) Interruption of cardiopulmonary resuscitation with the use of the automated external defibrillator in out-of-hospital cardiac arrest. *Annals of Emergency Medicine*, **42**, 449–457.

Woods SL, Sivarajan-Froelicher ES, Halpenny CJ, Underhill-Motzer S (eds) (2000) *Cardiac Nursing*, 4th edn. Philadelphia: Lippincott, Williams and Wilkins.

Wyatt JP, Illingworth RN, Clancy MJ, Munro P, Robertson CE (1999) *Oxford Handbook of Accident & Emergency Medicine*. Oxford: Oxford University Press.

Zerwic JJ (1999) Patient delay in seeking treatment for acute myocardial infarction symptoms. *Journal of Cardiovascular Nursing*, **13**(3), 21–32.

Chapter **27**

Medical emergencies

Tim Kilner

CHAPTER CONTENTS

INTRODUCTION

A substantial proportion of the ED nurse's workload involves dealing with patients who present with medical emergencies. Medical emergencies are many and varied, and it is beyond the scope of this chapter to consider them all. The main conditions are identified and the assessment and management detailed. It is, however, possible to provide initial management of any life-threatening medical emergency by making an assessment of, and interventions to support, the airway, breathing and circulation. Provided these are intact, baseline observations of pulse, respiration and blood pressure should be established. When coupled with effective communication, these 'routine' actions form the basis of care for the patient with a potentially life-threatening medical condition.

RESPIRATION

Respiration is a process that is fundamental to life itself. In the absence of external respiration, oxygen is not absorbed into the circulation and carbon dioxide is not removed from it. Such a state is clearly incompatible with life and is of an importance few would fail to acknowledge. The process of respiration is considerably more complex than external respiration alone (see Fig. 27.1). Respiration also takes place at a cellular level, known as internal respiration, where oxygen plays a fundamental part in cell energy production, or metabolism, with one of the by-products of this process being carbon dioxide. Internal and external respiration cannot sustain life without the existence of an adequate transport system which enables the oxygen absorbed by external respiration to be delivered to the cells to support internal respiration, and the removal of carbon dioxide produced

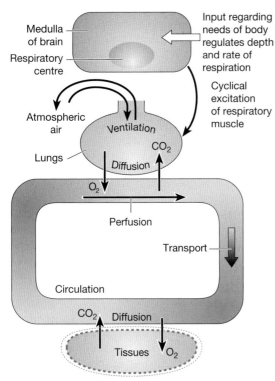

Figure 27.1 Process involved in respiration. (After Hinchliff et al. 1996.)

by internal respiration to the lungs for excretion by means of external respiration.

It is essential that assessment of the respiratory system takes into account *all* of these processes, as the presence of one process does not ensure that other processes are functioning. It is equally important that an assessment evaluates the adequacy of these processes and not just their presence or absence.

The mechanics of respiration

Inspiration occurs when intrathoracic pressure falls below atmospheric pressure. This fall in intrathoracic pressure is caused by an increase in the intrathoracic volume, which occurs when muscle contraction causes the rib cage to move upwards and outwards at the same time as the diaphragm is flattening. During normal inspiration it is the movement of the diaphragm that accounts for the greatest change in intrathoracic volume and not the expansion of the rib cage (Ganong 2003). The fall in intrathoracic pressure causes air to be drawn into the lungs.

Expiration occurs when the lungs recoil, at the end of inspiration, bringing the chest wall back to its pre-inspiratory position. The diaphragm domes, returning to its pre-inspiratory state. Air leaves the lungs by this passive process. Movement of gas is proportional to changes in volume. Therefore, small changes in volume will result in small movements of gas, with the risk that inspired air may only be moving in and out of the anatomical dead space, never reaching the site of gas exchange at the alveoli.

Assessment of the mechanics of respiration

For external respiration to be adequate, the chest wall must be intact, the thorax and diaphragm must be able to rise and fall and that movement must be sufficient to create a negative pressure which will draw air beyond the anatomical dead space and to the alveoli. Patient assessment should reflect this and at least include an assessment of the adequacy of respiratory volume by observing the extent and symmetry of chest expansion and recoil. Observation must also be made to ascertain whether the chest is moving symmetrically and to note if movement is in any way paradoxical.

Neural control of respiration

The rate, rhythm and volume of respiration are governed by the central nervous system, with the involuntary or automatic component being controlled by the respiratory centre in the medulla of the brain. There is a degree of voluntary control over respiration, for instance when an individual intentionally takes a deep breath, which is controlled by the cortex of the brain.

Chemoreceptors in the carotid and aortic body sense changes in blood pH. As the levels of carbon dioxide rise in the blood, the blood becomes more acid and impulses from the chemoreceptors to the respiratory centre increase. In response to this, the respiratory centre increases the respiratory rate. A similar process occurs in the brain where chemoreceptors in the medulla respond to changes in the pH of cerebrospinal fluid. Chemoreceptors are also responsive to a fall in blood oxygen concentrations, increasing impulses to the respiratory centre as the levels of oxygen fall.

In those individuals with chronic respiratory disease, the respiratory centre becomes unresponsive to the changes in carbon dioxide concentration. In these circumstances the falling oxygen concentrations become the main stimuli for respiration. Consequently the administration of high concentrations of inspired oxygen may lead to an increase in carbon dioxide retention, a decrease in respiratory rate and ultimately respiratory arrest. Administration of oxygen to those patients who may have chronic respiratory disease should be done with great care. This is considered further in respect of chronic obstructive pulmonary disease later in the chapter.

Assessment of respiratory control

Assessment should be made of the rate, rhythm and volume of respiration, as this may give an early indication of the increased carbon dioxide or decreased levels of oxygen in the blood. A further and often more striking indication of these physiological processes is the use of the accessory muscles of respiration in the neck, shoulders and abdomen. This is often associated with tracheal tug and recession of the sternum and intercostal muscles.

Bronchial tone

The tone of the bronchi and bronchioles is maintained by the smooth muscle contained within their walls.

Hypoxia

Hypoxia is regarded as being one of the leading causes of preventable death in the trauma patient, but it is often overlooked as a potential threat to life in the many patients who attend ED for reasons other than having sustained an injury. Hypoxia, or inadequate tissue oxygenation, falls broadly into four broad groups (see Box 27.1):

- hypoxic hypoxia
- anaemic hypoxia
- stagnant hypoxia
- histotoxic hypoxia.

Assessment of gas exchange

In recent years, there has been an increased reliance upon pulse oximetry in respiratory assessment. In many cases, this technology is helpful in identifying hypoxia. However, pulse oximetry must be used with caution as it has the potential to mislead (Moyle 2002). Pulse oximetry gives an indication of the degree to which the available haemoglobin is saturated with oxygen. The relationship between oxygen saturation and the amount of oxygen within the circulation is illustrated in graphical format as the oxygen dissociation–haemoglobin dissociation curve. Assuming that the relationship on this curve is normal for a given patient, Gibson (2003) suggests that an oxygen saturation of 90% represents a blood oxygen tension of 8 kPa. The normal range for arterial blood gasses are shown in Box 27.2.

A patient with carbon monoxide poisoning may well have an anaemic hypoxia whilst still presenting what appears to be a normal oxygen saturation on the pulse oximeter. Similarly, patients with other forms of hypoxic anaemia may have normal pulse oximetry readings because the pulse oximeter is a reflection of the degree of saturation of each red blood cell and not of the total oxygen content of the blood. Again

---

Box 27.1   Types of hypoxia

- **Hypoxic hypoxia**
  Oxygen is not available to haemoglobin in the red blood cells. This may occur when the patient is in an atmosphere which has a reduced oxygen content, although it is most likely to occur as a result of a decrease in respiratory rate and/or volume. If untreated, conditions such as pulmonary oedema or pneumonia lead to hypoxic hypoxia by preventing the diffusion of oxygen at the alveolar/capillary interface in the lungs.

- **Anaemic hypoxia**
  The oxygen-carrying capacity of the blood is reduced because of a lack of available haemoglobin. In the acute episode, this is likely to be due to hypovolaemia where haemoglobin is lost in proportion to the number of red cells lost. This type of hypoxia may also occur following chronic conditions where the number of red cells is normal but the haemoglobin is either reduced or not readily available, e.g. in iron deficiency anaemia and sickle cell anaemia. Following carbon monoxide poisoning, the carbon monoxide preferentially binds to the haemoglobin, preventing oxygen binding with the haemoglobin and thus resulting in anaemic hypoxia.

- **Stagnant hypoxia**
  This occurs as a result of failure of the circulatory system to transport oxygenated blood to the tissues. Normal diffusion occurs at the alveolar/capillary interface in the lungs, but inadequate circulation prevents the oxygen from being delivered to the tissues. This type of hypoxia is classically associated with physiological shock, be that cardiogenic, neurogenic, anaphylactic etc. This type of hypoxia may also occur at a local level where vascular obstruction causes a reduction in blood flow distal to the obstruction.

- **Histotoxic hypoxia**
  In this case, adequate concentrations of oxygen are transported to the tissues, but the cells are unable to utilize the oxygen. This type of hypoxia usually results from certain types of poisoning, classically cyanide poisoning.

pulse oximetry must be used with caution when there is probe movement or when peripheral perfusion is low, as recorded saturation may be inaccurate (Levine & Fromm 1995).

It must be remembered that pulse oximetry only provides information about the patient's oxygen saturation; it is not able to offer information regarding carbon dioxide in the blood. Consider the patient who is having an acute asthma attack and who has been given oxygen therapy by facemask. They may well have what may be regarded as satisfactory oxygen saturation, yet have inadequate ventilation with high and increasing levels of blood carbon dioxide. The most accurate way to assess the gaseous content of the circulating volume is by arterial blood gas analysis. Not only does this investigation provide information regarding respiratory gases in the circulation, but it is also a vital tool in the assessment of acid-base balance.

ASTHMA

Asthma has been described as a localized disease of the airways that results in episodes of increased airflow obstruction. While many of the 10% of children and 5% of adults in the population who have asthma are asymptomatic or are well controlled with medication, approximately 1500 people per year die from asthma (Newman-Taylor 2003). Acute asthma is characterized by an acute attack of bronchospasm in which the airways become swollen, constricted and plugged with mucous. The airflow obstruction, which characteristically fluctuates markedly, causes a mismatch of alveolar ventilation and perfusion and increases the work of breathing. Being more marked during expiration it also causes air to be 'trapped' in the lungs. Respiratory arrest may occur within a few minutes of the onset of a severe episode or death may occur from alveolar hypoventilation and severe arterial hypoxaemia in the patient exhausted by a prolonged attack. Severe airflow obstruction is manifested in the symptoms of shortness of breath, wheezing, chest tightness and a cough. Acute severe asthma may arise from absence of treatment or from inadequate or unsuccessful treatment and is life-threatening and should be considered a medical emergency.

In the non-asthmatic individual, there is a minimal reaction of the smooth muscle in the bronchial wall to stimulation by inhaled allergens such as the house dust mite, animal hair or pollen. Non-allergenic stimulants such as cold weather, cigarette smoke, anxiety and exercise also have a minimal effect on the reactivity of the smooth muscle. In the individual with asthma, reaction to such stimulation is exaggerated, a response termed bronchial hyperreactivity, which is thought to be associated with an inflammatory process.

Asthma can be broadly divided into two main types: allergic and non-allergic. Allergic asthma, as the name suggests, is triggered by allergens such as the house dust mite and others previously identified. This condition generally appears in childhood and may improve as the child reaches adolescence (Axford 1996). Conversely, non-allergic asthma is triggered by factors such as anxiety or cold weather, first presenting in middle age. The symptoms of non-allergic asthma tend to intensify in both severity and frequency as the individual becomes older (Axford 1996).

Attendance at the ED is usually precipitated by one of two events:

1. an acute event in the individual who has episodic asthma, i.e. who is symptom-free between distinct acute episodes; or
2. an acute increase in the severity of symptoms in the individual who has chronic asthma, where tightness and wheezing are present most of the time, if not controlled by regular medication.

Initially, the most obvious sign of asthma may be noisy respiration in the form of a wheeze, which is generally expiratory but can also be inspiratory. One must be cautious not to make false assumptions based upon this symptom, for, as Axford (1996) notes, 'all that wheezes is not asthma'. Wheezing is a sign of airway obstruction that may or may not be asthmatic in origin.

Assessment

A full and objective assessment is essential and should include a full history – it may not be possible to obtain this from the patient, if breathless. In cases of severe and life-threatening asthma, treatment should not be delayed in order to obtain a full history.

- The history should include:
  - onset of symptoms
  - duration
  - exacerbation

- medication history; beta blockers, aspirin and non-steroidal anti-inflammatory drugs may precipitate a severe asthma attack in some patients with asthma
- Observation
  - respiratory effort
  - use of accessory muscles
  - chest movement and symmetry
  - skin colour and appearance, such as sweating
  - respiratory rate, rhythm and depth
  - pulse
  - blood pressure
  - temperature (episode may have been precipitated by a chest infection).
- Palpation
  - degree of chest expansion
  - temperature of the skin
- Percussion – resonance of the chest
- Auscultation
  - quality of breath sound
  - degree of air entry
  - silence
- Peak expiratory flow rate
  - measured against predicted and actual normal for that individual
  - should not be done if the patient has signs of severe or life-threatening asthma (i.e. is unable to speak a complete sentence)
- Pulse oximetry – use with caution; remember it will not tell you the amount of carbon dioxide the patient is retaining
- Arterial blood gas analysis
- Chest X-ray.

From the assessment it will be possible to identify those patients with severe and life-threatening asthma who need immediate intervention (see Tables 27.1 and 27.2).

Management
Position the patient to sit upright to maximize ventilation. Patients may need high concentrations of oxygen or medication nebulized by an oxygen-driven

Table 27.1 Features of severe asthma. (After Greaves et al. 1997)

Adult	Child
Cannot complete sentences	Cannot talk or feed
Pulse >110 min	Pulse >140 min
Respiratory rate >25 min	Respiratory rate >50 min
Peak flow rate <50% of predicted	

Table 27.2 Features of life-threatening asthma. (After Greaves et al. 1997)

Adult	Child
Exhaustion	Reduced conscious level
Cyanosis	Agitation
Bradycardia	Cyanosis
Hypotension	Silent chest
Silent chest	Coma
Peak flow <33% of predicted	
Coma	

system. The drug regime recommended by the British Thoracic Society guidelines (British Thoracic Society 2004) includes nebulized salbutamol, and oral or i.v. steroids depending upon the mechanism and severity of the attack. In life-threatening asthma, ipratropium should be added to the nebulizer and expert advice must be sought. For children with moderate exacerbation bronchodilators may be given by inhaler using a spacer device. ED nurses must be familiar with the current British Thoracic Society guidelines on asthma and in particular the flow charts relating to the management of acute asthma in adults in ED and the management of acute asthma in children in ED. In addition to continued reassessment based upon the initial assessment, monitor the cardiac rhythm. Provide psychological care for patient and family in dealing with their stress and anxiety.

In the less severe episodes, it is important to check out the patient's understanding of the illness and management. It is not uncommon for some individuals with asthma to have a poor understanding of the purpose of their medication, when it should be taken and how to take it correctly. It is important to make use of such opportunities to provide some preventive care. It is also essential that appropriate follow-up is arranged to continue patient education and monitoring in the primary health-care setting. Patients with little understanding of their condition and medication regime will continue to attend EDs where their symptoms will be treated without resolving the underlying issues.

It is important to differentiate asthma from hyperventilation, as the presenting symptoms of both are dramatic and can easily be confused by the inexperienced nurse. A hyperventilating patient will be tachypnoeic but not tachycardic and will usually have oxygen saturation levels of 100%. Hyperventilation is associated with anxiety and responds quickly to rebreathing through a paper bag. Hyperventilating patients generally do not have a history of asthma.

CHRONIC OBSTRUCTIVE PULMONARY DISEASE

Chronic obstructive pulmonary disease (COPD) is a collective term for a number of chronic respiratory diseases, the most common of which are chronic bronchitis and emphysema (British Thoracic Society 1997).

Chronic bronchitis

Chronic bronchitis is most frequently seen in adults of middle age and beyond. It is characterized by a productive cough resulting from increased mucous secretion from hypertrophied mucus-secreting glands in the bronchi. The patency of the smaller bronchi is further compromised by inflammation of the mucosa. The cough and associated inflammation last for several months each year and occur on consecutive years.

Assessment

When the individual with chronic bronchitis attends the ED, it is usually because of an acute exacerbation of symptoms associated with a superimposed upper respiratory tract infection. Assessment of the individual will include:

- A full history, including past history as well as the history of the current episode
  - onset of symptoms
  - duration
  - exacerbation
- Observation
  - signs of chronic respiratory disease, e.g. clubbing of the fingers, barrel chest
  - respiratory effort
  - use of accessory muscles
  - chest movement and symmetry
  - skin colour
  - respiratory rate, rhythm and depth
  - pulse
  - blood pressure
  - temperature
- Palpation
  - degree of chest expansion
  - temperature of the skin
- Percussion – resonance of the chest
- Auscultation
  - quality of breath sound
  - degree of air entry
- Pulse oximetry – use with caution; remember many of these patients retain carbon dioxide which can result in fatal respiratory acidosis, even in the presence of adequate oxygen saturation. Pulse oximetry will not provide any information about elevated levels of carbon dioxide
- Arterial blood gas analysis – will be abnormal given the chronic respiratory disease and should be viewed in the light of the individual's actual or predicted normal
- Sputum sample – for microbiological examination (microscopy, culture and sensitivity)
- Chest X-ray.

Assessment of the patient is likely to reveal the following clinical features:

- purulent productive cough
- increased sputum volume
- dyspnoea
- tachypnoea
- wheezing
- respiratory distress and use of accessory muscles
- poor chest expansion
- cyanosis.

Management

Position the patient sitting upright to maximize ventilation. Oxygen should be given at a low concentration, initially no more than 28%; increased concentrations may be necessary if improvement does not occur, but this should be based on the results of arterial blood gas analysis. Whilst on oxygen the patient must be closely monitored for signs of respiratory depression. Antibiotics, bronchodilators and steroids should be given if asthma is an element in the acute episode. Where nebulized medication is indicated the British Thoracic Society (2004) recommend that a compressed air nebulizer should be used and the patient given supplemental oxygen by nasal prongs. In addition to continued reassessment based upon the initial assessment, the cardiac rhythm should be monitored. Arterial blood gas analysis must be carried out within the first hour of admission to the ED and results used to inform ongoing management of the patient. Psychological care for patient and family should be provided in dealing with their stress and anxiety

Emphysema

Dilatation of the alveoli reduces the functional surface area of the lung available for gas exchange. The mechanics of respiration are also compromised by the reduction of elasticity and recoil of the lung. As with other chronic respiratory conditions, emphysema is commonly seen in adults beyond middle age. The individual attends the ED with an increase in the severity of the symptoms, often associated with additional respiratory disease or infection.

Assessment should follow the format as for the patient with chronic bronchitis. Such assessment will reveal:

- dyspnoea
- quiet breath sounds
- overinflation of the chest
- forced expiration through pursed lips.

Management of the patient is much the same as that for chronic bronchitis.

PULMONARY OEDEMA

Although pulmonary oedema for many patients has its origins in the cardiac system, it is a manifest problem in the respiratory system.

Cardiac–related pulmonary oedema

The most common presentation of pulmonary oedema of cardiac origin seen in the ED is as a result of left ventricular failure which may or may not be secondary to acute myocardial infarction. Failure of the left ventricle leads to back-pressure in the pulmonary circulation. As the pressure builds, fluid is forced from the circulation first into the pulmonary interstitial spaces and then, with further increases in pressure, into the alveoli. This fluid within the interstitial spaces and the alveoli reduces the efficacy of gas exchange at the alveolar-capillary interface.

Other possible causes of pulmonary oedema

It is important to remember that pulmonary oedema is not a disease in itself but is merely a symptom of some other underlying pathology, e.g.:

- opiate overdose
- inhalation of toxic or irritant substances
- allergic reactions
- airway burns/inhalation injury
- circulatory volume overload (overinfusion)
- pulmonary embolism
- hypoalbuminaemia
- near drowning

Assessment

Onset is usually sudden with the individual attending the ED as symptoms worsen and respiratory function deteriorates. Assessment must focus upon the presenting symptoms, but must also aim to consider the possible underlying causes:

- A full history (past history as well as the history of the current episode)
  - onset of symptoms

  - duration
  - exacerbation
- Observation
  - airway
  - signs of possible underlying mechanisms, e.g. inhalation injury, substance misuse
  - respiratory effort
  - use of accessory muscles
  - chest movement
  - skin colour
  - respiratory rate, rhythm and depth
  - pulse
  - blood pressure
  - temperature
  - level of consciousness
- Palpation
  - degree of chest expansion
  - temperature of the skin
- Percussion – resonance of the chest
- Auscultation
  - quality of breath sound
  - degree of air entry
- Pulse oximetry – with caution
- Arterial blood gas analysis
- Chest X-ray.

Assessment is likely to reveal:

- dyspnoea
- orthopnoea
- tachypnoea
- exhaustion
- respiratory distress
- noisy respiration
- expectoration of frothy sputum.

Management
Management of the patient is dependent upon the underlying pathology, but will include securing the airway and positioning the patient upright to maximize ventilation. Provide high-concentration oxygen through a Hudson mask with reservoir bag at a flow rate of 10–15 L/min. Diuretics may reduce the fluid load from the circulation. Morphine/diamorphine, if not contraindicated, causes venous pooling, thus reducing venous return on loading on the heart. Opiates will also help in the reduction of anxiety, but one must be vigilant for signs of respiratory depression. Vasodilators in the form of nitrates, if indicated, also cause venous pooling. Catheterization should be considered and the patient's fluid output should be carefully monitored. Twelve-lead ECG should be performed to monitor any cardiac changes. In addition to continued reassessment based upon the initial assessment, monitor the cardiac rhythm. Psychological care

should be provided for patient and family in dealing with their stress and anxiety.

PULMONARY EMBOLISM

Pulmonary embolism is a common cause of respiratory-related death in the UK, with an estimated 30 000 deaths each year (Edwards et al. 1995). It is a commonly associated complication of deep vein thrombosis (DVT), where a fragment detaches from the thrombus to form an embolus (Fig. 27.2). The embolus flows through the circulation until it wedges in narrow branches of the arterial system, classically branches of the pulmonary artery. The pulmonary circulation becomes obstructed, which consequently reduces the efficacy of gas exchange and ventilation perfusion mismatch occurs.

Predisposition to pulmonary embolism, generally speaking, is determined by a predisposition to DVT, i.e.:

- sluggish circulation due to
  - bed rest
  - limb immobilization
  - heart failure/reduced cardiac output
- venous injury
  - trauma
  - venous cannulation
- increased coagulability
  - drugs, such as oral contraceptives
  - dehydration
  - polycythaemia
- increased age.

Emboli may arise from other mechanisms such as air, fat or amniotic fluid entering the circulation, but these are less common. Symptoms are related to the size of the area of lung affected, the rate of onset and the severity of the symptoms being determined by the size and number of emboli:

- Small emboli. These wedge in smaller vessels, close to the alveolar-capillary interface, and affect only a small area of lung.
- Medium emboli. These wedge in the larger branches of the pulmonary artery some distance from the alveolar-capillary interface. They affect a larger area of lung than do smaller emboli and result in a greater ventilation-perfusion mismatch.
- Large emboli. These wedge in the largest branches of the pulmonary artery, furthest away from the alveolar-capillary interface. They affect very large areas of the lung and result in a massive ventilation perfusion mismatch.

Assessment

A good assessment is vital, as the symptoms of pulmonary embolism are often confused with those of acute myocardial infarction:

- A full history, considering predisposition to and evidence of DVT, as well as the history of the current episode:
  - onset of symptoms
  - duration
  - exacerbation
- Observation
  - signs of possible underlying mechanisms, in particular DVT
  - respiratory effort
  - use of accessory muscles
  - chest movement
  - skin colour
  - respiratory rate, rhythm and depth
  - pulse
  - blood pressure
  - sputum
  - level of consciousness
- Palpation
  - degree of chest expansion
  - temperature of the skin
- Percussion – resonance of the chest
- Auscultation
  - quality of breath sound
  - degree of air entry
- Pulse oximetry – with caution
- Arterial blood gas analysis
- Chest X-ray
- 12-lead ECG.

Table 27.3 outlines the features of emboli of different sizes. An ECG may reveal an S wave in lead I, a Q

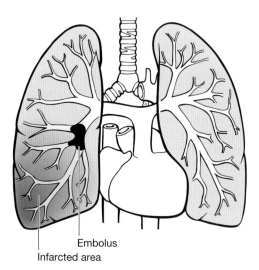

Embolus

Infarcted area

Figure 27.2 Pulmonary embolism.

Table 27.3 Features of pulmonary emboli

Small emboli	Medium emboli	Large emboli
Slow onset	Rapid onset	Sudden onset
Mild – moderate dyspnoea	Pleuritic chest pain	Dyspnoea
Fatigue	Dyspnoea	Chest pain
	Haemoptysis	Haemoptysis
		Tachycardia
		Compromised circulation
		Hypotension
		Cyanosis
		Reduced level of consciousness
		Unconsciousness

wave in lead III and an inverted T wave in lead III. The ECG may also be useful in excluding other diagnoses such as myocardial infarction and pericardial disease.

Management
Position the patient sitting upright to maximize ventilation. Administer high-concentration oxygen using a Hudson mask with reservoir bag at a flow rate of 10–15 L/min. Bloods should be taken for clotting screen. Anticoagulants, such as heparin, are often the only form of treatment given for massive pulmonary embolism. A thrombolytic such as alteplase may be indicated primarily in patients who are haemodynamically unstable (British Thoracic Society 2003).

ANAPHYLAXIS

An acute anaphylactic reaction is the result of a severe or overwhelming allergic or hypersensitivity reaction with sometimes fatal consequences. Symptoms will usually occur rapidly within minutes of exposure to the causative allergen, especially if given parenterally. Repeated administration of parental or oral therapeutic agents may also precipitate an anaphylactic reaction.

Commonly cited triggers include:

- antibiotics, e.g. penicillin or other penicillin derivatives
- bee or wasp stings
- insect or snake venom
- foodstuffs, e.g. nuts or shellfish.

Clinical features
The clinical features of anaphylactic shock may occur singly or in combination and may include respiratory distress, cyanosis, bronchospasm, laryngeal obstruction, circulatory collapse, hypotension, tachycardia, generalized erythema, urticaria, nausea, vomiting, abdominal pain and diarrhoea. Generally, the faster the onset of symptoms, the more life-threatening is the reaction.

Management
The priority is to secure and maintain the airway; intubation may be required especially if laryngeal oedema is present. If the patient is able to maintain an open airway, she/he should be administered supplemental oxygen by a face mask at a high flow rate of 10–15 L/min. Adrenaline slows the release of cellular chemical mediators and, additionally, causes vasoconstriction. It also has beneficial effects on myocardial contractility, peripheral vascular tone and bronchial smooth muscle. Adrenaline should be administered via the intramuscular route and NOT the intravenous route.

The ED nurse should be alert to the dangers of anaphylactic reactions and have knowledge of any relevant patient history. The nurse should avoid giving medication to patients with a known allergic disorder, such as hay fever or asthma, unless absolutely necessary. Ensure that prescribed medication is given by the most appropriate route; anaphylactic reactions are more likely to occur when drugs are given via the parenteral route.

NEAR DROWNING

Near drowning following submersion in water results from one of two main mechanisms: 'dry' drowning and 'wet' drowning. Dry drowning occurs following immersion in cold water, the cold water causing laryngospasm and vagal stimulation which leads to asphyxiation, hypoxia and cardiac arrest. Little or no water enters the lower airways or lungs and death is secondary to airway obstruction rather than pulmonary oedema (Morris 2003). More commonly, drowning and near drowning occur as a result of wet drowning. After a period of breath-holding following immersion, the individual is forced to inhale by reflex mechanism. Water is aspirated into the lungs along with the large volumes of water which have been swallowed. The inhaled water obstructs the lower airways and thus prevents adequate gas exchange. Consequently, the individual rapidly becomes hypoxic, which leads to unconsciousness and cardiac arrest (Knopp 1992).

Near drowning is often associated with other factors which complicate the individual's condition. In adults, as much as 25% of cases have been documented as being associated with alcohol use (Mills et al. 1995). Hypothermia is common in UK waters. This is inevitable when the water is below 10°C as body heat is lost despite the individual actively exercising (Greaves et al. 2005). Near drowning is frequently associated with head and neck injury, when individuals dive into shallow water or water which contains submerged objects.

Occasionally near-drowning victims can be asymptomatic; however, most present with mild dyspnoea, a deathlike appearance with blue or grey colouring, apnoea or tachypnoea, hypotension, heart rate as slow as 4 to 5 beats per minute or pulselessness, cold skin, dilated pupils known as fish eyes, hypothermia and vomiting (Morris 2003). Significant neurological impairment occurs in up to 25% of near-drowning patients. Neurological injury results from hypoxia and can lead to cerebral oedema and brain stem herniation. Approximately 20% of comatose patients recover completely (Emergency Nurses Association 1994). Hypothermia is an important clinical feature in determining outcome as it decreases the metabolic demands of the body, and severe cerebral hypoxia may be prevented or delayed. Acidosis is a common finding in near-drowning patients. Metabolic acidosis is primarily due to tissue hypoxia, but a respiratory component may be present following aspiration. Hypoxia and acidosis act as myocardial depressants and precipitate circulatory collapse.

Assessment

There are some physiological differences between near drowning in fresh water and that in salt water. These differences are functionally irrelevant in the early management of the individual in the ED. Assessment of the individual must ensure that due consideration is given to the mechanism of injury in respect of potential head and neck trauma. This should include:

- A full history
  - onset of symptoms
  - duration
  - exacerbation
- Observation
  - airway
  - signs of possible underlying factors; head and neck trauma, alcohol use
  - respiratory effort
  - use of accessory muscles
  - chest movement
  - skin colour
  - respiratory rate, rhythm and depth
  - pulse
  - blood pressure
  - temperature
  - level of consciousness
- Palpation
  - degree of chest expansion
  - temperature of the skin
- Percussion – resonance of the chest.
- Auscultation
  - quality of breath sound
  - degree of air entry
- Pulse oximetry – with caution
- Arterial blood gas analysis
- Chest X-ray.

The presentation of the individual following near drowning may be diverse, but is likely to include at least some of the following:

- head and neck trauma
- reduced level of consciousness – unconscious
- apnoea
- tachypnoea
- shallow respiration
- pulmonary oedema
- hypothermia
- arrhythmias
- asystole.

Symptoms may be delayed. Apparently well patients must be observed and reviewed over the subsequent 48 hours.

Management

- Airway management with cervical spine control
- High-concentration oxygen, with intermittent positive pressure ventilation if indicated
- Rewarming if indicated (see hypothermia)
- Management of arrhythmias
- Management of injuries
- Cardiac monitoring
- Continued reassessment based upon the initial assessment
- Psychological care for the patient and family in dealing with their stress and anxiety.

CARBON MONOXIDE POISONING

Carbon monoxide poisoning is the most common cause of poisoning in the UK, and is thought to cause 1000 deaths/year, of which approximately one-third result from self-poisoning (Robinson & Stott 1993). Carbon monoxide is a colourless, odourless, tasteless gas produced by incomplete combustion of organic material. Poisoning is usually associated with inhalation of smoke from fires in confined spaces, engine exhausts and faulty heating systems. It is often referred to as the silent killer as victims of accidental exposure often have no idea they are being poisoned, even when they develop severe symptoms. Consequently, victims are likely to remain in a life-threatening environment without realizing the dangers. Carbon monoxide combines more readily with haemoglobin than oxygen does – its affinity is more than 200 times that of oxygen. Once combined with carbon monoxide, haemoglobin is unable to bind with oxygen, resulting in a fall in PO_2 and an anaemic hypoxia.

Assessment

Assessment is largely dependent upon a clear history and a high index of suspicion, as symptoms in themselves may not be self-evident:

- A full history – has the individual been in a confined space in which carbon monoxide may be present? The history should include:
  - onset of symptoms
  - duration
  - exacerbation
- Observation
  - airway – soot, carbonaceous sputum as evidence of an inhalation injury
  - respiratory effort
  - use of accessory muscles
  - chest movement
  - skin colour – may look pink or flushed (cherry red appearance may not be evident)
  - respiratory rate, rhythm and depth
  - pulse
  - blood pressure
  - temperature
  - level of consciousness
- Auscultation
  - quality of breath sound
  - degree of air entry
- Pulse oximetry – can be extremely misleading, giving high readings even though the patient is hypoxic
- Arterial blood gas analysis.
- Bloods for carboxyhaemoglobin.

Presentation will depend upon the percentage of carboxyhaemoglobin present (see Table 27.4).

Management

The patient should be given high-concentration oxygen, with intermittent positive pressure ventilation if indicated. In the presence of 100% O_2 there is a 50% reduction of carboxyhaemoglobin in the first 20 minutes. Consider hyperbaric oxygen, which forces oxygen onto the haemoglobin and reduces the half-life

Table 27.4   Presentation of carbon monoxide poisoning

Carboxyhaemoglobin	Symptoms
<10%	No symptoms
10–20%	Headache
	Nausea
	Vomiting
	Loss of manual dexterity
21–40%	Confusion
	Lethargy
	ST depression on ECG
	Apathy – loss of interest in leaving dangerous environment, and therefore may be fatal
41–60%	Ataxia
	Convulsions
	Apnoea
	Coma
>60%	Usually fatal

of carbon monoxide as well as decreasing intercranial pressure and cerebral oedema (Driscoll et al. 1994). The indications for hyperbaric oxygen (Axford 1996) are:

- conscious patients with levels of carboxyhaemoglobin of >20%
- neurological symptoms other than headache at any time since exposure
- pregnancy
- cardiac arrhythmias.

RENAL DISORDERS

The renal system is an important system as it influences a large number of physiological processes, e.g. the control and maintenance of blood pressure, fluid and electrolyte balance, acid-base balance and excretion of by-products of metabolism.

Maintenance of blood pressure

Baroreceptors in the renal arterial system respond to a fall in blood pressure by stimulating the release of renin from the juxta-glomerular apparatus. The renin enters the bloodstream and acts upon angiotensinogen, produced in the liver to form angiotensin I. Angiotensin I is then converted to angiotensin II by angiotensin-converting enzyme (ACE) found mainly in the lungs and kidney. Angiotensin has a number of effects which raise blood pressure:

- acts directly on arterioles to cause vasoconstriction
- stimulates the circulation centre in the central nervous system resulting in vasoconstriction
- stimulates the thirst mechanism in the hypothalamus
- influences renal blood flow and the glomerular filtration rate by renal vasoconstriction
- stimulates the adrenal cortex to secrete aldosterone, which increases sodium reabsorption by the kidney and so causes water retention.

Fluid and electrolyte balance

A fluid deficit in the circulating blood volume is detected by the osmoreceptors, located in the hypothalamus. This causes the secretion of antidiuretic hormone from the posterior pituitary. This hormone stimulates increased water absorption in the kidney and this is supported by the effects of the renin-angiotensin pathway (described above).

Acid–base balance

In cases where the blood is acidotic the lungs play a major part in the reduction of the acidosis by the excretion of the acid-producing hydrogen ions in the form of carbon dioxide. However, the kidney provides a valuable additional role in the reduction of the hydrogen ion concentration. The kidney provides a back-up in the case of inadequate respiration; it removes acid produced by fat and protein metabolism which cannot be removed by the lungs and it allows bicarbonate to be reabsorbed to supplement that being used in buffering processes. Acid is excreted by the kidney in a buffered form.

Excretion of by-products of metabolism

Carbohydrates and fats are broken down to carbon dioxide and water and are excreted by means of processes as detailed previously. Many substances such as protein and amino acids contain nitrogen, which relies upon the kidney to excrete nitrogenous by-products in the form of urea, uric acid and creatinine.

Assessment of the renal system
The renal system gives an insight into many physiological processes and should not be underestimated when making a patient assessment. Likewise an assessment of the renal system should not be restricted to those patients with renal conditions. The assessment of these processes and of renal function is via the urine output in terms of volume, frequency and content. This may be achieved by accurate fluid balance measurement and recording at intervals appropriate to the patient's condition. Routine urine testing using reagent strips offers a wealth of information, as does a visual inspection of the urine, which is frequently undervalued in assessment.

URINARY TRACT INFECTION

Of the many conditions which are of renal or urinary tract in origin, few are seen in the ED. Where the patient does attend with an underlying renal or urinary tract pathology, it is generally because of pain rather than any other symptom, the most common conditions being urinary tract infection (UTI) and renal colic.

This is commonly caused by *E. coli* from faeces; other organism groups that cause UTI include *Proteus, Pseudomonas, Streptococcus, Staphylococcus epidermidis* and *Klebsiella* (Edwards et al. 1995). Following inoculation, organisms rapidly multiply in the ideal culture material of the urine. The individual will generally present at the ED complaining of pain on micturition.

Assessment
- A full history
  - onset of symptoms
  - duration
  - exacerbation
- Observation
  - skin colour
  - temperature
  - urine – colour, opacity, odour
- Midstream specimen of urine – for microscopy, culture and sensitivity.

  Symptoms of UTI include:

- dysuria
- frequency of micturition
- haematuria.

  In its advanced stages UTI may lead to infection of the kidney or kidneys in the form of pyelonephritis, which may present as:

- signs of UTI
- fever
- loin pain
- nausea
- vomiting.

Management
Management of the condition is based upon:

- antibiotics
- increased oral fluid intake
- patient education.

Renal colic

Renal colic is the most common presentation of renal calculi. It occurs most frequently between 20 and 50 years of age with a male:female ratio of 3:1. About 50% of patients have a single episode but the remaining 50% have recurrences within 5 years (Trevedi 1996, Nicholson 2004). Renal calculi are predominantly calcium in origin, although they may be calcium/ ammonium phosphate, urate or cystine. The calculi form in the kidney when the urine is saturated with the given solute and the kidney is unable to excrete it. The solute, in its crystalline form, deposits in the kidney causing pain. Pain is at its most intense when the calculi pass through the urinary tract.

Assessment
- A full history and pain assessment
  - onset of symptoms
  - duration
  - exacerbation
  - skin colour
  - temperature
  - urine – colour, opacity, odour, laboratory stick test. Urine should be filtered through filter paper to identify evidence of grit from the calculi
- Observation
- Midstream specimen of urine – for microscopy, culture and sensitivity.

The main feature identified by the assessment is likely to be pain; however, other features may be present:

- pain – unilateral pain radiates from the loin to left or right lower quadrants. Suprapubic pain may also be present. Pain may be sudden or intermittent in onset
- restlessness
- dysurea
- urgency
- frequency
- haematurea
- proteinurea
- UTI
- Management

- Analgesia – opiates, non-steroidal anti-inflammatory drugs
- Antispasmodics – atropine
- Anti-emetics
- Increase fluid intake – orally or i.v.
- Patient education – advise patient to increase fluid intake especially at night when urine normally concentrates.

DEHYDRATION – FLUID VOLUME DEFICIT

The mechanisms leading to dehydration are many and varied. It is likely that the patient will attend the ED with a condition resulting in dehydration rather than with dehydration per se. It is important to consider the processes involved in the underlying illness to identify the potential for dehydration. There are two main types of dehydration, depending on the type of fluid deficit, i.e. hypertonic, isotonic (Table 27.5).

In an effort to correct dehydration, patients may inadvertently overhydrate, leading to subsequent physiological disturbance. This is covered in Table 27.6.

Assessment
This should include:

- A full history, including past history as well as the history of the current episode:
  - onset of symptoms
  - duration
  - exacerbation
- Observation
  - respiratory effort
  - use of accessory muscles
  - chest movement
  - skin colour
  - respiratory rate, rhythm and depth
  - pulse
  - blood pressure
  - temperature
  - level of consciousness
  - urine – volume, colour and concentration
- Palpation
  - degree of chest expansion
  - skin temperature and elasticity
- Auscultation
  - quality of breath sound
  - degree of air entry
- Pulse oximetry (depending upon respiratory symptoms) – with caution
- Arterial blood gas analysis
- Chest X-ray.

THERMOREGULATION

The control of body temperature takes place in the hypothalamus in response to changes in core temperature, detected by thermoreceptors in the hypothalamus, skin and spinal cord. When the body temperature rises, the hypothalamus responds by

Table 27.5 Dehydration – fluid deficit. (After Paradiso, 1995)

	Hypertonic deficit	Isotonic deficit
Mechanism	Occurs when fluid is lost without the loss of electrolytes Extracellular fluid becomes concentrated and fluid moves from the intracellular compartment to the extracellular compartment	Occurs when fluid and electrolytes are in normal physiological proportions Extracellular and intracellular fluid remains unchanged
Possible causes	Severe GI infections, causing fluid loss and sodium concentration Increased insensible loss Low-volume, concentrated feeds (infants or nasogastric) Inability to access water (environmental isolation/entrapment loss of consciousness)	Diarrhoea and vomiting Increased urine output (renal disease, diuretics) Increased sweating Burns Haemorrhage Lack of fluid and electrolyte intake
Symptoms	Decreased skin elasticity Dry mucous membranes Hypotension Tachycardia Increased respiratory rate and volume Increased thirst Pitting oedema	Acute weight loss Dry mucous membranes Hypotension Tachycardia Increased respiratory rate and volume Decreased and concentrated urine output Sunken eyes Pleural effusion Pulmonary oedema Dependent oedema
Management	Water replacement Hypotonic i.v. fluids	i.v. replacement of isotonic fluids Blood and blood products Anti-emetics

increasing sweating, respiration and blood flow to the skin, via the autonomic nervous system. Normal human body temperature displays a circadian rhythm, ranging from 35.8°C (96.4°F) in the predawn hours to 37.3°C (99.1°F) in the late afternoon (Bickley & Szilagyi 2003) and body temperatures that exceed the norm of 37.0°C (98.6°F) are often observed in healthy people. Abnormal elevation of temperature (pyrexia) is categorized as hyperthermia or fever. Hyperthermia is the result of a failure of thermal control mechanisms. In fever, the thermal control mechanisms are intact.

When the temperature falls, the body aims to raise the body temperature by heat conservation and increased heat production. Heat is conserved by reducing the activity of the sweat glands, erection of the body hair and diverting the blood flow from the periphery to the core. Heat is produced by involuntary muscle activity in the form of shivering and by voluntary muscle activity such as stamping the feet.

Assessment of body temperature

Assessment of the body temperature is reliant upon thermometry, which has traditionally been by means of the clinical thermometer either orally, axillary or rectally. These methods often yield inaccuracies in temperature measurement as thermometers are often removed before an accurate temperature has been recorded. With the advent of electronic tympanic thermometers, this has become less of a problem. However, inaccuracies do occur if the ear canal is occluded by either wax or other debris. Again it is important not to discount the value of patient observation as a means of assessment.

Heat illness

Heat illness is inextricably linked to fluid and electrolyte balance. An increase in body temperature is controlled by an increase in sweating as a means of dissipating heat by evaporation. Increased sweating, although a relatively efficient way of reducing temperature, results in the loss of considerable amounts of fluid. Consequently, electrolyte concentrations, especially sodium, become deranged.

A number of factors predispose heat illness. These are rarely of significance individually, but pose a great risk in combination:

- high ambient temperature
- high humidity (humidity reduces effective evaporation through sweating)

Table 27.6 Overhydration – fluid excess. (After Paradiso, 1995)

	Hypertonic excess	Isotonic excess
Mechanism	Increased sodium concentrations with fluid volume remaining normal	Increase in fluid and electrolyte concentrations of normal physiological concentrations
	Extracellular fluid becomes concentrated with intracellular fluid moving into the extracellular compartment	No movement of fluid across the compartments
Possible causes	Intake of relatively large volumes of salt water	Excessive intake of isotonic fluids either orally or i.v.
		Abnormal fluid and electrolyte retention following renal disease
		Corticosteroid therapy
Symptoms	Circulatory overload	Circulatory overload
	Oedema	Oedema
	Increased cardiac output	Increased cardiac output
	Congestive cardiac failure	Congestive cardiac failure
	Pulmonary oedema	Pulmonary oedema
	Increased BP	Increased BP
	Full bounding pulse	Full bounding pulse
	Decreased level of consciousness	
	Muscle twitching	
	Fitting	
	Coma	
	Hypernatraemia	
Management	Management of underlying disease	Diuretics
	Removal of sodium with diuretics	Treatment of underlying disease, e.g. CCF i.v.
	Replacement of fluid lost by drug-induced diuresis	replacement of hypertonic fluids with caution

- exercise
- clothing which reduces the skin surface area available for evaporation.

Assessment

Good assessment is important to establish the type of heat illness which has occurred and to guide management:

- A full history, including past history as well as the history of the current episode:
  - onset of symptoms
  - duration
  - exacerbation
- Observation
  - airway
  - respiratory effort
  - use of accessory muscles
  - chest movement
  - skin colour
  - respiratory rate, rhythm and depth
  - pulse
  - blood pressure
  - temperature
  - level of consciousness

- Palpation
  - degree of chest expansion
  - temperature and elasticity of the skin
- Blood for urea and electrolytes.
- Pulse oximetry – with caution.

From the assessment, two conditions may be identified. These are heat exhaustion and heat stroke.

Heat exhaustion   The signs and symptoms are:

- loss of fluid and electrolytes
- slight increase in core temperature
- tachycardia
- headache
- dizziness
- sweating.

Heat stroke (life-threatening)   Signs and symptoms are:

- core temperature above 41°C
- heat increases beyond the body's ability to lose heat (beyond 42°C hypothalamic control of temperature is lost)
- sweating may be absent
- hot dry skin

- nausea and vomiting
- hypovolaemia
- hypokalaemia
- decreased level of consciousness – unconsciousness.

Management
Heat exhaustion

- Place in a cool environment, with gentle air flow.
- Remove clothing preventing heat loss.
- Replace isotonic fluid – orally if conscious and oriented and not vomiting; otherwise by the intravenous route.
- Tepid sponging and the use of a fan is not advocated as this causes peripheral vasoconstriction, pooling the blood to the core with a consequential rise in core temperature.

Heat stroke

- Secure the airway if indicated
- Administer high-concentration oxygen and assisted ventilation if required.
- Remove clothing
- Carry out active cooling – consider immersion in cool water, taking into account potential airway and breathing problems. Spraying the skin with cool water in the presence of air flow may be a more practical intervention to reduce body temperature through evaporation
- Carry out intravenous fluid replacement and correction of electrolyte imbalance.

NERVOUS SYSTEM

The brain is highly intolerant to a fall in oxygen and glucose levels and is therefore highly sensitive to changes in its blood flow. This sensitivity is manifest in changes in the level of consciousness and subtle signs such as confusion or disorientation. As the brain is responsible for the control and regulation of many vital functions, such as respiration, cardiac output or movement, by means of the somatic or autonomic nervous system, symptoms may be manifest in these systems or processes.

Neurological assessment

As with all assessment, neurological assessment is about the interpretation of trends in clinical signs and not single observations viewed in isolation. One of the most important and informative signs is the level of consciousness. The accepted tool for this assessment is the Glasgow Coma Scale.

Headaches

Although headaches, when accompanied by other neurological signs, may be an indication of some underlying condition, they are infrequently life-threatening in themselves (Goadsby 2003). Headaches with no other neurological signs fall broadly into three main groups: tension, migraine and cluster. In order to differentiate between the three and to identify any serious underlying conditions, a full assessment is essential, with great emphasis being placed upon the history:

- A full history: including past history as well as the history of the current episode:
  - location of pain
  - type of pain
  - severity/intensity of pain
  - onset of pain
  - duration of pain
  - frequency of pain
  - context in which pain occurs
  - what exacerbates or relieves pain
  - other associated neurological symptoms
  - health history – has the individual experienced these headaches previously?
  - current medication – especially over-the-counter medications taken for symptom relief, vasodilators or caffeine-containing drugs
  - allergies
  - diet – including intake of caffeine
  - alcohol and substance use
  - smoking.
- Observation
  - signs of possible underlying mechanisms, substance misuse for example
  - skin colour
  - respiratory rate, rhythm and depth
  - pulse
  - blood pressure
  - temperature
  - level of consciousness (GCS)
  - photophobia
  - neck stiffness.

Tension headaches

These are associated with stress and can often be associated with identifiable causes, such as increase in workload, financial pressures and bereavement. Pain is usually slow in onset, often increasing in intensity over a number of hours and is described as a dull or nagging ache. Generally the pain is generalized and described as a band around the head, rather than focused in a specific area. Tension headaches are frequently chronic as the underlying stress may be chronic.

Management is based upon managing the stress through relaxation techniques and addressing underlying problems where possible. In the immediate term, pain relief may be achieved with simple over-the-counter analgesics as appropriate in the light of current medication history. Ensure that analgesics do not contain caffeine.

Migraine

Migraine may be described as a headache with associated symptoms such as photophobia or sensitivity to movement. However, visual disturbances and aura only occur in about 15% of sufferers. At the onset the pain is unilateral and is accompanied by nausea, vomiting, numbness of hands, face and tongue, weakness and clumsiness. The pain is described as throbbing or pounding and is often intensified by light. Common migraine has similar clinical features, but without the aura, individuals often being awoken from sleep by the pounding headache.

Individuals often find the symptoms less intense if they are able to lie down in a quiet darkened room. Analgesia, especially containing codeine, may help in symptom relief but should be preceded by an anti-emetic. Analgesia alone is of little benefit, as reduced gastric motility prevents its absorption. If vomiting is severe, consideration should be given to administering the anti-emetic per rectum.

The majority of migraine sufferers experience their first episode before the age of 30 and so any individual who presents with a first attack over the age of 40 should be viewed with suspicion and carefully investigated.

Cluster headaches

Cluster headaches refer to repeated episodes of headaches occurring several times a day and lasting between 30 minutes and 2 hours, clusters lasting from 1 to 4 months followed by a period of remission. Pain can occur at any time, but often follows a pattern and frequently occurs an hour after falling asleep. The pain is described as a stabbing, boring pain, which causes the individual to be restless, pacing the floor rather than going to bed. Vomiting is not common. Trigger factors have been linked with alcohol and vasodilators in particular. Treatment is based on analgesia, which is best taken prophylactically prior to expected episodes.

Headaches with associated neurological symptoms

Serious neurological illness may manifest in the form of headaches, but is likely to be accompanied by other neurological signs. Brain tumours, for example, are often associated with fitting and focal neurological signs. The form of the focal signs is dependent upon the site of the tumour, but may include changes in mood, memory, balance, motor function, gait and coordination. The most serious indication of underlying pathology is failing vision and or reducing levels of consciousness. Again, a thorough history is important in order to establish trends; single occurrences are open to misinterpretation.

Any headache associated with other neurological symptoms must be treated with suspicion and the patient referred immediately.

Subarachnoid haemorrhage

Spontaneous subarachnoid haemorrhage generally results from the rupture of an intercranial aneurysm on a major artery in the circle of Willis. The patient generally presents with sudden onset of an intense headache which may initially be frontal or occipital, but eventually becomes generalized. The blood in the subarachnoid space leads to irritation and neurological signs such as drowsiness, confusion, neck stiffness, photophobia, convulsions and loss of consciousness. Depending upon the location of the bleed, the individual may have aphasia, hemiparesis or hemiplegia.

Management is focused on supporting the vital functions in terms of airway, breathing and circulation. Particular attention should be given to the monitoring of the blood pressure, as a raised blood pressure may increase the degree of bleeding.

Cerebrovascular accident and transient ischaemic attacks

Ischaemic brain injury

The most frequently observed types of brain ischaemia seen in the ED are transient ischaemic attacks and ischaemic stroke. In both cases, ischaemia leads to focal loss of cerebral function. As the name suggests, the symptoms of the ischaemia are short-lived, lasting less than 24 hours, the actual ischaemia being shorter in duration than this. When symptoms last more than 24 hours, death occurs from what is thought to be a cerebral vascular event alone (Lott et al. 1999).

In most cases stroke is ischaemic in origin leading to infarction. There are, however, a smaller number of instances where stroke is haemorrhagic in origin, resulting from either a primary intercerebral bleed or a subarachnoid haemorrhage in the remaining (Warlow 1996).

Assessment

- A full history
  - onset of symptoms
  - duration
  - exacerbation
- Observation
  - skin colour, appearance
  - respiratory rate, rhythm and depth
  - pulse
  - blood pressure
  - temperature
  - Glasgow Coma Scale.

The modes of presentation of both transient ischaemia and stroke differ little other than in the duration of the symptoms. Symptoms vary depending upon the area of brain affected:

- hemiparesis
- hemiplegia
- dizziness
- dysarthria
- dysphagia
- dysphasia
- ataxia
- visual disturbances
- confusion
- reduced level of consciousness
- unconsciousness.

Management

As with subarachnoid haemorrhage, management is focused upon supporting the vital functions in terms of airway, breathing and circulation. Particular attention should be given to monitoring of the blood pressure, as a raised blood pressure may increase the degree of bleeding.

Epilepsy

Epilepsy in itself is not a medical emergency; however, there are a number of mechanisms which may make it so, the most common being injury sustained during a convulsion and several seizures following on from the previous in quick succession – status epilepticus. This is more common at the extremes of age, with over 50% of all cases occurring in children and a disproportionately high incidence in those over 60 years of age. It also occurs most commonly in patients with no previous history of epilepsy (Wilkes 2004).

Neurones within the brain communicate in a systematic way. During a seizure, discharge from the neurones is chaotic, often manifesting in a tonic-clonic fit, but it may manifest in many other ways. During the tonic phase, the individual loses consciousness, this being accompanied by muscle contraction causing the body to become stiff, jaw to be clenched, air to be forced out of the lungs and possibly incontinence. The tonic phase is followed by the clonic phase which is characterized by rhythmic contractions of the limbs and trunk – convulsions.

Normally when convulsions cease, the individual is drowsy, confused and may have a headache. The main danger for the individual in such circumstances is from injury when falling to the ground or colliding with objects or from having objects forced into the mouth by unwitting 'helpers'. It is important to establish if the fit is related to epilepsy or if it is a symptom of some other condition such as head injury or subarachnoid haemorrhage. Status epilepticus, where as one seizure ends another immediately commences, is a potentially life-threatening condition requiring immediate intervention to break the cycle. Status epilepticus has a significant mortality (2–4%) and morbidity (10%) with irreversible neurological damage (Appleton 1994). The mainstay of management is securing the airway, administration of oxygen, assessment of respiratory and cardiac function and the administration of either lorazepam or diazepam intravenously (Scottish Intercollegiate Guidelines Network 2003).

GLUCOSE REGULATION

Two of the hormones secreted by the pancreas, insulin and glucagon, have an important function in the maintenance of blood glucose levels. Insulin is secreted in response to elevated blood glucose levels, its function being to promote the storage of glucose by facilitating its uptake by the cells and by the synthesis of glycogen in the liver, renal cortex and the muscles. Consequently, these actions reduce blood glucose.

Unlike insulin, the stimuli for glucagon release are hunger and a low blood sugar level, the net effect of its release being to raise the blood sugar level. This is achieved by the glycogenolysis, the conversion of stored glycogen into glucose. In addition, glucose is synthesized from lactate, amino acids and glycerol.

Assessment of blood sugar

Patient observation and a nursing history may provide an indication that the patient has an altered blood sugar. The use of single drop of blood laboratory sticks is a rapid and accurate method of providing objective confirmation of your observations. This should always be followed up with a laboratory test of a larger sample of blood drawn by venepuncture. Such assessments should also be considered for those patients who have an altered level of consciousness and where a raised or lowered blood sugar cannot be excluded.

Diabetes mellitus

Diabetes mellitus is a condition whereby the cells are unable to access and utilize glucose taken in through the diet, due to either a lack of insulin or ineffective insulin. A lack of naturally occurring insulin is referred to as type 1, commonly known as insulin-dependent diabetes mellitus (IDDM), which generally first appears in childhood. Where naturally occurring insulin is present but is ineffective, the condition is termed type 2, commonly known as non-insulin-dependent diabetes mellitus (NIDDM). This often first appears in later life. As a consequence of the cells' inability to access the glucose, it remains in the circulation, with some being excreted by the kidneys. In the absence of effective glucose metabolism, the body begins to metabolize fats.

Three main conditions occur in diabetes which may present a threat to life: hypoglycaemia, diabetic ketoacidosis (DKA) and hyperglycaemic hyperosmolar state (HHS) also known as hyperosmolar non-ketotic state (HONK). HHS replaces the older terms, 'HONK coma' and 'HONK', because mild to moderate ketosis is commonly present in this state and alterations of sensoria may be present without coma (English & Williams 2003).

Hypoglycaemia occurs in all types of diabetics and non-diabetics and occurs when there is a lowered plasma level of glucose. Diabetic ketoacidosis almost only ever occurs in type 1. In the presence of uncontrolled hyperglycaemia metabolism of lipids occurs, resulting in the production of large amounts of ketones and an associated metabolic acidosis (English & Williams 2004). Hyperglycaemic hyperosmolar state most commonly occurs among type 2 diabetics and is associated with often very high blood glucose levels, frequently without the production of ketones and the associated acidosis.

Assessment

Assessment of the neurologically impaired patient is important regardless of the suspected mechanism:

- A full history
  - onset of symptoms
  - duration
  - exacerbation
- Observation
  - skin colour, appearance
  - respiratory rate, rhythm and depth
  - pulse
  - blood pressure
  - temperature
  - odour on the breath

- Reagent strip blood test for glucose
- Formal blood sample for laboratory blood glucose measurement
- Assessment for dehydration.

Hypoglycaemia

Symptoms and signs

- Blood glucose of less than 3.0 mmol/L
- Rapid in onset in IDDM, where synthetic insulin intake oversupplies glucose intake or where there is an increased glucose demand
- Slower in onset in NIDDM.

Early signs

- weakness
- sweating
- tachycardia
- palpitations
- tremor
- irritability
- confusion
- amnesia
- visual disturbance.

Later signs

- unconsciousness
- fitting.

All individuals with a reduced level of consciousness, especially if associated with alcohol, should routinely have blood glucose measured by use of a reagent labstick.

Management
The conscious individual

- Fast-acting sugar in the form of a drink, e.g. sugar in tea or coffee, soft drink – not diet/low calorie. It is important to note that metformin is a sucrose inhibitor, therefore sugar in the form of glucose is required for patients on this medication.
- Longer-acting sugar, e.g. a sandwich or biscuits.

The unconscious individual

- Maintain the airway
- Support breathing
- Glucagon by injection – converted into glucose by the body; benefits are temporary and so it must be followed up with oral long-acting sugar when consciousness returns and the individual is able to protect his own airway
- 50% glucose intravenous infusion – must be into a large vein as hypertonic fluids are highly irritant.

Diabetic ketoacidosis

Symptoms and signs

- Blood glucose persistently above 15 mmol/L
- Usually type 1, but can occasionally be type 2
- Osmotic diuresis – water following glucose excreted by the kidney
- Thirst
- Polyuria
- Oliguria
- Fatigue
- Warm dry skin
- Nausea
- Vomiting
- Electrolyte imbalance
- Loss of consciousness.

Management

- Airway management as required
- Support of breathing
- Rehydration with i.v. isotonic fluids
- Insulin – guided by measured blood glucose
- Correction of electrolyte imbalance.

HAEMATOLOGY

The blood has a number of important functions, many of which impinge on other systems and processes. It plays a vital role in the transportation of respiratory gases, maintenance of body temperature, acid-base balance, fluid and electrolyte balance and immunity. Blood, by volume, is predominantly plasma, in which are suspended red blood cells, white blood cells and platelets. Red blood cells are predominantly involved in the transportation of oxygen by means of the haemoglobin. The red cells are produced in the bone marrow and remain in the circulation for about 120 days. Changes in blood concentration, infection and some drugs are known to easily damage the relatively fragile red blood cells.

White cells are produced in the bone marrow and are considerably less numerous than the red blood cells. The white cells are of three main types: granulocytes (neutrophils, eosinophils and basophils), lymphocytes and monocytes.

Collectively these cells form the basis of the body's defence system. Platelet formation also takes place in the bone marrow; 60–75% of platelets stay in the circulation and the bulk of the remainder are found in the spleen (Hinchcliff et al. 1996). Platelets are predominantly involved in clotting processes.

The plasma, as well as being a transport medium for the red cells, white cells and platelets, contains a number of salts and proteins. The proteins have a wide range of functions, including maintaining the osmotic pressure of the blood, clotting and immunity.

Haematological assessment

Much of the assessment may be based upon patient observation and the nursing history. However, much information may be gained from the appropriate haematological and biochemical tests and the interpretation of the results.

Sickle cell disease

Although commonly viewed as affecting only black people, sickle cell disease is in fact also seen in Mediterranean, Middle Eastern and Indian communities (Franklin 1990). Sickle cell disease is thought to have evolved over a considerable time in malaria-endemic areas, as a defence against malaria. The evolutionary changes have resulted in a change in the structure of the haemoglobin, which in sickle cell disease can lead to a change in the shape of the red blood cell to form the classically sickle-shaped blood cell, and these changes are at a genetic level, accounting for the hereditary element of sickle cell disease (Davies & Oni 1997).

The most commonly occurring crisis experienced by sufferers of sickle cell disease is painful crisis and this accounts for over 90% of hospital admissions for patients with sickle cell disease (Brozovic et al. 1987). Sickle cells can cluster together causing occlusion of small blood vessels. Such obstruction reduces the blood flow to the distal tissues and causes the acute pain. It is the acute pain which precipitates the attendance at the ED, but it is essential that an adequate assessment is made to identify factors which may have triggered the episode, such as:

- reduced oxygenation – often following exercise
- cold or excessive heat
- dehydration
- fever
- infections
- stress.

Assessment

Assessment will include:

- A full history, including past history as well as the history of the current episode:
  - onset of symptoms
  - duration
  - exacerbation
- Observation
  - respiratory effort
  - use of accessory muscles

- chest movement and symmetry
- skin colour
- respiratory rate, rhythm and depth (respiration may be compromised if sickling occurs in the pulmonary circulation)
- pulse
- blood pressure
- temperature
- Glasgow Coma Scale as sickling in cerebral vessels can lead to ischaemic stroke
- Palpation
  - degree of chest expansion
  - temperature of the skin
- Auscultation
  - quality of breath sound
  - degree of air entry
- Pulse oximetry – with caution
- Chest X-ray.

Clinical features

These include severe pain which commonly starts in the limbs, but may occur in the back and chest. Other clinical features may be associated with the precipitating factors, such as dehydration.

Management

This includes rapid and adequate analgesia, usually requiring opiate analgesics. These should not be delayed by undertaking a detailed examination (Department of Health 1993). Intravenous fluids are particularly important for patients with renal involvement and the aim should be to generate urine output in excess of 100 ml/h (McLaren 2004). Seek specialist advice from the haematologist. As well as pain relief, ensure the patient is warm and able to rest. Oxygen therapy should be given if indicated; however, oxygen will be of little or no benefit to most individuals in sickle cell crisis as the problem is associated with obstructed blood flow and not oxygenation of that blood. It is highly recommended that each department has a policy for managing individuals with sickle cell disease and information on where to access specialist advice and support locally.

Neutropaenic pyrexia

One of the major causes of fevers in cancer patients is infection, especially in relation to neutropaenia. Fever in the neutropaenic cancer patient represents an absolute emergency, since undetected and untreated infections in neutropaenic patients can progress quickly (Bosnjak 2004). Fever in a neutropaenic cancer patient may signify a life-threatening infection and in a cancer patient should be considered indicative of infection until proven otherwise and appropriate assessments should be instituted immediately.

Assessment

Clinical evaluation of an infection-related fever includes a complete history and physical examination with careful attention to inspection of the skin, all body orifices, fingerstick and venepuncture sites, biopsy sites, and skin folds (e.g. breasts, axilla, groin). The perirectal area should also be assessed, since a history of haemorrhoids places neutropaenic patients (especially those with leukaemia) at particular risk for infection. Assessment should include the respiratory, gastrointestinal, urinary and neurological systems. Patients should be checked for abdominal distension and tenderness. Cultures should be obtained from each port and lumen, as well as from a peripheral vein.

Management

All neutropaenic cancer patients should be considered to be at risk for infection and, once febrile, should be treated immediately with antimicrobials, without waiting for clinical and/or microbiological documentation of infection (Bosnjak 2004): this is known as empirical antibiotic therapy. Empirical antibiotic treatment of all neutropaenic patients at the onset of fever continues to be controversial. However, it also remains the key aspect of infection management. The specific composition of the empirical antibiotic regimen also remains subject to change, which is due to the changing pattern of pathogens, the emergence of antibiotic-resistant organisms, the appearance of the new clinical entities, the availability of new drugs and the improved models for patient's infection risk categorization (Bosnjak 2004). While there is a general consensus that empirical therapy is appropriate, there is no consensus as to which antibiotics or combinations of antibiotics should be used.

CONCLUSION

In the modern ED, a 'medical emergency' can range from a full cardiac arrest to a GP referral patient with an exacerbation of a chronic condition. This chapter has considered the more common medical conditions which may result in ED attendances. The ED nurse plays an important role in identifying and alleviating symptoms and conditions which can be debilitating for the patient. While many medical conditions are chronic, the exacerbation of these conditions may require the patient to attend ED for subsequent admission. The provision of supportive care can alleviate the suffering and disruption caused by these medical emergencies.

References

Appleton R (1994) *The Nursing Times Guide to Epilepsy*. Basingstoke: Macmillan.

Axford J (1996) *Medicine*. Oxford: Blackwell Science.

Bickley LS, Szilagyi PG (2003) *Bates' Guide To Physical Examination And History Taking*, 8th edn. Philadelphia: Lippincott, Williams & Wilkins.

Bosnjak S (2004) Treatment of a febrile neutropenic patient. *Archives of Oncology*, **12**(3), 179–181.

British Thoracic Society (2004) *The British Guideline on the Management of Asthma*. Edinburgh: BTS & SIGN.

British Thoracic Society (2003) British guidelines on the management of suspected acute pulmonary embolism. *Thorax*, **58**, 470–484.

British Thoracic Society (1997) British Thoracic Society Guidelines for the management of chronic obstructive pulmonary disease. *Thorax*, **52**(Suppl. 5), S1–28.

Brozovic M, Davies SC, Brownell AI (1987) Acute admissions of patients with sickle cell disease who live in Britain. *British Medical Journal*, **294**, 1206–1208.

Davies SC, Oni L (1997) Management of patients with sickle cell disease. *British Medical Journal*, **315**, 656–660.

Department of Health (1993) *Report of a Working Party of the Standing Medical Advisory Committee on Sickle Cell, Thalassaemia and other Haemoglobinopathies*. London: HMSO.

Despopoulos A, Sibernagi I (1986) *Color Atlas of Physiology*. New York: Thième.

Driscoll P, Gwinnutt P, LeDuc Jimmerson C, Goodall (1994) *Trauma Resuscitation: The Team Approach*. Basingstoke: Macmillan.

Edwards CRW, Bouchier IAD, Haslet C, Chilvers ER (1995) *Davidson's Principles and Practice of Medicine*, 17th edn. Edinburgh: Churchill Livingstone.

Emergency Nurses Association (1994) *Emergency Nursing Core Curriculum*, 4th edn. Philadelphia: WB Saunders.

English P, Williams G (2004) Hyperglycaemic crises and lactic acidosis in diabetes mellitus. *Postgraduate Medical Journal* **80**, 253–261.

Franklin I (1990) *Sickle Cell Disease: A Guide for Patients, Carers and Health Workers*. London: Faber & Faber.

Ganong WF (2003) *Review of Medical Physiology*, 21st edn. Connecticut: Appleton & Lange.

Gibson GJ (2003) Respiratory function tests. In: Warrel DA, Cox TM, Firth JD, eds. *Oxford Textbook of Medicine*. Oxford: Oxford University Press.

Goadsby PJ (2003) Headache (chronic tension-type). *Clinical Evidence Concise*, **9**, 269–270.

Greaves I, Hodgetts T, Porter K (2005) *Emergency Care: A Textbook for Paramedics*, 2nd edn. London: WB Saunders.

Hinchcliff S, Montague S, Watson R (1996) *Physiology for Nursing Practice*, 2nd edn. London: Baillière Tindall.

Knopp RK (1992) Near drowning. In: Rosen P, Barkin RM, Braen G, et al., eds. *Emergency Medicine: Concepts and Clinical Practice*. St Louis: Mosby Year Book.

Levine RL, Fromm RE (1995) *Critical Care Monitoring: From Pre-hospital to the ICU*. St Louis: Mosby.

Lott C, Hennes HJ, Dick W (1999) A medical emergency. *Journal of Accidental Emergency Medicine*, **16**(1), 2–7.

McLaren H (2004) Anaemia. In: *Textbook of Emergency Medicine*, 2nd edn. (eds P Cameron, G Jelinek, AM Kelly, L Murray, AFT Brown, J Heyworth) Edinburgh: Churchill Livingstone.

Mills K, Morton R, Page G (1995) *Colour Atlas and Text of Emergencies*, 2nd edn. London: Mosby-Wolfe.

Morris J (2003) Environmental emergencies. In: Newberry L, ed *Sheehy's Emergency Nursing: Principles and Practice*, 5th edn. St Louis: Mosby.

Moyle J (2002) *Pulse Oximetry*. 2nd edn. London: British Medical Journal Publishing Group.

Newman Taylor AJ (2003) Endocrine disorders. In: Warrel DA, Cox TM, Firth JD, eds. *Oxford Textbook of Medicine*. Oxford: Oxford University Press.

Nicholson P (2004) Renal colic. In: *Textbook of Emergency Medicine*. 2nd edn. (eds P Cameron, G Jelinek, AM Kelly, L Murray, AFT Brown, J Heyworth) Edinburgh: Churchill Livingstone.

Paradiso C (1995) *Fluids and Electrolytes*. Philadelphia: JB Lippincott.

Robinson R, Stott R (1993) *Medical Emergencies: Diagnosis and Treatment*, 6th edn. Oxford: Butterworth Heinemann.

Scottish Intercollegiate Guidelines Network (2003) *Diagnosis and Management of Epilepsy in Adults: A National Clinical Guideline*. Edinburgh: Scottish Intercollegiate Guidelines Network.

Trevedi BK (1996) Nephrolithiasis. *Postgraduate Medicine*, **100**(6), 3–78.

Warlow (1996) Cerebrovascular disease. In: Weatherall DJ, Ledingham JGG, Warrell DA, eds. *Oxford Textbook of Medicine*, 3rd edn. Oxford: Oxford University Press.

Wilkes GJ (2004) Seizures. In: *Textbook of Emergency Medicine*. 2nd edn. (eds P Cameron, G Jelinek, AM Kelly, L Murray, AFT Brown, J Heyworth) Edinburgh: Churchill Livingstone.

Chapter 28

Surgical emergencies

Valerie Small

CHAPTER CONTENTS

INTRODUCTION

The management of patients presenting with surgical emergencies relies upon rapid assessment, the formulation of an accurate working diagnosis and timely appropriate management to reduce overall morbidity and mortality. The emergency nurse may be the first person to assess the patient, and therefore finely tuned assessment skills are vital. To ensure patient assessment is safe and thorough, the skills of inspection, auscultation, palpation and percussion should be utilized appropriately during patient consultations. Some of the physical examination skills described in this chapter will require both instructions in the technique and repeated practice to achieve a proficient level of competence. This chapter will describe non-traumatic surgical emergencies of the abdominal and pelvic regions in adults, according to the following classification: acute abdomen, vascular and genitourinary emergencies.

ANATOMY AND PHYSIOLOGY OF THE ABDOMEN

A comprehensive knowledge of the anatomy and physiology of the abdomen is vitally important for the emergency nurse to assist in the rapid assessment and initiation of treatment for patients who present with a surgical emergency. The external and internal anatomy of the abdomen is broadly described in Chapter 8 (Abdominal Injuries). The anatomy and physiology of specific abdominal organs are outlined throughout this chapter.

Oesophagus

This muscular tube extends from the pharynx to the stomach. It is about 25 cm long and lies in front of the vertebral column and behind the trachea within the mediastinum. The oesophagus transports food from the pharynx, and upper and lower oesophageal sphincters regulate the movement of food into and out of the oesophagus. Lubrication of the food is provided by mucous glands coating the inner surface of the oesophagus.

Stomach

The stomach is a 'J'-shaped organ lying under the diaphragm in the epigastric, umbilical and left hypochondrial regions of the abdomen. The most superior part of the stomach is called the fundus. The largest part is the body, which has a convex area laterally called the greater curvature and a concave area medially called the lesser curvature. The final part of the stomach is the pylorus, which provides the opening into the first part of the small intestine. The muscular coats of the stomach consist of three layers: a longitudinal outer layer, a middle circular layer and an inner oblique layer of muscle fibres. The lining mucosa of the stomach is arranged into folds called rugae. These folds allow the stomach to stretch, and they disappear as the stomach is filled. The cells in the stomach produce mucus, hydrochloric acid, intrinsic factor, regulatory hormones and pepsinogen, which is involved in protein digestion.

The small intestine

The small intestine is about 6 m in length and is composed of three parts: the duodenum, the jejunum and the ileum. The duodenum is about 25 cm long, the jejunum is 2.5 m long and the ileum is 3.5 m long. The duodenum nearly completes a 180° arc which contains the head of the pancreas. The common bile duct from the liver and the pancreatic duct both empty into the duodenum. The surface area of the duodenum is greatly increased by tiny projections called villi, which are covered by columnar epithelium. The villi are about 1 mm high, and with around 10–40 mm^2 the surface area is greatly increased for absorption of nutrients. About 9 L of water enter the small intestine each day, most of which is reabsorbed, with only about 1 L reaching the large intestine. The jejunum and the ileum are similar in structure to the duodenum. The junction between the ileum and the large intestine is the ileocaecal sphincter which has a one-way valve.

The large intestine

The large intestine is responsible for the elimination of food residue and the maintenance of water and electrolyte balance. It consists of the caecum, colon, rectum and anal canal. The caecum is the first part of the large intestine and has a 9 cm long blind tube called the appendix attached. The colon is about 1.8 m long, consisting of ascending, transverse, descending and sigmoid colons. The lining of the large intestine contains many mucus-producing goblet cells and columnar cells which reabsorb water. About 1 L of water enters the large intestine each day, but only about 100 ml is lost in the faeces – the rest is reabsorbed. The circular muscle layer is complete, with an incomplete longitudinal layer of muscle. Contraction of this longitudinal layer gives the colon a pouched appearance called haustra. The rectum is a straight muscular tube running from the sigmoid colon to the anal canal. This canal is about 3 cm long and is the final part of the digestive tract.

Peritoneum

The abdominal cavity is lined by a serous membrane called the parietal peritoneum, with the organs being covered by the visceral layer of the peritoneum. There is a potential space between these two layers called the peritoneal cavity, which contains serous fluid. A small amount of fluid in the peritoneal cavity allows the abdominal organs to move freely. The intestines are supported in the abdominal cavity by a fan-like structure of connective tissue called the mesentery. The mesentery connecting the lesser curvature of the stomach to the liver and diaphragm is called the lesser omentum. The greater omentum connects the greater curvature of the stomach to the transverse colon and the posterior abdominal wall. The greater omentum also covers the front of the abdominal organs. It contains a lot of adipose tissue and looks like a fatty apron hanging over the organs. If infection occurs in the peritoneum, the greater omentum tries to wall off the infection by surrounding it, to prevent its spread. The mesenteries contain blood and lymphatic vessels and nerves that supply the abdominal organs.

Abdominal organs which lie against the posterior abdominal wall have their anterior surface covered by peritoneum and are described as retroperitoneal organs. These are the duodenum, pancreas, ascending colon, rectum, kidneys, adrenal glands and the bladder.

Abdominal wall

The abdominal wall is composed of skin, fascia and four pairs of flat, sheet-like muscles called rectus abdominis, external and internal oblique and transverse abdominis. The linea alba is a tough, fibrous band of tissue which stretches from the sternum to the symphysis pubis and is made up of the aponeurosis of the abdominal muscles. Part of the external oblique muscle forms the inguinal ligament, which runs from the anterior superior iliac pubic tubercule. Just superior to the medial end of this ligament is the superficial inguinal ring which is the outer opening of the inguinal canal. This canal contains the spermatic cord and the ilio-inguinal nerve in males and the round ligament of the uterus and the ilio-inguinal nerve in females. The posterior abdominal wall is composed of the bones of the lumbar spine and the hip bones, along with the psoas, quadratus lumborum and iliacus muscles.

NURSING ASSESSMENT OF THE ACUTE ABDOMEN

The clinical approach to patients with surgical emergencies is the same as that of any emergency. An initial overview is accomplished rapidly to evaluate that the airway is patent and protected, that air exchange is adequate, and that the patient has adequate systemic perfusion. The tools for evaluating abdominal complaints are: patient history, physical examination, imaging studies, and laboratory tests. Once airway, breathing and circulation have been assessed and appropriate interventions to correct any abnormalities have been performed, the emergency nurse may proceed to gather the history of the presenting complaint. According to the literature the most common pitfall in evaluating abdominal pain is the failure to obtain a sufficiently detailed and accurate history (Newton & Mandavia 2003).

History

The essential elements of the history are to determine

- The nature, onset, location and radiation of the abdominal pain
- The presence and sequence of onset of associated symptoms such as fever, nausea, vomiting, urinary symptoms, and pelvic symptoms (in women)
- Pertinent history related to bowel movements, appetite, weight changes, and menstrual history
- Previous medical history of similar episodes, prior medical and surgical history, and current medication use. Alcohol intake, tobacco use and known allergies should also be ascertained
- Social history related to occupation, family history, activity level, and recent foreign travel.

To establish a full clinical picture, the emergency nurse may further ascertain the following:

- **Appetite**. Has there been a recent alteration in dietary habits? Does the patient avoid certain foods for any reason? Is there any difficulty in swallowing; is there any sensation of food sticking

in the throat or chest? Has there been any change in the patient's weight? Do the patient's clothes still fit? Is the abdomen bloated?
- **Tongue**. The state of the tongue gives some indication of the state of hydration of the body. Patients who have been ill for some time with a gastrointestinal problem frequently have a fluid and electrolyte deficit. A dry brown tongue may be found in any severe illness, uraemia or acute intestinal obstruction. Additional longitudinal furrows may indicate dehydration
- **Skin**. Any change in skin colour, bruising or itching may be as a result of liver disease
- **Bowel habits**. Is there any constipation, diarrhoea, blood or mucus in the stool?
- **Energy**. Are there any feelings of lethargy or changes in mental status?

Pain assessment

Abdominal pain is due to:

- Contraction of muscle tissue
- Irritation of the mucosa
- Stretching of an organ
- Inflammation of the peritoneum
- Irritation of nerves in the area.

The body is programmed to appreciate pain from areas under voluntary control and the skin. We are therefore not able to appreciate the precise location of the source of visceral pain. In pain originating in the heart, for example, impulses pass along the dermatomes of T1-T4, so the patient experiences pain across the chest and down the arms. Pain may therefore be referred to a site far from its origin; for instance, pain from the spleen may be referred to the left shoulder due to irritation of the phrenic nerve. There are several aspects to consider when assessing a patient's pain, which can be usefully remembered by the mnemonic TROCARS (see Box 28.1).

GENERAL PRINCIPLES OF PATIENT ASSESSMENT AND ABDOMINAL EXAMINATION

Begin the assessment of the gastrointestinal tract by examining the patient's hands to discover signs of disease (see Table 28.1). Next examine the patient's eyes for pale conjunctiva as this is indicative of anaemia. Enlarged lymph nodes may be found in the supraclavicular fossa, suggestive of secondaries from a gastric carcinoma.

For the purposes of specific examination the abdomen can be divided into either four quadrants (Fig. 28.1) or nine regions (Seidel et al. 1987). To divide

Table 28.1   Hand examination

Clinical finding	Cause
Pallor	Anaemia
Clubbing	Cirrhosis
	Crohn's disease
	Ulcerative colitis
Palmar erythema	Liver disease
Spoon-shaped nails	Iron deficiency

the abdomen into quadrants draw an imaginary line from the xiphoid process of the sternum through the umbilicus to the symphysis pubis, draw a second perpendicular line across the abdomen through the umbilicus. This divides the abdomen into quadrants: right upper quadrant, right lower quadrant, left upper quadrant and left lower quadrant and is the most common method of mapping the contents of the abdomen.

In order to perform the abdominal examination satisfactorily it is essential to have a good light source and the patient should be made as relaxed as possible. Patient privacy and a full explanation of the procedure will assist in making the patient comfortable. The patient should be placed in a supine position with the head resting on a small pillow and the arms resting by the sides. In some cases the patient may be more comfortable with a small pillow under the knees, to help relax the abdominal muscles. Although it is necessary to expose the area from the sternum to the pelvis, the patient should be kept as warm as possible during the procedure, which should be performed quickly and efficiently. The patient should be examined from his right side, in a gentle manner, with warm hands and short fingernails.

Inspection

Inspection can reveal important information, including the presence of distension, masses, surgical scars, discoloration by ecchymosis (Cullen's and Grey-Turner's signs), and skin abnormalities such as spider angiomata, petechiae, jaundice and rashes. Look for any visible peristalsis and pulsations. Pulsation of the abdominal aorta may be observed in thin patients or in those with an aortic aneurysm. The location of operation scars may give clues as to the type of surgery previously performed. The abdomen is normally symmetrical, and may be asymmetrical due to bowel obstruction, hernia or spinal deformity. It is useful to try to visualize the underlying organs during the examination. For example, asymmetry of the lower abdomen may be due to a distended bladder, masses of the ovary, uterus or colon. Distended veins around the umbilicus signify portal hypertension. Generalized distension of the abdomen may be due to one of the five Fs:

- fat
- fluid
- faeces
- flatus
- foetus.

The abdomen should move freely with respiration, but this will be diminished or absent in generalized peritonitis.

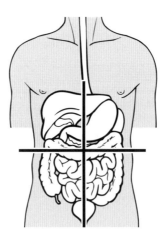

Right upper quadrant

Right lobe of liver
Gallbladder
Pylorus
Duodenum
Head of pancreas
Upper right kidney

Right lower quadrant

Lower right kidney
Cecum
Appendix
Ascending colon
Right fallopian tube (female)
Right ovary (female)
Right ureter
Bladder (distended)

Left upper quadrant

Left lobe of liver
Spleen
Stomach
Left kidney
Body of pancreas
Splenic flexure of colon

Left lower quadrant

Descending colon
Sigmoid colon
Left fallopian tube (female)
Left ovary (female)
Left ureter
Bladder (distended)

Figure 28.1   Abdominal contents.

Auscultation

Auscultation should precede palpation as the latter can induce peristalsis artificially. Bowel sounds are regarded as the least helpful element of the abdominal examination because reflex ileus can occur with virtually any painful abdominal condition and might persist for some time, even with intra-abdominal catastrophes (Newton & Mandavia 2003). The emergency nurse may gain valuable experience from listening to many normal abdomens to establish a baseline. Initially, it is best to listen using the diaphragm of the stethoscope to the right of the umbilicus. Bowel sounds should be checked for at least 1 minute in all four quadrants, before declaring that they are absent. Absent bowel sounds are a feature of paralytic ileus, late obstruction and generalized peritonitis.

In an obstructed patient, the absence of bowel sounds suggests strangulation or ischaemia. In small bowel obstruction the bowel sounds are exaggerated initially, with frequent low-pitched gurgles, rising to become high-pitched tinkling sounds as peristalsis increases above the obstruction. The presence of these sounds coincides with the peristalsis and the colicky abdominal pain suffered by the patient. In between these painful episodes, the bowel is quiet. The bowel is also hyperactive in gastroenteritis and severe diarrhoea.

Normally, blood flow along arteries cannot be heard using a stethoscope. However, when the vessel becomes diseased the resultant turbulence, as the blood flows over atheromatous plaques, produces soft high-pitched sounds called bruits. These bruits may be heard using the bell of the stethoscope over a diseased aorta and renal, hepatic, splenic or femoral vessels. Check the aorta by listening in the mid-epigastric region above the umbilicus. Renal bruits may be heard in this area, and additionally in the flanks or posteriorly over the kidneys. Femoral bruits may be heard in the groin. Bruits are heard even if the patient changes position.

Percussion

Light percussion is performed to determine the presence of masses, enlargement of an organ or abdominal distension. The middle finger of the left hand is placed on the area to be percussed, and the back of its middle phalanx is struck with the tip of the middle finger of the right hand. The percussing finger should be bent, so that when the blow is delivered its terminal phalanx is at right angles to the metacarpal bone it is striking. Tympany is the normal percussion note and is a hollow resonant sound heard over the abdomen, apart from over the solid organs. Dull percussion notes will be heard over dense organs such as the liver and spleen, tumours or over a fluid-filled bladder.

Palpation

Palpation is saved for last and should be performed gently, beginning with the quadrant most remote from the patient's pain, moving towards the painful area. Deep palpation and the classically described test for rebound tenderness have limited utility and might be misleading (Newton & Mandavia 2003). If the patient is not relaxed, the abdominal muscles will tense, making examination impossible. Using a warm hand flat on the abdominal wall, gently palpate all four quadrants. Palpation of specific organs requires practice, and further description is beyond the scope of this chapter. Check for the presence and equality of the femoral pulses, and assess the femoral and inguinal lymph nodes for tenderness or enlargement.

Vomit

The strongest stimuli for vomiting are irritation and distension of the stomach. Nerve impulses are transmitted to the medulla, and returning impulses to the upper gastrointestinal organs, diaphragm and abdominal muscles. The stomach is then squeezed between the diaphragm and the abdominal muscles. Prolonged vomiting will lead to loss of gastric juice and fluid. This can lead to disturbance in fluid and acid-base balance. If bleeding is severe, the vomit may look like pure blood or it may be dark with clots. Bleeding may be altered to a dark brown or black colour by gastric juice. The dark colour is due to the conversion of haemoglobin into haematin. The altered blood is sometimes compared to 'coffee grounds'. Blood in vomit may have been swallowed from mouth injuries or epistaxis. Vomit may have a faecal odour in advanced intestinal obstruction.

Faeces

Black stools may be due to the presence of blood or iron. Bleeding high in the intestinal tract produces offensive 'tarry' stools. If bleeding is from the large intestine, the blood may be less mixed with the faeces and may be seen as streaks. Stools may be pale in obstructive jaundice, diarrhoea or malabsorption.

Shock

Shock is a condition which results from inadequate blood supply to the tissues, leading to a decreased supply of oxygen and other nutrients, which are essential to maintain the metabolic needs of the body. Without oxygen, the cells shift from aerobic to anaerobic metabolism. Anaerobic metabolism is a less efficient method of extracting energy, and the cells begin to use up their stores of adenosine triphosphate (ATP) faster than they can be replaced. This disturbs the cell electrolyte balance, causing sodium to be retained and potassium lost. Excessive sodium in the cell means that it becomes waterlogged. This immediately affects the cells of the nervous system and myocardium leading to depression of their function. The water that leaks into the cells is coming from the interstitial space and will be replaced from the intravascular space, causing further hypovolaemia. Anaerobic metabolism produces large quantities of acid. This increase is detected by the brain, which increases the respiratory rate to reduce the carbon dioxide level and correct the imbalance.

As the supply of oxygen and nutrients fails to meet the demand, the body responds by activating compensatory mechanisms to improve perfusion to the vital organs. As the blood volume decreases, the peripheral blood vessels constrict due to sympathetic stimulation, which increases peripheral resistance and raises the blood pressure. As a result the patient looks pale and has cold clammy skin. As perfusion of the vital centres in the brain is reduced, the patient becomes anxious and restless.

The increase in peripheral resistance may be detected clinically by a rise in the diastolic blood pressure. Eventually as the body loses the battle, the systolic pressure will begin to fall. Reduced blood flow to the kidney, because it is not a vital organ as far as the body is concerned, causes the release of certain chemicals which increase sodium retention, increase water retention and increase vasoconstriction. The release of adrenaline causes glycogen to be broken down to supply the additional glucose needed and as a result an increased blood sugar level will occur.

The management of the patient who has lost blood or body fluids is the most important aspect of dealing with surgical emergencies. It is vital that the condition is recognized and treated promptly to reduce both morbidity and mortality. Rapid volume repletion is indicated in patients with severe hypovolaemia or hypovolaemic shock; delayed therapy can lead to ischaemic injury and possibly to irreversible shock and multiorgan failure. The management of the patient with haemorrhage may be surgical, or in certain cases conservative. Clinical symptoms include tachycardia, hypotension, peripheral vasoconstriction, oliguria and a narrowed pulse pressure in the absence of jugular venous distension or pulmonary oedema. Monitoring of vital signs and nursing observations are of vital importance and should be carried out at least quarter-hourly. Accurate measurement of intake and all output including

vomiting will assist in assessing adequate tissue perfusion. Hourly urinary output of approximately 1 ml/kg per hour is indicative of effective circulating volume.

Management principles

It is important to provide emotional support for the patient, since fear and anxiety can aggravate the condition.

- Administer oxygen via a non-rebreather mask at 12–15 L/min.
- Initiate intravenous fluid replacement. Two large-bore cannulae, 14 or 16 gauge, should be placed in the antecubital fossa and well secured to provide an adequate flow rate. Blood should be drawn for baseline laboratory investigations including blood group and cross-match. The choice of replacement fluid depends in part upon the type of fluid that has been lost: as an obvious example blood components are indicated in patients who are bleeding (Scott 2004). In general an initial bolus of 1–2 L of isotonic saline is recommended and is the preferred solution in managing patients with severe volume depletion not due to haemorrhage. Both isotonic saline solutions (crystalloid) and colloid-containing solutions are used to replace extracellular fluid deficit, but research has shown that saline solutions are as safe and effective in expanding the plasma volume as colloid and are much less expensive (Scott 2004). Following the administration of a fluid bolus it is important to assess the patient's response by rechecking vital signs and assessing the patient's general condition. The rate of flow is usually slowed as the blood pressure increases: too rapid an increase in blood pressure can cause further bleeding. In extreme cases of haemorrhage or haemorrhagic shock it may be necessary to give the patient O-negative blood (universal donor), while awaiting type-specific blood. Fluids may be given rapidly using a pressure device, but should be warmed to prevent inducing hypothermia. Hypothermia results in decreased tissue extraction of oxygen from haemoglobin and impaired cardiac contract. Hypothermia also causes problems with blood clotting due to disruption of cellular enzymes and platelets, and increased fibrinolysis. An arterial line should be placed in all patients who fail to respond promptly to initial fluid resuscitation.
- Provide prescribed analgesia
- Prepare the patient for surgery where indicated
- The patient may be positioned with the legs slightly elevated to increase venous return to the heart and so increase blood pressure

- Gastric distension can lead to vomiting; inserting a gastric tube will allow decompression of the stomach and provide a sample for testing
- Inserting a urinary catheter will allow accurate fluid balance and provide evidence of successful fluid volume replacement
- Monitor the temperature to determine hypothermia, or pyrexia due to infection.

ACUTE ABDOMINAL EMERGENCIES

Bowel obstruction

Obstruction to the passage of contents may occur in the small or large bowel and is a serious life-threatening condition. Obstruction of the small bowel is more common because the ileum is the narrowest segment, and therefore more easily obstructed. Obstruction of the large bowel tends to develop more slowly and is associated with a high mortality rate (Biondo et al. 2004). The most common cause of small bowel obstruction is postoperative adhesions, with hernias being the second most common cause. Adhesions are bands of scar tissue following inflammation which can constrict the intestine. Other causes of bowel obstruction are:

- volvulus – twisting of bowel more common in the elderly
- intussusception – segment of intestine prolapsed into an adjacent part, usually in infants
- mesenteric embolus – interferes with blood supply, foreign bodies (e.g. drug smugglers swallowing packages), faecal impaction, tumours
- paralytic ileus – peristalsis may be interrupted by disturbance of the nerve supply following peritonitis, pancreatitis, shock, spinal cord lesions, or after abdominal surgery
- inflammatory bowel disease (Crohn's disease).

Pathophysiology

Obstruction of the bowel causes fluid, gas and air to collect near the obstruction site. The bowel tries to force its contents past the obstruction by increasing peristalsis. This causes damage to the intestinal mucosa, which results in further swelling at the site. This increased pressure exceeds venous and capillary pressure, causing reduced blood supply to the bowel. As the bowel wall swells, instead of performing its normal function in this area, it starts to secrete water, sodium and potassium, leading to dehydration. Gas-forming bacteria collect in the area and aggravate distension by fermentation, which produces more gas. If untreated, the interruption of the blood supply

to the bowel will lead to gangrene, perforation of the bowel and peritonitis. Patients who develop septicaemia in these cases have a 70% mortality rate (Emmans 1993).

Assessment

Obstruction of the small bowel is commonly associated with sudden onset of colicky abdominal pain radiating over the whole abdomen. Appendicitis is characterized by a dull pain in the right lower quadrant, accompanied by an elevated temperature. The pain of pancreatitis is constant, not colicky, and the pain of diverticulitis usually occurs in the left lower quadrant and may be accompanied by blood in the faeces (Clemings et al. 1990). In large bowel obstruction, the pain has a more gradual onset. In small bowel obstruction there is vomiting of gastric juice, mucus and bile in high obstructions. If the obstruction is in the ileum or large bowel, the patient may vomit faecal contents. This loss of fluid by vomiting and increased intestinal secretion leads to severe dehydration and electrolyte imbalance. The extravasation of plasma from the capillaries adds to the accumulation of fluid in the intestines, which compresses the veins, reducing venous return and contributing to the shock.

The patient will display the classic features of shock as previously described; rapid weak pulse, restlessness, low blood pressure and cold, clammy skin. There is constipation and no flatus is passed. The patient suffers abdominal distension due to the accumulation of gas and fluids, with active tinkling bowel sounds initially, progressing to absent bowel sounds as peristalsis diminishes. The stretched weakened intestinal wall becomes permeable to organisms and perforation of the bowel may lead to peritonitis. Obstruction of the large bowel is less acute, with complete constipation (obstipation) and slowly developing distension; diarrhoea may be present with partial obstruction. The pain is described as colicky, with vomiting and dehydration occurring later.

Investigations

Blood should be sent for full blood count, electrolytes, amylase, glucose and cross-match. A raised WCC can be an indicator of infection, which can suggest perforation or even ensuing sepsis and possible bacterial translocation as the gut becomes so distended that the bowel contents are able to pass through its membranes (Hughes 2005, Bratt-Wyton 1998). Abdominal radiographs in both the supine and upright positions may reveal bowel distortion and distension, with air or fluid levels. In small bowel obstruction, a central gas shadow may be seen, with no air in the large bowel. In large bowel obstruction, gas can be seen proximal to the blockage but not distal to it.

Management

The most life-threatening problem for this patient is fluid volume deficit and therefore the initial priorities are to treat the shock due to the hypovolaemia and to prevent further complications. Administer 100% oxygen via a non-rebreather mask at 12–15 L/min. Initiate large-bore intravenous infusions, using crystalloids such as normal saline. A nasogastric tube should be inserted to decompress the stomach, as fluid shifts can be more severe as the bowel becomes decompressed. Accurate recording of fluid balance and vital signs is essential. Assist the patient into a comfortable position, and give prescribed analgesia and antibiotics, which reduce the risk of sepsis if the bowel perforates.

In less urgent cases of large bowel obstruction, the patient may be given an enema to attempt to clear the obstruction. Intestinal obstruction other than paralytic ileus is treated surgically. In some cases, it may be possible to delay surgery to improve the patient's general condition, but if there is evidence of compromised blood supply to the intestines, emergency surgery is indicated. If the bowel is strangulated or if there is gross distension, surgery should take place within 1 hour to avoid perforation.

The extent of the surgery required will depend upon the cause of the obstruction. Simple adhesions may be divided, but if the blood supply to the bowel has been interrupted, the bowel is checked for viability and, if gangrenous, will require resection with anastomosis or a stoma. Stomas may be temporary or permanent.

Ileus is most often associated with intraperitoneal or retroperitoneal infection; it may be produced by mesenteric ischaemia, arterial or venous injury or after intra-abdominal surgery. Gastric and colonic motility disturbances after abdominal surgery result from abdominal manipulation. The small bowel is rarely affected, with motility and absorption returning to normal within a few hours of operation. The large bowel may remain inert for 48 to 72 hours. Symptoms include abdominal distension, vomiting, obstipation and cramp. Treatment is usually conservative and involves nasogastric suction to reduce distension. Intravenous fluids to correct electrolyte deficiencies are essential; the condition usually resolves gradually.

Peritonitis

This is a life-threatening condition due to inflammation of the visceral and parietal peritoneum (Hughes 2005). The most serious causes of peritonitis are perforation of a viscus into the peritoneal cavity, trauma, infected peritoneal blood, foreign bodies, strangulating intestinal obstruction, pelvic inflammatory disease, mesenteric thrombosis or embolism. This chemical and bacterial invasion causes an inflammatory response, with depressed intestinal motility and distension of the bowel with gas and fluid.

Pathophysiology

The peritoneal cavity is a closed sac, which normally contains a little fluid to allow the abdominal organs to move freely. The great omentum is a sheet of peritoneum which is reflected off the stomach and hangs down in front of the intestines like a curtain. If peritonitis occurs, the great omentum tries to wall off the infection by surrounding it, to prevent spread of infection. The peritoneum is remarkably resistant to infection and unless contamination continues from an uncontrolled source, tends to heal with treatment Box 28.1.

Assessment

The symptoms of peritonitis depend on the virulence and extent of the infection. In a previously well patient the sudden onset of abdominal pain is either localized if the process is confined by viscera or omentum, or generalized if the entire peritoneal cavity is involved. The patient usually lies very still and looks unwell. The abdomen is distended, rigid like a board and there is rebound tenderness, with absent bowel sounds. Signs of shock may be present (tachycardia, pallor, sweating, low blood pressure), along with pyrexia, nausea and vomiting. Respirations may be shallow due to interference by extreme abdominal distension. The peritoneal membrane becomes oedematous, with loss of protein and electrolyte fluid into the peritoneal cavity aggravating the shock. If peritonitis is not treated promptly and effectively, multisystem failure occurs rapidly (Hughes 2005).

Box 28.1 Assessing abdominal pain using mnemonic TROCARS
T Timing - duration of the pain
R Radiation - does the pain go anywhere else?
O Occurrence - when does the pain start?
C Charateristics - colicky, sharp, dull
A Aggravating factors - food, exercise
R Relieving factors - rest, medicines
S Site and Severity - location and pain score

Investigations

Plain abdominal radiographs in both supine and upright positions may show distension of both small bowel and colon, or air under the diaphragm. As little as 20 ml of air will produce a gas shadow between the liver and the diaphragm. Blood should be sent for full blood count, glucose, electrolytes, amylase (to exclude pancreatitis), arterial blood gas and group and cross-match.

Management

The treatment of peritonitis primarily involves treatment of the underlying disease; therefore early diagnosis is imperative. Two large-bore intravenous cannulae should be inserted and intravenous crystalloid fluids (either normal saline 0.9% or Hartmann's solution) should be commenced to treat hypovolaemia; blood transfusion may be commenced to treat shock and replace the protein lost in the inflammatory response in the peritoneum. 100% oxygen should be administered via a non-rebreather mask, at 12–15 L/min. A nasogastric tube should be passed to decompress the stomach and relieve distension. The use of antibiotics is advocated prior to results of cultures being available, with third-generation cephalosporins being regarded as the most safe and effective treatment. Immediate surgery is nearly always indicated for patients with peritonitis arising from appendicitis, perforated peptic ulcer, or diverticulitis. Acute pancreatitis and pelvic inflammatory disease (PID) are exceptions.

Appendicitis

This is a common cause of acute abdominal pain and is the commonest surgical emergency. The overall lifetime occurrence is approximately 12% in men and 25% in women (Old et al. 2005). It is more common in children, adolescents and young adults. Accurate and early diagnosis is essential to minimize morbidity. Prompt surgical treatment may reduce the risk of appendix perforation. The case-fatality rate is reported to be >1% in non-perforated cases, which rises to 5% or higher when perforation occurs (Old et al. 2005).

Several factors are claimed to predispose the patient to appendicitis, including:

- faecoliths – hard pellets of faeces
- food residues
- enlargement of lymphoid tissue in response to a viral infection in children.

All of these causes will lead to blockage of the appendix, allowing secretions to collect.

Pathophysiology

The appendix is a narrow blind tube which is attached to the inferior part of the caecum. It has no known physiological function, and if diseased it can be removed. Inflammation begins in the mucosa after a breach in the epithelium, allowing the entry of bowel bacteria. The appendix is a blind tube, and if secretions cannot pass the obstruction they will accumulate, causing enlargement and pain. The resulting infection leads to ulceration of the mucosa, which eventually spreads, causing peritonitis. Inflammation can cause the greater omentum to become adherent to the appendix in an attempt to wall off the infection. If the area has time to be walled off and the appendix then ruptures, an abscess will form. However, the build-up of pressure within the wall can lead to the distal part of the appendix becoming gangrenous and perforating, causing generalized peritonitis, before it has time to be walled off.

Assessment

Typical signs and symptoms of acute appendicitis appear in >50% of patients: they complain of sudden onset of epigastric or peri-umbilical pain followed by brief nausea and vomiting after a few hours. The pain is described as steady, persistent or constant by the patient. As the inflammation spreads through the walls of the appendix, involving the parietal peritoneum, it becomes confined to the right lower quadrant (Old et al. 2005). Pain is aggravated by coughing, and on rectal examination there is increased pain on the right side. There may be rebound tenderness in the right lower quadrant, although rebound tenderness in other areas suggests that the appendix has perforated and caused peritonitis. The patient may also exhibit a low-grade pyrexia of 38–39°C. The patient will try to avoid sudden movements, which increase the pain, and may keep the right thigh flexed to provide pain relief.

The following signs may demonstrate the pain of appendicitis:

- McBurney sign – tenderness on palpation in an area about 2 inches from the anterior superior iliac spine on a line with the umbilicus (the single most important sign)
- Aaron's sign – pain or distress in the area of the heart or stomach when McBurney's point is palpated
- Rovsing sign – pain in the right lower quadrant with palpation of the left lower quadrant
- Psoas sign – pain in the abdomen on hyperextension of right thigh (often indicates retroperitoneal retrocaecal appendix)

- Obturator sign – pain on internal rotation of right thigh (pelvic appendix)
- Dunphy's sign – increased pain in right lower quadrant with coughing.

Investigations

If the diagnosis of appendicitis is clear from the history and physical examination no further testing is required and prompt surgical referral is warranted (Old et al. 2005). When diagnosis is not clear options include observation and limited diagnostic tests. Blood should be sent for full blood count which may reveal a leucocytosis. Leucocyte count is raised above 10 000 in 90% of cases. Other blood tests may include glucose, amylase (to exclude pancreatitis) and electrolytes. Females with lower abdominal pain should always have their beta human chorionic gonadotrophin (B-HCG) checked, to help exclude ectopic pregnancy. A urine specimen may help to exclude urinary tract infection or urinary calculi as a cause of the pain. Imaging studies are cost-effective if a definitive diagnosis can be made and observation in a hospital can be avoided; however, outcome studies to date suggest that imaging has a small part to play in assessing atypical presentations of appendicitis (Old et al. 2005).

Differential diagnosis

- right-sided lobar pneumonia or pleurisy
- perforated ulcer
- acute cholecystitis
- intestinal obstruction
- gastroenteritis
- acute salpingitis.

Management

Initiate intravenous fluids to re-hydrate the patient. Keep patient fasting. Provide prescribed analgesia. Preoperative intramuscular or intravenous antibiotics should be commenced, with third-generation cephalosporins the preferred choice. If the condition is still located within the appendix, and it has not perforated, an appendectomy is performed. If it has progressed to peritonitis, the patient may be managed conservatively with antibiotics and intravenous fluids and surgery arranged at a later stage to remove the appendix.

The appendix may be removed by open appendectomy or laparoscopic appendectomy. The laparoscope is particularly useful in young women to allow widespread visualization of the abdomen and pelvis. This allows differentiation of appendicitis from gynaecological disease with minimally invasive surgery. The laproscope also reduces hospital stay by decreasing postoperative ileus because the tissues are handled less. There are fewer adhesions and there is less scarring from smaller incisions.

Acute pancreatitis

Acute pancreatitis has become increasingly common in Western countries in recent years (Munoz & Katerndahl 2000, Goldacre & Roberts 2004, Meadows 2005). It is a protean disease capable of wide clinical variation and may be classified as mild, involving minimal organ dysfunction with uneventful recovery, or severe, leading to necrosis and multisystemic organ failure and death (Goldacre & Roberts 2004).

Pancreatitis is an inflammatory process in which pancreatic enzymes autodigest the gland (Khoury & Deeba 2005). Recurrent attacks are referred to as chronic pancreatitis and both forms of disease present in the emergency department with acute clinical findings. Studies report that acute pancreatitis remains a disease with a high mortality rate. It is reported that death rates in the first month after admission are 30 times higher than in the general population of the same age; there have been no significant improvements in fatality rates since the 1970s (Mann et al. 1994, Goldacre & Roberts 2004).

Pathophysiology

The pancreas is located in the retroperitoneal space but as it does not have a capsule inflammation can spread easily. In acute pancreatitis, parenchymal oedema and peripancreatic fat necrosis occur first, leading to a process known as acute oedematous pancreatitis. The inflammatory process may remain localized in the pancreas, spread to regional tissues, or involve remote organ systems. Local complications of severe disease include pseudocyst, abscess and pseudoaneurysm formation (Mitchell et al. 2003).

Acute pancreatitis has numerous causes; however, two of the common causes are biliary tract obstruction related to cholelithiasis and alcohol abuse (Munoz & Katerndahl 2000, Goldacre & Roberts 2004).

Attacks of acute pancreatitis in biliary disease are the result of temporary impaction of a gallstone in the sphincter of Oddi: although the precise pathogenic mechanism is unclear, the literature suggests that the obstruction of the pancreatic duct in the absence of biliary reflux can increase ductal pressure, triggering extravasation of enzymes into the parenchyma, leading to acute pancreatitis.

Long-term alcohol abuse or alcohol intake >100 g/ day over several years cause the protein of pancreatic enzymes to precipitate within small pancreatic ductules. In time, protein plugs accumulate, inducing additional histological abnormalities. At the ductal level ethanol increases the permeability of ductules which allow enzymes to reach the parenchyma, resulting in organ damage. On the cellular level ethanol leads to intracellular accumulation of digestive enzymes; the premature activation of pancreatic enzymes results in leaks out of the ducts into the pancreatic acinar cells, causing auto-digestion of the gland (Munoz & Katerndahl 2000).

Oedema or necrosis and haemorrhage are prominent gross pathological changes. Tissue necrosis is caused by activation of several pancreatic enzymes, including trypsin and phospholipase A2. Haemorrhage is caused by extensive activation of pancreatic enzymes, including pancreatic elastase, which dissolves elastic fibres of blood vessels. In oedematous pancreatitis inflammation is usually confined to the pancreas, resulting in a mortality rate > 5%. Where there is severe necrosis and haemorrhage, inflammation is not confined to the pancreas and the mortality rate ranges from 10% to 50%.

Pancreatic exudate containing toxins and activated pancreatic enzymes permeates the retroperitoneum and sometimes the peritoneal cavity, inducing a chemical burn and increasing the permeability of blood vessels. This causes extravasation of large amounts of protein-rich fluid from the systemic circulation into 'third spaces', producing hypovolaemia and shock. On entering the systemic circulation these activated enzymes and toxins increase capillary permeability throughout the body and may reduce peripheral vascular tone, thereby intensifying hypotension. Circulating activated enzymes may also damage tissue directly: e.g. phospholipase A2 is thought to injure alveolar membranes of the lungs, leading to acute respiratory distress syndrome (ARDS).

Incidence and causes of acute pancreatitis

The incidence of acute pancreatitis in the UK has been reported to be as high as 38 per 100 000 per year and increasing; about 25% of patients develop severe or life-threatening complications and require support in high-dependency or intensive-care units (O'Reilly & Kingsnorth 2004, Mergener & Baillie 1998). Biliary tract disease and alcoholism account for 80% of hospital admissions for acute pancreatitis; the remaining 20% are attributed to other conditions. See Table 28.2 (Munoz & Katerndahl 2000).

Assessment

Acute pancreatitis may be difficult to diagnose as the signs and symptoms are common to many illnesses (Munoz & Katerndahl 2000, Mitchell et al. 2003). In acute pancreatitis abdominal pain may develop

---

Table 28.2   Minor causes of acute pancreatitis

- Medications (e.g. azathioprine, corticosteroids, sulfonamides, thiazides, frusemides, non-steroidal anti-inflammatory, methyldopa and tetracyclines)
- Viral infections (e.g. mumps, cytomegalovirus, hepatitis virus, Epstein-Barr virus and rubella)
- Structural abnormalities of the pancreatic duct (e.g. stricture, cancer)
- Structural abnormalities of the common bile duct (e.g. choledochal cyst, sphincter of Oddi stenosis)
- Peptic ulcer disease
- Abdominal or cardiopulmonary surgery which may insult the gland by ischaemia
- Endoscopic retrograde cholangiopancreatography (ERCP)
- Vascular disease (especially severe hypotension)
- Trauma to the abdomen or back resulting in sudden compression of the gland
- Hypercalcaemia (almost always due to hyperparathyroidism)
- Hyperlipidaemia
- Renal transplantation
- Heredity pancreatitis
- Intestinal parasites such as ascaris which can block pancreatic outflow
- Idiopathic

---

quickly, is frequently devastating in severity, fluctuates very little in intensity and usually persists for at least several days. Abdominal pain is located in the epigastric region or in the right upper quadrant radiating to the back or flank. The pain is classically described as constant, dull and boring and is worse when the patient is supine. The discomfort may lessen when the patient assumes a sitting or foetal position; however, coughing, vigorous movement and deep breathing may accentuate or aggravate pain. A heavy meal or drinking binge may trigger the pain and onset of symptoms. Nausea and vomiting are present in 75–90% of patients (Munoz & Katerndahl 2000). The patient will appear acutely ill and diaphoretic, and pulse rate will be elevated usually between 100 to 140 beats/min. Respirations may be shallow and rapid and blood pressure may be transiently high or low, with significant postural hypotension. Temperature may be normal or even subnormal in the first instance but may increase to 37.7–38.3°C within a few hours. The patient may also present with jaundice and dehydration. Examination of the lungs may reveal limited diaphragmatic excursion and evidence of atelectasis. About 20% of patients experience upper abdominal distension caused by gastric distension or a large pancreatic inflammatory mass displacing the stomach anteriorly. Abdominal tenderness always occurs and is usually isolated to the upper abdomen; it may be associated with mild to moderate muscular rigidity in that region. The entire abdomen rarely exhibits severe peritoneal irritation in the form of rigid board-like abdomen. Bowel sounds may be hypoactive. Rectal examination usually discloses no tenderness and stool usually tests negative for occult blood. The literature suggests that acute pancreatitis should be considered in the differential diagnosis of every acute abdomen (Munoz & Katerndahl 2000). The differential diagnosis of acute pancreatitis would include perforated gastric and duodenal ulcer, mesenteric infarction, intestinal obstruction, ectopic pregnancy, dissecting aneurysm, biliary colic, appendicitis, diverticulitis haematoma of abdominal muscles or spleen. In comparison the abdominal pain associated with choledocholithiasis tends to last for several hours rather than days. Pain associated with a perforated ulcer or mesenteric ischaemia may also develop quickly and is characteristically very severe, but nausea and vomiting are usually mild and disappear soon after the onset of pain. Pain associated with intestinal obstruction tends to increase and recede in a pattern similar to labour pains.

Investigations

Laboratory tests cannot confirm a diagnosis of acute pancreatitis but can support the clinical impression (Mitchell et al. 2003). Laboratory tests include full blood count, in particular white cell count, blood for group and cross-match, serum amylase, serum lipase, blood glucose, urea and electrolyte and liver function tests. The literature suggests that the expected rise in serum amylase levels in patients with pancreatitis may not always be seen as in cases of coexisting conditions such as hypertriglyceridaemia; conversely a rise in serum amylase can occur as a result of numerous non-pancreatic conditions (Mergener & Baillie 1998, Mitchell et al. 2003). Serum lipase concentration rises within 4 to 8 hours of an episode of acute pancreatitis, peaks at 24 hours and returns to normal after 8 to 14 days, making it a useful diagnostic method in patients presenting late, e.g. >24 hours after the onset of pain. An elevated trypsin level has a better likelihood ratio for detecting pancreatitis than the amylase level and is reported as the most accurate serum indicator for acute pancreatitis; however, this test is not widely available and is therefore not routinely used (Munoz & Katerndahl 2000). Imaging studies such as chest X-ray may be indicated if pleural effusion is suspected. Plain abdominal radiograph and ultrasound may reveal the presence of air under the diaphragm, or gas shadows secondary to bowel distension, but the most reliable imaging modality in the diagnosis of acute pancreatitis is computed

tomography (Mergener & Baillie 1998, Munoz & Katerndahl 2000).

Prediction of the severity of the attack at the time of admission can prove difficult; however, several scoring systems with clinical, laboratory and radiological criteria have been developed (British Society of Gastroenterology 1998, Balthazar 2002, Mitchell et al. 2003).

The Ranson scoring system aims to estimate the severity of acute pancreatitis but has limitations in that it is recorded over two days and therefore the score is only valid after 48 hours post admission (Meadows 2005) (Table 28.3). A Ranson score of 0–2 has a minimal mortality rate, a Ranson score of 3–5 has a 10%–20% mortality, with scores higher than 5 having a mortality rate of more than 50% and being associated with more system complications. The Glasgow Criteria (British Society of Gastroenterology 1998) have been validated in the UK and are recommended for initial assessment. If three or more criteria occur over the initial 48 hours following admission this indicates severe acute pancreatitis (Table 28.4).

Table 28.3 Ranson's (1982) criteria of severity in acute pancreatitis

At admission	Age > 55 years
	WBC > 16 000/mm^3
	Glucose > 200 mg/dl
	LDH > 350 IU/L
	AST >250 U/L
During initial 48 hours	Hct decrease of >10%
	BUN increase of > 5 mg/dl
	Ca <8 mg/dl
	PaO_2 <60 mmHg
	Base deficit >4 mEq/L
	Fluid sequestration >6 L

Table 28.4 Glasgow scoring system for the initial prediction of severity in acute pancreatitis

Age	>55 years
White blood cell count	>15 × 10^9/L
Glucose	>10 mmol/L
Urea	>16 mmol/L
PaO_2	<60 mmHg
Calcium	<2 mmol/L
Albumin	<32 g/L
Lactate dehydrogenase	>600 units/L
Asparate/alanine aminotransferase	>100 units/L

An imaging grading system has been developed by Balthazar (2002) to evaluate abdominal computerized tomography scan results (Table 28.5). The chance of infection or death in grades A or B is almost nil but this increases in C and D and in patients graded E there is a 50% increased incidence of infection with a mortality of 15%.

Management

The majority of patients presenting to the emergency department are treated conservatively and approximately 80% respond to such treatment. The patient should have baseline observation of vital signs and a pain score recorded by the emergency nurse. A large-bore 14g cannula should be inserted and a rapid infusion of crystalloid commenced. Laboratory and radiological investigations should be initiated immediately to assist with establishing a diagnosis. A nasogastric tube is indicated where vomiting is protracted or if obstruction is seen on the abdominal radiograph; studies have shown that the use of nasogastric tube with suction is no longer advocated as routine therapeutic measure as it has not demonstrated a decrease in symptom mortality or hospital stay (Tenner & Banks 1997, Munoz & Katerndahl 2000). A urinary catheter should be inserted in order to record and closely monitor fluid intake and output. Analgesics such as pethidine or meperidin are recommended to relieve pain and are often accompanied by an antiemetic in preference to morphine, as morphine may cause spasm of the sphincter of Oddi, which has the potential to worsen the condition (Mergener & Baillie 1998). High-flow oxygen 100% is administered through a non-rebreather mask at 12–15 L/min with continuous assessment of oxygen saturation. The role of antibiotics in the management of early acute pancreatitis is controversial (Munoz & Katerndahl 2000) but antibiotic therapy may be commenced in severe cases associated with septic shock, in other conditions such as cholangitis or when CT scan indicates that there are fluid collections in the pancreas. The preferred antibiotics are those secreted by the biliary system such as ampicillin and third-generation cephalosporin.

Table 28.5 Balthazar CT grading system for staging acute pancreatitis

Grade A – Normal pancreas
Grade B – Focal of diffuse gland enlargement
Grade C – Peripancreatic inflammatory changes
Grade D – Fluid collections in a single location
Grade E – Multiple fluid collections, gas in or near pancreas.

VASCULAR DISORDERS

Oesophageal varices

These refer to the localized dilatation of veins in the lower oesophagus, due to the impairment of portal blood flow through the liver.

Pathophysiology

In patients suffering from cirrhosis of the liver, the blood flow from the portal vein meets resistance in the damaged organ. This increased resistance causes back pressure into the veins that normally empty into the portal system. The veins most affected are those at the lower end of the oesophagus. The veins become weak and varicosed, lifting the mucosa so that they protrude into the oesophagus, where they can be damaged by passing food, coughing, vomiting or straining. Patients with liver disease may also have abnormal blood clotting, which exacerbates the problem. Bleeding from these veins can be both dramatic and fatal; because of the high pressure within the vascular bed, hypovolaemia occurs quickly. The mortality rate for each bleeding episode is 30%; if underlying conditions remain untreated 70% of patients who develop haemorrhage die within one year of the initial bleeding episode (Gow & Chapman 2001).

Assessment

The patient may have a history of alcohol abuse and ascites, without abdominal pain. Painless haematemesis is suggestive of varices. Haematemesis following peptic ulceration may cause significant vomiting of bright-red blood, but is usually accompanied by abdominal pain. In bleeding, there may be a dramatic haematemesis, occasionally preceded by feelings of dizziness, as the bleeding into the stomach causes the blood pressure to fall. There may be a history of previous episodes. Features of portal hypertension are splenomegaly and ascites. Some of the blood will pass through the intestinal tract and will appear later as melaena. Patients with portal hypertension may be asymptomatic until they suddenly suffer catastrophic haemorrhage.

Investigations

Full blood count, electrolytes, glucose, gases, clotting factors and liver function tests should be requested.

Management

This life-threatening condition is one of the most complex emergency conditions to manage as the patient requires prompt aggressive resuscitation. The patient and relatives will require significant emotional and psychological support also as haemorrhage is generally profuse and is extremely frightening for all concerned.

In massive haemorrhage, the patient may lose consciousness and therefore airway clearance will be a priority. Ensure that there are adequate receivers and working suction to hand, as bleeding can be sudden and profuse. Provide 100% oxygen via a non-rebreather mask at 12–15 L/min. Establish at least two large-bore intravenous lines and be prepared to give large quantities of 5% dextrose. Saline should be avoided as this may worsen ascites. Blood should be drawn for immediate group and cross-match for six units of blood (O-negative can be used initially). A central line should be inserted to monitor the central venous pressure as a guide to fluid replacement along with a urinary catheter to monitor output and maintain accurate fluid balance records. Prevention of encephalopathy and aspiration are important measures during resuscitation; therefore obtunded and actively bleeding patients should have endotracheal intubation to prevent aspiration (Bornman et al. 1994). Urgent endoscopy is essential to confirm the presence of oesophageal varices but should only take place in a well-equipped specialist centre after the patient has been adequately resuscitated.

Balloon tamponade

A Sengstaken triple-lumen or a Minnesota quadruple lumen tube may be inserted orally to apply pressure to the bleeding veins and to allow aspiration from the stomach and upper oesophagus (see Fig. 28.2). Applied by an experienced team, balloon tamponade can achieve control of variceal bleeding in up to 90% of cases, with acceptably low morbidity (Bornman et al. 1994). If time permits, the tube may be chilled

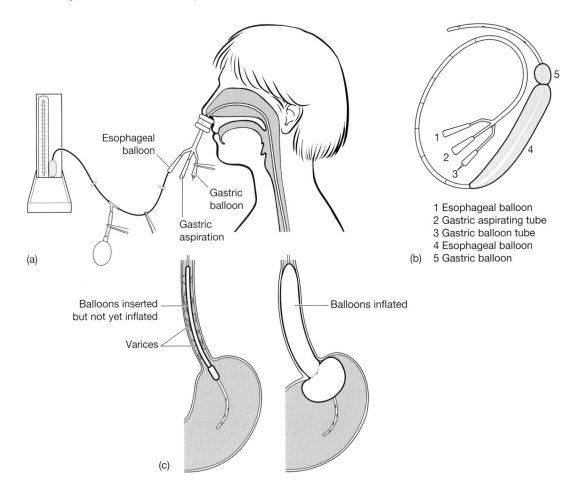

1 Esophageal balloon
2 Gastric aspirating tube
3 Gastric balloon tube
4 Esophageal balloon
5 Gastric balloon

Figure 28.2 Use of Sengstaken tube.

prior to insertion as this makes the tube more rigid and aids insertion. Insertion of the tube is a fairly unpleasant procedure for the patient, but many patients will be sedated and intubated to allow the clinician to have more control over the airway. The patient will need to be placed in the left lateral decubitus position to allow for tube placement although the tube can be placed while the patient is supine. The tube can remain in position for up to 12 hours. Leaving the tube in excess of 12–24 hours carries a significant risk of oesophageal necrosis, oedema, ulceration and perforation. Inflation of the oesophageal balloon will make swallowing difficult for the patient, and suction may be required (Christensen 2004). Suction should be available before, during and after removal of the tube. The emergency nurse should maintain a vigilant assessment of the patient's respiratory status after the tube has been inserted. If signs of respiratory distress or obstruction develop, the nurse should immediately cut away the valves from the end of the tube and remove it (Smith & Fawcett 2004). Care should be taken to ensure that the correct balloons are inflated and deflated. Inadequate inflation will be ineffective at controlling bleeding, while excessive pressures will cause tissue damage. As soon as the tube is placed the balloons are inflated and a portable chest X-ray is carried out to confirm the position of the tube. X-ray should be repeated every four hours as long as the tube is inflated to assess position and balloon size; progressive decline in balloon size indicates a leak and the balloon must be re-inflated. Inflation of the oesophageal balloon should always be done under pressure control with a manometer. Manometer pressure should read between 25 and 40 mmHg and the balloon should be deflated every two hours for ten minutes and then re-inflated. Regular monitoring of the patient's vital signs and fluid balance should be maintained to assess the effectiveness of the tube at achieving haemorrhage control.

Pharmacological control

Vasoactive drugs to control variceal bleeding have been used for 40 years. Vasopressin is still the most widely used agent and is best administered by continuous intravenous infusion at a rate of 0.4 U per min. This may be given to produce arterial vasoconstriction, which will reduce the amount of blood entering the portal system. Potentially serious cardiac complications (which occur in 15% of patients) and plasminogen activator and factor VIII release (which may aggravate coagulopathy) are important factors limiting the use of vasopressin alone (Gow & Chapman 2000). Terlipressin, the triglycyl synthetic analogue of vasopressin, given in a bolus injection

has a longer therapeutic action (4 hours vs. 40 mins) and there are no cardiac side-effects.

Somatostatin does not cause systemic vasoconstriction: its action is on the smooth muscle of splanchnic vessels, resulting in a reduction in splanchnic and hepatic blood flow. The efficacy of somatostatin to control variceal bleeding has been tested in studies against vasopressin and proved in some studies to be more effective at reducing bleeding and transfusion requirements (Saari et al. 1990).

Endoscopic sclerotherapy

In this technique a coagulating substance is injected into the varices, which seals the bleeding veins by coagulation and is the primary method of treatment (Smith & Fawcett 2004). The patient will require repeated treatments at regular intervals for a few years. Severe complications of injection sclerotherapy include:

- haemorrhage
- aspiration
- oesophageal perforation
- portal vein thrombosis.

Percutaneous transhepatic portal vein embolization

This may be done under X-ray control to insert embolic material directly into the blood vessels. Emergency surgery carries considerable risk and it is preferable to stabilize the patient's condition and undertake surgery when bleeding is controlled. Various options are available:

- a portacaval shunt – this makes an anastomosis between the portal vein and the inferior vena cava
- a splenorenal shunt
- a mesocaval shunt between the superior mesenteric vein and the inferior vena cava
- a transoesophageal ligation of the bleeding vessels

Surgery will reduce the risk of further ruptured varices, but will not resolve the underlying liver disease. Other procedures involve oesophageal transection and anastomosis, or ligation of bleeding veins. In patients with oesophageal varices, there is a 60–80% recurrence over 2 years, with 20% mortality during each further episode of bleeding.

Abdominal aortic aneurysm

An aneurysm is a focal dilatation of a blood vessel which has been weakened by atheroma. The normal aorta is approximately 2 cm in diameter: aneurysm is diagnosed in cases where dilation is in excess of 3 cm. The commonest site for aneurysms is the aorta, although they can occur elsewhere, such as the common iliac vessels.

Pathophysiology

The largest-diameter arteries, such as the aorta, have a greater proportion of elastic tissue and a smaller proportion of smooth muscle compared with other arteries. Elastic arteries are stretched when the ventricles of the heart pump blood into them. The elastic recoil prevents blood pressure from falling rapidly and maintains blood flow while the ventricles are relaxed. As the arteries become smaller, they undergo a gradual transition from having walls containing more elastic tissue than smooth muscle to having walls with more smooth muscle than elastic tissue. This allows these arteries (radial, brachial etc.) to have a greater degree of vasoconstriction and vasodilatation, allowing them to alter blood flow according to local demands.

Arteries are composed of three layers. From the inside to the outer wall the layers are:

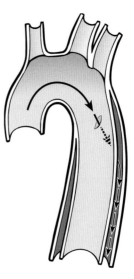

Figure 28.3   Dissecting aortic aneurysm.

- tunica intima – an endothelium composed of simple squamous cells and a small amount of connective tissue
- tunica media – the middle layer consists of smooth muscle arranged circularly around the blood vessel
- tunica adventitia – composed of connective tissue

The walls of the arteries undergo changes as they age, mainly in the large elastic arteries such as the aorta, coronary arteries serving the heart and carotid arteries serving the brain. Atherosclerosis refers to the deposition of material in the walls of arteries to form plaques. This fatty material contains cholesterol and may be replaced by connective tissue and calcium deposits. Atherosclerosis increases resistance to blood flow, as the deposits reduce the internal diameter of the arteries. The rough plaques attract passing platelets, which adhere to them, increasing the chances of thrombus formation. As the tunica media becomes weakened, the wall of the aorta begins to bulge.

The aneurysm may form a sac or it may separate through the layers of the vessel, called a dissecting aneurysm, without a visible dilatation (see Fig. 28.3). Dissecting aneurysms can spread for some distance along the aorta and affect other organs, such as the kidneys. Aneurysms can also send off emboli to distant sites. Risk factors for rupture relate to the size of the dilatation and range from 4–5 cm = 0.5–5% to >8 cm = 30–50%. Contributing factors for rupture include hypertension, chronic obstructive airway disease, diabetes, smoking, family history, ratio to adjacent normal aorta, rapid expansion. Fatal rupture is

commoner among women than men, although there is a higher instance of aneurysm in men, of the order of 5:1. Some authors estimate that 4–8% of all patients older than age 65 have an AAA (Rogers & McCormack 2004). The rate of expansion is estimated to be 10% per year. Mortality following rupture of an AAA is more than 90%, with many people dying before reaching hospital. In comparison, mortality rates following emergency repair are approximately 50%, and following elective AAA repair are between 5 and 10% (Bick 2000, Galland 1998).

Assessment

Abdominal aortic aneurysms tend to affect middle-aged to elderly people. There may be a history of atherosclerosis and the patient may have suffered a previous myocardial infarction or stroke or may have peripheral vascular disease or chronic obstructive pulmonary disease (Bick 2000). If the aneurysm is pressing on other structures, there may be abdominal pain radiating to the back or groin. There may be few initial indications that the patient has an aneurysm, until it is large and causes pressure on other structures, or it starts to leak. The immediate problem is of sudden abdominal pain and collapse. Patients with a dissecting aneurysm may complain of a sudden tearing or ripping pain. There is no history of haematemesis, which tends to exclude oesophageal varices or perforated ulcer.

The patient has signs of hypovolaemic shock, pale, cold, clammy skin and rapid respirations. The blood pressure may be low with an accompanying tachycardia. Physical examination may reveal a pulsatile mass in the centre of the abdomen, and in extreme cases pulsation may be visible. A pulsatile mass can be found in 80–90% of patients (Drake 1993). The patient's femoral pulses may be weak or absent. Impaired blood supply to a limb may lead to 'blue toe syndrome', which is a classical manifestation of AAA in 5% of patients. This presentation may cause an ischaemic, painful extremity or cyanotic toes due to atheroembolism. Emboli may also involve the mesenteric and renal arteries, leading to intestinal ischaemia, haematuria and renal failure (Rogers and McCormack 2004).

Differential diagnosis
- pancreatitis
- renal colic
- biliary disease
- musculoskeletal back pain

The classic triad of AAA (abdominal aortic aneurysm) therefore is abdominal or back pain, hypotension, and a pulsatile abdominal mass.

Investigations
Blood should be cross-matched urgently – initially at least 10 units in anticipation of surgery. Also request full blood count, amylase, glucose, gases and clotting studies. Further investigations should be tailored to the clinical condition of the patient. Chest and abdominal X-rays waste time in unstable patients who need urgent intervention. Ultrasound can be performed in the emergency department, allowing continual monitoring of the patient in a controlled environment. CT scan is time-consuming and involves moving the patient to the X-ray department. Angiography provides very detailed information and is best reserved for stable patients.

Management
A senior surgeon should be involved early in the care of these patients, and in unstable patients limited investigations should be undertaken prior to surgery. Provide 100% oxygen via a non-rebreather mask at 12–15 L/min. Initiating large-bore intravenous access with two 14-gauge cannulae and controlled fluid resuscitation are critical for a patient with an aneurysm.

The patient's systolic blood pressure should be maintained <90 mmHg to decrease the pressure of ventricular systole against the fragile aorta. Attempting to increase blood pressure beyond this range may rupture the aneurysm, with fatal consequences

for the patient. Fluids should be warmed to prevent hypothermia and coagulopathy. Frequent monitoring of the patient's vital signs and fluid balance are essential to detect subtle changes in the patient's condition. Analgesia can be administered intravenously and titrated according to the patient's response. The analgesia of choice is morphine, as non-steroidal anti-inflammatories may induce renal failure. Antibiotics may be prescribed to reduce postoperative infection. Surgery may involve an endovascular repair which involves an endograft being inserted to replace the diseased aorta. Timely surgery is crucial: operative mortality for unrupted aneurysm is less than 5%, whereas emergency surgery after rupture is greater than 50%. Morbidity rates are between 15 and 30%, with a five-year survival rate of 60%. The mortality rate in untreated patients is 100% (Rogers & McCormack 2004, Bick 2000).

Arterial embolism

Occlusion of an artery may follow external compression, thrombosis or embolism. This deprives the tissues of vital blood supply. An embolus is a mass of material which can lodge in a blood vessel, occluding the lumen and obstructing the blood flow. This may have been introduced from outside the body or it may have arisen from within. Most often it is a thrombus which has become dislodged from the wall of a blood vessel.

Pathophysiology
Emboli travel along blood vessels until they reach a point where the vessel diameter stops them from going any further. The effect on the tissue supplied by that vessel depends upon the presence of collateral circulation to that area. The most common emboli are derived from thrombi in the circulatory system. Thrombi can develop in peripheral blood vessels due to atheroma, aortic aneurysms or trauma. Thrombi in the arterial system can form within the heart on areas of dead myocardium, where the circulating platelets are exposed to the rough collagen, thus encouraging clot formation. Atrial fibrillation causes blood to stagnate in the heart, allowing thrombi to form. Emboli from the right side of the heart or the veins cause pulmonary embolism, while emboli from the left side can travel to the brain, viscera or limbs.

If the occlusion has been gradual, collateral circulation will have developed, so that blood is able to flow around the occlusion. However, if the occlusion is sudden, there will be no collateral vessels, and blood flow will stop at the occlusion. The resulting ischaemia may cause necrosis, gangrene and loss of the limb if circulation is not restored quickly. In the case of the abdominal organs, death of a small part of the kidney will leave a scar, whereas death of a small area of the bowel will lead to perforation and peritonitis. Thromboses tend to occur in association with atheroma at areas of turbulent blood flow, such as at the bifurcation of arteries.

Assessment

The limb may feel cold to the touch compared with the other limb, and the skin may appear pale or cyanosed. Peripheral pulses below the obstruction disappear. In the lower limb, the following peripheral pulse sites may be assessed: femoral popliteal, posterior tibial and dorsalis pedis.

The likely findings can be remembered as the six Ps:

- pain – this may be sudden and severe in embolic episodes, or occur over several hours in the case of thrombosis; it is aggravated by flexion and extension of the limb
- pulseless – with decreased or absent capillary refill – this is a very late sign
- pallor – the limb will look pale
- paraesthesia – the patient may complain of tingling sensations in the limb
- perishing cold – the limb feels cold to the touch
- paralysis – there is loss of function due to the decreased blood supply to the nerves and muscles.

Investigations

Blood should be sent for full blood count, electrolytes, glucose and clotting studies as a baseline prior to treatment. Assess blood flow in the limb using Doppler or angiography. ECG and chest X-ray are also required.

Management

Provide 100% oxygen via a non-rebreather mask at 12–15 L/min. Establish intravenous access in the unaffected limb. Keep the limb warm and in a dependent position to encourage vasodilatation. Carry out regular monitoring of vital signs and distal pulses in the affected limb, as well as cardiac monitoring and pulse oximetry in the normal limb. Provide prescribed analgesia; anticoagulants may also be prescribed, such as heparin 15 000 units every 12 hours.

Surgery should be undertaken as soon as possible, and is most effective within 6–12 hours of occlusion. Embolectomy may be carried out under local or general anaesthesia. In some cases, more advanced surgery requiring patch grafting of the blood vessels may be required. In the case of arterial reconstruction, the percentages of limbs saved in survivors are 80% in femoropopliteal bypass grafts and 60% in femorotibial bypass grafts.

GENITOURINARY DISORDERS

Retention of urine

Pathophysiology

The urethra exits the bladder inferiorly and anteriorly near the entrance of the two ureters. The ureters and bladder are lined with transitional epithelium which is specialized to stretch as the volume of urine increases. The walls of the ureter and bladder have smooth muscle, and waves of muscle contraction propel the urine along from the kidneys to the bladder. Contraction of muscle in the bladder will force urine to flow along the urethra to exit the body.

At the junction of the urethra and bladder, the smooth muscle of the bladder forms the internal sphincter. The external sphincter is skeletal muscle surrounding the urethra as it extends through the pelvic floor. These sphincters regulate the flow of urine through the urethra. Enlargement of the gland causes stretching and distortion of the urethra, which obstructs the bladder outflow. The bladder muscle enlarges in an attempt to overcome the obstruction, causing high pressures to be generated. Eventually the bladder becomes dilated and the muscle hypotonic.

Assessment

Urinary retention in younger men is relatively rare, occurring in seven in every 1000 patients aged 40 to 59 years. The risk rises dramatically in men aged 70 to 79 years with moderate to severe lower urinary tract symptoms; they have a five-year cumulative incidence of more than 13.8%. Urinary retention may be acute or chronic (Wareing 2004). Urinary retention may develop in males with previous symptoms of prostatic obstruction (hesitancy, poor stream, dribbling). Benign prostatic enlargement occurs most often in men over the age of 60 years. Retention may be precipitated by constipation, 'holding on too long', infection, neurological disease or postoperatively. Chronic retention is relatively painless, and although the bladder is distended it is not tender because the distension is more gradual. There may be a history of frequency, with overflow incontinence usually at night. The patient may present with severe lower abdominal pain or discomfort, a palpable distended bladder, and feeling the need to pass urine but unable to do so. The nurse should consider the last time of voiding, intake and output and relevant history. In addition, vital signs to establish a baseline should be checked.

Investigations

Urine, when available, should be taken for culture and routine analysis. Blood should be sent for full blood count, renal profile and acid phosphatase (a marker of disease activity). Further investigations will be arranged at a later time (ultrasound, urine flow rates etc.).

Management

Patients with retention of urine can be quite distressed and will need reassurance. It may be possible to overcome the retention by ensuring privacy for the patient and altering his position if possible. Warm baths and letting the patient listen to running water may help; however, in a number of cases the patient will require catheterization, by either the transurethral or suprapubic method.

If retention has been acute, not more than 1000 ml of urine should be drained initially, and then 300 ml each hour until the bladder is empty (Royle & Walsh 1992, Wareing 2004). Sudden decompression of the bladder can result in an inflow of blood to the area and some capillary bleeding. The sudden emptying of an over-distended bladder can result in an atonic bladder wall. The suprapubic route may be chosen when there is trauma to the urethra or when it has proved impossible to pass a urethral catheter. It is a surgical procedure and, in common with urethral catheterization, requires aseptic technique. It may be performed under local or general anaesthesia. The catheter is sutured in place and taped to the abdomen to reduce traction on the tube.

Urinary catheters

Although urinary catheterization is seen as a last resort for urinary retention, it remains a common procedure for short-, medium- and long-term management. The urethra may become inflamed in response to the materials used in the manufacture of the catheter. This risk increases as the catheter is left in over several weeks. Short-term indwelling catheters currently available include plastic or PVC material, which should not be left in place longer than 14 days; other short-term catheters include latex-based catheters coated with Teflon, and these may remain in situ up to 28 days. Silicone catheters could be left in situ for up to 12 weeks. Recent developments include hydrogel-coated latex and all-silicone catheters, which are reported to be more biocompatible than previous materials (Pomfret & Tew 2004). The use of hydrogel in the manufacture of indwelling catheters has improved patient care and reduced the incidence of bacterial adherence and catheter encrustation (Pomfret & Tew 2004).

Bypassing of urine around the catheter can be an alarming and distressing experience for the patient (Mayes et al. 2003). Patients with larger catheters tend to experience more bypassing problems than those with smaller catheters (Winn 1996, Pomfret & Tew 2004). Catheters with smaller balloons allow the catheter tip to sit lower in the bladder, leaving less residual urine. The main rule, therefore, is to choose the smallest catheter that will drain adequately and cause minimal urethral trauma (Wilson 2001).

- 12–14 Ch/Fg for clear urine
- 14–16 Ch/Fg for urine containing debris
- 18+ Ch/Fg for urine containing haematuria and clots.

In tandem with choosing a small catheter size, balloon infill volume should be the smallest volume that will retain the catheter in the bladder; adult catheters may have 10, 20 or 30 ml balloons. It may be concluded that where bypassing is a problem, inserting larger catheters or adding water to the balloon is not the solution; in fact it is likely to irritate the bladder further. It is not necessary to try to occlude the urethra by using a large catheter. The urethral folds will normally close upon themselves. Urinary catheters often become encrusted and blocked by crystalline *Proteus mirabillis* biofilms; in some early studies carried out it has been reported that when retention balloons were inflated using the anti-bacterial solution Triclosan that there was a decrease in the formation of biofilms on catheter surfaces, reducing the incidence and frequency of catheter blockages (Stickler et al. 2003, Pomfret & Tew 2004).

Discharge advice

Adequate provision for the discharge of patients from emergency departments is recognized as a priority for all those concerned with the quality of care offered to patients. Although patients with retention of urine may have previous experience of catheter insertion, it is vital that the nurse ensures adequate after-care arrangements (Dunnion & Kelly 2005). It is sometimes assumed that patients do not ask questions because they know all the answers! Do not assume that the patient has received adequate education in the management of his condition. The nurse should ensure that the patient, and in certain cases the carers, understands the importance of adequate fluid intake to sustain the urine output and hydration, as well as the routine care of the catheter. There have been a number of studies into the efficacy of performing meatal cleansing with a variety of cleansing agents: none has proven to reduce the level of bacteriuria (Pomfret & Tew 2004). Daily cleansing of the catheter/meatus junction with soap and water to remove mucopus is all that is required (NICE 2003). Patients should have some point of contact in the community if they experience problems.

Torsion of the testis

Torsion of the spermatic cord involves twisting of the testis and epididymis on their axis. It is a urological emergency and must be differentiated from other complaints of testicular pain, because delay in diagnosis can lead to loss of the testicle.

Pathophysiology

The scrotum is divided into two by a connective tissue septum which separates the testes. Beneath the skin of the scrotum there is a layer of loose connective tissue and a layer of smooth muscle called the dartos muscle. In cold temperatures the dartos muscle contracts, causing the skin of the scrotum to become firm and wrinkled and thus reducing its overall size. At the same time, extensions of the abdominal muscles, called cremaster muscles, which extend into the scrotum, contract. The testes are then pulled nearer to the body and their temperature is raised. During warm weather the process is reversed and the testicles descend away from the body, which lowers their temperature. If the testes become too cold or too warm, the normal sperm production does not occur.

The outer part is a white connective tissue capsule. Part of the capsule extends to the interior of the testis, dividing it into about 250 lobules with tubules in which sperm cells develop. Interstitial cells secrete the hormone testosterone. Sperm cells move from these tubules to the epididymis, where they mature in a few days and develop their capacity to function as sex cells. The vas deferens passes from the epididymis via the inguinal canal through the abdominal wall to the prostate gland. The urethra is a passage for both urine and male reproductive fluids. While semen is passing through the urethra, a reflex causes the urinary sphincter muscles to contract, stopping urine from passing from the bladder to the urethra.

Torsion of the testis is due to an anatomic abnormality in which the testicle is not attached to the scrotum (see Fig. 28.4) The congenital anomaly is present in approximately 12% of males, 40% of whom have the abnormality in the contralateral testicle (Rupp & Zwanger 2005). Torsion produces an initial occlusion of the venous return from the testis, although the arterial supply continues for some time. There follows congestion of the testis, with haemorrhagic infarction as the arterial system becomes impaired. The infarction produces a shrunken, fibrotic testis. Toncich (2004) notes that the extent and rapidity of the damage depends on the degree of torsion, i.e. the number of turns.

- Incomplete torsion (<360°) may not completely obstruct arterial flow

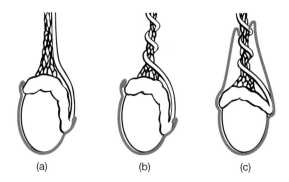

Figure 28.4   Testicular torsion.

- One turn (360°) causes necrosis in 12–24 hours
- Two or more (>720°) causes necrosis in less than 2 hours because arterial flow is completely obstructed (Herbener 1996).

Assessment

Torsion is often precipitated by exertion which causes contraction of the cremaster muscle producing the torsion. The patient is usually 15–30 years old, with sudden onset of pain in one testis. Pain may radiate up to the abdomen, the original site of the testicles in the embryo. Nausea and vomiting are common, and on examination the patient is found to have a hot swollen testis.

Differential diagnosis

- Epididymitis
- Testicular tumour
- Trauma
- Hydrocele

Investigations

Use of a Doppler on the spermatic cord is an attempt to measure arterial blood flow to the involved testis. While absence of blood flow obviously supports the diagnosis, the presence of blood flow does not exclude torsion. Ultrasound may be helpful, although most would agree that if there is a doubt it is best to perform surgical exploration.

Management

The patient may be in considerable pain and will require both emotional support and prescribed analgesia. Surgery should be performed as soon as possible, and viability depends on the number of twists and the time taken to untwist the testis (Toncich 2004). A salvage rate of 100% is found in patients if the testis is untwisted within four hours; after six to eight hours the salvage rate markedly decreases.

Informed consent will include an explanation by the surgeon that the testis may have to be removed if it is found to be non-viable at operation, as well as an explanation that both testes will be fixed by suturing. As torsion is a bilateral phenomenon in 40% of individuals, so the uninvolved testis will be fixed to the scrotum during the operation to prevent subsequent torsion. If the testis is viable at operation, it is sutured to the scrotal wall, and if it is deemed unsalvageable it is removed.

PREOPERATIVE PREPARATION

The length of time available for the preparation of the patient for surgery will depend upon the patient's clinical condition. The chief objective is to ensure that the patient goes to surgery in the best physical and psychological condition. There will be some overlap between the medical and nursing input in the preparation of the patient.

Psychological

While surgical procedures and their preparation may be relatively routine for staff in the emergency department, the need for surgery may come as quite a shock to patients and their relatives, with little time for psychological preparation. Jaworski & Wirtz (1995) noted that during an acute crisis the patient may seem to understand, but information and instructions may have to be repeated. It has been shown that providing patients with information preoperatively leads to more favourable postoperative outcomes (Hayward 1975, Mackintosh & Bowles 1997). It has also been demonstrated that informing patients about anticipated pain and giving them some control over the pain experience decreased apprehension, increased pain tolerance and resulted in earlier discharges (Hayward 1975, Vorshall 1980, Carr 1990, Mackintosh & Bowles 1997). Even where the patient's condition is grave and surgery is being undertaken as a desperate last measure, it remains important to be truthful to both patients and their relatives without unduly frightening them.

Consent

The word consent literally means 'to feel together' that something should be done (Curtin 1993). In today's legal and ethical climate, patient involvement is so important that treating a patient without adequately informing him/her about the treatment is considered negligence, and treatment without consent is considered battery. When signing the consent form, the patient should be rational and not under the influence of drugs or alcohol that may impair comprehension.

As far as the law is concerned there is no specific requirement that consent should be given in a particular way; however, consent in writing is by far the best method for all procedures involving risk. Besides explaining treatments and alternatives in terms the patient understands and specifying who will perform the procedure, the provider must invite and answer his/her questions (Dunn 1999). It is important that the nurse is present during the surgeon's explanation to the patient to allow for continuity. It is, however, not the nurse's responsibility to explain the procedure: the nurse's role in obtaining informed consent is to advocate for the patient: protect his/her rights, preserve their dignity, identify fears, and determine the level of understanding and approval of the care to be given. Keep in mind that each patient's response is unique and based on personality, education level, emotional makeup, and intellectual capacity. To verify that your patient has received enough necessary information to give consent, ask him/her to state in his/her own words what information has been given. If any doubts exist about the level of patient understanding or decision-making capacity the surgeon or healthcare provider should be notified (Dunn 1999).

In an emergency, where the patient's life is in danger and the patient is not able to consent, the doctor may proceed and do what is required without formal consent. This is rarely necessary, and even in the unconscious patient consent should be sought where possible from the next of kin.

Skin preparation

Kjonniksen et al. (2002) conducted a systematic literature review and found there was strong evidence to recommend that when hair removal is considered necessary, shaving should not be performed. Instead a depilatory or electric clipping, preferably immediately before surgery, should be performed.

Nursing issues in preoperative preparation

In emergencies, preparation is limited to the essentials but there are many opportunities for the emergency nurse to ensure that the patient has adequate physical and psychological support prior to urgent operative intervention.

The following list identifies some important nursing considerations, both practical and psychological, which may be tailored to the individual patient:

- Patient privacy and confidentiality
- Family issues such as young or aged dependants addressed
- Notification of relatives.

- Informed consent – patient has reached age of consent (16 years)
- Spiritual needs addressed (minister of religion or appropriate other)
- Psychological preparation (post-operative anxieties, altered body image, phobias)
- Non-pharmacological pain control (warm packs)
- Prescribed pharmacological pain control
- Allergy status established
- Identification and removal where appropriate of prosthetics, cosmetics and jewellery, including body piercing
- Adequate intravenous access
- Oral hygiene and gastric decompression using nasogastric tube where appropriate
- Appropriate laboratory tests such as blood for group and cross-match, full blood count, renal and liver profiles
- Urine testing to detect diabetes, impaired renal function or pregnancy
- Catheterization when strict fluid monitoring is required
- Patient identification bracelet to correspond with clinical record
- Clinical records should include recent vital signs,

fluid balance, drug history, allergy history, property list and any other relevant information such as contact telephone number for next of kin

In more controlled circumstances additional information may be gathered on the patient's condition through

- Radiological investigations
- Electrocardiograph
- Special investigations specific to the patient's condition.

CONCLUSION

An emergency is defined as a serious condition requiring immediate treatment. The management of surgical emergencies in this chapter covers the full spectrum of patients, from those suffering the discomfort of urinary retention to life-threatening conditions such as aortic aneurysm. With the exception of trauma very few conditions warrant immediate surgery, and a period of resuscitation and stabilization is of considerable benefit to the patient and remains the key to ensuring the best outcome for the patient.

References

Balthazar E.J (2002) Staging of acute pancreatitis. *Radiological Clinics of North America*, **40**(96), 1199–1209.

Bick C (2000) Abdominal aortic aneurysm repair. *Nursing Standard*, **15**(3), 47–52.

Biondo S, Pares D, Frago R et al. (2004) Large bowel obstruction: predictive factors for postoperative mortality. *Diseases of the Colon and Rectum*, **47**(11), 1889–1897.

Bornman PC, Krige JE, Terblanche J (1994) Management of oesophageal varices. *Lancet*, **343**, 1079–1084.

Bratt-Wyton R (1998) Interpretation of routine blood tests. *Nursing Standard*, **13**(12), 42–48.

British Society of Gastroenterology (BSG) (1998) UK Guidelines for the Management of Acute Pancreatitis. *GUT*, **42**(suppl 2), S1–S13.

Carr BCJ (1990) Post-operative pain: patient's expectations and experiences of post-operative pain. *Nursing Research*, **20**(1), 26–31

Christensen T (2004) The treatment of oesophageal varices using a Sengstaken-Blackmore tube: considerations for nursing practice. *Nursing in Critical Care*, **2**, 58–64.

Clemings L, Duda J, Duda J (1990) Gastrointestinal emergencies. In: Kitt S, Kaiser J, eds. *Emergency Nursing: A Physiological and Clinical Perspective*. Philadelphia: WB Saunders.

Curtin LL (1993) Informed consent: cautious, calculated candor. *Nursing Management*, **24**(4), 18–20.

Drake T (1993) Aortic aneurysm and aortic dissection In: Markovchick VJ, Pons PT, Wolfe RE, eds. *Emergency*

Medicine Secrets, 3rd edn. Philadelphia: Hanley & Belfus.

Dunn D (1999) Exploring the grey areas of informed consent. *Nursing*, **29**(7), 41–47.

Dunnion ME, Kelly B (2005) From the emergency department to home. *Journal of Clinical Nursing*, **14**, 776–785.

Emmans LS (1993) Bowel disorders. In: Markovchick VJ, Pons PT, Wolfe RE, eds. *Emergency Medicine Secrets*. Philadelphia: Hanley & Belfus.

Galland RB (1998) Problems associated with aortic surgery. *Care of the Critically Ill*, **14**(2), 51–55.

Gilchrist BF, Lobe TE (1992) The acute groin in paediatrics. *Clinical Paediatrics* **31**, 488–496.

Goldacre MJ, Roberts SE (2004) Hospital admission for acute pancreatitis in an English population, 1963–98: database study of incidence and mortality. *British Medical Journal*, **328**, 1466–1469.

Gow PJ, Chapman RW (2001) Modern management of oesophageal varices. *Postgraduate Medicine Journal*, **77**(904), 75–81.

Hayward J (1975) *Information: A Prescription Against Pain*. London: Royal College of Nursing.

Herbener TE (1996) Ultrasound in the assessment of the acute scrotum. *Journal of Clinical Ultrasound*, **24**, 405–421.

Hughes E (2005) Caring for the patient with an intestinal obstruction. *Nursing Standard*, **19**(47), 56–64.

Jaworski MA, Wirtz KM (1995) Spinal trauma. In: Kitt S, Selfridge-Thomas J, Proehl J, Kaiser J, eds. *Emergency*

Nursing: A Physiological and Clinical Perspective. Philadelphia: WB Saunders.

Kjonniksen I, Andersen BM, Sondenaa VG, Segadal L (2002) Preoperative hair removal – a systematic literature review. *AORN (Association of Perioperative Registered Nurses),* **75**(5), 928–939.

Mackintosh C, Bowles S (1997) Evaluation of a nurse-led acute pain service. Can clinical nurse specialists make a difference? *Journal of Advanced Nursing,* **25**(1), 30–37.

Mann DV, Hersjman MJ, Hittinger R, Glazer G (1994) Multicentre audit of death from acute pancreatitis. *British Journal of Surgery,* **81**, 890–893.

Mayes J, Bliss J, Griffiths P (2003) Preventing blockage of long-term indwelling catheters in adults: are citric acid solutions effective? *British Journal of Community Nursing,* **8**(4), 172–175.

Mergener K, Baillie J (1998) Fornightly review: Acute pancreatitis. *British Medical Journal,* **316**, 44–48.

Mitchell RMS, Byrne MF, Baillie J (2003) Pancreatitis. *The Lancet,* **361**(9367), 1447.

Munoz A, Katerndahl DA (2000) Diagnosis and management of acute pancreatitis. *American Family Physician,* **62**(1), 164–174.

Newton E, Mandavia S (2003) Surgical complications of selected gastrointestinal emergencies: pitfalls in management of the acute abdomen. *Emergency Medical Clinics of North America,* **21**(4), 873–907.

NICE (2003) *Prevention of Healthcare-associated Infection in Primary and Community Care.* London: National Institute for Clinical Excellence.

Old JL, Dusing, RW, Yap W, Dirks J (2005) Imaging for suspected appendicitis. *American Family Physician,* **71**(1), 71–78.

O'Reilly DA, Kingsnorth AN (2004) Management of acute pancreatitis. *British Medical Journal,* **328**, 968–969.

Pomfret I, Tew LE (2004) Urinary catheters and associated UTIs. *Journal of Community Nursing,* **18**(9), 15–20.

Ranson JH (1982) Etiological and prognostic factors in human acute pancreatitis: a review. *American Journal of gastroenterology,* **77**(9), 633–638.

Rogers RL, McCormack R (2004) Aortic disasters. *Emergency Medicine Clinics of North America,* **22**(4), 887–908.

Royle JA, Walsh M (1992) *Watson's Medical and Surgical Nursing,* 4th edn. London: Baillière Tindall.

Saari A, Klvilaakso E, Inberg M et al. (1990) Comparison of somatostatin and vasopressin in bleeding oesophageal varices. *American Journal of Gastroenterology,* **85**, 804–807.

Scott RA (2004) Shock. In: *Textbook of Adult Emergency Medicine,* 2nd edn. P Cameron, G Jelinek, AM Kelly, L Murray, AFT Brown, J Heyworth (eds). London: Churchill Livingstone.

Seidal HM, Ball JW, Dains JE, Benedict GW (1987) *Mosby's Guide to Physical Examination.* St Louis: CV Mosby Co.

Smith GD, Fawcett T (2004) Oesophageal varices. *Gastrointestinal Nursing,* **2**(5), 33–39.

Stickler DJ, Jones GL, Russell AD (2003) Control of encrustation and blockage of Foley catheters. *The Lancet,* **361**, 1435–1437.

Tenner S, Banks PA (1997) Acute pancreatitis: non-surgical management. *World Journal of Surgery,* **21**, 143–148.

Toncich G (2004) The acute scrotum. In: *Textbook of Adult Emergency Medicine,* 2nd edn. P Cameron, G Jelinek, AM Kelly, L Murray, AFT Brown, J Heyworth (eds). London: Churchill Livingstone.

Vorshall B (1980) The effects of pre-operative teaching on post operative pain. *Topics in Clinical Nursing,* **2**(1), 39–43.

Wareing M (2004) Urinary retention: Issues of management and care. *Emergency Nurse,* **11**(8), 24–27.

Wilson J (2001) *Infection Control in Clinical Practice,* 2nd edn. London: Baillière Tindall.

Winn C (1996) Basing catheter care on research principles. *Nursing Standard,* **10**(18), 38–40.

Chapter **29**

Gynaecological and obstetric emergencies

Orla Devereux

INTRODUCTION

This chapter considers women's health in both pregnant and non-pregnant patients. Although many of the principles of management are similar, significant anatomical differences exist, and many of the signs and symptoms have different implications. Conditions relating to female reproduction form a relatively small part of ED work; however, many women actively choose ED for both emergency care and preventative intervention. As well as its physical implications, for many patients an obstetric or gynaecological condition can be distressing and value-laden. This chapter seeks to equip the ED nurse to rapidly assess the patient's condition and intervene appropriately. It will provide an outline of relevant anatomy and physiology before identifying conditions commonly treated in ED.

ANATOMY AND PHYSIOLOGY

The female reproductive organs consist of:

- uterus
- ovaries
- fallopian tubes
- vagina
- external genitalia

They are situated outside the peritoneal cavity (see Fig. 29.1).

The uterus is located in the anterior pelvis above the bladder. It is a pear-shaped organ with thick walls, made up of three layers: an outer serous membrane, a middle layer of smooth muscle, and the mucosal inner layer of endometrium, which is extremely vascular. The top of the uterus is called the fundus; it is the height of this which is measured to determine the gestation of pregnancy (see Fig. 29.2).

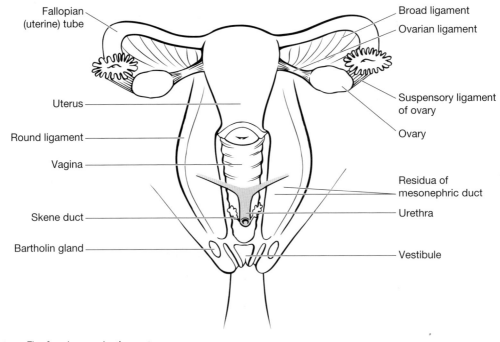

Figure 29.1 The female reproductive system.

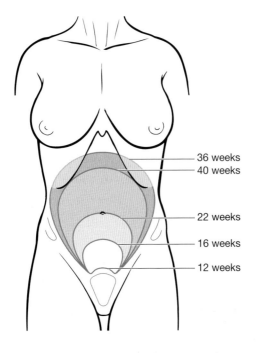

Figure 29.2 Change in fundal height during gestation.

The neck of the uterus is called the cervix. This opens into the vagina, the opening of which is called the os. The status of the os is an important consideration in assessing bleeding in early pregnancy. The ovaries sit bilaterally to the uterus, on the lateral pelvic wall, and are connected to the uterus by fallopian tubes. The fallopian tubes have a funnel-like opening below the ovaries, which collects the ova and transports them by peristalsis to the uterus. The tubes are made up of smooth muscle and mucous membrane. The vagina is an elastic tube leading to the external genitalia. There are two small glands either side of the vaginal opening called Bartholin's glands which can be prone to cyst formation in some women.

During child-bearing years, the female reproductive cycle varies in length between 21 and 35 days, but for most the average cycle is 28 days. The cycle consists of ovulation and menstruation, and is governed by changes in hormone levels. The first 5–7 days of the cycle represent menstruation. This is followed by a 7–8 day follicular phase preparing the endometrium for implantation of a fertilized egg. At around days 14–15 of the cycle, ovulation occurs. Once the ovum is released from the follicle, the luteal phase then commences: the collapsed follicle becomes an endocrine gland called the corpus luteum. It secretes oestrogen and progesterone to support the egg if fertilized. If the egg is not fertilized the luteal phase is responsible for the degeneration of the corpus luteum, after which the thickened lining of the endometrium sheds and the cycle begins again. If the egg is fertilized, the corpus luteum continues to secrete hormones until about 3 months into the pregnancy when the placenta takes over.

Fertilization of the ovum takes place in the fallopian tube, and during the first few days it passes slowly towards the uterus while a series of cell divisions take place forming a mass of embryotic cells. The embryo reaches the uterus between 3 and 5 days after fertilization. It then begins to implant into the uterine wall by about days 6–7 after fertilization. The placenta forms around where the embryo is embedded and, after a few weeks, begins to provide oxygen and nutrients to support fetal growth for the rest of the pregnancy. By 5 weeks after implantation the fetal heart is pumping well, and nutrients pass from the maternal blood supply across the placental membrane to nourish the fetus. The pregnancy is divided into trimesters of growth: in the first the internal organs develop; in the second the fetus grows in length and systems begin to mature; and in the last trimester the fetus fattens out and builds up reserves for birth. Physiological changes in pregnancy are plentiful, and an overview of key changes is given in Box 29.1; however, a detailed description is beyond the scope of this text and only those changes related to emergency care in ED will be discussed.

EMERGENCY CARE OF THE NON-PREGNANT WOMAN

History

Obtaining an accurate history is vital to establish the severity of a patient's condition. Because of the personal nature of gynaecological complaints, the nurse should ensure that assessment is carried out in private and in a sensitive and non-judgemental manner. Box 29.2 highlights the information that should be obtained.

Assessment

General assessment of the woman with a gynaecological condition should include baseline observations of pulse, respiration, blood pressure and temperature to detect signs of shock or infection. The level of pain should be determined, together with the exact location. Gentle abdominal examination will assist in this.

Box 29.1   Physiological changes in pregnancy

Cardiovascular
- Blood vascular increases by 30%
- Red cell mass rises by 20%
- Plasma increases by up to 50%
- Peripheral resistance decreases, reducing diastolic BP in the first and second trimesters
- Heart rate increases by up to 20 beats/min
- CVP falls by 65% by term
- Cardiac output increases by up to 30%

Respiratory
- Oxygen consumption increases by 20%
- Respiratory rate increases
- Pulmonary function alters, residual capacity decreases, minute volume increases by 40–50% and tidal volume increases

Renal
- Renal plasma flow and glomerular filtration rate increase steadily throughout pregnancy to a 50% greater capacity by term
- Speed of urine formation increases
- Water and sodium reabsorption rates are increased

Gastrointestinal
- Smooth muscle relaxes, and therefore gastric emptying is faster
- Intestines are relocated into the upper abdomen
- Acid regurgitation is common

Endocrine
- Base metabolic rate increases by up to 25%
- Anterior pituitary hypertrophy occurs
- Thyroid hypertrophy occurs

Other
- Anaemia develops because of rapid increase in iron requirements
- Cell-mediated immunity is depressed
- Autoimmunity disease eases during pregnancy

If clinically indicated, a vaginal examination should be carried out once, either by the nurse or, more commonly, by the doctor. Assessment should include urinalysis to detect a urinary tract infection as a primary cause of pain. Initially this can be diagnosed by the presence of leucocytes, protein and blood in urine, but culture and sensitivity should follow to ensure appropriate antibiotic therapy. A pregnancy test should also be carried out routinely to exclude unknown pregnancy. Abdominal pain is often the

---

Box 29.2 History related to gynaecological assessment

- Duration of symptoms
- Type and location of any pain
- Is there any redness of itching?
- Date of last menstrual period, and duration
- Was menstrual period normal?
- Is there any possibility of pregnancy?
- Is the patient sexually active? What (if any) contraception is being used?
- Is there any abnormal vaginal discharge or bleeding? If so, what is the discharge like?
- How heavy is bleeding, i.e. how often are pads or tampons being changed?
- Past history of pregnancy
- Coexisting medical problems/drug therapy
- Is there a history of assaults?

---

primary reason women with gynaecological complaints attend ED (Gondeck 1998). Conditions causing acute abdominal pain are shown in Box 29.3.

Menstrual pain

Mid-cycle pain

This is known as Mittelschmerz disease and is a benign, transient mid-cycle pain occurring at or after ovulation. Pain is usually unilateral and lasts 24–48 hours. Some women experience this every month as part of their usual cycle; for others it is an unexpected pain sometimes associated with per vaginal (PV) bleeding which causes enough discomfort and anxiety for the patient to seek emergency health care. Mittelschmerz pain is thought to be caused by a combination of local irritation due to blood, follicular fluid and prostaglandins released after ovulation, and increased peristalsis in the fallopian tubes (Hinchliff et al. 1996). At this time, most women experience microscopic PV bleeding, a few regularly have overt bleeding and most women

---

Box 29.3 Causes of acute abdominal pain in gynaecology

- Menstrual cycle
  - mid-cycle pain
  - menstruation
- Ovarian cyst
- Pelvic inflammatory disease (PID)

---

will have an occasional mid-cycle PV bleed. This is due to a temporary fall in hormone levels between the follicular and luteal phases of the menstrual cycle. Bleeding usually lasts only a few hours.

Mittelschmerz disease is diagnosed by relating the type of pain to the stage of the woman's menstrual cycle. It should only be diagnosed once other causes, such as ovarian cyst and pelvic inflammatory disease, have been ruled out (Reedy & Brucker 1995). The condition is self-limiting, and therefore treatment involves symptom control and education. Non-steroidal anti-inflammatory drugs (NSAIDs), such as ibuprofen, are usually the most effective analgesia. The patient should be made aware of the cyclical nature of the condition, and the possibility of recurrence.

Dysmenorrhoea

In most cases, dysmenorrhoea (period pain) is self-diagnosed and treated at home; however, when symptoms are unusually severe, some women seek emergency care. Two types of dysmenorrhoea exist: primary and secondary dysmenorrhoea. In the former, uterine spasm involves A nerve fibres, responsible for acute pain, and C nerve fibres responsible for chronic and referred pain (Golub 1992); (see also Ch. 24). Primary dysmenorrhoea is most common in adolescents and young women who have not had children.

Secondary dysmenorrhoea is more common in women over 30 with gynaecological problems such as endometriosis. In both types of dysmenorrhoea, the patient will have crampy, low abdominal pain either at onset of menses or 24 hours prior to onset. The woman may have referred pain in the back and legs. Associated symptoms include breast tenderness, nausea/vomiting, diarrhoea and headache, all due to rapid hormonal changes.

Diagnosis should be made only after other causes of pain and bleeding have been excluded. Management revolves around symptom control, and the condition is self-limiting. NSAIDs are the analgesia of choice because they inhibit intrauterine synthesis of prostaglandin (Weissmann 1991) as well as decreasing pain. Small quantities of alcohol are effective in the treatment of dysmenorrhoea because it reduces oxytocin and vasopressor activity, therefore reducing uterine spasm. Ethically, however, this method of pain control should only be advocated for women who understand the potential dangers of alcohol ingestion and are legally old enough to use it (Reedy & Brucker 1995). Discharge information should include the commonality of dysmenorrhoea and, in the case of secondary dysmenorrhoea, information and advice about the predisposing condition.

Ovarian cyst

These usually result from a dysfunction in the menstrual cycle, when a collection of fluid forms around the corpus luteum. Cyst formation is more common in endometriosis and most are benign and self-limiting. In some instances, the cyst increases in size and becomes symptomatic at about 5 cm diameter (Lichtman & Papera 1990). Eventually, if growth persists, bleeding, rupture or torsion can occur. Ovarian cysts are uncommon in women using oral contraception (Selfridge-Thomas 1997).

Assessment

The patient will have abdominal pain, worse on the affected side, with possible guarding on examination. Onset of pain is usually during the latter half of the menstrual cycle or the week prior to menses where the cycle is regular. The patient will experience prolonged menstruation. If a small cyst ruptures, the fluid collected in it is reabsorbed without any clinical evidence. Rupture of a large cyst can cause potentially life-threatening hypovolaemia.

Assessment of vital signs should be ongoing, as a mild tachycardia can quickly deteriorate into severe hypotension and shock in ovarian cyst rupture. Prior to rupture, a large cyst can twist around the vascular pedicle, causing ovarian torsion. This is identified by a sudden onset of intermittent but sharp pain. Nausea or vomiting is an early sign of ovarian torsion.

Management

Cysts not causing haemodynamic compromise tend to be managed conservatively with follow-up investigation from a GP or gynaecological clinic. If adequate pain control cannot be achieved, hospital admission should be considered. If the patient has mild to moderate signs of hypovolaemia, intravenous fluid support should be established, and laparoscopic surgical decompression of the cyst should be considered. In cases of severe hypotension or torsion, fluid resuscitation and urgent surgical intervention are necessary. These women will need both information and psychological support during a time which potentially threatens their fertility.

Pelvic inflammatory disease

Pelvic inflammatory disease (PID) is an increasing gynaecological problem, with approximately 20% of female infertility attributed to it (Reedy & Brucker 1995). It is also linked to an increase in ectopic pregnancy. PID is a generic term used to describe infection of the pelvic peritoneum, connective tissue and reproductive organs – most commonly the fallopian tubes (also termed salpingitis). PID results from:

- sexually transmitted diseases (STDs), particularly gonorrhoea and chlamydia
- termination of pregnancy
- childbirth with assisted delivery
- gynaecological surgery.

The use of intrauterine devices for contraception does not increase the risk of PID except in the 20 days following their insertion (Farley et al. 1992). Sexually transmitted diseases are the most common cause of PID, especially caused by *C. trachomatis* and *N. gonorrhoeae*. The infection occurs in the genital area and spreads along mucosal surfaces, causing transient bouts of inflammation. Infection tends to settle in fallopian tubes, causing scar tissue and adhesions. This makes ovum passage more difficult and increases the likelihood of ectopic pregnancy because the fertilized egg is unable to pass to the uterus and implants in the tube. PID is most common in young women with multiple sexual partners, young age at first sexual intercourse or high frequency of sexual intercourse, and within that group has a higher incidence in women from lower socioeconomic groups (Bryan 2004, Wolner Hanbseen 1991). The most common age group is 15–19 years of age (Selfridge-Thomas 1997), which has considerable implications for future health care and fertility therapy, as women with PID are at increased risk of chronic pelvic pain, ectopic pregnancy and infertility.

A patient with PID will present with moderate to severe abdominal pain, worse with walking, urination, bowel action and intercourse. She may be tachycardic and will be pyrexic. If STD is the cause, the patient will have a thick vaginal discharge. If pelvic abscess or peritonitis is developing, the patient will also have nausea or vomiting. Lichtman & Parera (1990) highlighted three grades of PID (see Box 29.4).

Management

Pain relief is a priority for management of all types of PID. The strength of analgesia needed will vary depending on the severity of infection and the patient's individual perceptions of her condition. Grade I infection can be treated with broad-spectrum

Box 29.4	Grades of pelvic inflammatory disease
Grade I	Infection confined to tube(s) or ovary(s)
Grade II	Infection complicated by abscess or tissue mass
Grade III	Infection spread beyond pelvis due to a ruptured abscess. Peritonitis is commonly present

antibiotics, usually cefotaxime or tetracycline, and the patient can be discharged and followed up in the STD clinic. Grade II conditions warrant hospital admission for i.v. antibiotics. Grade III PID is uncommon, but necessitates hospitalization and surgical intervention as well as antibiotic therapy.

If the woman is pregnant or has not responded to, or complied with, oral antibiotics, hospital admission should be considered. If the patient is discharged from ED, it is essential that she has appropriate health education to enable her to recognize a recurrence and get treatment. This is important in reducing potential long-term health problems, such as infertility. If the PID originates from an STD, the patient's partner should be encouraged to attend an STD clinic and advice should be given about the use of barrier methods of contraception during intercourse.

Bartholin's cyst

The Bartholin's glands lie on either side of the vagina and secrete fluid onto the surface of the labia. In normal health these cannot be seen or palpated. If the duct becomes blocked, a small cyst forms; these are usually benign and self-limiting. They can, however, become infected with *E. coli* or STDs such as gonorrhoea. If infection occurs, the labium becomes inflamed and oedematous to the extent that the patient may have difficulty walking. This is a painful and distressing condition, which is resolved by early excision and drainage of the cyst. This is usually performed as an in-patient. Antibiotic therapy is also indicated (Walters 1992).

Sexually transmitted disease

Patients may present to ED because of its relative anonymity compared with GP attendance. Many people are still unaware of the existence and accessibility of STD clinics. Broadly, common symptoms of STD are genital irritation or pain, infection, discharge and sometimes bleeding. Specific symptoms and management are shown in Table 29.1.

The role of the ED nurse in caring for patients with STDs is twofold: first, to provide immediate therapy to resolve the acute episode with appropriate STD clinic follow-up; and second, to provide non-judgemental health education aimed at preventing the spread of STDs. All direct sexual contacts of the patient should be advised to have a health check. It is not possible for the ED nurse to personally follow up patient contacts, but the nurse can support the patient in informing a current partner, and information can then be cascaded to anyone else who may be involved. Patients should refrain from sexual activity until the infection is clear. Advice about barrier contraception should also be given (Wright 1999).

Emergency contraception

Postcoital contraception is available in the form of oral oestrogen-based pills taken within 72 hours of intercourse or an intra-uterine contraceptive device (IUCD) which needs to be inserted within 5 days of intercourse.

Oestrogen-based pills

Oestrogen-based pills work by a combination of pituitary influence and action on the ovary and endometrium. The luteal phase of the menstrual cycle is shortened. The endometrial biochemistry is also altered to make it hostile to implantation. The way the pill works is important in differentiating between contraception which prevents pregnancy and drugs which induce abortion, which the oestrogen pill does not.

Many patients need this differentiation spelt out for long-term peace of mind. Before the postcoital pill is prescribed, it is important that the patient is aware of

Table 29.1   Sexually transmitted disease

Organism	Incubation	Symptoms	Discharge	Treatment
Neisseria gonorrhoea	3–5 days	Dysuria	Yellow	Cefotaxime
Chlamydia trachomatis	5–10 days	Urethral itching	Mucopurulent vaginal discharge	Tetracycline
Trichomonas vaginalis	1 week	Vaginal itching	Thin, frothy, greenish, foul-smelling	Metronidazole
Gardinerella vaginalis	5–10 days	Itching	Thin, white, fishy odour	Metronidazole
Candida albicans	Variable	Inflammatory itching	Thick white discharge	Clotrimazole
Herpes simplex II	2–12 days	Painful, genital lesions	–	Acyclovir
Genital warts	1–6 months	Wart - type lesions on genitals spreading up genital tract	–	Paint with 5% acetic acid

the risks associated with its use. The patient must be warned that a small teratogenic risk exists if the fetus survives, similar to continued use of daily oral contraception pills. As yet, however, oestrogen teratogenesis has only been proved where repeated high doses are used in early pregnancy (Stevens & Kenney 1994). It is advisable to document that this information was given to the patient.

Administration of the drug is in two doses, which should be taken within 72 hours of unprotected intercourse. Nausea and vomiting are significant side-effects of oral postcoital contraception and some doctors prefer to prescribe prophylactic antiemetics with the pill. Follow-up care should be sought around 3 weeks after postcoital contraception. It is because these facilities are not available in ED that some consultants choose not to offer emergency postcoital contraception. Most women will commence menses within 21 days of the postcoital pill. If this does not happen, a pregnancy test should be performed; however, the failure rate of the postcoital pill is less than 5% (Stevens & Kenney 1994). The patient should be advised about contraception in the short term while still in ED. The patient must also be advised to use barrier methods of contraception for the rest of this cycle as the postcoital pill alters the timing of ovulation. Longer-term contraception will be discussed in the follow-up check. It should also be noted that, because the postcoital contraceptive pill prevents uterine implantation, it does not preclude ectopic pregnancy. The patient should be advised of the symptoms of ectopic pregnancy and advised to seek medical care should these be experienced.

Intrauterine contraceptive device

The IUCD may be used up to 5 days after ovulation, or after unprotected intercourse if the date of ovulation is not known. It also works by preventing implantation, and failure is rare. There are disadvantages to its use in nulligravida women because of pain associated with insertion. It is not ideal for women with existing pelvic infection as it could exacerbate this. Irregular vaginal bleeding is also common after IUCD insertion. The advantage of this method is that it provides longer-term contraception. The use of prophylactic antibiotics may be considered for women who are at increased risk of sexually transmitted infection if an IUCD is to be inserted before results of tests are available (FFPRHC 2004, French et al. 2004).

SEXUAL ASSAULT

Rape and sexual assault are violent crimes. Police forces are increasingly caring for physically injured survivors of rape in dedicated rape suites equipped for the privacy and comfort of women who have been assaulted. ED departments should have a rape protocol that has been discussed with the local police force and rape support groups. This should ensure that the patient's best interests are served in terms of both immediate health care and her subsequent ability to produce evidence to prosecute the assailant. ED nurses should attempt to reinstate the patient's perception of control over what happens to her. Unless associated injuries prevent it, the patient should be encouraged to give explicit consent, either written or verbal, for any investigations or examination she undergoes.

Statistics for 2004/2005 show that there were over 13 000 reported offences of rape of a female in the UK. It is believed that this represents only a fraction of actual assaults (Walby & Allen 2004).

The decision to report sexual assault is entirely that of the patient, and ED staff must support that decision and plan care around it. Box 29.5 shows care paths for reporting and non-reporting of sexual assault. If the patient does not have significant physical injury, it may be appropriate to obtain a full history with the police if the patient wishes to report the attack. This is simply to prevent the patient having to describe the incident several times, which can be unnecessarily distressing. The decision to take a joint history should be the patient's. Box 29.6 highlights the essential information needed.

It is important that any potential forensic evidence is preserved. This is equally important in a patient who is unconscious or who has significant physical injury. A paper sheet should be placed under the

---

Box 29.5   Reporting/non-reporting sexual assault care paths. (After Holloway 1994)

Incident reported to police
- Police officer allocated to support patient
- Examination carried out by forensic medical examiner (FME)
- Entrance to victim support scheme
- Police statements obtained
- Police officer support throughout court case

Incident not reported
- Medical examination by senior A&E doctor
- Support agency contacted
- Follow-up at STD clinic
- Nurse support throughout
- Retain option of police involvement

Box 29.6   Obtaining a history from a survivor of sexual assault

- Establish the date, time and location of the attack
- Circumstances of assault:
    - where injured, i.e. in mouth, skin, breast, anus, vagina
    - was a condom used?
    - removal or damage to clothing by assailant
    - number of assailants
    - drugs/alcohol used
    - any associated physical injuries
- Action taken after assault:
    - cleaned teeth, mouthwash gargled
    - wash/shower/bath
    - changed clothes
    - urinated/bowels opened
    - changed tampon/pad
    - subsequent sexual intercourse
- Alcohol/drugs (prescribed or recreational) taken prior to the attack or since
- Previous sexual intercourse, if within 2 weeks
- Menstrual stage, date of last period and usual method of birth control if of child-bearing age
- Medical and obstetric history

take on this role whether or not the patient intends to prosecute, although Kelly (2002) notes that the vast majority of survivors (both female and male) express a preference for a female forensic examiner. The first priority must lie in protecting the patient from further humiliation and distress and, on those grounds alone, one examination is good practice. For evidence to be submissible, the examination, evidence collection and documentation should follow local police policy. The primary role of the ED nurse is in supporting the patient and assuring her privacy and safety until examination can take place. Box 29.7 shows what evidence should be collected and how it should be preserved.

Once the medical examination has been carried out, the patient needs to be advised about pregnancy risk and offered emergency contraception if appropriate. The patient should also be offered follow-up STD screening and it is imperative she has either actual contact with a rape survivors' support counsellor or contact telephone numbers for later use should she wish to do so. Rape trauma syndrome (RTS) is experienced by most sexual assault survivors in some form (Burgess & Holmstrom 1974). Good, sensitive, non-judgemental care immediately following the attack can help to reduce the impact of RTS. It is important that ED nurses understand the progression of this syndrome, both for immediate care of attack survivors and to help recognize and rationalize associated symptoms of patients some time after the assault. Box 29.8 outlines the stages of RTS. In the US an emerging trend is the use of Specialist Forensic Nurses, trained in the collection of forensic evidence, photo documentation and legal testimony. These clinicians are dedicated

patient to collect debris if possible; otherwise linen used should be saved. A mobile patient should be asked to stand on a paper sheet while undressing so that debris can be saved. Physical examination should be carried out at once by a forensic medical examiner (FME) (Holloway 1994). In some areas, the FME will

Box 29.7   Forensic evidence from survivors of sexual assault. (After Stevens & Kenney 1994)

- Observe and document the condition of clothing, i.e. damaged, stained, debris attachment to it. Clothing should be placed in a paper bag for dry storage
- Full medical examination, documenting injuries in detail; provide photographs if possible
- Obtain following samples:

Sample	Collect in	Store in
Blood group/DNA profile	EDTA bottles	Fridge
Blood alcohol	Fluoride oxadate bottle	Fridge
Saliva/sperm group	Universal container	Fridge
Urine/drugs/alcohol screen	Sodium fluoride	Fridge
Skin swabs	Plastic tube	Freezer
Vaginal/cervical swabs	Plastic tube	Freezer
Anal swabs	Plastic tube	Freezer
Loose hairs/debris	Plastic bag	Dry storage
Fingernail clippings	Plastic bag	Dry storage
Tampon/sanitary towel	Plastic bag	Freeze

to the care of survivors of sexual and domestic violence, liaising with medical and nursing staff, police social services and support agencies (Markowitz et al. 2005).

Domestic abuse is the violence perpetrated by one adult against another with whom they have or have had a sexual relationship. This violence may be physical, sexual and/or emotional (RCM 2005). The women's aid organization has found that there are increasing numbers of women and children seeking refuge from domestic abuse. In 2004/05 196 205, women and 129 193 children were provided with refuge-based services in the UK (Williamson 2006). Based on findings of the British Crime Survey of 22 643 women and men aged 16–59, Walby & Allan (2004) found that inter-personal violence is both widely dispersed and it is concentrated. It is widely dispersed in that some experience of domestic violence (abuse, threats or force), sexual victimization or stalking is reported by over one-third (36%) of people. It is concentrated in that a minority, largely women, suffer multiple attacks, severe injuries, and experience more than one form of inter-personal violence and serious disruption to their lives.

The practice of efficient patient processing in ED departments may obscure subtle signs of abuse, which may not be picked up until the woman presents with more serious physical injuries (Olshansky 2002). The confidential enquiry into maternal deaths (CEMACH 2004) found that 14% of the women whose deaths were assessed had a history of domestic violence which was either self-reported to healthcare professionals or was known to health and social services. This is believed to be a conservative estimate of the true prevalence of violence among these women, and ED nurses should be vigilant to the signs of abuse and the local services available to these patients.

EMERGENCY CARE OF THE PREGNANT WOMAN

History

As with other aspects of healthcare, an accurate history of events leading to ED attendance is imperative. In the case of a pregnant patient, a full obstetric history should be obtained as well as the history of the presenting complaint. Box 29.9 highlights the information needed for an obstetric history.

Assessment

General assessment should include baseline observations of pulse, blood pressure, respirations and

Box 29.9   Obtaining an obstetric history

- Number of previous pregnancies
  - terminations
  - miscarriages
  - live births – combinations in pregnancy, delivery, postnatal care
- This pregnancy
  - gestation
  - antenatal care
  - PV bleeding to date
  - other complications
  - ultrasound scans
  - fetal abnormality tests

Most patients receiving antenatal care in the UK have patient held notes which contain a detailed account of their obstetric history.

temperature to detect signs of shock, infection or pre-eclampsia. Routine urinalysis should also be carried out for glucose and protein. The progress of the pregnancy should be assessed in terms of the height of the fundus compared with estimated gestation, and after about 14–16 weeks fetal heartbeat should be assessed. Any vaginal discharge or bleeding should only be assessed in terms of type, quality and odour. Vaginal examination should only be carried out if it is necessary to determine the state of the cervical os or to identify causes of fresh vaginal bleeding. During assessment and care, maternal health should be paramount whatever the gestation of the fetus.

Miscarriage

Miscarriage is also termed 'spontaneous abortion' and describes the delivery of a non-viable fetus before 24 weeks' gestation. There are six types of miscarriage and these are listed in Table 29.2.

Miscarriage is extremely common and up to 20% of confirmed pregnancies spontaneously abort (Miscarriage Association 1996). Where a cause is investigated, pathological abnormalities with the fetus or placenta are commonly found (Creasy & Resnick 1993). Immunological incompatibility with the father, maternal infection, substance misuse and malnutrition have also been linked with spontaneous abortion (Reedy & Brucker 1995).

Despite the relative commonness of miscarriage, it can be devastating for the woman and her partner. Apart from the physical pain associated with miscarriage, the woman and her family are grieving for the loss of a baby, the dreams and plans they will have had for that baby, and their identity as a family (Duncan 1995). It is essential that ED nurses recognize the enormity of this loss and do not attempt to trivialize it

with comments like 'you can have another', or by functional care avoiding conversation about the miscarriage. Parents want their loss acknowledged and it is much better for the nurse to express condolences for the loss of their baby (Standing 1997).

Assessment

This should revolve around maintaining maternal health, as little can be done to alter fetal prognosis (Regan 1992). The patient's haemodynamic stability should be assessed, in terms of heart rate, respirations and blood pressure, as well as blood loss. When enquiring about blood loss, the nurse should seek to establish quantity in terms of the number of pads used per hour. The type of loss should also be noted, whether it is fresh or dark blood, and whether clots or tissue have been passed. This will help to determine the category of miscarriage occurring.

The amount and location of pain should be established, and appropriate analgesia given. A urine sample should be obtained to confirm pregnancy and to rule out urine infection as a cause of bleeding. Blood should also be taken to confirm rhesus status in case the patient is rhesus negative and anti-D serum is required. A vaginal examination will confirm the status of the cervical os, rule out a vaginal source for bleeding and identify any products of conception in the cervix or vagina. An ultrasound scan should be organized to confirm clinical findings, i.e. to identify a potentially viable pregnancy or retained products of conception. For humanitarian reasons, this should be done as soon as possible, as most patients and their partners need confirmation of a visible heartbeat to believe that everything is all right or, more commonly, they need the reinforcement that their baby is dead, or has been miscarried, in order to come to terms with their loss.

Table 29.2 Categorization of miscarriage

Type	Bleeding	Passed tissue	Cervical os	Pain	Size of uterus
Threatened	Slight	No	Closed	Mild	Normal for gestation
Inevitable	Moderate–heavy	No	Open	Moderate–severe	Normal for gestation
Incomplete	Heavy	Yes	Open with tissue present	Severe	Smaller than expected for gestation
Complete	Slight	Yes	Closed	Mild	Smaller than expected for gestation
Missed	None	No	Closed	Nil	Smaller than expected for gestation
Septic	Varies, foul odour often accompanies loss	Sometimes	Open	Moderate–severe High temperature	Normal or small for dates

Management

In most cases of miscarriage, ED care revolves around symptomatic management and psychological support. If the patient shows signs of hypovolaemia, intravenous fluid replacement should be commenced. Adequate analgesia should be given, particularly if the pregnancy is not viable. If the miscarriage has been an incomplete or missed abortion, the patient should be prepared physically and emotionally for an evacuation of retained products of conception (ERPC) in theatre. Psychological support for both the woman and her partner is important throughout their stay in ED, as the initial handling of their loss will impact on the grieving process they must work through (see also Ch. 13).

The use of the term 'spontaneous abortion' should be avoided at this time, as many people associate abortion with voluntary termination of pregnancy. Miscarriage, on the other hand, is seen as involuntary (Reedy & Brucker 1995). Using the term abortion can therefore cause unnecessary distress.

The length of the gestation may alter physical symptoms, but it does not alter emotional ones. All patients should be offered contact numbers for support groups or specialist counsellors. It is also useful to reinforce their need to grieve, and identify times which may be hard, such as the period around the baby's estimated delivery date. This helps the patient and her partner to legitimize their feelings. Some hospitals offer bereavement counselling and a book of remembrance for babies; others also offer the services of the hospital chaplain.

Ectopic pregnancy

This occurs when a fertilized ovum implants somewhere other than the endometrium. The most common site is the fallopian tube (Blackburn & Loper 1992), but implantation can also occur in the ovaries and abdominal cavities (see Fig. 29.3).

A diagnosis of ectopic pregnancy should be considered in all women of childbearing age presenting with abdominal pain or an unexpected collapse (Moulton & Yeats 2004). The incidence of ectopic pregnancy is about 0.5–1% of pregnancies (Stevens & Kenney 1994). This ratio has risen over the last decade and indications are that it will continue to rise with the increase in PID and IUCD use (Stovall & Ling 1992). The use of oral postcoital contraceptives and some fertility treatments also appear to increase the risk of ectopic pregnancy. Ectopic implantation appears to occur because of delay in passage of the fertilized egg. This passage is induced by muscular contraction and ciliary activity. If the fallopian tubes are damaged due to adhesions following infection, the ciliary activity is reduced and the egg cannot pass into the uterus, so it implants in the tube. Hormonal changes of the corpus luteum continue as, physiologically, the pregnancy is still viable at this stage. As a result, the uterus grows and softens as it would with a normal uterine pregnancy. The products of conception continue to expand, causing pain and vaginal bleeding in a 'spotting' form. It is usually at this stage that the woman seeks health intervention. If left unchecked, the products of conception will continue to grow until rupture of the tube occurs and devastating haemorrhage follows.

Assessment

Most patients will give a history of abdominal pain, sometimes unilateral or generalized lower abdomen and pelvic pain. The patient usually has intermittent vaginal bleeding or spotting and, as a result, may or may not be aware that she is pregnant. Most embryos die within 6–12 weeks of gestation due to lack of

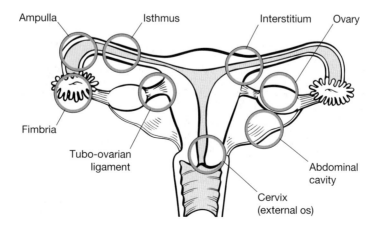

Figure 29.3 Sites of implantation of ectopic pregnancies.

placental development. For this reason, most women with ectopic pregnancy suffer a lot less nausea than those with a uterine pregnancy with a healthy developing placenta. Once the embryo dies, endometrium is shed and a large PV bleed ensues. This is different to the potentially life-threatening haemorrhage which occurs with a ruptured fallopian tube. The degree of haemodynamic compromise determines the urgency of intervention, and therefore accurate assessment of basic haemostasis is vital. Slight tachycardia would be expected because of the emotion and anxiety attached to ectopic pregnancy, but bradycardia together with an increase in respirations and postural and persistent hypotension should be treated seriously. As part of the assessment, a urine sample should be taken to confirm pregnancy, and an ultrasound scan will show the location of pregnancy after about 6 weeks' gestation. Table 29.3 highlights the clinical differences between a threatened miscarriage and an ectopic pregnancy.

Management

Early management revolves around symptom control and psychological support. Pain relief and routine intravenous access should be established via two large-bore cannulae. Blood samples are sent for group and cross-match beta HCG full blood count and coagulation studies. If the woman demonstrates signs of shock, fluid replacement should commence. Once the diagnosis has been made, using transvaginal/abdominal ultrasound and blood/urine HCG levels, treatment is prescribed dependent on the patients' haemodynamic status and gestation of pregnancy. In most instances, both haemodynamically stable and unstable patients can be managed by laparoscopy (RCOG 2004).

Medical management of ectopic pregnancy reduces the need for surgical intervention in women who are haemodynamically stable and at an early stage of the pregnancy. This involves the use of cytotoxic intramuscular methotrexate, single dose, administered using special safety precautions for its preparation, administration and disposal. As the embryo is one of the fastest growing cells in the body the proliferating trophoblastic tissue is very sensitive to the action of methotrexate, causing cell death and dissolution. Close monitoring of beta HCG levels by the gynaecological team is required to ensure this treatment has been successful (Miller & Griffin 2003). Local injections of prostaglandins and laparoscopic injections of hyperosmolar glucose solutions have also been used successfully with fewer side-effects. Conservative surgical management involves the removal of the conceptus via laparoscopic salpingostomy, conserving the fallopian tube. In cases where the conceptus has implanted within the fimbrial region of the fallopian tube, fimbrial evacuation may be considered (Moore 1998). These procedures carry an increased risk of future ectopic pregnancies because of scarred tissue. If salpingostomy is not possible, the fallopian tube is removed to prevent tubal rupture, with obvious implications for future fertility.

If ectopic rupture is suspected, the patient should be considered to have a life-threatening condition. Ruptured ectopic pregnancy is the highest single cause of maternal death (Rita 1998). Death usually occurs as a result of uncontrolled haemorrhage. This is because occult bleeding into the abdominal cavity

Table 29.3 Differential diagnosis of ectopic pregnancy vs. threatened miscarriage. (After Stevens & Kenney 1994)

Symptom	Ectopic Nature	Percentage of patients affected	Threatened miscarriage Nature	Percentage of patients affected
Abdominal pain	General or affected side	90	Midline, crampy	10
Shoulder tip pain		26		None
General abdominal tenderness	General	45	Usually non-tender	
	Lower	25		
	Unilateral	30		
Vaginal bleeding	Light/spotting	64	Light	100
Amenorrhoea		75		90
Uterus size	Normal	80	Right for dates	100
Shock		17		None
Dysuria		11		None
Rectal pain		9		None

can occur as well as PV loss; therefore, blood loss can be underestimated. The patient compensates initially, then becomes rapidly shocked. It is important to commence vigorous fluid resuscitation. Urgent surgical intervention is necessary to preserve maternal life. The woman and her partner's psychological needs should not be overlooked. As well as the physical distress, they are also coming to terms with the loss of their baby and the threat to future fertility that surgery brings. The nurse needs to acknowledge, not minimize, these feelings. A full description of psychological care and appropriate follow-up is given in the section on miscarriage.

As the mortality rate for deaths from ectopic pregnancy continues to rise, the confidential enquiry into maternal and child health 2000–2002 found that of those who died as a result of ectopic pregnancy, 66% were assessed as having had some form of substandard care. As a result the Royal College of Obstetricians and Gynaecologists set out recommendations for emergency departments (CEMACH 2004). They advised that ectopic pregnancy should be excluded in all women of childbearing age with unexplained abdominal pain. Furthermore all clinicians, including undergraduate medical and nursing students, need to be made aware of the typical and atypical presentations of ectopic pregnancy and how it may mimic gastrointestinal disease (CEMACH 2004).

Pre-eclampsia/eclampsia

Pre-eclampsia, or pregnancy-induced hypertension, occurs in about 7% of pregnancies (Stevens & Kenney 1994). Its causes have not been proven, but several theories exist, the most common being that susceptibility to eclampsia is a hereditary trait linked to a recessive gene (Chesley 1985). Other theories link eclampsia to a possible immunological cause where an antigenic reaction to the fetus causes maternal symptoms. Historic linkage of eclampsia to socioeconomic status has no foundation in research (Reedy & Brucker 1995). Women most susceptible to pre-eclampsia/eclampsia are those at either end of the child-bearing age range, i.e. younger than 16 or older than 35 years of age. It is most common in first pregnancies and in those women expecting twins or more, and there appears to be a familial link. Women with pre-existing health problems, such as diabetes and chronic hypertension, are more susceptible to pre-eclampsia.

The disease usually has a gradual onset, the pre-eclampsia phase. Because of good antenatal screening, most patients are identified and treated early. Therefore, the use of ED for care in the pre-eclampsic phase is uncommon, but it is important to understand the disease process in order to treat life-threatening eclampsia in ED. Pre-eclampsia has a multisystem impact (see Box 29.10).

Box 29.10   Multisystem impact of pre-eclampsia/eclampsia

Cardiovascular
- Hypertension – increased peripheral resistance
- Damage to blood vessels – vasopression traumatizes vessels and induces coagulopathy
- Haemorrhage – due to reduced platelets

Haematological
- Thrombocytopenia – results from coagulopathy and reduces platelets and fibrinogen activity
- Abnormal clotting
- Disseminating intravascular coagulopathy

Renal
- Impaired glomerular function – glomerular filtration rate (GFR) and renal blood flow are increased in pregnancy; with pre-eclampsia a decrease occurs
- Proteinuria – due to renal impairment
- Sodium/potassium retention – contributes to oedema
- Acute renal failure

Neurological
- Headache – due to cerebral oedema. In severe cases cerebral infarct/haemorrhage may occur
- Hyperreflexia – nerve-end irritation due to vasospasm
- Visual disturbance – due to retinal oedema; can lead to retinal detachment
- Convulsions – late sign of eclampsia

Respiratory
- Pulmonary oedema – due to cardiovascular and renal complications
- Haemorrhage – due to thrombocytopenia

Hepatic
- Abnormal liver enzymes
- Periportal haemorrhage – secondary to other system changes
- Infarction
- Rupture

Placental/fetal
- Placental infarction
- Abruptio placentae
- Fetal intrauterine growth retardation
- Fetal death

Pre-eclampsia

A triad of symptoms exists:

- hypertension – 30 mmHg or more above the woman's usual systolic BP or 15 mmHg above her usual diastolic BP
- proteinuria
- oedema – where this is present in the face or upper limbs it is of greater concern. Lower limb oedema, particularly of the feet or ankles, is usually mechanical in nature

If any two of these symptoms are present, the woman is considered to have pre-eclampsia. Persistent hypertension should be treated, and initially close maternal and fetal monitoring will necessitate admission.

Eclampsia

This is usually defined as the onset of seizures in pregnancy occurring after 21 weeks gestation or within 10 days of delivery. It is accompanied by at least two of the following signs: hypertension, proteinuria and oedema. Later signs include thrombocytopenia of raised aspartate amino transferase. Eclampsia is one of the main causes of maternal deaths, occurring in approximately 1 in 2000 pregnancies (Munro 2000). Prior to fitting, most patients complain of headache, visual disturbance, shortness of breath or right hypochondriacal pain. They may also have oliguria and appear confused. These symptoms are all derived from the physiological processes described in Box 29.10. While some women present in ED at this stage, more appear as emergency admissions once fitting has commenced. Staff should be alert to the possibility of a concealed pregnancy in young women who have no previous history of seizures. Eclampsic fitting is life-threatening to both the mother and fetus. It must be brought under control rapidly using small doses of diazepam, 10 mg i.v. repeated up to five times. It is administered in this manner to prevent fetal depression. Intravenous infusion of chlormethiazole or phenytoin should also be considered. Occasionally, short-term ventilation and paralysis may be necessary. Other presentations of impending eclampsia include severe right hypochondriacal pain and shock as a result of hepatic rupture.

Urgent laparotomy is indicated to control haemorrhage and preserve maternal life. In these circumstances, however, it has a mortality of about 70%. Symptoms of disseminating intravascular coagulopathy (DIC) accompany about 7% of eclampsic conditions (Stevens & Kenney 1994). Once pre-eclampsia reaches this stage, or fitting has occurred, urgent preparation to deliver the fetus should be made. Delivery usually resolves maternal symptoms, although in some cases they may persist for up to 10 days (Reedy & Brucker 1995). The baby has a greater chance of survival even if delivered premature.

Abrupto placentae

This is more commonly treated in obstetric units than in ED departments. It occurs as a result of premature separation of the placenta from the uterine wall. Haemorrhage and blood usually track between the uterus and placental membranes, causing PV bleeding and pain. Bleeding can be occult in about 10% of cases, and therefore diagnosis should not be made simply by the presence of PV bleeding. A pelvic ultrasound should be used to confirm diagnosis. Predisposing factors include substance misuse, pre-eclampsia, a maternal age of 35 or more, multiple gestation and as a result of trauma.

Emergency childbirth

The majority of births are normal deliveries requiring little assistance and the duration of labour is usually long enough for the woman to seek maternity care. Occasionally, however, it is necessary to deliver a baby in ED, if there is insufficient time to reach the delivery unit. The most common causes of emergency childbirth include multiparous women with precipitous (rapid) deliveries and adolescent girls who successfully conceal their pregnancy until they present with abdominal pains or do not recognize the signs of active labour. Some women in pre-term labour may also have precipitous deliveries. Child protection issues may be raised in cases where a woman whose child may be at risk may choose to avoid traditional routes of maternity care and travel to a hospital outside of their area, presenting to emergency departments in labour (McLoughlin 2001).

Labour can be described as a process by which the fetus, placenta and membranes are expelled through the birth canal. Normal labour begins spontaneously at approximately 40 weeks' gestation, referred to as 'term', with the fetus presenting by the head or 'vertex' (Bennet & Brown 1990). Box 29.11 outlines the stages of labour.

First-stage labour management

The nurse's role in the care of a woman facing imminent childbirth is to provide physical and emotional support in a calm, relaxed manner. The nurse should obtain enough information to assess the woman's immediate circumstances:

- What parity is the woman?
- At what gestation is the pregnancy?

Box 29.11 The three stages of labour

- **First stage**
  This is the longest phase during which the body prepares for delivery. The cervix effaces then dilates. There is usually a pink, mucous 'show' as this begins, and the amniotic membranes rupture as the cervix dilates. If this has not already occurred, contractions gradually increase in frequency and intensity. Transition to second stage occurs once the cervix is fully dilated to 10 cm. This phase usually lasts several hours, however the time reduces with the number of pregnancies.

- **Second stage**
  This is from full dilation until after delivery of the baby. During this phase, the baby's head travels down the birth canal. When it reaches the outlet, it flexes to present occiput first. This is a complicated but natural process. The visible occiput is termed 'crowning' and highlights the imminence of delivery. The head is followed by the shoulders, then the trunk and legs. This usually lasts up to 1 hour.

- **Third stage**
  This is from the delivery of the baby until complete delivery of the placenta and membranes and control of haemorrhage.

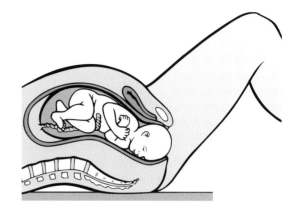

Figure 29.4 Cross-sectional view of crowning.

- What signs of onset of labour has she experienced?
- Has she a history of precipitous labour?
- What are the frequency and duration of the contractions?

The assistance of a midwife, obstetric and neonatal team should be obtained immediately, and provision for the imminent birth should be made. Signs of imminent childbirth include:

- the mother experiences tension, anxiety and intense contractions
- blood 'show' as a result of rapid dilation of the cervix
- bulging or gaping of the anus as a result of descent of the fetal presenting part
- bulging or fullness of the perineum
- 'crowning' of the fetal head at the introitus, which occurs when the fetal skull escapes under the pubic arch and no longer recedes (Fig. 29.4)
- the mother saying 'the baby is coming'.

In multiparous women, the last sign is symptomatic of imminent birth; however, in primiparous women, birth may take up to 30 minutes. Birth is near when the head stays visible between contractions. The mother should be made to feel in control, protecting her dignity, and should be kept informed of all that is happening. Her partner should be included as a source of constant support and encouragement to the mother at this time. The mother should be encouraged to adopt a position which is most comfortable for her, which is usually sitting on the trolley with her back well supported with pillows or a foam wedge. Nitrous oxide is the preferred method of pain relief when birth is imminent and the mother should be encouraged to inhale the gas while she is feeling the contractions. As well as providing pain relief, it is also an effective means of providing extra oxygen to both the mother and the fetus. Neither shaving, urinary catheterization or enema administration are required (Priestly 2004).

Baseline recordings of maternal temperature, pulse, respirations and blood pressure should be obtained. The fetal heartbeat is also recorded and may be auscultated using a fetal stethoscope or fetal Doppler when the head is presenting. The fetal heart sounds are more commonly located close to the midline below the umbilicus. The normal fetal heart rate is between 120 and 160 beats/min. A further assessment of fetal condition includes observation of the amniotic fluid or 'waters'; these are normally straw-coloured, but they may become green as a result of meconium.

Second-stage labour management
The attending nurse/midwife should open a sterile delivery set and wash the woman's vulva with sterile swabs and warmed antiseptic solution. With the next contraction, the woman should be encouraged to inhale deeply and bear down to facilitate the delivery. The nurse should place his/her fingers over the advancing head to prevent expulsive 'crowning',

which may result in perineal tearing and a heightened risk of intraventricular haemorrhage to the newborn infant (Fig. 29.5). As the fetal head advances and gradually distends the perineal tissue, the mother should be encouraged to pant to facilitate a controlled delivery and reduce maternal trauma. Once the baby's head emerges, the nurse should slip a finger over the occiput to feel if the cord is round the baby's neck. If this has happened, the cord should be released either by slipping it over the head or, if this is unsuccessful, by applying two artery forceps 2–5 cm apart and cutting the cord between them.

The nurse should continue to support the head, taking care not to put any traction on it (Fig. 29.6). Mucus should be removed with a sterile swab, but the eyes should not be cleansed due to the risk of infection. At the next contraction, the anterior shoulder should be delivered by gentle downward traction of the head. Then the baby should be raised and the posterior shoulder will deliver rapidly, followed by the trunk and legs. The baby should be dried and

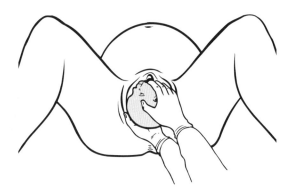

Figure 29.5 Hold infant's head gently in both hands.

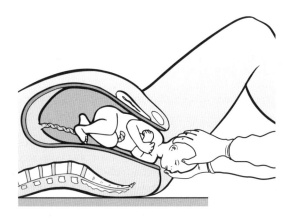

Figure 29.6 Carefully support infant's head as it is born.

placed in a warm towel, as a cold baby has an increased oxygen consumption and cold babies more easily become hypoglycaemic and acidotic; they also have an increased mortality (Advanced Life Support Group 1997). The newborn baby should be allowed to lie on the bed or be placed on the mother's abdomen, allowing her to see and touch the baby. The umbilical cord should be clamped and cut if this has not already been done and syntometrine given intramuscularly to the mother. This contains oxytocin and ergometrine. The oxytocin provides marked uterine contraction after approximately 3 minutes but is short-lived, and as its effects begin to wear off the ergometrine begins to act and provide longer-lasting uterine contractions, reducing the risk of postpartum haemorrhage (Greaves et al. 1997).

The time of the delivery and those involved in it should be recorded accurately. The Apgar score should also be recorded. This is a numerical scoring system used to assess the newborn baby's condition at 1 minute after birth and reassessed again after 5 minutes. While Kelnar et al. (1995) stress that assessment at 1 minute is important, it has been shown that an assessment at 5 minutes is much more reliable as a predictor of death during the first 28 days of life and of the child's neurological state and risk of major handicap at the age of 1 year (Nelson & Ellenberg 1981, Rehnke et al. 1987). The factors assessed are heart rate, respiratory rate, muscle tone, reflex response to stimulus, and colour. A score of 0–2 is given to each sign in accordance with the guideline in Table 29.4. A normal infant in good condition at birth will achieve an Apgar score of between 7 and 10. A score below 7 indicates some degree of asphyxia which requires some form of resuscitation (Michie 1990).

Third-stage labour management

The third stage of labour is from delivery of the baby to delivery of the placenta and usually takes about 5–20 minutes. A sterile receiver should be placed between the woman's thighs to collect any blood lost, and the umbilical cord is placed in the receiver. Once the signs of placental separation are observed, i.e. lengthening of the umbilical cord, a fresh gush of blood and contraction of the uterus causing the fundus to rise to the level of the umbilicus, the mother should be asked to bear down as for delivery to expel the placenta and membranes. Once delivered, the placenta should be examined for completeness. The fundus of the uterus may be massaged to promote contractions, expel blood clots and control haemorrhage. The woman's vagina and perineum should be examined for tearing which may require suturing. The mother's temperature, pulse and blood pressure

Table 29.4 Apgar scores

Factor	Score		
	0	1	2
A = appearance (colour)	Blue	Blue limbs, pink body	Pink
P = pulse (heart rate)	Absent	<100 beats/min	>100 beats/min
G = grimace (muscle tone)	Limp	Some flexion	Good flexion
A = activity (reflexes irritable)	Absent	Some motion	Good motion
R = respiratory effort	Absent	Weak cry	Strong cry

should be recorded and her lochia, i.e. PV loss, observed. The baby should also be examined, weighed and have a rectal temperature taken. Two identity bands should also be placed on the baby. Both mother and baby should then be transferred to the nearest maternity unit for post-natal care.

Postpartum haemorrhage

Postpartum haemorrhage occurs in 3–5% of pregnancies and accounts for almost 10% of maternal deaths (Beischer & Mackay 1986). It can be described as any bleeding from the genital tract which adversely affects the mother's condition following the birth of a baby, up to 6 weeks post-delivery. A blood loss of 500 ml or more at delivery is regarded as post-partum haemorrhage, irrespective of maternal condition.

There are two types of postpartum haemorrhage:

- Primary postpartum haemorrhage, which occurs within the first 24 hours post-delivery.
- Secondary postpartum haemorrhage, which occurs at any time after the first 24 hours, up to 6 weeks post-delivery, but most commonly occurs between 7 and 14 days postpartum. It can be described as bleeding in excess of the normal lochial loss and may be associated with retained placental tissue or uterine infection.

Assessment

History should include the following information:

- duration of symptoms
- quantity of bleeding in terms of number of pads used per hour
- type of blood loss, i.e. red, brown clots
- type of pain
- location of pain
- date of delivery and any subsequent period/PV bleeding
- any infection
- any trauma
- other related medical history.

The woman will have an enlarged, 'boggy', uterus. On palpation the uterus will feel soft, distended and lacking in tone. The fundal height will rise above the umbilicus as a result of retained blood in the uterus preventing uterine contraction. A low-grade pyrexia, rising pulse and falling blood pressure characterize postpartum haemorrhage, together with lower back and abdominal pain, and general restlessness.

Sanitary pads should be checked to evaluate the amount of bleeding and note the presence or absence of clots or odour.

Management

The aim of ED management is to control haemorrhage and maintain blood volume. Blood should be taken for group and cross-match, and large-bore i.v. lines for warmed crystalloids and blood should be established. Oxygen should also be administered. An i.v. injection of ergometrine or syntometrine may be given in order to cause uterine contraction, which assists in haemorrhage control. If the uterus is palpable, it may be massaged to enable it to contract and expel any clots. The presence of retained products of conception should be excluded on pelvic ultrasound. If debris is found or haemorrhage is not controlled, urgent evacuation of retained products of conception (ERPC) should be performed in theatre.

CONCLUSION

This chapter has considered the common gynaecological and obstetric reasons for presentation to ED. Many of these conditions have a life-long impact on the patient and her family, in terms of either physical or, more commonly, psychological well-being. It is imperative that ED staff are sensitive to the needs of the woman and her partner, and can offer privacy and compassionate, non-judgemental care. Inappropriate assessment or intervention can have catastrophic consequences. The information provided in this chapter should enable the nurse to make an informed assessment and plan therapeutic care for this emotionally and physically vulnerable group.

References

Advanced Life Support Group (1997) *Advanced Paediatric Life Support: A Practical Approach*. London: BMJ.

Beischer NA, Mackay EV (1986) Ante natal care: education of the patient. In: Beischer NA, ed. *Obstetrics and the Newborn*, 2nd edn. London: Baillière Tindall.

Bennett RV, Brown LK (1990) The first stage of labour: physiology and early care. In: Bennett RV, Brown LK, eds. *Myles Textbook for Midwives*. Edinburgh: Churchill Livingstone.

Blackburn S, Loper D (1992) *Maternal, Fetal and Neonatal Physiology*. Philadelphia: WB Saunders.

Bryan S (2004) Pelvic inflammatory disease. In: Cameron P, Jelinek G, Kelly AM, Murray L, Brown AFT, Heyworth J, eds. *Textbook of Adult Emergency Medicine*, 2nd edn. Edinburgh: Churchill Livingstone.

Burgess A, Holmstrom L (1974) *Rape: Victims of Crisis*. Maryland: RJ Brady.

Confidential Enquiry into Maternal and Child Health (CEMACH) (2004) *Why mothers Die 2000–2002*. 6th Report. London: Royal College of Obstetricians and Gynaecologists.

Chesley L (1985) Hypertensive disorders in pregnancy. *Journal of Nurse-Midwifery*, **30**(2), 99–104.

Creasy R, Resnick R (1993) *Maternal Fetal Medicine*. Philadelphia: WB Saunders.

Duncan D (1995) Fathers have feelings too. *Modern Midwife*, **5**(1), 30–31.

Faculty of Family Planning and Reproductive Health Care (2004) The copper intrauterine device as long-term contraception. *Journal of Family Planning and Reproductive Health Care*, **30**(1), 29–42.

Farley TM, Rosenberg MJ, Rowe PJ, Chen JH, Meink O (1992) Intrauterine devices and pelvic inflammatory disease: an international perspective. *Lancet*, **339**, 785–788.

French K, Ward S, McRae J, Nash T (2004) Emergency contraception, *Nursing Standard*, **18**(42), 49–53.

Golub S (1992) *Periods*. Newberry Park: Sage.

Gondeck J (1998) Gynecologic emergencies. In: Newberry L, ed. *Sheehy's Emergency Nursing: Principles and Practice*, 4th edn. St Louis: Mosby.

Greaves I, Hodgetts T, Porter K (1997) Childbirth. In: Greaves I, Hodgetts T, Porter K, eds. *Emergency Care: A Textbook for Paramedics*. London: Baillière Tindall.

Hinchliff S, Montague S, Watson R (1996) *Physiology for Nursing Practice*, 2nd edn. London: Baillière Tindall.

Holloway M (1994) Care of the sexually assaulted woman. *Emergency Nurse*, **2**(3), 18–20.

Kelly L (2002) *A Research Review on the Reporting, Investigation and Prosecution of Rape Cases*. London: HMCPSI.

Kelnar CJH, Harvey D, Simpson C (1995) *The Sick Newborn Baby*, 3rd edn. London: Baillière Tindall.

Lichtman R, Papera S (1990) *Gynecology: Well Woman Care*. Norwalk, CT: Appleton & Lange.

Markowitz JR, Steer S, Garland M (2005) Hospital-based intervention for intimate partner violence victims: a forensic nursing model. *Journal of Emergency Nursing*, **31**(2), 166–170.

McLoughlin AMP (2001) Unexpected birth in A&E departments. *Accident and Emergency Nursing*, **9**, 242–248.

Michie MM (1990) The baby at birth. In: Bennett RV, Brown LK, eds. *Myles Textbook for Midwives*. Edinburgh: Churchill Livingstone.

Miller JH, Griffin E (2003) Methotrexate administration for ectopic pregnancy in the Emergency Department: one hospital's protocol/competencies. *Journal of Emergency Nursing*, **29**(3), 240–244.

Miscarriage Association (1996) *Why Did it Happen to Us? A Summary of Causes, Tests and Treatment*. Wakefield: Miscarriage Association.

Moore L (1998) Ectopic Pregnancy. *Nursing Standard*, **12**(38), 48–55.

Moulton C, Yates D (2004) *Obstetric, Gynaecological Genitourinary and Perinal Problems. Emergency Medicine*, 2nd edn. London: Blackwell Science Ltd.

Munro PT (2000) Management of eclampsia in the Accident and Emergency Department. *Journal of Accident and Emergency Medicine*, **17**(1), 7–11.

Nelson KB, Ellenberg JH (1981) Apgar scores as predictors of chronic neurologic disability. *Pediatrics*, **68**, 36–44.

Olshansky E (2002) Emergency care of women who were abused was driven by the prevailing practice pattern of effective patient processing. *Evidence Based Nursing*, **5**(1), 29.

Priestly S (2004) Emergency delivery. In: Cameron P, Jelinek G, Kelly AM, Murray L, Brown AFT, Heyworth J, eds. *Textbook of Adult Emergency Medicine*, 2nd edn. Edinburgh: Churchill Livingstone.

Reedy N, Brucker M (1995) Emergencies in gynecology and obstetrics. In: Kitt S, Selfridge-Thomas J, Proehl JA, Kaiser J, eds. *Emergency Nursing: A Physiologic and Clinical Perspective*, 2nd edn. Philadelphia: WB Saunders.

Regan L (1992) Managing miscarriage. *The Practitioner*, **236**, 1513, 374–378.

Rehnke M, Carter RL, Hardt NS et al. (1987) The relationship of Apgar scores, gestational age and birthweight to survival of low birthweight infants. *American Journal of Perinatology*, **4**, 121–124.

Rita S (1998) Obstetric emergencies. In: Newberry L, ed. *Sheehy's Emergency Nursing: Principles and Practice*. St Louis: Mosby.

Royal College of Obstetricians and Gynaecologists (2004) *The Management of Tubal Pregnancy* (Guideline 21). London: RCOG.

Royal College of Midwives (RCM) *Position Paper No. 19a, Domestic Abuse in Pregnancy*. London: RCM.

Selfridge-Thomas J (1997) *Emergency Nursing: An Essential Guide for Patient Care*. Philadelphia: WB Saunders.

Standing J (1997) Miscarriage in ED: a review of the literature. *Emergency Nurse*, **5**(5), 25–29.

Stevens L, Kenney A (1994) *Emergencies in Obstetrics and Gynaecology*. Oxford: Oxford University Press.

Stoval R, Ling F (1992) Some new approaches to ectopic pregnancy. *Contemporary Obstetrics and Gynaecology*, **35**(5), 35–70.

Walby S, Allen J (2004) *Domestic Violence, Sexual Sssault and Stalking: Findings from the British Crime Survey*. London: Home Office Research, Development and Statistic Directorate.

Walters BA (1992) Caring for the patient with a disorder of the reproductive system. In: Royle JA, Walsh M, eds. *Watson's Medical-Surgical Nursing and Related Physiology*, 4th edn. London: Bailliière Tindall.

Weissmann G (1991) The actions of NSAIDs. *Hospital Practice*, **26**, 60–76.

Williamson E (2006) *Women's Aid Federation of England 2005 Survey of Domestic Violence*. London: Women's Aid Federation.

Wolner Hanbseen P (1991) Incidence and diagnosis of acute salpingitis. *Contemporary Obstetrics and Gynaecology*, **36**(2), 67–72.

Wright S (1999) Sexually transmitted diseases. *Nursing Standard*, **13**(46), 37–42.

Chapter 30

Ophthalmic emergencies

Janet Marsden

INTRODUCTION

A significant proportion of the workload of the ED is made up of patients with ophthalmic problems, ranging from 6% (Edwards 1987) to 8%. Tan et al. (1997) found a lack of basic ophthalmic training for ED SHOs leading to a lack of confidence on their part in the management of eye emergencies. This lack of confidence on the part of junior doctors is reflected in the nursing teams of many EDs and, combined with the apparent health of many ophthalmic patients, can lead to inappropriate management in the ED.

Being able to see and make a visual assessment of surroundings is taken for granted by most people and the sudden decline in or loss of sight is an extremely frightening experience. In ED, patients attend with acute and chronic ophthalmic conditions of varying degrees of severity. For some, immediate intervention can be sight-saving. This chapter will equip ED nurses to assess, identify and initiate care for patients with common ophthalmic conditions. Knowledge of the anatomy and physiology of the eye and surrounding structures will aid nurses in using mechanism of injury, signs and symptoms to assess the patient's condition. The chapter will address ophthalmic conditions in terms of assessment findings, which can be broadly categorized into two groups:

- trauma
- non-traumatic red eye.

ANATOMY AND PHYSIOLOGY OF THE EYE (FIG. 30.1)

Orbit

The orbit is a large bony socket which contains the eyeball or globe with its associated muscles, nerves,

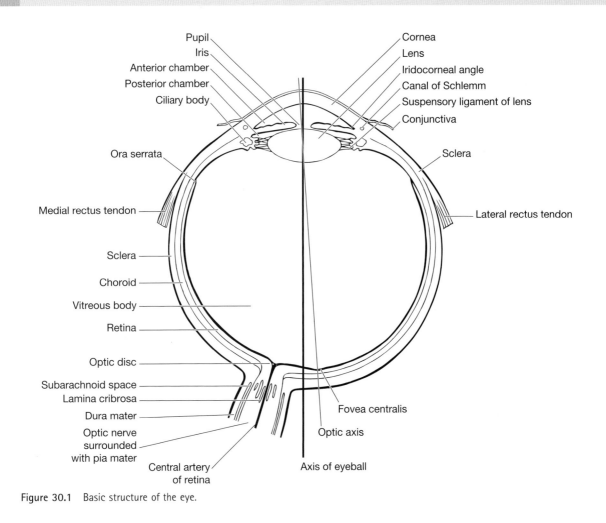

Figure 30.1 Basic structure of the eye.

blood vessels, fat and most of the lacrimal apparatus. Each of the two orbits is roughly pyramidal in shape with the apex lying posteriorly. The orbit is made up of seven individual bones: the maxilla, palatine, zygoma, sphenoid, frontal, ethmoid and lacrimal bones.

Eyelids

The lids are layered structures covered on their outer surfaces by skin and on their inner surfaces by conjunctiva (see Fig. 30.2). In between is subcutaneous tissue, the orbital septum of which thickens within the lids to form fibrous tarsal plates which give structure to the lid. The upper lid contains the levator muscle and the lower contains the inferior tarsal muscle, which retracts it. The lids are maintained in position by the medial and lateral canthal tendons which attach to the periosteum. The lids are closed by the orbicularis muscle.

Within the lid structure are a number of glands. Tarsal or Meibomian glands are arranged perpendicular to the lid margin on the conjunctival surface of the tarsal plate; when blocked and infected, these are known as chalazia (singular, chalazion). The eyelashes are more numerous on the upper lid than on the lower. Sebaceous and modified sweat glands open into each lash follicle – infection produces a hordeolum or stye.

Behind the lashes is the join between the conjunctiva and the skin of the lids. This is known as the grey line because of its relative avascularity. The lids protect the eye by preventing contact with foreign bodies and by preventing drying of the cornea and

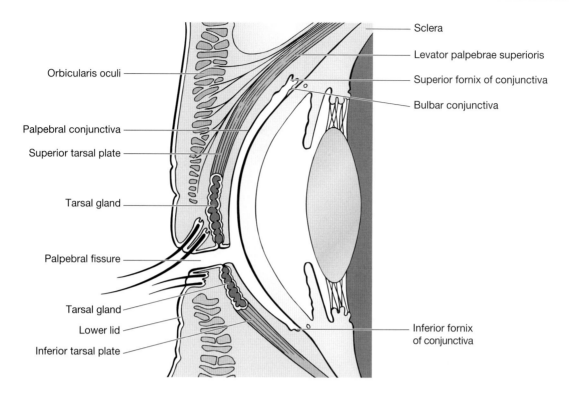

Figure 30.2   Lids and conjunctival formices.

conjunctiva. Lid closure and blinking help to spread the tear film over the front of the eye and move it into the lacrimal drainage apparatus.

Lacrimal system

The tear film is composed mainly of watery fluid from the lacrimal gland (99%), which is situated in the lacrimal fossa of the frontal bone in the orbit. The other important components of the tear film are mucin from the conjunctival goblet cells and oil from the Meibomian (tarsal) glands and the glands of Möll and Zeiss. The tear film is distributed over the surface of the eye by gravity, capillary action of the puncta and canaliculi and the eyelids. The tears leave the eye by evaporation and by way of the puncta, the upper of which takes around 30% of the unevaporated tears and the lower around 70% From the puncta, the tears flow into the canaliculi, into the common canaliculus and then into the lacrimal sac and through the nasolacrimal duct (see Fig. 30.3).

Conjunctiva

The conjunctiva is a thin, transparent mucous membrane lining the inner surface of the eyelid (palpebral conjunctiva), reflecting back on itself at the upper and lower fornices and covering the sclera as far as the corneoscleral junction (bulbar conjunctiva). The conjunctiva is adherent to the lid and rather less so to the Tenon's capsule overlying the sclera. It is most adherent at the corneoscleral junction (limbus). The conjunctiva is quite mobile in the fornices and over the globe and can absorb a large volume of fluid and become oedematous. The epithelium of the conjunctiva is continuous with the corneal epithelium. It contains goblet cells which secrete mucus. The main body of the conjunctiva is connective tissue housing blood vessels, nerves and other glands.

Cornea

The transparent cornea forms the anterior one-sixth of the globe. Its curvature is higher than that of the rest of the globe and it is the main structure responsible for the refraction of light entering the eye. It is an avascular structure which is nourished by the aqueous humour, the capillaries at its edge and from the tear film. Microscopically, it consists of five layers:

- The epithelium – consists of five layers of cells centrally, 10 or more at the limbus. Running

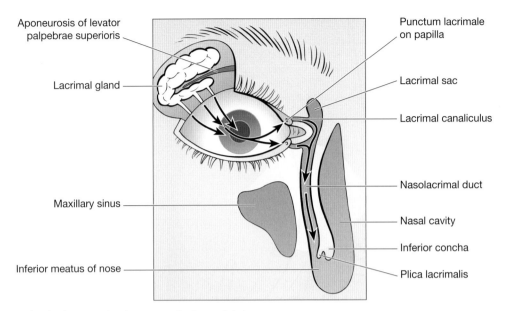

Figure 30.3 Lacrimal system showing tear production and drainage.

between the cells are the nerve endings of sensory nerve fibres, which are sensitive mainly to pain. The epithelium regenerates by the movement of cells from the periphery towards the middle.

- Bowman's layer – is acellular and consists of collagen fibres.
- Substantia propria or stroma – comprises 90% of the thickness of the cornea. It is transparent and fibrous, and is made up of lamellae of collagen fibres arranged parallel to the surface. This arrangement ensures corneal clarity.
- Descemet's membrane – a strong membrane which is the basement membrane of the endothelium.
- Endothelium – a single layer of flattened cells which plays a major role in controlling the hydration of the cornea by a barrier and active transport method. Loss of endothelial cells leads to corneal oedema and lack of clarity.

Sclera

Sclera forms the posterior five-sixths of the eye. It is 1 mm thick posteriorly and thinnest (0.3 mm) immediately posterior to the insertion of the recti muscles. The sclera forms the 'white' of the eye; its outer surface is smooth, except for where the six orbital muscles are attached. It is perforated posteriorly by the optic nerve at an area known as the lamina cribrosa. In this area, the sclera forms a meshwork rather than a solid structure to allow nerve fibres and the central retinal artery and vein to pass through it. The sclera is weakened at this point. Raised intraocular pressure can make the lamina cribrosa bulge outwards, producing a cupped disc.

The sclera is composed of two main layers: the episclera, a loose connective tissue which provides most of the nutritional support of the sclera via a vascular plexus; and the main body of the sclera, which is a dense fibrous tissue that is relatively avascular. The function of the sclera is to protect the intraocular contents and preserve the shape of the globe, maintaining the placement of the optical system. It provides the insertion for the muscles.

The uveal tract

The uveal tract is composed of the iris, the ciliary body and the choroid. The iris is a thin-pigmented diaphragm with a central aperture or pupil. It is located between the cornea and the lens. The pupil varies in size from 1 to 8 mm and differs in size on the two sides in 25% of 'normal' people. The iris divides the anterior segment into anterior and posterior chambers. Its periphery is attached to the ciliary body. The colour of the iris is produced by pigment in melanocytes within its structure. The main body of the iris consists of highly vascular connective tissue; it also contains nerve fibres, the muscle of the sphincter pupillae and the dilator pupillae. The sphincter forms a ring of smooth muscle around the pupil. When it contracts in bright light and during accommodation, the pupil constricts. The dilator is a thin layer of muscle extending from the iris root to the sphincter pupillae. When the dilator pupillae contracts in low-intensity light and during sympathetic activity such as fear, the pupil enlarges.

The ciliary body is continuous with the choroid and the margin of the iris. It contains the ciliary muscle used to change the shape of the lens during accommodation. Its outer, pigmented layer is continuous with the retinal pigment epithelium. Its inner, non-pigmented layer produces aqueous humour. The lens attaches to the ciliary body by a suspensory ligament whose fibres are known as zonules.

The choroid is a thin, soft, brown coat covering the inner surface of the sclera. It extends from the optic nerve to the ciliary body at the ora serrata. The inner surface of the choroid is firmly attached to the pigment layer of the retina. The main body of the choroid is a vascular layer, the choriocapillaris, which supplies nutrition to the external half of the retina and the macula. Its outer layer consists of larger vessels and collecting veins.

The angle and aqueous

The anterior segment of the globe is divided into two chambers. The anterior chamber lies between the cornea and the root of the iris. At the periphery of the anterior chamber is a junction between the cornea, sclera, ciliary body and iris, known as the angle. Within this angle is the trabecular meshwork. The posterior chamber is a slit-like cavity between the back of the iris and the ciliary processes and lens.

Aqueous humour is a clear fluid which fills both of these chambers. It is formed by the ciliary processes of the ciliary body. From the ciliary processes, the aqueous flows through the pupil into the anterior chamber and from there through the trabecular meshwork into a sinus, the canal of Schlemm. From this structure, it drains into the aqueous veins and into the general circulation. There is a continuous dynamic production and drainage of aqueous which supplies the metabolic needs of the lens and cornea. Pathologically high pressure, such as glaucoma, is usually due to reduced outflow of aqueous and causes damage to the retina.

The lens

The lens is a transparent, biconvex structure situated behind the iris and in front of the vitreous. It is flexible and kept in position by suspensory ligaments attached to the ciliary body. The convexity of its anterior surface is less than that of its posterior surface and it contributes to the refractive power of the eye. The lens consists of a capsule, an epithelial layer on its anterior surface and the lens fibres. The capsule is elastic and encloses the whole lens. The lens fibres constitute the main part of the lens. Epithelial cells change to become lens fibres throughout life. No cells are lost and therefore the centre of the lens becomes denser and less pliable over time. With age, the nucleus becomes dense and yellow; if it becomes opaque, it is known as a cataract.

When in its normal state, the lens is designed to focus light onto the retina. In order to focus on a near object, the lens must become more powerful. Contraction of the ciliary muscle moves the ciliary body forwards. This relieves pressure on the fibres of the zonule and allows the lens to relax and become more spherical. At the same time, the sphincter pupillae contracts, allowing light to enter through the thickest part of the lens. Light from a near source is therefore enabled to focus on the retina. This is known as accommodation and the amount of accommodative power possible reduces as the lens becomes less flexible with age, resulting in the need for 'reading glasses' in middle age.

Retina

The retina is the nervous coat of the eye and the internal layer of the globe. It is a thin, transparent membrane, continuous with the optic nerve and extending to the ora serrata behind the choroid. The retina consists of a pigmented layer next to the choroid which absorbs light and releases vitamin A, which is necessary for the functioning of the photoreceptors. The neural retina consists of photoreceptors and then a number of layers of nerve cells which serve to amplify and transmit the impulses from the photoreceptors to the optic nerve and from there to the brain.

Two types of photoreceptor are present within the retina: 'rods', which allow vision in dim light and in black and white; and 'cones', which are adapted to bright light and can resolve fine detail and colour. Rods are absent at the fovea and rise rapidly in numbers towards the periphery of the retina. Cones are most dense at the fovea and reduce in number towards the periphery. Light impinges on the photoreceptors, producing a chemical reaction which results in an electrical impulse. This is amplified by the various nerve cells and synapses in the neural retina and transmitted through the nerve fibre layer to the optic nerve.

Vitreous

The vitreous body fills the posterior segment of the eye. It is a clear, jelly-like substance consisting of a collagen framework with hyaluronic acid. Collagen fibrils attach the vitreous to the retina at the ora serrata and the optic disc. Its function is to transmit light and to contribute slightly to the resolving power of the eye. It supports the posterior surface of the lens and assists in holding the neural part of the retina in place against its pigment layer.

ASSESSING OPHTHALMIC CONDITIONS

History

Establishing the exact history of a patient's condition is fundamental to making an accurate diagnosis. The history of the presenting problem should include:

- How long the patient has had symptoms for and whether they are getting worse
- Rapidity and mode of onset (see Box 30.1: determining the mechanism of injury)
- Degree, type and location of pain
- Is vision reduced and to what degree?
- Has the patient had this, or a similar problem before?
- Are there any concurrent systemic problems?
- Is the patient photophobic?
- Is there any discharge or watering?
- Does the patient wear glasses/contact lenses?

Discussion of systemic problems and medication is important as it can point to possible ophthalmic problems. For example, there is a link between ankylosing spondylitis and uveitis, and a link between rheumatoid arthritis and dry eyes, and there are many ophthalmic side-effects of systemic drugs. The assessing nurse needs to investigate any pre-existing ophthalmic or other medical conditions. Of particular importance are conditions such as glaucoma, iritis and blepharitis; systemic conditions such as diabetes and rheumatoid arthritis; and any drug therapy, as all of these may affect the health of the eye.

Visual acuity

Assessment of visual acuity should be undertaken at initial assessment for any ophthalmic patient, before

---

any other investigations or treatment, except irrigation or instillation of topical anaesthetic. The patient's affected or poorer seeing eye should be tested first, and the other occluded with a card or the patient's hand. Any distance glasses should be worn. He should be asked to read down from the top of the Snellen chart, making an attempt at all possible letters. Visual acuity should be recorded as:

Distance at which the eye is being tested (usually 6 m)/
    Last line read by the patient

The number for this line is indicated on the Snellen chart, just above or just below the letters. If part of a line only is read, this may be recorded as the line above plus the extra letters, or the line below minus the missed letters. For example, if the patient reads the '12' line except for one letter, at 6 m, it should be recorded as 6/12 − 1.

If the patient's vision appears poor (less than 6/9), a pinhole (a small hole in a card or a commercial pinhole) can be held in front of the eye to negate the effects of any refractive error. The visual acuity should be recorded with and without pinholes and a note should be taken of whether distance glasses or contact lenses are worn. If the patient is unable to read the top letter, the distance should be reduced until the patient can see the top letter on the chart, i.e. 5/60, 4/60, etc. to 1/60. If the patient cannot see the top letter at 1 m, it should be ascertained whether he can count fingers (CF), see hand movements (HM) or just perceive light (PL) at 1 m. Lack of light perception is recorded as NPL. Normal visual acuity is 6/6, but normal visual acuity *for the patient* may be less for a variety of reasons.

Problems in accurate visual acuity assessment may occur if the patient does not speak English or is not able to read. Strategies to overcome this may include:

- using a recognition chart so that the patient may match letters or shapes
- obtaining the services of an interpreter or family member to translate for the patient
- with children, using picture tests such as the Kay picture test and making the procedure into a game – this will usually encourage greater cooperation.

Patients who are in pain should have a drop of topical anaesthetic instilled so that any corneal pain is alleviated and the patient can cooperate more fully with the procedure, thus achieving an accurate visual acuity. Patients sometimes feel that this is a test that they have to pass and 'cheat' by looking through their

---

> **Box 30.1   Determining mechanism of injury**
>
> - Chemical involvement – identify type of chemical substance.
> - Force of injury and size of projectile
> - Possibility of penetration – may be small and high speed
> - What first aid has taken place?

fingers etc. It should be explained that the nurse is attempting to obtain an accurate assessment of their vision and that it is important that they are not tempted to make it seem better than it really is.

Examining the eye

Eye examination must be systematic. It is very easy to assume a diagnosis from the history and, in that way, miss less obvious problems. The eye should be examined from the 'outside' – the eye position and surrounding structures – working 'in' to consider the globe itself. Considerations for a thorough eye examination are given in Box 30.2.

Remember to compare the findings with the normal eye. What appears to be an abnormality may be bilateral and normal for the patient.

Equipment to aid assessment

An adequate eye assessment can be performed with minimal equipment. A bright light source, such as a pen torch or adjustable light, is essential for examination of the eye. Ophthalmoscopes are useful for retinal examination, but not for general examination as they only produce a small spot of light. Magnification is a useful aid, particularly in the hunt for foreign bodies. A hand-held magnifier, head loupe or ring light can be used. Cotton buds are used to evert the eyelids, remove foreign bodies and during irrigation.

Fluorescein drops or strips which stain damaged epithelial tissue are useful in examining abrasions. The stain is inserted and then the eye is viewed through a cobalt blue filter, as a penlight attachment, slit lamp or ophthalmoscope filter. While slit lamps (a binocular microscope for eye examination) offer the optimum provision for examination, they are expensive and not vital to initial assessment. Topical anaesthetic, such as tetracaine 1% or oxybuprocaine 0.4%, should be available in single-dose applications for pain relief and to facilitate examination. Proxymetacaine stings less on initial application and may be preferable, especially in children (Andrew 2006).

Contact lenses

If the patient is wearing contact lenses, the lens should be removed from the injured eye, or from both eyes if inflammation or swelling is present. If possible, the patient should remove his own lens; each contact lens wearer develops his own way of doing it.

Box 30.2   Systematic eye examination

The eyes
- Are they in their normal position for the patient?
- Is there any enophthalmos/exophthalmos?
- Is movement normal?

The lids
- Position – look for entropion (lid turning inwards) and ectropion (lid turning outwards)
- Integrity – look for lacerations
- Lash line – is it intact; are there any ingrowing lashes/crusting/infestation?
- Swelling – the whole or part of the lid/pointing onto the lid margin/one or both lids

Conjunctiva
- Intenrity – look for lacerations
- Structure – is it smooth or are there follicles or papillae?
- Other features – conjunctival cysts, pterygia, pingueculae
- Inflammation – is it generalized or local?
- Subconjunctival haemorrhages
- Discharge – type

- Fornices (both lower and subtarsal area) – concretions or foreign bodies

Cornea
- Integrity – lacerations, abrasions, ulcers
- Clarity
- Foreign bodies

Anterior chamber
- Depth (the distance between the curved cornea and the iris) – generally equal in both eyes
- Contents, e.g. red blood cells – inflammation is difficult to see without a slit lamp

Iris
- Colour – may be dull if there is inflammation in the anterior chamber
- Integrity – iris changes may occur in both blunt and penetrating trauma
- Position – a deviated pupil may indicate a perforated eye
- Size and shape – smaller or larger than the fellow eye; round or oval?
- Reaction – to light and to near objects

Removal of lenses

To remove hard lenses, the nurse should stretch the skin of the eyelid by pulling gently in a lateral direction from the outside corner of the patient's eye. Once the skin is stretched, the nurse should push the upper and lower lids together using a finger from each hand. This movement catches the edges of the lens and breaks its suction to the cornea. Once this happens, the lens will fall out (see Fig. 30.4). Alternatively, the nurse could put a (washed) index finger on the lens and gently move away from the cornea. The lids can then be used to lever the edge of the lens away from the cornea, and as the adhesion to the cornea breaks, the lens can be gently removed (Stollery et al. 2005).

Hard lenses can also be removed using a specifically designed suction cup. The cup should be soaked in saline and then gently pressed against the contact lens. This forms a stronger suction than that of the lens to the cornea. The lens can then be lifted away from the eye. Other suction extractors must be squeezed before applying to the lens. The lens should be put into a labelled container with normal saline. If any significant corneal infection is present, such as an ulcer or abscess, the lens must be kept for microbiological culture.

Removal of soft lenses is demonstrated in Fig. 30.5.

Triage decisions

Similar to other illness and injury, ophthalmic conditions vary considerably in severity and urgency. Using the Manchester Triage Group guidelines (Mackway-Jones et al. 2005) eye complaints can be prioritized as follows:

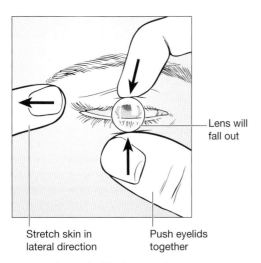

Figure 30.4 Removal of hard contact lenses.

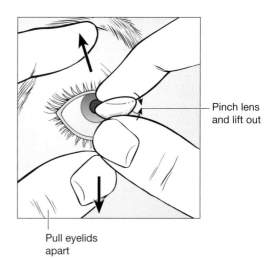

Figure 30.5 Removal of soft contact lenses.

- Priority one (red) – acute chemical eye injury; failure to act to dilute or neutralize chemical agents results in increased tissue damage and can lead to vascular damage and ischaemia and is therefore sight-threatening.
- Priority two (orange) – severe pain, penetrating eye injury or acute complete loss of vision. These presentations have the potential to be sight-threatening or result in further damage if not treated promptly.
- Priority three (yellow) – moderate pain, reduced visual acuity or unclear/inappropriate history.
- Priority four (green) – recent mild pain, red eye, foreign body sensation diplopia recent problem/injury.
- Priority five (blue) – chronic complaint without acute exacerbation.

OCULAR BURNS

Ocular burns may be divided most commonly into chemical, thermal and radiation (UV) burns.

Chemical burns

These are the most urgent category of ocular burns and causes may include alkalis, acids or solvents. Alkali burns are caused by substances such as sodium or potassium hydroxide, used as cleaning agents; calcium hydroxide, found in plaster and mortar; and ammonia, which is found in fertilizer and used in liquid form. Alkalis rapidly penetrate corneal tissue, combining with lipids in cell membranes, which results in cell disruption and tissue softening. A rapid rise in the pH in the anterior chamber may damage intraocular structures, and damage to vascular channels leads to ischaemia. Acids are less penetrating, and most damage is done during and soon after exposure. Acid substances combine with tissue, forming barriers against deeper penetration and localizing damage to the point of contact, although they can still be devastating. Acid burns are often due to car battery (sulphuric) acid or more complex organic and inorganic compounds. Solvent burns, although very painful, usually cause only transient irritation and damage. Thermal and/or contusion injuries due to the temperature or pressure of the chemical may be superimposed on the chemical injury (Marsden 1999a).

Primary management

A prompt and effective response to a chemical injury is vital to minimize tissue damage. One of the main determinants of ultimate outcome is duration of contact (Waggoner 1997), and as Glenn (1995) suggested, the initial treatment given by the nurse in the case of chemical eye injury may have more impact on the final vision than any subsequent care by the ophthalmologist.

Irrigation   The initial treatment involves copious irrigation to dilute the chemical and remove particulate matter. Irrigation should commence immediately, using whatever source is available. Herr et al. (1991) found no difference in the efficacy of irrigation fluids and therefore, in the ED, the irrigating fluid of choice is normal saline (0.9%) administered via a giving set to provide a directable and controllable jet. Sterile water is also used. The eyelids should be held open and contact lenses removed. A drop of topical anaesthetic should be instilled prior to irrigation to assist in patient compliance and minimize pain. All aspects of the cornea and conjunctiva (exposed by everting the upper lid) should be thoroughly irrigated. All particulate matter should be removed, by wiping with a cotton-tipped applicator if necessary.

Any delay in irrigation adds to the contact time and increases the risk of more severe injury. It is best to assume that any previous irrigation is inadequate and carry out adequate irrigation when the patient presents, unless a significant time has elapsed (hours) between injury and presentation. Specific irrigation time and fluid volume depend on the nature of the chemical and its physical state as well as the patient's condition. Waggoner (1997) suggested that it is impossible to over-irrigate a chemically injured eye and recommended irrigation for 15–30 minutes and one to two litres of saline is generally sufficient.

The use of pH paper to check for adequate irrigation may be debated. In alkaline injury in particular, the chemical leaches out of the eye for a number of hours after injury, thus altering the pH. Delay in therapy of a number of hours until the pH is back to normal will delay healing. It is useful though if used before irrigation to determine the type of chemical involved and again later to check any progress in returning to a normal pH (7.4 is the normal pH of the conjunctival sac) (Forrester et al. 1996). It must be remembered that a chemical may have a neutral pH and still cause injury. Ultimately, indicator paper is no substitute for adequate irrigation. Following irrigation, the patient's visual acuity should be checked.

Ophthalmic management

All but the most trivial chemical injuries should be referred to an ophthalmologist. The eye may look deceptively normal due to tissue blanching and ischaemia, which needs urgent assessment and treatment.
Ophthalmic management usually includes:

- mydriatics, which are used to dilate the pupil, reduce pain due to ciliary spasm and prevent adhesions between the iris and the lens (posterior synechiae)
- topical antibiotics – prophylactic use prevents secondary infection
- topical steroids to reduce and control inflammation
- admission to hospital may be required.

Solvent injury

This may be seen after staining with fluorescein as punctate stains on the cornea. They may be treated with a mydriatic drop to dilate the pupil and chloramphenicol ointment to prevent secondary bacterial infection and aid comfort. They usually resolve very quickly.

Thermal burns

These usually involve damage to the lids and are often associated with facial burns. Treatment is similar to that of thermal burns elsewhere on the body. Thermal burns range from very mild corneal injury which may be treated as an abrasion, with dilatation of the pupil and chloramphenicol ointment, to devastating injury such as that caused by molten metal which may require reconstruction of the globe and surrounding structures. Thermal burns involving the lids should be referred due to the possibility of aberrant healing, leading to lid closure and mobility problems (see also Ch. 10).

Radiation burns

These are likely to be caused by ultraviolet light in the form of sun lamps or from welding equipment. The symptoms are similar, ranging from mild discomfort to severe pain, photophobia and lacrimation. The condition is usually bilateral and symptoms are delayed by 6–10 hours. Topical anaesthetic drops may be used to facilitate examination but should not be given to the patient to use at home. Treatment may include dilatation of the pupil and topical chloramphenicol ointment. The most affected eye may be double padded. The condition resolves spontaneously within 24–36 hours.

Patients who have been using a MIG welder may need a fundal check if there is any residual loss of visual acuity after epithelial healing. The intensity of the light produced by this type of equipment may cause retinal burns (Marsden 1999b).

PENETRATING TRAUMA

Penetrating injuries and intraocular foreign bodies may cause eye damage by:

- disruption of the ocular tissues at the time of injury
- introduction of infection
- scar tissue formation (corneal, disrupting vision, retinal detachment caused by contracting scars inside the eye)
- reaction of the eye to foreign bodies – from organic material introducing infection or inflammation and from the deposition of pigments caused by degrading metal foreign bodies.

Large penetrating eye injuries are very obvious, but small perforations may be easily missed. The eye may look intact if the perforation is small and the wound may be sealed by iris tissue. It is very important, therefore, that a systematic eye examination is carried out and the particular circumstances of the incident are ascertained (Marsden 1996). Corneal perforations always leave a full-thickness scar, even if it is very small. Scleral perforations may be masked by overlying subconjunctival haemorrhage.

The use of Seidel's test may help to identify a full-thickness laceration. This involves instilling a drop of fluorescein into the eye and watching for dilution of it from escaping aqueous. The cobalt blue filter will identify dark tracks in the bright fluorescence, from escaping aqueous.

Patients with penetrating trauma should be referred urgently to an ophthalmologist. Wounds with retained foreign bodies should be protected with a rigid shield such as a cartella shield or a gallipot. Retained foreign objects should not be removed from the eye. In the case of other penetrating injuries, the eye should be covered with a single pad, so no pressure is applied to the eye, and a cartella shield if possible. The patient should be cared for lying flat or sitting at around 30 degrees in order to reduce the possibility of further injury or loss of ocular contents. After consultation with the ophthalmologist, a single drop of unpreserved antibiotic drop (a chloramphenicol minim) instilled in the eye may be useful. Preserved drops or ointments should not be used as both are toxic to intraocular tissues. There should never be an occasion when both eyes are covered. This can lead to extreme distress and disorientation.

LID TRAUMA

The eyelids must be intact, in the correct position and without any disruption to their structure and function in order that the eyes are protected effectively. Repair of lid trauma may be a planned activity rather than an emergency procedure due to the good vascularization of the lids and associated structures. Lid trauma, unless very superficial, should be referred to ophthalmologists, who are best able to achieve the necessary functional and cosmetic results for the patient.

MAJOR CLOSED TRAUMA

A direct blow to the eye from a blunt missile such as a clenched fist, squash ball or champagne cork may produce one or a combination of the following:

- ecchymosis (or black eye)
- hyphaema
- dislocation of the lens
- iridodialysis
- traumatic mydriasis or miosis
- traumatic uveitis
- traumatic angle recession
- posterior segment problems such as retinal oedema (commotio retinae), choroidal rupture and retinal detachment.
- blow-out fracture of the orbital floor or nasal wall
- orbital apex trauma and optic nerve injury
- retrobulbar haemorrhage.

Patients with reduced vision following blunt trauma should be referred to an ophthalmologist.

It is important to recognize the possibility of ocular involvement after indirect trauma such as base of skull fractures, as well as from more direct trauma where the eyes themselves do not appear to be involved. Any apparent loss or reduction of vision after trauma should be taken very seriously and the patient should be referred to an ophthalmologist urgently in order to reduce preventable vision loss.

Ecchymosis

Ecchymosis is more commonly known as a 'black eye'. It results from a blow to the orbit which leads to bruising and oedema of the eyelids. In itself, it is a relatively minor injury, treated with ice packs to relieve swelling. The force needed to cause this sort of injury may cause contusion or concussion injuries to any or all of the structures within the eye, as well as orbital rim or floor fractures. It is important, therefore, that the eye and surrounding structures are assessed carefully. The patient may be able to assist in opening the lids enough for the clinician to be able to assess the eye.

Hyphaema

Traumatic hyphaema may only be detectable with a slit lamp, when red blood cells may be seen floating in the anterior chamber, or alternatively it may be visible with the naked eye, when blood may fill the whole of the anterior chamber. The signs and symptoms of hyphaema are:

- history of trauma
- reduced visual acuity
- reddish haze present diffusely through the anterior chamber, a settled layer of blood inferiorly or complete filling of the anterior chamber
- pain – due to raised intraocular pressure and other eye injury
- pupil irregular or poorly reactive
- drowsiness – particularly in children.

Admission may be necessary in the treatment of hyphaema in children, and in the treatment of large hyphaema with raised intraocular pressure in adults, but generally patients are advised to rest at home. Daily intraocular pressure monitoring by an ophthalmologist is usual, and treatment with agents such as acetazolamide, glycerol or mannitol may be indicated if the intraocular pressure is raised.

Patients who need to be transported to an ophthalmic unit should be transported sitting upright to allow the blood cells to settle and the visual axis to clear as pigment from haemolysed red blood cells may permanently stain the corneal endothelium and reduce vision.

Luxation or subluxation of the lens

A patient with a total dislocation of the lens or a partial dislocation (subluxation) can also present to ED. It may be the result of trauma, hereditary, or associated with certain syndromes, such as Marfan's syndrome (Stollery et al. 2005). Vision will be disturbed, but the degree of visual disturbance will depend on the degree of dislocation; if 25% or more of the zonules of the lens are ruptured, the lens is no longer held securely behind the iris. The signs and symptoms of luxation or subluxation of the lens are:

- deepening of the anterior chamber due to tilting of the lens posteriorly – the anterior chamber may be shallow if the lens moves anteriorly
- pupil block – this may occur if the lens occludes the pupil
- a tremulous iris (iridodonesis).

The patient should be referred to an ophthalmologist. In general, if no complications occur, dislocated lenses are best left untreated. If complications do occur, such as raised intraocular pressure, these are treated before lens extraction is attempted, as surgery in these instances is difficult.

Iridodialysis

This is the disinsertion of the iris base from the ciliary body and it is often associated with hyphaema. No immediate treatment is undertaken. Whether or not surgical intervention is undertaken depends on the effect of iridodialysis on visual acuity after a suitable recovery period.

Traumatic mydriasis or miosis

This may be present after blunt trauma. Additionally, the pupil may react only minimally to light, or not at all, and may have an irregular shape. This deformity is indicative of complete or partial rupture of the iris sphincter. It may be permanent or transient.

Traumatic uveitis

A mild inflammatory reaction of the iris and/or ciliary body is frequently seen after blunt trauma. The patient complains of aching in the eye and cells, and flare may be seen in the anterior chamber. Treatment is as for any uveitis, i.e. dilatation and topical steroids by an ophthalmologist.

Angle recession

Angle recession refers to a separation or posterior displacement of the tissues at the anterior chamber angle at the site of the trabecular meshwork. At least 20% of patients with a hyphaema have some degree of angle recession and are followed up, as secondary glaucoma may eventually follow damage to the trabecular meshwork.

Cataract

A cataract is an opacity of the lens of the eye. It prevents light entering the lens properly and causes dimness of vision. When the structure of the lens is altered, e.g. as a result of a blunt (contusion) injury from a squash ball, aqueous enters the lens substance, causing it to swell and become cloudy. Contusion cataracts may occur as an immediate or long-term consequence of blunt trauma.

Posterior segment problems

A number of posterior segment problems may result from blunt trauma. Their common feature from the patient's perspective is a reduction in visual acuity which may be relatively temporary, usually a matter of weeks, or permanent. It is not possible to give the patient an accurate prognosis for vision initially as this may take some time and early referral to the ophthalmologist is important.

Orbital fractures

The orbits are each composed of seven bones, the thinnest of which are the lamina papyracea over the ethmoid sinuses, along the medial wall, and the maxillary bone on the orbital floor.

Medial orbital fractures

The lacrimal secretory structures, especially the naso-lacrimal duct, may be damaged and the medial rectus muscle may be trapped within fractures of the medial wall of the orbit.

Orbital floor fractures

These are often referred to as 'blow-out fractures' and are produced by transmission of forces through the bones and soft tissues of the orbit by an object such as a ball or fist. Fractures may be complicated by fat and muscle entrapment which limit ocular motility, causing double vision. They are often found by plain X-rays, but CT scans are used to investigate them further. Symptoms resolve without surgery in almost 85% of patients, as oedematous tissues usually settle, freeing muscles and allowing correct motility (Egging 1998). Signs and symptoms of orbital floor fracture include:

- diplopia
- enophthalmos
- surgical emphysema
- infraorbital anaesthesia

Orbital fractures are not considered an ocular emergency unless visual involvement or globe injury is present. Discharge instructions should include cautions about Valsalva's manoeuvres, such as straining at stool and nose blowing. Antibiotics should be prescribed to prevent orbital cellulitis as air from sinuses contaminates orbital tissue.

Orbital apex trauma and optic nerve injury

Orbital apex fractures may result from both direct, non-penetrating trauma or from penetrating trauma such as large foreign bodies A number of syndromes have been defined to describe different presentations which depend on the degree of injury to vascular and neural structures within the orbital apex.

Optic nerve injury may occur, often due to traumatic optic neuropathy from indirect trauma (such as fractures of the base of the skull). The nerve may be compressed by haematoma, damaged by foreign body or fracture, resulting in anything from minor trauma to the nerve to transection. Injury to the cranial nerves present in the orbit will present as double vision in injury to the III, IV and VI nerves and as sensory disturbance to the areas supplied by the trigeminal nerve (V). Visual acuity should be checked repeatedly in this group of patients and any reduction should prompt immediate referral to an ophthalmologist (Marsden 2006).

Retrobulbar haemorrhage

This may occur from direct or indirect trauma to the orbit and progress rapidly, resulting in pain, proptosis of the globe, lid and conjunctival swelling and congested conjunctival vessels with sub-conjunctival haemorrhage. An ophthalmologist should be involved immediately if the globe begins to proptose after trauma and CT or MRI scan may be required urgently. Visual acuity should be checked very frequently as reduction in acuity suggests compression of the optic nerve, and emergency decompression of the haemorrhage by lateral canthotomy (a horizontal incision at the lateral canthus, through skin and conjunctiva and then through the lateral canthal tendon, under topical anaesthetic) will be required to relieve this.

MINOR TRAUMA

The vast majority of eye injuries are relatively minor and involve the anterior segment only. It is important, however, to bear in mind the possibility of more major trauma and not to rule it out without a comprehensive examination. If it is assumed that the eye injury is likely to be trivial, sight-threatening injuries may easily be missed. The degree of pain following eye trauma is not a good indication of the severity of the injury. Corneal abrasions can be extremely painful, whereas a sight-threatening perforating injury may be virtually painless.

Traumatic subconjunctival haemorrhage

This is common after a variety of injuries and is, in itself, relatively minor. Fluorescein should be used to rule out a conjunctival laceration. The condition is self-limiting and does not require treatment. A traumatic subconjunctival haemorrhage which extends backwards so that the posterior border is not visible may be an indication of significant orbital trauma and may warrant further investigation if the history and other signs and symptoms are indicative of this. The patient should be reassured that the haemorrhage will resolve, usually over a period of weeks.

Corneal abrasion

Corneal abrasions are very common as the corneal epithelium is easily damaged. The damage to the cornea exposes superficial corneal nerves, causing tearing, eyelid spasms and pain. The degree of pain may be considerable and visual acuity is likely to be reduced. Providing the deeper layers of the cornea are not involved, there should be no visual impairment after the abrasion has healed. Topical anaesthetic may be needed in order to examine the eye effectively. The eye should be stained with fluorescein, and the extent of the abrasion documented.

Eye pain is difficult to control. The pain associated with a breach in the corneal epithelium has a component of ciliary muscle spasm which can be relieved, along with a degree of the patient's pain, by the use of a dilating drop such as cyclopentolate 1%. Topical non-steroidal anti-inflammatory (NSAI) drops provide a significant degree of effective pain relief for patients with corneal pain and are usually prescribed four times daily (Brahma et al. 1996, Fechner & Teichmann 1998, Rhee & Pyfer 1999).

Any breach in the corneal epithelium places the eye at risk of infection. A prophylactic antibiotic is necessary and chloramphenicol is usually the antibiotic of choice. Short courses of topical chloramphenicol do not appear to cause systemic side-effects (Besamusca & Basteinsen 1986, Gardiner 1991, Consumer's Association 1997) and it is considered to be a very safe drug, widely used throughout ophthalmology in the UK. In the treatment of corneal abrasions, this is often prescribed in ointment form, as this provides a lubricant layer over the eye, which enables the lid to slide over the damaged epithelium, and is therefore much more comfortable for the patient. As the antibiotic is for prophylaxis rather than treatment of infection and the ointment base is for comfort, there

is no need to prescribe a 'course' of antibiotics. When the abrasion is healed, the patient will know as the pain will have resolved. At that point, the antibiotic treatment may be stopped. Corneal abrasions generally heal within 48–72 hours. Abrasions which appear slow to heal or involve loose epithelium should be referred to an ophthalmologist.

In some instances, the cornea is at particular risk of infection, slow healing or recurrent abrasion. This is particularly the case in human, animal or vegetable material scratches. It is important, therefore, that the patient uses the antibiotic ointment at night for a period of 3–4 weeks to prevent this occurring. Follow-up visits are not usually necessary unless the abrasion is particularly large, involves the deeper layers of the cornea or the patient is a child.

Conjunctival abrasion and foreign body

Foreign bodies do not often penetrate the conjunctiva and are therefore easily wiped off using a moistened cotton bud after instillation of topical anaesthetic. The resulting (and any concurrent) abrasion may be treated with antibiotic ointment. A pad is not usually necessary and the degree of pain experienced is much less than with corneal trauma.

Subtarsal foreign body

In this case, the patient often presents with a foreign-body sensation and a history of something falling or blowing into the eye. Management involves everting the upper lid using a moistened cotton-tipped swab. Any foreign material trapped underneath the lid may be wiped off with the swab. The eye should then be stained with fluorescein to rule out any corneal abrasion. If corneal abrasions are present, they are often linear, superficial and quite characteristic of this type of injury. If the corneal injury is minimal, a stat dose instillation of antibiotic ointment is usually sufficient. If larger abrasions are present, they should be treated as corneal abrasions.

Corneal foreign body

These commonly occur from grinding wheels and other industrial machines, from DIY and even wind-borne materials. The patient may present with a foreign-body sensation, especially when opening or closing the eye. Superficial foreign bodies are often easily removed with a moistened cotton bud after instillation of topical anaesthetic. Dry cotton buds should not be used as they can stick to the corneal epithelium, which is moist, and this may result in a large abrasion, complicating the injury.

Impacted corneal foreign bodies need to be removed using the edge of a hypodermic needle (most commonly 21 g) held tangentially to the cornea with the hand supported on the patient's cheek or nose. The needle may be mounted on a cotton bud or syringe for easier manipulation. After the initial removal of the foreign body, a rust ring often remains which must be removed completely. This is easier after 24–48 hours of treatment with antibiotic ointment and referral to an ophthalmic unit is recommended

Removal of corneal foreign body with a needle is a procedure which must be carried out with extreme care. It is quite possible to penetrate the cornea with a needle and corneal scarring will result if the deeper layers of the cornea are damaged. This can cause visual problems if it involves the visual axis. It is therefore important that if the ED possesses a slit lamp, it is utilized for the removal of corneal foreign bodies so that both a high degree of magnification and support for the patient's head are possible. ED staff may feel most comfortable removing only peripheral foreign bodies and referring on central ones. If in any doubt, the patient should be referred to an ophthalmic unit.

After removal of the foreign body, treatment is as for a corneal abrasion. Many patients have repeat visits for removal of corneal foreign bodies and treat them as something of an occupational hazard, although opportunities should still be taken to reinforce the need for adequate eye protection as it is most unlikely that one foreign body would penetrate the eye while another stayed on the cornea. X-ray examination is only indicated if there is a definite history of a high-speed foreign body hitting the eye, such as a hammer and chisel, and no foreign body can be found.

EYEPADS

There is no evidence that padding the eye enhances healing; however, for many patients, padding can make the eye much more comfortable. The decision to pad the eye of a patient with a corneal abrasion should therefore be accompanied by the advice that if the pad makes the eye more comfortable, it can be left in place, without disturbance for 24 hours and then removed and antibiotic treatment commenced. If the pad makes the eye less comfortable, it may be removed and antibiotic ointment commenced immediately. In this way, those patients who can be helped by padding, are, and others are not made worse by the indiscriminate application of eyepads (Marsden 2006).

A single pad will not keep the eye closed and further damage to the cornea may be caused by the surface of the pad. If padding is required, the following method should be used:

Fold one pad in half and place over the closed eyelids after instilling the necessary medication. Place the second pad, flat, over the first and secure with two or three pieces of tape (see Fig. 30.6). It is unnecessary to pad an eye merely because topical anaesthetic has been used. Anaesthetic drops last for only around 20–30 minutes and the risk of the patient sustaining any further injury because of the topical anaesthetic drop is minimal (Cheng et al. 1997)

The ED nurse should not pad the eye of a patient who is driving home. If the patient leaves the eyepad

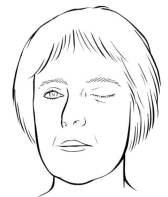

Eye closed after instillation of antibiotic ointment

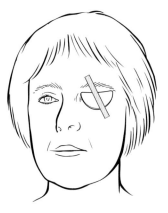

Single folded pad over the closed lid and taped down – ensures the patient cannot open his eye under the pad

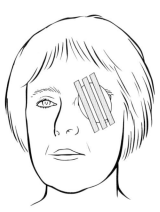

Second pad – open (unfolded) over the first and taped firmly to the face

Figure 30.6   Use of eye pads.

on and drives anyway, he is breaking the law, invalidating his insurance and is a danger to other road users. A drop of topical anaesthetic will facilitate driving home safely and the patient may then pad the eye at home.

EYEDROPS

Topical anaesthetic drops are a very valuable tool for examination purposes. They 'magically' remove all the patient's pain and he may be very keen to have some to take home so that this pain-free state may continue. Unfortunately, topical anaesthetic drops also inhibit epithelial healing. The patient will be pain-free, but the epithelial defect will not heal (Andrew 2006).

Topical non-steroidal anti-inflammatory drugs (NSAIDs) have been evaluated for use in corneal pain (Brahma et al. 1996) and found to be extremely useful. Their use does not appear to delay healing and no adverse effects have been found. A number of NSAIDs are available in eye drop form, including diclofenac sodium, flurbiprofen sodium and ketorolac trometamol.

Mydriatic and cycloplegic drops, such as cyclopentolate, dilate the pupil and paralyse accommodation. The patient's near vision is therefore blurred for a period. This does not mean that the patient should not drive. If he feels safe to do so, there is nothing to stop him driving, as the legal standard for driving only includes distance vision and distance vision is not affected by dilatation. Near vision, which is affected, is not used to any great extent for driving. However, he should be warned that, if it is a bright day, he may be quite dazzled by sunlight and should wear sunglasses and take extreme care.

Steroid drops should not be prescribed in the ED as the effects of steroids on the eye in a misdiagnosed condition can be catastrophic.

RED EYE

Ophthalmic trauma is fairly easy to recognize with the aid of a history and a brief eye examination. However, ophthalmic medical problems are, on the whole, less easily diagnosed and therefore may be dealt with less well than other problems. The differential diagnosis of the red eye (Marsden 2006) is shown in Table 30.1.

Subconjunctival haemorrhage

Patients may present with a spontaneous subconjunctival haemorrhage. The patient may not have noticed any irritation and is often prompted to attend by others noticing the haemorrhage, which presents as a deep red patch of blood under the conjunctiva. It may be quite small and circumscribed or may be severe enough for the conjunctiva to protrude like a 'bag of blood'. Providing there is no history of trauma, no treatment is needed except reassurance. Patients with clotting disorders or those on anticoagulants may be prone to repeat episodes. Subconjunctival

Table 30.1 Differential diagnosis of the red eye

	Conjunctivitis	Uveitis	Glaucoma	Corneal ulcers
Lids	? Swollen follicles, papillae if allergic	Normal	Normal	May be swollen
Conjunctiva	Injected	Injected	Injected	Injected
Cornea	? Punctate staining	Normal, bright reaction	Very hazy	Opacity/stains with fluorescein
Anterior chamber	Deep	Deep	Shallow or flat	Deep
Iris	Normal	May look muddy	May be difficult to see	Normal
Pupil	Normal	Slight miosis (compared with fellow) sluggish	Fixed, oval, semi-dilated	Usually normal, may be slightly sluggish
Pain	Gritty	Deep pain in eye	Severe pain in and around eye and head	Gritty
Discharge	Pus/watery /sticky in morning	May water	No	May water
Photophobia	If severe	Yes	No	Not usually
Systemically	? Flu-like symptoms (URTI)	Well	Nausea, vomiting, severe abdominal pain, dehydration	Well

haemorrhages will take up to 3 weeks to resolve and the blood may spread under the conjunctiva and actually appear worse before it begins to resolve.

Blepharitis

This chronic eyelid condition is very common. The patient is likely to present with gritty, sore eyes and red-rimmed eyelids with crusting, which may be mild to very severe, along the lid margin – the lash line. Treatment involves regular lid cleaning, using a cotton bud dipped in a solution of baby shampoo and water to 'scrub' the lid margin along the lash line to remove all the crusts. When the condition is acute, antibiotic ointment should be rubbed into the lid margin after lid hygiene two to four times a day. As this is a chronic condition, lid cleaning should continue even after the symptoms have resolved, or the condition will recur. Occasionally, punctate staining may occur at the corneoscleral junction. This is marginal keratitis, an inflammatory change. The patient should be referred to an ophthalmologist.

Conjunctivitis

Inflammation of the conjunctiva is by far the most common cause of red eyes. Bacterial conjunctivitis in adults is uncommon (Tullo & Donnelly 1995) and most conjunctivitis in adults is viral. Conjunctivitis in children is more likely to be bacterial.

Bacterial conjunctivitis

The patient is likely to present with a red, irritable eye, describing the sensation as 'gritty' rather than painful. Discharge is likely to be purulent and profuse, and the lashes may be coated with it. There will be no corneal staining with fluorescein. Treatment is usually with a broad-spectrum antibiotic such as chloramphenicol or fucidic acid, applied topically in the form of drops. Drops are often prescribed quite frequently during the first 48 hours; for example, in the case of chloramphenicol drops, 2-hourly application would not be unreasonable.

Health education information, particularly on how to control the spread of infection, should be given and the nurse must ensure that the patient understands how to use his medication before leaving the department. Information on how to keep the lids clean and free from discharge may be needed, e.g. using cooled, boiled water and cotton wool or tissues, especially by parents of small children who may also need extra help instilling the prescribed medication effectively. Patient education should also, where appropriate, incorporate discussion of cross-contamination through eye make-up, pillows and towels (Egging 1998).

Viral conjunctivitis

Viruses, often types of adenovirus, are by far the most common cause of conjunctivitis in adults. Once again, the patient is likely to complain of a gritty sensation, but the discharge is much less likely to be purulent than profuse watering, with stickiness often only in the morning when the watery discharge has dried and the lids are stuck together. If the lid is everted, the conjunctiva covering it will appear very bumpy rather than smooth. These 'bumps' are follicles and are inflamed lymphoid tissue. This roughness of the conjunctiva is what makes the eye feel so gritty and irritable. The patient with viral conjunctivitis often complains of dryness, along with a watery eye. The tears, although profuse, are inadequate in quality and dry up very quickly; the eye responds to the irritation and dryness by producing more. There may be punctate erosions on the cornea when stained with fluorescein.

Some types of adenovirus, of which there are about 30, cause upper respiratory tract infection and this, when combined with an eye infection, is known as pharyngoconjunctival fever. The patient may feel generally unwell with flu-like symptoms and the preauricular lymph node may be enlarged. Treatment of viral conjunctivitis is based on controlling the symptoms. Unless the eye is particularly sticky, antibiotics are not indicated. Artificial tears may help to control the feeling of dryness and irritation and these may be used very frequently, e.g. every 30 minutes. A bland ointment such as simple eye ointment may also be helpful. Cold compresses on the lids may ease the irritation of this very distressing condition The patient should be aware that viral conjunctivitis may persist for 3–6 weeks and the symptoms of dryness may last much longer.

Adenoviral conjunctivitis is a condition with symptoms out of all proportion to its relative clinical importance. Once the symptoms have peaked, however, the patient may be said to be no longer an infection risk. Adenovirus is highly infectious and infection control is of paramount importance, both for the patient and for the department. Hand washing is the first line of defence in infection control and is vital to stop the spread of viral conjunctivitis. Swabs to identify specific organisms are not required. Results do not change treatment and the swab is both painful and costly.

Chlamydial conjunctivitis

A patient presenting with a unicoular, chronic conjunctivitis causing only mild symptoms may have a chlamydial infection. A swab should be taken for culture and chlamydial identification and the patient referred to genito-urinary medicine if the swab proves positive.

Allergic conjunctivitis

Allergic conjunctivits is very common and presents acutely in two distinct ways. Firstly, the patient may have red eyes with itching and watering and an appearance of large bumps (papillae) on the subtarsal conjunctiva. This presentation is particularly common during spring and summer – the 'hay fever' season – and may also be associated with a runny nose, sneezing etc. Treatment is with systemic antihistamines and/or topical antihistamine treatment such as emadastine. Topical mast cell stabilizing drops such as sodium cromoglicate are of little value in an acute exacerbation but may be useful if used throughout the whole of the 'hay fever' season by patients who are aware that they are likely to develop allergic conjunctivitis.

The second allergic presentation is an acute and frightening atopic reaction which involves massive swelling of the conjunctiva (chemosis) which the patient often describes as 'jelly' on the eye. This is usually due to the patient rubbing the eye with an allergen present on the hand or finger, and common allergens include some plant juices and cat hairs, although it is unlikely that the particular allergen will be identified. This condition is completely self-limiting and requires no treatment unless the chemosis is severe and protruding from the closed lids. In this case, lubricant drops may be helpful to prevent drying. Adequate reassurance is needed and, if the reaction is severe, the patient may need to be monitored for systemic effects of the allergen.

Anterior uveitis (also known as uveitis, iridocyclitis, iritis)

Uveitis is an inflammatory condition of part or all of the uveal tract (iris, ciliary body and choroid) which may be associated with systemic disease such as ankylosing spondylitis but which is often idiopathic. It may also occur secondary to trauma. The most common presentation is anterior uveitis (inflammation of iris and ciliary body, also commonly known as iritis). Common presenting symptoms are photophobia, pain due to iris and ciliary spasm, conjunctival redness (injection), which may be more marked around the corneoscleral junction (limbus), and decreased visual acuity. The reduction in vision is due to protein and white blood cells (part of the inflammatory response) in the anterior chamber. The pupil, because of spasm and inflammation, is likely to be small (miosed)

compared with the unaffected eye and may react sluggishly. There will be a clear reflection of light when a light is shone onto the cornea, demonstrating the lack of corneal involvement, and there will be no staining with fluorescein. Prompt referral to an ophthalmologist is required and treatment is with topical corticosteroids, and mydriatics to dilate the pupil to reduce inflammation and prevent adhesions of the iris and lens.

Acute glaucoma

In acute glaucoma, the outflow of aqueous in the eye is obstructed by the peripheral iris covering the trabecular meshwork. The pressure inside the eye increases rapidly as aqueous continues to be produced, resulting in the sudden onset of severe pain, due to the increased intraocular pressure, and blurred vision due to corneal oedema. Haloes may be seen around lights. The pain is not likely to be localized in the eye, but may involve the whole head and may be accompanied by nausea, vomiting and abdominal pain. Patients are usually elderly and are likely to be hypermetropic (long-sighted). On examination, the patient's eye will be red and the reflection of light from the cornea will be very diffuse, demonstrating that the cornea is oedematous. The pupil is likely to be semi-dilated, oval and fixed.

Acute glaucoma is an ophthalmic emergency and the patient should be referred to an ophthalmologist urgently, including emergency ambulance transportation if necessary. Prolonged raised ocular pressure at this level will cause permanent loss of vision, which may be severe and will occur quickly. Treatment involves the use of carbonic anhydrase inhibitors, such as acetazolamide intravenously, constriction of the pupil once the pressure has reduced and, eventually, laser treatment when the pressure is back to normal. In the ED, analgesia and antiemetics may be required. Occasionally, patients present having coped with these symptoms for some time and may be dehydrated due to prolonged vomiting, and rehydration may therefore be necessary. A great deal of explanation, reassurance and care are needed by these ill and often terrified patients.

Corneal ulcers

There are three main types of corneal ulcer which are likely to be seen in the ED. All should be referred to an ophthalmic unit because differentiation between the different types of corneal ulcer is sometimes difficult and the treatment is completely different.

Bacterial ulcers occur as 'fluffy' white demarcated areas on the cornea which stain with fluorescein. They are caused by a number of organisms, some of which, e.g. *Pseudomonas*, are very difficult to treat. All need a number of investigations to be carried out, such as Gram stain and culture, which will be done in the ophthalmic unit without delay. Patients may be treated with frequent antibiotic drops on either an outpatient or, if the infection is severe, an in-patient basis. Delay in treatment of infected corneal ulcers can result in devastating intraocular infection.

Marginal ulcers appear as ulcerated areas which stain with fluorescein and are usually close to the limbus. They are part of a hypersensitivity response by the eye to staphylococcal exotoxins and are usually treated with steroid eye drops by an ophthalmologist.

Viral ulcers caused by herpes simplex virus are known as 'dendritic' ulcers because of their branching, tree-like shape when stained with fluorescein. They are treated with acyclovir eye ointment, again only by an ophthalmologist.

HEALTH PROMOTION

Many patients with ophthalmic conditions are only seen for a short period in ED, before either discharge or referral, and there is therefore limited time to advise patients. It is important, however, that patients leave the department with a basic knowledge of their condition, in order to understand the importance of drug treatment and follow-up requirements and instruction on correct eyedrop instillation and side-effects of any drug therapy. Patients with newly diagnosed conditions should also be aware of recurring symptoms which should prompt them to seek early treatment.

Many activities in the home and workplace cause eye injuries, due to equipment, materials, chemicals and radiation. Patients with such injuries should be encouraged to wear eye protection or to check that any equipment already in use is of a suitable standard. All eye protection should conform to British Standard BS 2092 requirements. Children, in particular, are vulnerable to eye injuries. Parents need sympathetic health education to minimize the risks of sight-damaging injury (Kutsche 1994).

CONCLUSION

While ocular emergencies do not present a threat to the patient's life, sight is precious and the ED nurse can have a critical impact on a patient's vision. Once lost, vision cannot be replaced, and therefore knowledge of the management of the most common ophthalmic conditions will assist the nurse in protecting sight and promoting health.

References

Andrew S (2006) Pharmacology. In: J Marsden, ed. *Ophthalmic Care*. Chichester: Wiley.

Besamusca F, Bastiensen L (1986) Blood dyscrasias and topically applied chloramphenicol in ophthalmology. *Documenta Ophthalmologica*, **64**, 87–95.

Brahma AK, Shah S, Hillier VF, McLeod D, Sabala T, Brown A, Marsden J (1996) Topical analgesia for superficial corneal injuries. *Journal of Accident and Emergency Medicine* **13**, 186–188.

Consumer's Association (1997) *Drugs and Therapeutics Bulletin*, **35**(7), 49–52.

Cheng H, Burdon MA, Buckley SA, Moorman C (1997) *Emergency Ophthalmology*. London: BMJ.

Edwards RS (1987) Ophthalmic emergencies in a district general hospital casualty department. *British Journal of Ophthalmology*, **71**, 938–942.

Egging D (1998) Ocular emergencies. In: Newberry L, ed. *Sheehy's Emergency Nursing: Principles and Practice*, 4th edn. St Louis: Mosby.

Fechner PU, Teichmann KD (1998) *Ocular Therapeutics*. New Jersey: Slack.

Forrester J, Dick A, McMenamin P, Lee W (1996) *The Eye: Basic Sciences in Practice*. London: WB Saunders.

Gardiner F (1991) Chloramphenicol: a dangerous drug? *Acta Haematologica*, **85**, 171–172.

Glenn S (1995) Care of patients with chemical eye injury. *Emergency Nurse*, **3**(3), 7–9.

Herr RD, White GL, Bernhisel K et al. (1991) Clinical comparisons of ocular irrigation fluids following chemical injury. *American Journal of Emergency Medicine*, **9**, 228–231.

Kutsche PJ (1994) Ocular trauma in children. *Journal of Ophthalmic Nursing and Technology*, **13**(3), 117–120.

Mackway-Jones K, Marsden J, Windle J (2005) *Emergency Triage*, 2nd edn. London: BMJ.

Marsden J (1996) Ophthalmic trauma in accident and emergency. *Accident and Emergency Nursing*, **4**(1), 54–58.

Marsden J (1999a) Ocular burns. *Emergency Nurse*, **6**(10), 20–24.

Marsden J (1999b) Painless loss of vision. *Emergency Nurse*, **6**(9), 13–18.

Marsden J (2006) The care of patients presenting with acute problems. In: Marsden J, ed. *Ophthalmic Care*. Chichester: Wiley.

Rhee DJ, Pyfer MF eds (1999) *The Wills Eye Manual*, 3rd edn. Philadelphia: Lippincott, Williams and Wilkins.

Stollery R, Shaw M, Lee A (2005) *Ophthalmic Nursing*, 3rd edn. Oxford: Blackwell Science.

Tan MMS, Driscoll PA, Marsden JE (1997) Management of eye emergencies in the accident and emergency department by senior house officers: a national survey. *Journal of Accident and Emergency Medicine*, **14**, 157–158.

Tullo AB, Donnelly D (1995) Conjunctiva. In: Perry JP, Tullo AB, eds. *Care of the Ophthalmic Patient*, 2nd edn. London: Chapman and Hall.

Waggoner MD (1997) Chemical injuries of the eye: current concepts in pathophysiology and therapy. *Survey of Ophthalmology*, **41**(4), 275–313.

Chapter **31**

Ear, nose and throat emergencies

Tim Kilner

INTRODUCTION

Ear, nose or throat (ENT) conditions presenting at the emergency department (ED) are often trivialized, even though some can subsequently become life-threatening. For those patients who attend the ED with an ENT disorder, the onset of symptoms is likely to be acute, but the nurse should be alert to the fact that the current episode may also be a feature of a chronic condition. It is also important to be alert to the danger of viewing the patient only in terms of the presenting symptoms.

It is often the case that such conditions are accompanied by systemic illness precipitated by local infection. Equally important is the fact that the individual may have psychological, social and emotional needs as well as the presenting pathophysiological needs. This may be obvious in the case of an individual who has hearing loss as a direct result of being in close proximity to the seat of an explosion, but may be less apparent in the individual whose hearing loss results from wax impaction, but who is concerned that she may be becoming permanently deaf.

This chapter broadly examines ENT conditions in terms of infection, trauma and foreign bodies. The nursing care of patients is discussed in relation to presenting conditions.

THE EAR

The attendance at the ED department of a patient with an ear-related problem is usually precipitated by one or more of the following symptoms:

- pain
- discharge from the ear
- hearing loss
- foreign bodies in the ear canal
- direct trauma to the external structure of the ear.

Anatomy of the ear

The ear is divided into three sections: external, middle and inner ear (see Fig. 31.1). The outer ear funnels sound into the middle ear, which serves to transmit the sound to the auditory apparatus of the inner ear. The external ear consists of the aurical (or pinna), ear canal and tympanic membrane. The S-shaped ear canal is approximately 2.5–3.0 cm long and terminates at the tympanic membrane. The canal is lined with glands that secrete cerumen, a yellow waxy material that lubricates and protects the ear. Ear wax, sloughed off skin cells and dust may impair sound transmission through the outer ear, especially if a plug of wax attaches to the eardrum. The bone behind and below the ear canal is the mastoid part of the temporal bone. The lowest portion of this, the mastoid process, is palpable behind the lobule (Bickley & Szilagyi 2003).

The tympanic membrane (or eardrum) is a thin, translucent, pearly grey oval disc separating the external ear from the middle ear. It can easily be observed with an otoscope. The tympanic membrane vibrates and moves in and out in response to sound. The middle ear is an air-filled cavity containing three tiny bones, the ossicles, which are individually called the malleus (hammer), the incus (anvil) and the stapes (stirrup), so named because of their appearance. The malleus is attached to the tympanic membrane by a set of ligaments. The incus is attached to the malleus and they move as one. The stapes attaches to the oval window, the membrane separating the middle and inner ear. When the tympanic membrane vibrates in response to sound, the malleus and incus are displaced, and the stapes vibrates against the oval window continuing the transmission of sound. The pharyngotympanic tube, formerly known as the Eustachian tube, which connects the middle ear with the nasopharynx, allows the passage of air to equalize pressure on either side of the tympanic membrane. The inner ear is composed of several fluid-filled chambers encased in a bony labyrinth in the temporal bone. The semicircular canals are also important for balance.

Presentation to ED may be prompted by a single symptom, such as hearing loss resulting from wax impaction. The patient may alternatively have multiple symptoms, resulting from, for example, an ear infection where pain, discharge and hearing loss may be present in combination with systemic illness.

Infections of the ear

Acute otitis externa

The external auditory meatus is a canal-shaped structure which extends from the external opening of the ear to the tympanic membrane. The integrity of the canal is protected from pathogens by its lining. The lateral one-third is composed of skin which is a continuation from the concha, which is the depression in the centre of the shell-shaped external structure of the ear – the pinna. The lining continues as an epithelial layer, protecting not only the medial two-thirds of

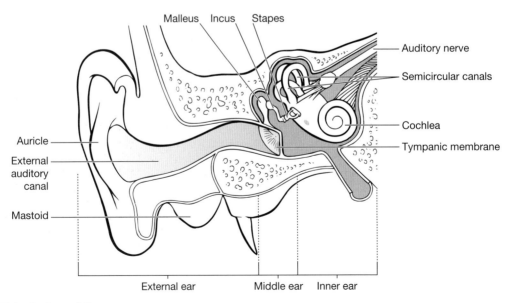

Figure 31.1   Anatomy of the ear.

the external auditory meatus but also the tympanic membrane.

The protective lining of the external auditory meatus may be easily breached by direct trauma, although pre-existing dermatological conditions, typically eczema and psoriasis, as well as external mediators such as maceration by water, may influence the resilience of the lining (Ludman 1997).

Clinical evidence and management   Acute otitis externa is essentially a localized or diffuse infection of the lining of the external auditory meatus commonly associated with organisms such as *Pseudomonas aeruginosa, Staphylococcus epidermides, Staphylococcus aureus* and *Streptococcus pyogenes* (van Balen et al. 2003). Acute otitis externa frequently occurs following bathing or swimming when the external auditory meatus is cleaned out using the corner of a dirty towel. For this reason it is often referred to as 'swimmer's ear'. Infection may be diffuse within the external auditory meatus or it may be focal in the form of a local swelling known as a furuncle, which may be extremely painful. Taking swabs for microbiological studies may not be well tolerated by the patient. It is essential that careful preparation of the patient takes place before any attempt is made to take a swab, especially if the individual is a child. Attempts to take a swab from an uncooperative child should be avoided as there is a risk that the tympanic membrane may be perforated by the swab if the child moves her/his head.

As the external auditory meatus contains no mucus-secreting cells, discharge from the ear is minimal; however, any discharge which does occur is usually thick and foul-smelling infected wax. The canal may also contain cell debris, which is unlikely to cause hearing loss, but may contribute to the intense irritation the individual may experience.

Treatment is based upon cleaning and drying the external auditory meatus. This should only be done after examination of the ear canal to determine the integrity of the tympanic membrane. Following cleansing of the external auditory meatus, topical medication containing steroids may be instilled. The type of medication is dependent upon the infecting organism, i.e. fungal or bacterial infection.

Acute otitis externa largely results from identifiable causes and therefore lends itself to prevention strategies. The focus of much of the nursing care may revolve around prevention of future exposure by identifying high-risk behaviour and educating those individuals in ways of reducing the risks, such as keeping the ear clear of any water. O'Donoghue et al. (1992) suggested that certain occupational groups may be exposed to the risk of acute otitis externa. Typically these are individuals who work in occupations where they are required to wear inserts in their ears, such as telephonists and workers using internal ear defenders, as well as healthcare workers sharing a communal stethoscope.

Although these individuals are at risk, the likelihood of subsequent infection may be reduced through careful history-taking and appropriate health education regarding aural hygiene and cleansing of equipment. Single-operator use should also be advocated, thus reducing the risks of the individual infecting others and re-infecting themselves. Patients should be provided with the advice and support necessary for them to instil any prescribed medication.

Acute otitis media
An acute infection of the middle ear, that is, medial to the tympanic membrane, may cause pain, a feeling of pressure, or fullness, in the ear and hearing loss, the symptoms being caused by infective material splinting the tympanic membrane. Discharge from the external ear may be present, but in order for this to occur, the tympanic membrane must have been damaged, usually as a result of the increased pressure causing perforation.

Clinical evidence and management   Acute otitis media is often associated with systemic illness and pyrexia (Ludman 1997), which may be attributed to the otitis media alone or occur in conjunction with coincidental upper respiratory tract infection. Acute otitis media is characterized by rapid onset of ear pain, headache, tinnitus, hearing loss, and nausea or vomiting. Infants and young children may present with irritability, crying, rubbing or pulling the ear, restless sleep and lethargy (Olson 2003). Children are often prone to acute otitis, with up to 30% of those presenting with otitis media being children under three years of age (O'Neill 1999), as the infection frequently results from upper respiratory tract infection of bacterial or viral origin (Strome et al. 1992).

Uncomplicated otitis media may be treated with systemic antibiotics, supported by analgesia with antipyretic properties, although the benefits of early antibiotic therapy are questionable. Little and colleagues (2001) suggest that in most cases involving children antibiotics only provide symptomatic benefits after the first 24 hours, at which time symptoms are generally resolving. Serious complications, such as meningitis, mastoiditis, intracranial abscess, permanent hearing loss and neck abscess can develop as a result of otitis media (Olson 2003).

If the tympanic membrane has perforated, it is often the painful result of otitis media, trauma or foreign body insertion and is associated with loss of hearing. The individual should be advised to keep the ear dry and prevent water entering the ear. However, the ear should not be packed, and the patient should be advised not to do this at home, as it may prevent the discharge draining from the ear. More than 90% of tympanic membrane perforations heal spontaneously and management includes antibiotics, analgesia, and antipyretics (Olson 2003). In some cases, where the tympanic membrane is intact, the infective material may cause the membrane to bulge, which also causes pain and loss of hearing. In such cases, admission to hospital is required in order that the tympanic membrane may be surgically perforated under general anaesthetic and grommets inserted to allow the discharge to drain out freely.

Mechanical obstruction

Impacted wax

The lateral one-third of the external auditory meatus contains cells which secrete a waxy substance called cerumen, the purpose of which is to act as a defence against dust and other foreign material entering the external auditory meatus.

Clinical evidence and management Cerumen may build up in the external auditory meatus, causing mechanical obstruction, which may be exacerbated by cleaning the ear with cotton-tipped buds. Such activities often cause cerumen to be pushed deep into the canal, causing impaction against the tympanic membrane. Obstruction in either case may cause a reduction in hearing, but rarely causes complete deafness. Impacted cerumen is often hard and resistant to removal by syringing alone; thus, in the ED the most appropriate management is to initiate a regime to soften the cerumen using commercially available ear drops.

Patient education involves self-administration with advice to contact their GP in 2–3 weeks to arrange for ear syringing. Ear syringing is rarely indicated in the ED department. Poor technique and failure to take adequate precautions may cause the patient serious harm; it is therefore imperative that ear syringing is carried out by a nurse who is suitably trained in the technique.

Foreign bodies

Clinical evidence

Older children and adults may present with a history of having a foreign body in the ear. Young children have a tendency to put foreign bodies in their ears, but as they often do not disclose this information,

the nurse should be suspicious of children who present with earache, hearing loss and discharge from the ear. Small insects may also crawl into the ear canal and become trapped, causing a great deal of discomfort if still alive and buzzing.

Management

Foreign bodies may be removed using a variety of techniques, by individuals with the appropriate skills (Davies & Benger 2000). Care should be taken to ensure that this process does not impact the foreign body further in the ear, causing trauma to the external auditory meatus and the tympanic membrane. If the object is not retrieved at the first attempt, the patient should be referred to the ENT department.

If the tympanic membrane is intact and the foreign body is not vegetable in nature, then syringing the external auditory meatus with warm water may flush the foreign body out. However, this should only be carried out by those skilled in the technique. If the foreign body is vegetable matter, this technique should be avoided as it is likely to cause the foreign body to swell and impact in the external auditory meatus.

Where insects have entered the external auditory meatus causing the patient severe distress, Barkin & Rosen (1994) suggest that the insects should be killed in situ by the instillation of alcohol or 2% lidocaine into the external auditory meatus, prior to removal. For patients whose personal convictions dictate that no harm befalls the insect, the use of penlight may attract a live insect out of the ear canal. Analgesic and/or antibiotic treatments should be prescribed as necessary. Safe removal of a foreign body from the external auditory meatus requires a skilled operator and a cooperative patient, which is not always possible to achieve in the ED department. If in any doubt, the patient should be referred to the ENT department.

Perforation of the tympanic membrane

Perforation of the tympanic membrane may be caused by two main mechanisms – either direct or indirect trauma. In both cases the symptoms are much the same, i.e. hearing loss, pain and possibly bleeding from the external auditory meatus.

Direct trauma

This is commonly caused by the insertion of objects either to clean the ear or to relieve itching, although any object inserted into the external auditory meatus has the potential to cause tympanic perforation. Objects frequently used are cotton-tipped buds and hair grips. In most cases, the ruptured tympanic membrane will heal spontaneously in 1–3 months (Strome et al. 1992); however, ENT opinion should be sought. Pain relief and prophylactic antibiotics may be required, especially if the mechanism of injury includes contamination by water or a foreign body.

This provides the ED nurse with a health education opportunity in terms of prevention of subsequent episodes particularly in relation to aural hygiene. The importance of keeping the ear dry at all times must be stressed. A protective cotton plug coated with petroleum jelly will enable the patient to shower safely; however, swimming and generally getting the ears wet should be avoided.

Indirect trauma

Perforation of the tympanic membrane may be caused by high pressure transmitted along the external auditory meatus to the tympanic membrane. This barotrauma to the tympanic membrane results from significant changes in atmospheric pressure causing air trapped in the external ear canal or behind the tympanic membrane to expand or contract enough to rupture the eardrum. This pressure may be generated by such forces as a slap to the ear, flying, diving or exposure to an explosion. Pressures of as little as 15 kPa on the tympanic membrane may cause it to rupture (Mellor 1997), although in the explosion scenario some individuals will be protected from these pressures because of the orientation of the external auditory meatus to the blast wave (Maynard et al. 1989). As it is unlikely that data will be available regarding blast wave pressure, all individuals who have been in close proximity to an explosion should be carefully assessed and referred to the ENT department if appropriate.

Although tympanic membrane rupture may be seen in isolation from other injuries following an explosion, the nurse should be aware of other injuries which may have occurred, such as lung and gastrointestinal injury, which may be covert in nature. The nurse should also be aware of the emotional and psychological crisis the patient will be experiencing, not only from the incident itself, be it explosion or assault, but also from anxieties about the permanency of hearing loss and the problems associated with communication. As perforation of the tympanic membrane may be caused by a slap to the ear, such injuries in children may be resultant of a non-accidental injury.

External trauma

Wounds to the external ear or pinna in most cases may be closed by conventional wound closure methods. However, if the cartilage of the pinna is involved, scrupulous wound cleansing is required, as any

subsequent infection is likely to lead to permanent deformity of the pinna (Wardrope & Smith 1992). Blunt trauma to the pinna, commonly occurring in contact sports, may result in haematoma formation. The haematoma, if untreated, may lead to the necrosis of the underlying cartilaginous skeleton of the pinna. O'Donoghue et al. (1992) advocate early incision and drainage as the most appropriate course of action in order to reduce morbidity. This is likely to require a general anaesthetic, and therefore referral to the ENT department is pertinent.

There is an increasing trend of cosmetic piercings of the upper one third of the pinna which puncture the cartilage. Hanif and colleagues (2001) report how infections following such piercings can result in auricular perichondritis.

THE NOSE

Anatomy and physiology

The nose is a structure with a bony and cartilaginous skeleton which is attached to the skull via the frontal bone and the maxilla. It is a vascular structure whose prime functions are to interface with the respiratory system, to warm, filter and moisten inhaled air and to act as a sense organ involved in the enjoyment of food and the detection of danger in the case of smoke and gas (O'Donoghue et al. 1992). The upper third of the nose, where the frontal and maxillary bones form the bridge, is bony (see Fig. 31.2).

Foreign bodies

A foreign body in the nose usually occurs in children and they often will be accompanied by parents who are distressed and anxious about their child's well-being.

Clinical evidence and management

Usually the child will have told the parents that she/he has put something up her/his nose, or the parents will have noticed that the child has a purulent discharge from one nostril. Unilateral discharge is highly suggestive of a foreign body in the nose; however, children are not averse to placing foreign bodies in each nostril, resulting in a bilateral discharge.

The removal of a foreign body in the nose follows the same rules as the removal of a foreign body in the ear. The child should be seated in a dental chair or on a parent's lap in a semi-recumbent position. Initial assessment and history should ascertain the type of foreign body present, how long it has been in the nostril and whether there has been any bleeding or discharge. Careful explanation and instruction regarding the procedure for removal are required and psychological

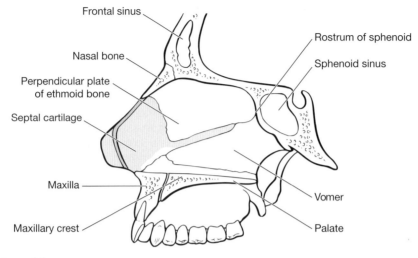

Figure 31.2 Anatomy of the nose.

support for both parents and child is essential both for humanitarian reasons and to gain their cooperation during the procedure. Removal can be attempted using some topical anaesthetic spray, a ring curette or alligator forceps (Olson 2003). Care should be taken to prevent damage to the highly vascular nasal septum and mucosa during removal of a nasal foreign body. If the child is too distressed, the foreign body is too far into the nostril or there is any evidence of trauma to the nostril already, then the child should be referred to the ENT surgeon (Reynolds 2004).

Epistaxis

Epistaxis is often seen as a relatively minor problem in the ED department. However, something as simple as a nose bleed can quickly turn into a life-threatening condition if it is not treated swiftly and correctly (Moulds 1992). Most nose bleeds come from ruptured blood vessels on the nasal septum. Epistaxis can commonly occur in (Budassi-Sheehy 1990):

- children
- adults, usually aged 50–80 years, with hypertension
- patients with blood dyscrasias
- patients on anticoagulant/aspirin treatment
- patients with alcoholism
- patients with allergies
- patients with recent nasal trauma – often following an assault.

Clinical evidence and management

The patient will present with active bleeding from the nose, or a recent history of bleeding which may have

stopped. The leading cause of epistaxis is nose picking, otherwise known as digital manipulation or 'epistaxis digitorum' (Joyce 1991). The main aim of treatment is to stop the epistaxis. If the bleeding is from the anterior end of the septum – Littles' area – bleeding can usually be alleviated by seating the patient upright and advising her to hold the front soft part of the nose very firmly (Reynolds 2004). The patient's head should be tilted forward over a bowl.

This compression must be applied for at least 30–40 minutes without interruption (Walsh & Kent 2000). The use of ice can be helpful for its vasconstricting action; however, toleration may be a problem for children and the elderly. The patient should be encouraged to expectorate blood rather than swallow it, as this can lead to vomiting, which makes measurement of blood loss difficult. Haematemesis is also very anxiety-provoking for the patient.

If the bleeding is from the posterior part of the nose, indicated by continuous bleeding after compression or as seen on examination, the patient may need to have the nose packed or the area cauterized. In this case, the patient is usually referred to the ENT surgeon. If it is to be done in the ED department, a spray of cocaine solution (2.5–10%), a good head light and mirror, silver nitrate sticks and nasal packing are needed.

If the patient is hypertensive on presentation an antihypertensive, such as nifedipine, may need to be administered.

Occasionally, the patient with an epistaxis may need resuscitative care due to blood loss. The siting of a large-bore intravenous line and commencement of replacement fluid, monitoring of vital signs, and taking of blood for a full blood count and cross-match are necessary in this case (Bird 1999). All patients with epistaxis have the potential to become shocked if bleeding is not stopped. Initial assessment involves an estimate of the amount of bleeding, the length of time active bleeding has been taking place and any previous relevant medical history. Physical assessment of the patient should always include monitoring of vital signs.

Nasal fracture

This is the most common facial fracture, usually caused by blunt trauma and commonly seen in the ED patient who has been assaulted (Walsh & Kent 2000). Clinically, the injury can usually be recognized immediately afterwards by the distortion from normal shape, although this soon becomes obscured by soft tissue swelling (Ludman 1997).

Clinical evidence and management

There will be a history of trauma to the nose, swelling deformity and occasionally epistaxis. It is important to examine the nose for any evidence of cerebrospinal fluid (CSF), rhinorrhoea and any indication of fractures to the cribiform plate. Normal CSF is clear and slightly yellow, but CSF nasal drainage is frequently mixed with blood. Gisness (2003) describes septal haematoma as a bulging, tense bluish mass that feels doughy when palpated. Septal haematomas should be urgently drained to prevent airway obstruction and necrosis of the septal cartilage. Paige & Barlett (2000) state that untreated septal haematoma causes a permanent nasal deformity known as a saddle deformity.

Generally, little can be done for patients following a fracture of the nose until 5–10 days after the initial injury, due to soft tissue swelling. The patient should therefore be referred to the ENT outpatients department. Since the nasal bones will become firmly set within 3 weeks of the injury, the need for treatment should be assessed after a week, and, if necessary, reduction under general anaesthetic will be planned for the following week. X-rays are often requested for medicolegal reasons, but are not strictly necessary (see also Chapter 9).

Rhinorrhoea

Otherwise known as a 'runny nose', this is caused by excess mucus being produced by an inflamed nasal mucosa.

Clinical evidence and management

The patient presents with a runny nose or the sensation of something dripping down the back of the throat. The discharge may be clear or purulent (O'Donoghue et al. 1992). The causes are:

- allergy
- infection
- foreign body
- underlying tumour.

The patient may need to have a foreign body removed. If an allergy is suspected, antihistamines may be prescribed, and advice should be given on avoidance of common allergens, i.e. grass/tree pollen, dust and cat or dog fur. The patient may also need to be referred to an allergy clinic. Infective rhinosinusitus may need treatment with antibiotics. If a tumour is suspected, urgent referral to ENT will be necessary.

Advice, explanation and health education regarding the taking of antihistamines (whose main side-effect is drowsiness) and antibiotics should be given to the patient. If the rhinitis is viral in origin, antibiotics will have little or no effect, and they should therefore not be seen as a panacea for this, or any other, condition.

Allergic rhinitis

This can be seasonal or perennial. The symptoms are those of sneezing, nasal obstruction and rhinorrhoea. There is often itching of the nose, eyes and palate, accompanied by loss of smell, rhinorrhoea and episodes of sneezing. Secondary symptoms such as headache and facial pain may also occur due to nasal congestion (Stearn 2005). Evidence of associated allergic diseases, such as asthma and eczema, should also be sought as there is a high correlation between the conditions. Bousquet et al. (2001) note that some 80% of asthma patients also suffer from allergic rhinitis. Patients should be advised to avoid common allergens as much as possible, such as grass/tree pollen, cat or dog fur and house dust, especially in the early morning and later afternoon/early evening when pollen counts are at their highest. Wearing sunglasses, spectacles or contact lenses (if appropriate) may also be beneficial in reducing eye symptoms. Patients should be given antihistamines and advised to see their GP for further prescription of any topical decongestants and for referral to a local allergy clinic.

Sinusitis

Sinusitis is an inflammatory, and usually infective, condition of the paranasal sinus, which is associated with approximately 90% of viral infections of the upper respiratory tract. Complications of untreated or inadequately treated acute sinusitis include chronic sinusitis, orbital abscess, meningitis, brain abscess, cavernous sinus thrombosis and osteomyelitis of the maxillary or frontal bones (Olson 2003, Kumar 2004).

Clinical evidence and management

The main symptoms a patient can present to the ED are sneezing, headache and facial pain which are worse when bending forward, and a recent history of upper respiratory tract infection. Maxillary toothache without obvious dental cause may also occur. The patient may be very worried about her/his sinusitis headache. A set of baseline observations of pulse, blood pressure, temperature and respirations will aid diagnosis. This, along with a clinical history, may help to rule out other diagnoses such as hypertension or subarachnoid haemorrhage.

Treatment usually involves prescription of a broad-spectrum antibiotic. Advice can be given to take analgesia and to use a decongestant spray. The patient should be advised to see her/his GP if symptoms persist, as referral to the ENT department may be necessary. Complications of sinus disease include meningitis, orbital extension and brain abscess (Kumar 2004).

THE THROAT

Anatomy and physiology

The throat, or pharynx, consists of the nasopharynx, oropharynx and laryngopharynx. It is a funnel-shaped tube that starts at the internal nares (nasal passages) and extends to the level of the cricoid cartilage. Its wall is composed of skeletal muscles and lined with mucous membrane. The central portion (oropharynx) provides a common passage for air, drink and food (Bickley & Szilagyi 2003). Pharyngeal constrictor muscles propel food or liquid into the oesophagus. These muscles are also responsible for the gag reflex, which is controlled by the cranial nerves. The larynx helps to prevent aspiration, assists in coughing and serves as the organ for speech.

Airway obstruction

Many patients who attend the ED with either an apparently trivial throat condition or more severe conditions are potentially at risk of airway obstruction. Thus the potential for a life-threatening condition to be overlooked is ever-present, unless there is a high index of suspicion and a rigorous assessment of these patients takes place (see also Chapter 2).

Airway obstruction can be partial or complete and is dynamic in nature. In the case of oedema, where the airway may initially be partially obstructed, it can progress rapidly to complete obstruction as the oedema progresses. Relatively large foreign bodies inhaled into the airway may well rapidly obstruct it, while oedema of the airway in response to an allergic reaction may obstruct it in a more progressive manner.

Should the airway become compromised, by whatever means, patency must be achieved as a matter of urgency, in order for ventilation to occur. Airway management should initially be in the form of basic techniques, such as positioning the patient and the Heimlich manoeuvre where the obstruction is caused by a foreign body. The Heimlich manoeuvre is not recommended for infants because of poor protection of the upper abdominal organs (American Heart Association & International Liaison Committee on Resuscitation 2000).

Circumstances such as complete obstruction by an impacted foreign body or rapidly progressing oedema may dictate the early use of advanced techniques, such as endotracheal intubation, cricothyrotomy and surgical airway. Oxygen should be administered to all patients with actual and potential airway obstruction. Admission must be considered for observation of patients whose airway has been compromised and where deterioration is a possibility.

A number of events can compromise the airway. If these are dealt with effectively, complete obstruction can be prevented. These events will be discussed under the headings traumatic, infective and reactive.

Oral cavity

Trauma

Trauma to the oral cavity can cause a great deal of tissue swelling. Extensive bleeding can occur because of the vascular nature of the region, which is why lacerations to the tongue can bleed dramatically. Teeth can be dislodged or broken and inhalation can occur. Fracture of the mandible may also cause problems and these are dealt with in Chapter 9. Injuries to the oral cavity are common in young children (Zimmermann et al. 2006).

A visual assessment is vital in determining the extent of any injury. Suction may be required to enable visual assessment to take place. Blind suction should be avoided as this can exacerbate trauma and increase the likelihood of additional problems, such as vomiting. X-rays can be of benefit in suspected fractures or in locating lost teeth when inhalation is suspected. Where an assault has occurred, photographs may be of use for medicolegal purposes. Bleeding from tooth sockets can usually be arrested with haemostatic agents and slight pressure. Antibiotics may be prescribed prophylactically.

It is essential that anxiety is reduced by reassuring the patient at the time of initial assessment. In the case of children, injuries frequently appear worse than they really are, especially when bleeding is profuse, and parents require as much reassurance as the children. Not all lacerations in the mouth will require sutures. Small lacerations, particularly to the inside of the lip, will usually heal well without intervention, other than advice on oral hygiene and the use of medicated mouth washes. Similarly, lacerations of the tongue bleed profusely, but they too usually heal well. Sutures inside the oral cavity should be soluble so that removal is not required. Those patients with extensive lacerations in the oral cavity will require appropriate referral. External cold compresses may be helpful in reducing swelling.

Infective

Infections of the oral cavity most commonly involve the teeth and gums and referral to a dentist may be the most appropriate action.

Clinical evidence and management   Abscesses of the teeth may need drainage and/or antibiotic therapy, which is most appropriately carried out by a dental practitioner. Frequently the most appropriate course of action is to refer the patient to her/his GP, but in the interim the patient may be prescribed antibiotics and analgesia. Patient education may focus upon the safe and efficacious use of prescribed medication.

Reactive

Reactions occur as a result of exposure to foreign substances to which the body has developed an allergy, resulting in a local or systemic allergic reaction which in severe cases may manifest as anaphylactic shock.

Aetiology of anaphylactic shock   Anaphylaxis is a severe acute allergic reaction causing hypotension and collapse. It generally follows from exposure to a foreign protein to which the patient has been previously sensitized. The individual becomes sensitized to the allergen by the production of antibodies in response to this exposure. These bind to basophils in the blood and sensitize the cells. Common sensitizing substances are antibiotic medication, especially penicillin and pencillin derivatives, bee stings, foodstuffs such as peanuts and non-steroidal anti-inflammatory medications. When the allergen re-enters the body, this stimulates the release of mediators of anaphylaxis, e.g., histamine, serotonin, slow-release substances of anaphylaxis (SRS-A) and platelet-activating factors (PAF), which result in cellular damage.

Clinical evidence of anaphylactic shock

Physiological changes include:

- increased blood capillary permeability – causing localized oedema
- smooth muscle contraction (bronchioles)
- increased gastric secretion
- increased mucus secretion
- inhibited coagulation.

These changes may result in some or all of the following symptoms:

- wheezing
- urticaria
- pruritis
- stridor
- respiratory difficulty
- tachypnoea
- hypotension
- collapse.

Symptoms can occur within minutes of ingestion, with the allergen gaining rapid access to the circulatory system through the digestive tract and activating mast cells in the mouth, throat, lungs, skin, abdomen and other tissues and organs (Crusher 2004). Management is based on positioning of the patient in the supine position and the administration of adrenaline via the intramuscular route. This is supported with high-flow oxygen to combat potential hypoxia. Where adrenaline is administered, the patient should be admitted for a period of observation. If possible, the allergen should be identified to enable the patient to avoid this in the future.

Those patients with mild reactions and who are discharged home require advice on the safe and efficacious use of any prescribed medications, most likely antihistamine tablets. Specifically they should be warned of the sedative effects of this type of medication and thus the implications for driving and operating machinery while taking the medication. Subsequent exposure to an unidentified allergen may cause a more severe reaction which could be potentially fatal. It is crucial that these patients are offered advice on identifying the allergen which caused the reaction. This is perhaps best achieved by referral to their own GP who may arrange appropriate tests and support.

Pharynx

Swelling in this region is more likely to compromise the airway than in the oral cavity because of the smaller diameter of the lumen of the airway. This is highly significant in children, where as little as 1 mm of oedema may cause 75% occlusion of the airway.

Traumatic

Clinical evidence   External as well as internal trauma may cause oedema in this region. People who have attempted suicide by hanging or strangulation and those involved in accidents involving strictures around the neck account for a proportion of this group of patients. In cases of strangulation and hanging where the patient is unable to self-advocate, for whatever reason, consideration should be given to any medicolegal implications, and where appropriate the police may need to be informed. Victims of road traffic accidents may also suffer trauma to this region of the body which can be easily overlooked in the presence of more obvious injuries, highlighting the importance of thorough primary and secondary surveys. Where neck injuries are apparent, the possibility of trauma to the internal structures should be considered.

Inhalation injury due to hot gases and flames may be present in burn-injured patients. Signs of inhalation injury from hot substances are not always evident, but a useful sign to look for is singed nostril hairs. If the gas was hot enough to damage these hairs then airway damage should be expected. Similarly, the ingestion of corrosive substances may also cause burns and swelling to the pharynx area. Inhalation of small foreign bodies, such as fish bones, rarely causes airway obstruction, but they can be troublesome, causing irritation, increased salivation and coughing because they are lodged in the pharynx. Patients should be advised that fish bones can often scratch the side of the throat on the way down, leaving them with the feeling that the foreign body is still there.

Management   The airway is the number one priority. Careful and accurate assessment of the patient and the extent of injuries must be carried out early. If the patient is conscious, a history of the event and mechanism of injury will give an indication of the stresses involved. Signs of airway obstruction such as noisy breathing should be noted and monitored for deterioration. Admission is essential where there is a degree of swelling which is likely to increase, leading to the airway becoming compromised.

For patients with small foreign bodies in their pharynx, X-ray examination may be helpful and could reveal radio-opaque objects. A plain lateral soft-tissue X-ray of the neck can provide valuable information about tissue swelling.

Infective

Clinical evidence   There will be a number of patients attending the ED department with simple sore throats. They often only need reassurance and simple advice, possibly with referral to their GP if symptoms persist. There will be some adults among them with a peritonsillar abscess that will require further intervention. Children are less likely to complain of a sore throat but often go off their food and generally feel unwell and are pyrexial. These children may present with dysphagia, a wheeze or stridor and will need careful assessment. The possible cause of these symptoms is epiglottitis, which is a potentially fatal inflammation of the epiglottis and pharynx as a result of infection. McEwan et al. (2003) report an age range of presentation between 6 months and a little over 10 years.

Management   Peritonsillar abscesses in need of drainage will require the attention of the ENT team. The patient should be referred as soon as the diagnosis has been made. As a general anaesthetic may be required, the patient should be kept nil by mouth, and unnecessary examination of the throat should be avoided as this is likely to be very uncomfortable.

Children with epiglottitis will require urgent assessment and admission by the paediatric team. It is essential that the child is kept calm and is not distressed, that examination in ED is kept to a minimum, and that insertion of instruments, such as thermometers or tongue depressors, should not take place, as this may cause the epiglottis to be pushed onto the larynx, thus occluding the airway completely. Endotracheal intubation should only be carried out by those who are extremely experienced in these techniques. If the airway becomes occluded then patency should be ensured by means of cricothyrotomy.

CONCLUSION

This chapter has examined the care of the individual who attends the ED department with a condition relating to the ear, nose or throat. For practical purposes, care has been artificially described in terms of specific conditions, when in reality many of the identified conditions form only a part of a broader clinical picture. Care should encompass the psychological, emotional and social needs of patients and their families. What may be regarded as a minor condition to the ED nurse is often a terrifying experience for the affected individuals.

The key element in care with these individuals, as with all aspects of ED care, is communication. Patients who attend the emergency department with an acute ENT condition are often regarded as having a trivial condition, yet many of these conditions have the potential to become life-threatening. Patients who have traumatic injuries are rightly given high priority and are treated aggressively, yet the preventable causes of death in both groups of patients are the same, i.e. hypoxia and hypovolaemia – hypoxia resulting from a foreign body impacted in the airway, and hypovolaemia resulting from epistaxis. People die from acute ENT conditions and, in many instances, these deaths are preventable. The ED nurse has a critical role to play in reducing the number of these preventable deaths.

References

American Heart Association & International Liaison Committee on Resuscitation (2000) *Pediatric Basic Life Support*, **46**, 301–341.

Barkin RM, Rosen P (1994) *Emergency Paediatrics: A Guide to Ambulatory Care*, 4th edn. St Louis: Mosby.

Bickley LS, Szilagyi PG (2003) *Bates' Guide to Physical Examination and History Taking*. 8th edn. Philadelphia: Lippincott, Williams & Wilkins.

Bird D (1999) Managing epistaxis in A&E. *Emergency Nurse*, **7**(3), 10–13.

Bousquet J, van CauwenbergeP, Khaltaev N (2001) Allergic rhinitis and its impact on asthma. *The Journal of Allergy and Clinical Immunology*, **108**(5), s147–s333.

Budassi-Sheehy S (1990) *Mosby's Manual of Emergency Care*. St Louis: CV Mosby.

Crusher R (2004) *Anaphylaxis Emergency Nurse*, **12**(3), 24–31.

Davies P, Benger J (2000) Foreign bodies in the nose and ear: a review of techniques for removal in the emergency department. *Journal of Accident and Emergency Medicine*, **17**, 91–94.

Gisness C (2003) Maxillofacial trauma In: Newberry L, ed. *Sheehy's Emergency Nursing: Principles and Practice*, 5th edn. St Louis: Mosby.

Hanif J, Frosh A, Marnane C, Ghufoor K, Rivron R, Sandhu G (2001) High ear piercing and the raising incidence of perichondritis of the pinna. *British Medical Journal*, **322**, 906–907.

Joyce SM (1991) Epistaxis. In: Hamilton GC, Sanders AB, Strange GR, Trott AT, eds. *Emergency Medicine: An Approach to Clinical Problem Solving*. Philadelphia: WB Saunders.

Kumar S (2004) Ear, nose and throat. In: *Textbook of Emergency Medicine* (2nd edn) (eds P Cameron, G Jelinek, AM Kelly, L Murray, AFT Brown, J Heyworth). Edinburgh: Churchill Livingstone.

Little P, Gould C, Williamson I, Moore M, Warner G, Dunleavey J (2001) Pragmatic randomised controlled trial of two prescribing strategies for childhood acute otitis media. *British Medical Journal*, **322**, 336–342.

Ludman H (1997) *ABC of Otolaryngology*, 4th edn. London: BMJ.

Maynard RL, Cooper GJ, Scott R (1989) Mechanisms of injury in bomb blasts and explosions. In: Westaby S, ed. *Trauma Pathogenesis and Treatment*. Oxford: Heinemann Medical Books.

McEwan J, Giridaran W, Clarke R, Shears P (2003) Paediatric acute epiglottitis: not a disappearing entity. *International Journal of Pediatric Otorhinolaryngology*, **67**, 317–321.

Mellor S, Dodd K, Harmon J Cooper G (1997) Ballistics and other implications of blast. In: Ryan J, Rich N, Dale R, Morgans B, Cooper G (eds) *Ballistic Trauma: Clinical Relevance in Peace and War*. London: Arnold.

Moulds A (1992) Managing a nosebleed. *Practice Nurse*, **4**(18), 467–473.

O'Donoghue GM, Bates GJ, Narula AA (1992) *Clinical ENT: An Illustrated Textbook*. Oxford: Oxford University Press.

O'Neill P (1999) Clinical evidence: acute otitis media. *British Medical Journal*, **319**(7213), 833–835.

Olson C (2003) Dental, ear, nose and throat emergencies. In: Newberry L, ed. *Sheehy's Emergency Nursing: Principles and Practice*, 5th edn. St Louis: Mosby.

Paige K, Barlett S (2000) Facial trauma and plastic surgical emergencies. In: Fleischer O, Ludwig S, eds. *Textbook of Emergency Pediatric Medicine*. 4th edn. Philadelphia: Lippincott, Williams & Wilkins.

Reynolds T (2004) Ear, nose and throat problems in Accident and Emergency. *Nursing Standard*, **18**(26), 47–53.

Stearn R (2005) One airway, one disease. *Primary Health Care*, **15**(2), 31–34.

Strome M, Kelly JH, Fried MP (1992) *Manual of Otolaryngology Diagnosis and Therapy*, 2nd edn. Boston: Little, Brown.

van Balen F, Smit W, Zuithoff P, Verheij T (2003) Clinical efficacy of three common treatments in acute otitis externa in primary care: randomised controlled trial. *British Medical Journal*, **327**, 1201–1205.

Walsh M, Kent A (2000) *Accident & Emergency Nursing – A New Approach*, 4th edn. Oxford: Butterworth Heinemann Ltd.

Wardrope J, Smith JAR (1992) *The Management of Wounds and Burns*. Oxford: Oxford University Press.

Zimmermann CE, Troulis MJ, Kaban LB (2006) Pediatric facial fractures: recent advances in prevention, diagnosis and management. *International Journal of Oral Maxillofacial Surgery*, **35**(1), 2–13.

PART 7

Practice issues in emergency care

PART CONTENTS

Chapter 32

People with learning disabilities

Margaret Sowney & Michael Brown

INTRODUCTION

There is an increasing recognition of the need to respond to and meet the health needs of vulnerable groups within society. There are a range of people who may, for a variety of reasons, be vulnerable and this includes people with learning disabilities, children, people with mental health problems, people with acquired brain injury and those with dementia. Nurses who work in emergency care are often the first point of contact with healthcare services for patients and are in a good position to ensure that the needs of vulnerable patients are appropriately assessed and responded to in a person-centred way. In order to respond appropriately it is necessary for these nurses to have an appreciation and overview of the key health and care needs of vulnerable patients – this is important, as their needs are often different and distinct, requiring specific responses and actions.

PEOPLE WITH LEARNING DISABILITY IN SOCIETY

People with learning disabilities are an integral part of society and need to be recognized and valued as equal citizens. It is estimated that as a group they form almost 2% of the overall population across the United Kingdom, totalling some 1.5 million. It is further estimated that prevalence rates per thousand of the general population indicate that there will be 3 to 4 persons with severe learning disabilities and 25 to 30 with milder learning disabilities.

Across the world a range of definitions are used when referring to this population. The term learning disability has been adopted within the UK and refers to people with cognitive impairments that impact significantly upon their development. Other terms used across the world include developmental disability, mental handicap and mental retardation. Increasingly the term intellectual disability is being adopted; however, irrespective of the current terminology used it is generally agreed that the term learning disability relates to:

- a significantly reduced ability to understand new or complex information, to learn new skills
- a reduced ability to cope independently and
- which started before adulthood, with a lasting effect on development
  (Department of Health 2001a).

A learning disability is a disorder that covers a spectrum of the population and is frequently referred to as mild, moderate, severe or profound. The level of cognitive impairment increases with the severity of learning disability, thereby affecting a person's ability to understand new or complex information, learn and develop skills and use them independently. In order to be considered as a learning disability it is generally accepted that the disorder usually occurs on or around the time of birth and certainly before the age of 18.

There is a wide range of causes that result in the development of a learning disability. These can be conceptualized as occurring pre-natally, prior to birth peri-natally, during birth and post-natally following birth.

Pre-natal issues

Some of the causes of learning disability are preventable, highlighting the need for access to genetic counselling and effective nutrition, including vitamin supplements. For example, folic acid taken prior to and up to the 12th week of pregnancy is known to help prevent neural tube defects. The management of pre-existing health conditions such as diabetes is important.

Additionally there is a range of lifestyle issues such as smoking, alcohol and drug misuse that can have an impact and result in learning disability. Environmental risk factors include exposure during pregnancy to infections such as rubella (German Measles), cytomegalovirus and genitourinary infections such as syphilis.

Peri-natal issues

Peri-natally, at or around the time of birth, there are risk factors that can result in learning disability. There is increasing evidence that premature and low-birth-weight babies are at risk from developmental delay and that some will have a learning disability of a nature that will require ongoing additional support. Trauma during birth can occur and factors such as breach presentations and asphyxia can be causes. Therefore good maternal care is necessary along with access to health education.

Post-natal issues

Post-natally, good nutrition is necessary to support healthy growth and development. Social deprivation and abuse require preventive interventions to promote growth and development. There are also a number of infections that are common in childhood that carry a risk of brain damage, such as gastroenteritis, meningitis and encephalitis. Environmentally, trauma and injury resulting from falls and accidents such as car injuries can result in brain damage and learning disability.

CHANGING POLICY AND LEGISLATIVE DIRECTIONS

The four countries of the UK all have clear policy frameworks regarding the care and support of people with learning disabilities:

- Scotland – The Same as You? (Scottish Executive 2000)
- England – Valuing People (Department of Health 2001)
- Wales – Fulfilling the Promises (Welsh Assembly 2002)
- Northern Ireland – Equal Lives (Department of Health, Social Services and Public Safety 2004).

Collectively these policies are seeking to bring about change and improvement in the lives of children, adults and older people with learning disabilities that support and enable them to contribute as equal and valued members of society. These changes and developments are important, as people with learning disabilities have not been valued and respected. Today, however, there is a clear shift in focus for the care and support of this group towards community inclusion, which is bringing about the closure of long-stay institutions across the country (Scottish Executive 2003).

In addition to the clear policy frameworks that have been developed, there are specific pieces of legislation that are particularly relevant that impact on the lives of people with learning disability. The Disability Discrimination Act (1995) is particularly significant as this legislation makes it explicitly illegal to discriminate against a person with a disability, including those with learning disabilities. The Act requires all public services, including health services, to make a *reasonable adjustment* to enable people with disabilities to access services. Also of significance is the Human Rights Act (1998) and it is relevant from a number of perspectives. The Act contains articles that seek to protect the rights of citizens in areas such as the right to life, the right to marriage, the right to freedom of expression and the right to freedom from discrimination. It is important that healthcare professionals in emergency care have an understanding of the implications and potential impact on their practice and care.

As a result of cognitive impairment some people with learning disabilities may experience capacity difficulties that impact upon their ability to make decisions about certain aspects of their life. Healthcare procedures and treatments can have important implications for a patient and there may be particular difficulties for some people with learning disabilities regarding their comprehension and understanding and as a result their capacity to give informed consent. In Scotland the Adults with Incapacity (Scotland) Act (2000) provides a clear framework to support people with capacity issues, including people with learning disabilities.

THE HEALTH PROFILE OF PEOPLE WITH LEARNING DISABILITIES

As a group, people with learning disabilities have a differing health profile when compared to the general population and as a result particular responses are required. Additionally they have higher health needs, many of which frequently go unrecognized and unmet. This has a significant impact on their health and well-being and contributes to their need to access healthcare services and to premature death.

The health needs of people with learning disabilities can be complex and brings many into contact with all aspects of the healthcare system. For some their need for ongoing healthcare will be life-long in order to manage and limit the consequences of a range of chronic health conditions found within this population. There are a range of health issues experienced by this group that frequently require them to access emergency care services, and therefore all nurses require an overview and understanding of the care needs, not only those who work in specialist services (Scottish Executive 2002).

People with learning disabilities have the same everyday health needs as the general population, such as requiring treatment, investigation and management of conditions such as asthma and diabetes. The notion of everyday health needs includes access to emergency care services, as people with learning disabilities experience accidents and trauma as do the general population. Collectively therefore nurses in emergency care will encounter people with learning disabilities and need to be able to respond appropriately, yet many report feeling poorly prepared to meet the needs of this group (McConkey & Truesdale 2000, Iacono & Davis 2003, Sowney & Barr 2006a).

It is relevant to reflect on healthcare education programmes, where it is clear that few health care professionals have received any significant education or clinical experience in assessing and meeting the distinct health needs of this population and as a consequence they lack confidence in providing care (Slevin & Sines 1996). It is therefore apparent that many healthcare professionals, including nurses in emergency care, are not well prepared to respond effectively to this group of patients (Brown 2005). It is not, however, acceptable to fail to respond due to a lack of confidence and experience, and the role of continuing practice development and education programmes is important and all should incorporate a focus on the needs of people with learning disabilities (NHS Education for Scotland 2004a).

AN EVOLVING EVIDENCE BASE OF HEALTH NEEDS

As a result of the overall improvements in health experienced by the general population, people with learning disabilities are living longer and into older age. Previously their life expectancy was significantly shorter. Now there is a new phenomenon, with more living on into older age, meaning there will be more people with learning disability in the future, many with complex care needs. This will mean that nurses in emergency care will see the full spectrum of people with learning disabilities, from those with a mild learning disability through to those with highly complex physical and mental disabilities related to old age.

Communication is the number one ranked problem experienced across the spectrum of the learning disability population. They experience a high prevalence of difficulty with comprehension, expression and pragmatic communication (Bartlet & Bunning 1997). Additionally, paid carers frequently overestimate their communication abilities (Purcell 1999). This overestimation is an important issue that needs to be taken into account when emergency care nurses are undertaking patient assessments, where they may rely on a carer for additional information and background about the person with learning disabilities.

People with learning disabilities experience higher prevalence rates of sensory impairment when compared with the general population. It is estimated that there is a 4% prevalence of visual problems experienced by people with a mild learning disability under 50 years old in comparison to 2 to 7% in the general population. The level of visual impairment increases with the level of learning disability, with a 21% prevalence rate of hearing impairment being experienced by those with mild learning disabilities under 50 years in comparison with 0.2 to 1.9% in the general population (Evanhuis et al. 2001). There is also a higher prevalence of hearing disorders in people with severe learning disability. These issues are particularly prevalent in people who have very severe learning disabilities and are frequently associated with a range of other health needs such as epilepsy, gastric disorders, cerebral palsy, hydrocephalus, respiratory disorders and immobility. Many will require tube feeding, increasingly via PEG tubes, some may need ventilation and routine suctioning, while others may have valves and shunts inserted due to blockage in the circulation of cerebrospinal fluid. Their presence needs to be considered when undertaking assessment in emergency departments.

Respiratory disease is the commonest cause of death in this population and is associated with pneumonia, often secondary to swallowing and aspiration problems (Hollins et al. 1998). In contrast to the general population, cardiovascular disease is the second commonest cause of death within this population. Cardiac abnormalities are a feature of specific syndromes such as Down's syndrome, and ongoing investigation, treatment and monitoring is required for such persons (Hollins et al. 1998). People with learning disabilities experience higher rates of gastric problems, including gastric oesophageal reflux disorder (GORD), oesophagitis and *Helicobacter pylori* infection. Complications can result from these problems and investigation and treatment are indicated (Böhmer et al. 2000).

Constipation is an important and frequent problem experienced by a significant number of people with learning disabilities, particularly those with severe learning disabilities, and is an issue that may bring some into contact with emergency services, yet it can be overlooked. Those most at risk are those with mobility problems, poor diets and fluid intake combined with medication for epilepsy and gastric problems (Böhmer et al. 2001). Assessment and diagnosis can prove challenging and patients with learning disabilities who are constipated may exhibit challenging behaviours due to their abdominal pain and discomfort.

People with learning disabilities experience a different pattern of cancer when compared to the general population. Gastric, oesophagus and gall bladder cancer are more prevalent in this population and there are higher levels of leukaemia experienced by people with Down's syndrome (Cooke 1997, Hasle 2000, Patja et al. 2001).

Within the learning disability population there are high rates of tooth and gum disease and an increased use of anaesthetics for examinations and treatment (Cumella et al. 2000). It is important for nurses undertaking assessments with people with learning disabilities to look beyond what may appear to be challenging behaviours, as closer review may indicate pain and distress associated with dental problems and this is an issue that needs to be excluded.

Epilepsy is extremely common in the learning disability population, with some 10 to 20% of people with mild learning disabilities experiencing seizures, moving to over 50% in those with severe and complex learning disabilities. This is in comparison with some 1% of the general population. The epilepsy presentation within the learning disability population is more complex than that experienced by the general population and there are higher levels of polypharmacy, complex seizure types and sudden unexplained death as a result of seizures (Sillanpaa et al. 1999). As a consequence of seizures, people with learning disabilities may require emergency treatment of status epilepticus, while some will experience injury and trauma that will also require attention from emergency care services.

As with the general population, people with learning disabilities experience accidents and orthopaedic problems associated with falls that will bring them into contact with emergency nurses. It is now recognized that women with learning disabilities have higher rates of osteoporosis and associated fractures. Additionally as a result of mobility, balance and gait problems people with learning disabilities experience accidents and fractures that are linked to their premature death (Center et al. 1998).

While there is an increasing recognition of the sexual health needs of people with learning disabilities, this is in an area requiring a higher focus. People with learning disabilities can be victims of sexual abuse, with an associated impact on their sexual healthcare. Additionally women with learning disabilities have a low uptake of cervical and breast-screening programmes targeted at the general population (Brown et al. 1995, Hollins 2002).

People with learning disabilities have a higher prevalence of psychiatric ill health and, as with their physical health needs, their mental health pattern differs when compared to the general population. This point is significant when linked with the communication difficulties that may be present and is an important factor that needs to be considered by emergency nurses when undertaking patient assessment. People with learning disabilities have a higher prevalence rate of schizophrenia, 3% compared to 1% in the general adult population (Lund 1985, Doody et al. 1998). Furthermore, depression was found in 22% of people with learning disabilities compared to 5.5% in the general adult population (Richards et al. 2001). Anxiety and panic disorders are common in the general population and are also experienced by people with learning disabilities of all ages, although the disorder may fail to be recognized in this population and be considered to be challenging behaviour, thereby affecting diagnosis and treatment (Patel et al. 1993, Moss et al. 2000).

Emergency nurses will be familiar with patients who self-injure. Self-injury is found in the learning disability population and is associated with autism, IQ, level of immobility and hearing difficulties. Prevalence rates of self-injury have been found to be as high as 17.4% in this population, with some 1.7% being of a severe and sustained nature (Collacott et al. 1998). Dementia is found in higher rates within the learning disability population and occurs at an earlier age. It is particularly common within people with Down's syndrome (Cooper 1997, Patel et al. 1993, & Holland 2000).

Autistic spectrum disorder is a life-long disability that affects the way a person communicates and relates to others around them. People with autism also experience problems and difficulties with social interaction as well as having altered capacity to understand emotional expressions. Autism may be associated with learning disabilities; however, it is important to recognize that autism covers a spectrum. Not all people with autism also have a learning disability. It is estimated that there are some 60 per 10 000 population of children with autistic spectrum disorder, though data are currently not available for the prevalence within the adult population. People with autistic spectrum disorder present with a range of additional health needs, including mental health, communication, epilepsy and some may experience problem behaviours (Public Health Institute of Scotland 2001, Medical Research Council 2001).

PEOPLE WITH LEARNING DISABILITIES AS HEALTH SERVICE USERS

People with learning disabilities are high users of all aspects of health services. Yet when compared with the general population their care episodes are shorter. Mencap (2004) suggest that on average 14% of the general population will require general hospital services: this is in comparison to 26% of people with learning disabilities. Therefore it becomes evident that all nurses irrespective of the clinical focus of their role will come into contact with people with learning disability as result of their health needs and the need to access health services. This contact is also likely to increase, as people with learning disabilities are now living longer and into old age, resulting in them also developing health needs associated with older age.

As a result of their health profile people with learning disabilities will come into contact with emergency services. However, their opportunity to access quality healthcare is dependent in part on emergency nurses' ability and willingness to learn and respond appropriately to their communication patterns, the number one ranked problem experienced by this population. The challenge then for nurses within this fast-moving environment is to find ways in which the needs of people with learning disabilities are both identified and met in equity with others who access the service.

REDUCING CHALLENGES IN ACCESSING SERVICES

Communication is a basic human right and a fundamental principle central to inclusion within society. It is a two-way process and all people use a variety of means to communicate, including both verbal and non-verbal means. Yet within society there is a significant dependence on verbal communication, leaving those with reduced or no verbal skills at a significant disadvantage in interacting in the world around them (Arnold & Boggs 1999).

DoH (1992) estimates that between 40 and 50% of people with learning disabilities experience some degree of difficulty with communication, with sensory impairments being more common in this population. Evidence consistently shows that poor communication is one of the key barriers experienced by people with learning disabilities in accessing quality health (Fox & Wilson 1999, Cumella & Martin 2000, PAMIS 2001, DHSSPS 2004, US Public Health Services 2002, Iacono & Davis 2003, Barr 2004).

For the health care professional, poor communication increases the challenges normally encountered in assessing the patient's needs, informing them of their current health status and seeking and gaining valid consent, all which are prerequisites in providing quality care. Thus it is crucial that nurses within the emergency department have a greater understanding of the communication difficulties experienced by people with intellectual disabilities, as a failure to communicate effectively can result in serious consequences. Primarily poor communication impacts on the nurse's ability to conduct an appropriate assessment of the individual's holistic needs, which in turn can have many negative consequences for the patient who has a learning disability, including:

- needs not being assessed and identified, thus not met
- an increased risk of harm due to non-compliance
- a greater risk of diagnostic overshadowing or differential diagnosis
- difficulties informing consent leading to a reluctance of staff to carry out previously identified care
- a reduction of patient involvement in discussions and decisions about healthcare
- reduction in opportunities to exercise the right to give or withhold consent.

ASSESSING NEEDS

Currently there is little documented evidence available on the experience of people with learning disabilities of the emergency department, although this situation is gradually changing. Houghton (2001) suggests that this dearth of information within the emergency care literature may indicate a lack of awareness of emergency nurses regarding the health needs of people with learning disabilities. What is more concerning is a misconception that the needs of people with learning disability are not associated with emergency care (Sowney and Barr 2006b). This is an issue that requires to be challenged, as it is now accepted that general hospital services can present significant risk to the lives and health of people with learning disabilities. The National Patient Safety Agency state that:

> 'People with learning disability may be more at risk of things going wrong than the general population, leading to varying degrees of harm being caused whilst in general hospitals'
> (National Patient Safety Agency 2004, p. 11)

The risk factors identified include a limited knowledge and understanding of the health needs, an increased prevalence and risk of dysphagia and aspiration pneumonia, barriers preventing equal access to healthcare, a lack of education and practice development opportunities, complex communication issues and misdiagnosis or no diagnosis.

Though the number of people with learning disabilities accessing emergency services is increasing, currently there is no mechanism for quantifying their attendance. Whilst the absence of these figures may actually be seen as a positive step towards inclusion, nurses within emergency care frequently ask the question 'how do we know if a person has a learning disability if there are no obvious signs?' There is no guaranteed way of gaining this understanding, particularly if the person has a mild learning disability and does not wish anyone to be a aware of this. However, there may be a few indicators of the presence of a learning disability, including:

- vagueness providing a history
- difficulties expressing current need
- slowness in answering questions.

It is important that the right of people to withhold this information is respected; however, if a nurse suspects that a person may have learning disability and may require some further support to aid their assessment, treatment and recovery, this understanding is then justified. During the patient assessment some broad general questions may then help clarify the situation, for example, 'do you have any contact with health care professionals?' In addition, following the provision of information throughout the whole process (whether verbal or written) nurses need to continually ask broad questions that will establish the individual's current understanding.

While emergency nurses are skilled at carrying out a rapid assessment of needs, this process is not, however, as straightforward when the patient has a learning disability and communication difficulties and as such some further issues require consideration.

Hospitalization regardless of the time involved is known to cause stress, which is often demonstrated in people with learning disabilities by heightened emotional responses and behaviours. These emotional responses, including fear, insecurity or physical discomfort, can impact on the individual's ability to express needs and understand information regarding their condition and their compliance with treatment. Although compliance is required for many of the interventions associated with examination, treatment and care, ineffective communication and inappropriate timing of interventions, particularly at the heightened emotional stage, can cause harm to the individual (Arnold and Boggs 1999).

People with learning disabilities often need more time to express their needs, particularly when they are ill, yet within emergency departments, where time is considered to be of the essence, affording extra time to encourage interaction is problematic (Walsh

& Dolan 1999). In order to conduct the assessment safely the emergency nurse must afford more time to the process of triage (Houghton 2001), which may be up to four times more than that required for a person without such disabilities. The challenge for nurses is to find out how the individual communicates, then investigate ways in which they can best communicate with each other to gain the appropriate information required for the assessment, rather than apportion blame for ineffective communication with people with learning disabilities. In doing so they can reduce the patient's distress, fear and insecurities, whilst facilitating opportunities for the nurse to inform the patient, thus increasing compliance with examination, treatment or care (Hayward 1975, Boore 1978).

Many people with learning disabilities who have little or no speech exhibit unusual behaviours as a way of communicating with others. Such behaviours can include rocking; head banging; increased flexion or extension and hypersensitivity to either sound or touch in their response to pain. However, as these messages are sent in a way that is quite different to what emergency nurses experience on a daily basis, there is a greater chance that these messages are misunderstood, being associated with learning disability and not a means of communicating a need. The danger in not understanding behavioural cues is a risk of diagnostic overshadowing and differential diagnoses.

An understanding of these two terms, diagnostic overshadowing and differential diagnosis, is particularly relevant in relation to assessing the health needs of people with learning disabilities. Diagnostic overshadowing occurs when clinicians, due to their limited knowledge and understanding of the differing presentations of illness in people with learning disabilities, assume that all clinical presentations and symptoms are as a result of the person's learning disability, as opposed to considering other possible physical or psychological underlying reasons (Jopp & Keys 2001). Clearly the consequences of diagnostic overshadowing could be potentially fatal for some people with learning disabilities as their true underlying health need will not be identified and treated. Furthermore the term differential diagnosis relates to the range of possible clinical diagnoses that may result from the patient's history and from assessment and investigation (Reiss et al. 1982). In relation to people with learning disabilities where communication can be impaired there is an increased possibility that the range of differential diagnoses is not explored fully, and the potential seriousness of the condition going unrecognized – the problem of misdiagnosis is

real and can have fatal consequences for persons with learning disabilities.

Thus, the assessment of healthcare needs, including pain, in people with learning disabilities can be very challenging. Pain presents itself in many ways and people have varying thresholds of pain; however, this is complicated further if the individual also has communication difficulties. Nonetheless, pain needs to be accurately assessed in people with learning disabilities through a comprehensive holistic approach informed by the use of appropriate pain assessment tools and where possible including information from a carer who is knowledgeable of the patient when well, thereby allowing a comparison with the presenting history. In addition to the knowledge of and skills in using various pain assessment tools the emergency care nurse also requires knowledge of how the perception of pain is verbalized and demonstrated in people with intellectual disabilities (Cumella & Martin 2000). Furthermore, the assessment of pain and the provision of adequate pain relief are also associated with the nurse's attitudes. Consequently, if nurses believe that people with learning disabilities experience pain differently to those who do not have learning disabilities, then the opportunity to receive appropriate pain relief is reduced, increasing the patient's experience of stress, anxiety and fear. However, while pain is a subjective experience, the opportunity to be pain-free must be seen by emergency nurses as a patient's priority.

The role of the families and carers in the assessment process is very important too, as they can provide essential support to the person with a learning disability, assisting them to express needs and make choices known. This is particularly so if the person has severe to profound learning disability with complex needs. Therefore it is both good practice and a duty of care for nurses within emergency care to work collaboratively with family members, demonstrating the value of their contribution, as well as showing a caring, respectful attitude towards the individual. Whilst the role of the carer in assisting with the provision of vital information cannot be underestimated, nurses *are*, however, responsible for using various skills to gain the information required to carry out a patient assessment, then to analyse the information, *judging* the value and worth (Sowney & Barr 2006b).

INVOLVING PEOPLE WITH LEARNING DISABILITIES

Involving people with learning disabilities in their care when they are acutely ill can be challenging. However, all patients need to be adequately informed of their health status to enable them to make informed decisions regarding their healthcare. Additionally the receipt of information in a format that is understood reduces fears and anxieties experienced by people with learning disabilities in acute general hospitals and increases opportunities for greater compliance and recovery. Evidence shows that informed people are better able to manage and cope with treatment and the effects of hospitalization and this is particularly important when working with vulnerable people.

People with learning disabilities may have difficulty understanding written information provided in general hospitals and frequently require the help of others to gain an understanding of the documents and their significance. Recent research on access to acute general hospitals has highlighted many areas of good practice within the emergency care environment in the development of various means of gaining and providing information to people with learning disabilities. This includes working guidelines and the development of more appropriate user-friendly leaflets and posters. Emergency nurses have an obligation to be aware of the good practice within their own area to facilitate good communication with people with learning disabilities.

CONSENT

It is impossible to consider communication difficulties experienced by people with learning disabilities without discussing the connection with the provision of valid consent. Central to the process of gaining valid consent is good communication; however, without the required information in a format that is clearly understood and accessible, people with learning disabilities remain passive in asserting control over their ability to self-determine and their own bodies.

The law recognizes the right of all adults to consent to examination, treatment and care and this includes people with a learning disability. Yet people with learning disabilities are often viewed by healthcare professionals as being incapable of making decisions and as such are frequently excluded from discussions and decisions regarding their healthcare (Hart 1999, Hutchinson 2005, Barr 2004, Mencap 2004, Sowney et al. 2006c). Such false beliefs regarding the capacity to maintain control over their own bodies reduces opportunities for people with learning disabilities to be empowered, increasing their passivity in decision-making. Evidence shows that parents and other relatives are often asked to consent on behalf of the an adult who has a learning disability, even though the law states that no one can give valid consent on behalf

of another adult. It is therefore important to distinguish between consent and assent from a relative or carer. A relative or carer assenting and agreeing with a course of action is not valid consent.

In order to give valid consent, individuals must first have the ability to understand, maintain and judge information and in addition communicate a choice to others (Wong et al. 1999). The support mechanism of using the relative/carer to assist with explanations is good practice by nurses; however, no decisions should be made by the relatives or carers regarding the treatment or care that has not been the patient's identified choice (Hart 1999). Healthcare professionals have both a legal and professional responsibility to obtain valid consent prior to the commencement of any examination, treatment or care and have a responsibility to ensure people with learning disabilities are empowered to make healthcare decisions (DoH 2001c, Welsh Assembly 2002, DHSSPS 2004, NMC 2004, NHS Health Scotland 2004). In addition, many investigations and treatments may be required within the emergency care environment and nurses must appreciate that valid consent for one aspect of care does not cover all other aspects of care. In addition nurses need to remember that consent is ongoing, being context-dependent, in that a person may have capacity to consent at one time and not at another (Dye et al. 2004). If, however, there is concern from the health care professional about an individual's capacity to consent this must be confirmed through a test of capacity.

In the absence of consent to examination, treatment and care within the emergency care environment, there is an increased risk of harm to the person with a learning disability from procedures being carried out by nurses without the full cooperation of the patient. Furthermore treatment without valid consent is unlawful. Similarly nursing staff can inadvertently cause harm through decisions not to act rather than to act, due to difficulties gaining valid consent (Barr 2004).

Emergency nurses need to be familiar with the issue of valid consent, having an understanding that both choice and control over healthcare decisions are key principles for all patients. In addition these aspects are central to the provision of inclusive services for people with learning disabilities (Scottish Executive 1999, DoH 2001c, Welsh Assembly 2002, NHS Health Scotland 2004, DHSSPS 2004).

Improving communication and facilitating valid consent

- Take a little extra time to communicate
- Seek other means of gaining and providing

information, verbal and non-verbal. Some people respond better to short phrases and pictures

- Be aware of good practice elsewhere to enhance communication with people with learning disabilities, such as the development of leaflets and posters more suitable to providing information to people with learning disabilities
- Always direct questions to and converse with the person with a learning disability first. Being valued and respected increases opportunities for trust
- Encourage relatives or carers to support the individual in communicating needs or decisions, not to do this for them
- Understand that behaviour is a means of communicating and expressing a need. It is not a symptom of a learning disability
- Use the guidelines on consent as a framework to aid decision making.

ADDITIONAL SUPPORT MODELS

The main focus of the work of emergency nurses is not with people with learning disabilities. However, they are a group who have significant health needs and have experienced institutional discrimination from healthcare professionals in the past (NHS Health Scotland 2004). While there are actions that can be taken by nurses in emergency care that will have a significant impact on the care experience of this group, there are times when people with learning disabilities require support beyond that which is available. Models of additional support are now being developed that see experienced learning disability nurses taking on liaison roles within general hospitals (Brown et al. 2005). These liaison models help to ensure that those with the most complex of care needs receive appropriate care and support and help to create a partnership between patients, their carers, acute care nurses and specialist in learning disability healthcare.

The focus of the liaison model may be on preadmission planning and assessments, thereby helping to ensure the appropriate care arrangements are in place. Alternatively there may be communication, consent or diagnosis concerns and the liaison nurse is well placed to help problem-solve and make referrals onto other specialists in learning disability health services. These new and innovative models of practice present an opportunity for research collaborations to determine their impact on health outcomes (Brown et al. 2005)

The UK is fortunate to have specialists in learning disability healthcare; however, this is not the case across the world. Frequently these specialists work as part of community learning disability teams and comprise a range of professionals, including learning disability nurses, speech and language therapists, occupational therapists, physiotherapists, dieticians, clinical psychologists and psychiatrists. Collectively they are a resource available to nurses and others in emergency care to assist in the assessment and identification of health needs, as well as providing specialist interventions and treatments to people with learning disabilities with complex needs. Today links are being established between emergency care professionals and specialist learning disability teams, with liaison nurses acting as the central coordinating point, thereby ensuring that the most appropriate care and support is available to this vulnerable group.

CONCLUSION

The learning disability population is increasing and ageing, with more living into older age with more complex health needs. Health care professionals in emergency care need to become familiar with the distinct needs of this group. As the evidence base of the health needs of people with learning disabilities evolves and is better understood, it becomes apparent that their health needs when compared to the general population are different. Failure to recognize and respond to their distinct pattern of health needs contributes to and results in their health inequalities that in turn contribute to premature death.

Central to effective care is the need to recognize the patterns of communication used by people with learning disabilities and the important role that relatives and carers can play in facilitating and enabling an accurate assessment and identification of needs. Models of additional support are being developed and it is incumbent on nurses within the emergency care environment to be aware of and communicate with specialist learning disability teams in order to reduce challenges in assessing and providing care to this vulnerable group.

References

Arnold E, Boggs K (1999) *Interpersonal Relationships: Professional Communication Skills for Nurses.* Philadelphia: WB Saunders Company.

Barr O (2004) Promoting access. The experience of children and adults with learning disabilities and their families/carers who had contact with acute general hospitals in the

WHSSB Area and the views of nurses in these hospitals. *A Report to the Western Health and Social Services Board.* Londonderry: WHSSB.

Bartlett C, Bunning K (1997) The importance of communication partnerships: a study to investigate the communication exchanges between staff and adults with learning disabilities. *British Journal of Learning Disabilities,* **25,** 148–153.

Beange H, McElduff A, Baker W (1995) Medical disorders of adults with mental retardation: a population study. *American Journal on Mental Retardation,* **99**(6): 595–604.

Böhmer CJ, Klinkenberg-Knol EC, Niezen-de Boer MC, Meuwissen SG (2000) Gastroesophageal reflux disease in intellectually disabled individuals: how often, how serious, how manageable? *American Journal of Gastroenterology,* **95**(8), 1868–1872.

Böhmer CJ, Taminiau JA, Klinkenberg-Knol EC, Meuwissen SG (2001) The prevalence of constipation in institutionalized people with intellectual disability. *Journal of Intellectual Disability Research,* **45,** 212–218.

Boore JRP (1978) *Prescription for Recovery.* London: Royal College of Nursing.

Brown H, Stein J, Turk V (1995) The sexual abuse of adults with learning disabilities. Report of a second two-year incidence survey. *Mental Handicap Research,* **8,** 3–24.

Brown M, MacArthur J, Gibbs S (2005) *A New Research Agenda: Improving General Hospital Care for People with Learning Disabilities.* Edinburgh: NHS Lothian.

Brown M (2005) Emergency care for people with learning disabilities: what all nurses and midwives need to know. *Accident and Emergency Nursing,* **13**(4), 224–231.

Center J, Beange H, McElduff A (1998) People with mental retardation have an increased prevalence of osteoporosis: a population study. *American Journal of Mental Retardation,* **103**(1), 19–28.

Collacott, RA, Cooper SA (1998) Epidemiology of self-injurious behaviour in adults with learning disabilities. *The British Journal of Psychiatry,* **173,** 428–432.

Cooke LB (1997) Cancer and learning disability. *Journal of Intellectual Disability Research,* **41,** 312–316.

Cooper SA (1997) Epidemiology of psychiatric disorders in elderly compared with younger adults with learning disabilities. *The British Journal of Psychiatry,* **170,** 375–380.

Cooper SA, Melville C, Morrison J (2004) People with intellectual disabilities: their health needs differ and need to be recognised and met. *British Medical Journal,* **239,** 414–415.

Cumella S, Ransford N, Lyons J, Burnham H (2000) Needs for oral care among people with intellectual disability not in contact with Community Dental Services. *Journal of Intellectual Disability Research,* **44**(Pt 1), 45–52.

Cumella S, Martin D (2000) *Secondary Healthcare for People with a Learning Disability.* London: Department of Health.

Department of Health (1992) *Mansell Report on Services for People with Learning Disabilities or Challenging Behaviours or Mental Health Needs.* London: Department of Health.

Department of Health (2001a) *Valuing People: A New Strategy for Learning Disability for the 21st Century.* London: Department of Health.

Department of Health (2001b) *Seeking Consent. Working with People with Intellectual Disabilities.* London: Department of Health.

Department of Health (2001c) *Reference Guide to Consent to Examination or Treatment.* London: Department of Health.

Department of Health, Social Services and Public Safety (2003) *Reference Guide to Consent to Examination Treatment or Care.* Belfast: DHSSPS.

Department of Health, Social Services and Public Safety (2004) *Equal Lives: Review of Policy and Services for People with Learning Disabilities in Northern Ireland.* Belfast: DHSSPS.

Doody GA, Johnstone EC, Sanderson TL, Owens DG, Muir WJ (1998) 'Pfropfschizophrenie' revisited. Schizophrenia in people with mild learning disability. *The British Journal of Psychiatry,* **173,** 145–153.

Dye L, Hendry S, Dougal J, Burton M (2004) Capacity to consent to participate in research: a reconceptualisation. *British Journal of Intellectual Disabilities,* **32**(3), 144–149.

Evenhuis HM, Theunissen M, Denkers I, Verschuure H Kemme H (2001) Prevalence of visual and hearing impairment in a Dutch institutionalised population with intellectual disability. *Journal of Intellectual Disability Research,* **45**(5), 457–464.

Fox D, Wilson D (1999) Parents expectations of general hospital admission for adults with learning disabilities. *Journal of Clinical Nursing,* **8,** 610–614.

Hart SL (1999) Meaningful choices: consent to treatment in general health care settings for adults with learning disabilities. *Journal of Learning Disability,* **3**(1), 20–26.

Hasle H, Clemmensen I, Mikkelsen M (2000) Risks of leukaemia and solid tumours in individuals with Down's syndrome. *Lancet,* **355,** 165–169.

Hayward J (1975) Information: a prescription against pain. London: Royal College of Nursing.

Holland AJ (2000) Ageing and learning disability. *The British Journal of Psychiatry,* **176**(1), 26–31.

Hollins S, Attard MT, von Fraunhofer N, McGuigan S, Sedgwick P (1998) Mortality in people with learning disabilities: risks, causes and death certification findings in London. *Developmental Medicine and Child Neurology,* **40,** 50–56.

Hollins S, Perez W (2000) *Looking after my Breasts.* London: Gaskell Press.

Houghton BM (2001) Caring for people with Down's syndrome in Accident and Emergency. *Nurse,* **9**(2), 24–27.

Howells G (1986) Are the medical needs of the mentally handicapped adults being met? *Journal of the Royal College of General Practitioners,* **36,** 449–453.

Hutchinson C (2005) Addressing issues related to adult patients who lack the capacity to give consent. *Nursing Standard,* **19**(23), 47–53.

Iacono T, Davis R (2003) The experience of people with developmental disability in Emergency Departments and hospital wards. *Research in Developmental Disability,* **24,** 247–264.

Jopp DA, Keys CB (2001) Diagnostic overshadowing reviewed and reconsidered. *American Journal on Mental Retardation*, **106**, 416–433.

Lund J (1985) The prevalence of psychiatric morbidity in mentally retarded adults. *Acta Psychiatrica. Scandanavica*, **72**(6), 563–570.

Medical Research Council (2001) *Review of Autism Research: Epidemiology and Causes*. London: Medical Research Council.

MENCAP (2004) *Trust me right! Better Healthcare for People with Intellectual Disabilities*. London: MENCAP.

McConkey R, Truesdale M (2000) Reactions of nurses and therapists in mainstream health services to contact with people who have learning disabilities. *Journal of Advanced Nursing*, **32**, 158–163.

Moss S, Emerson E, Kiernan C, Turner S, Hatton C, Iborz A (2000) Psychiatric symptoms in adults with learning disability and challenging behaviour. *The British Journal of Psychiatry*, **177**, 452–456.

National Patient Safety Agency (2004) *Understanding the Patient Safety Issues for People with Learning Disabilities*. London: National Patient Safety Agency.

NHS Education for Scotland (2004) *Getting it Right Together: the Implementation of Recommendations 16, 17 and 20 from Promoting Health, Supporting Inclusion Report*. Edinburgh: NHS Education for Scotland.

NHS Health Scotland (2004) *People with Learning Disabilities in Scotland: The Health Needs Assessment Report*. Glasgow: NHS Health Scotland.

Nursing and Midwifery Council (2004) *Code of Professional: Standards for Conduct, Performance and Ethics*. London: Nursing and Midwifery Council.

PAMIS (2001) *The Views of Family Carers on the Contribution of Nurses to the Care and Support of People with Profound and Multiple Learning Disabilities (PMLD)*. University of Dundee: PAMIS.

Patel P, Goldberg D, Moss S (1993) Psychiatric morbidity in older people with moderate and severe learning disability. II: The prevalence study. *The British Journal of Psychiatry*, **163**, 481–491.

Patja K (2000) Life expectancy of people with intellectual disabilities: a 35-year follow-up study. *Journal of Intellectual Disability Research*, **44**, 590–599.

Patja K, Eero P, Livanainen M (2001) Cancer incidents among people with intellectual disability. *Journal of Intellectual Disability Research*, **45**, 300–307.

Public Health Institute of Scotland (2001) *Autistic Spectrum Disorders. Needs Assessment Report*. Glasgow: Public Health Institute of Scotland.

Purcell M, Morris I, McConkey (1999) Communication between staff and adults with intellectual disabilities in naturally occurring settings. *Journal of Intellectual Disability Research*, **45**, 16–25.

Reiss S, Levitan GW, Szyszko J (1982) Emotional disturbance and mental retardation: diagnostic overshadowing. *American Journal of Mental Deficiency*, **86**, 567–574.

Richards M, Maughan B, Hardy R, Hall I, Strydom A, Wadsworth M (2001) Long-term affective disorder in people with mild learning disability. *The British Journal of Psychiatry*, **179**, 523–527.

Scottish Executive (2000) *The Same as You? A Review of Services for People with Learning Disabilities*. Edinburgh: The Stationery Office.

Scottish Executive (2002) *Promoting Health, Supporting Inclusion: The National Review of the Contribution of all Nurses and Midwives to the Care and Support of People with Learning Disabilities*. Edinburgh: The Stationery Office.

Scottish Executive (2003) *Home at Last? The Report on Hospital Closure Service Reprovision Sub Group – The Same As You?* Edinburgh: The Stationery Office.

Scottish Executive (2005) *A Good Practice Guide on Consent for Health care Professionals in NHS Scotland: A Draft Consultation*. Edinburgh: Scottish Executive Health Department.

Sillanpaa M, Gram L, Johannessen SI, Tomson T (Eds) (1999) *Epilepsy and Mental Retardation*. Stroud: Wrightson Biomedical.

Slevin E, Sines D (1996) Attitudes of nurses in general hospitals towards people with learning disabilties: influence of contact of graduate and non graduate status. A comparative study. *Journal of Advanced Nursing*, **24**, 1116–1126.

Sowney M, Barr O (2006a) The perceived challenges encountered by nurses in accident and emergency caring for adults with intellectual disabilities. *Journal of Advanced Nursing*, **55**(1), 36–45.

Sowney M, Barr O (2006b) The challenges for nurses communicating with and gaining valid consent from adults with intellectual disabilities within the accident and emergency care service. *Journal of Clinical Nursing*, **15**(1), 1–9.

Sowney M, Brown M, Barr O (2006c) Caring for people with learning disabilities in emergency care. *Emergency Nurse*, **14**(2), 23–30.

US Public Health Service (2001) *Closing the Gap: A National Blueprint to Improve the Health of Persons with Mental Retardation. Report of the Surgeon Generals Conference on Health Disparities and Mental Retardation*. Washington DC: US PHS.

Van Schrojenstein Lantman-de Valk HM, van den Metsemakers AM, Maaskant MAM, Haveman M, Urlings H, Kessels A, Crebolder H (1997) Prevalence and incidence of health problems in people with intellectual disability. *Journal of Intellectual Disability Research*, **41**, 42–51.

Walsh M, Dolan B (1999) Emergency nurses and their perceptions of caring. *Emergency Nurse*, **7**(4), 24–31.

Welsh Assembly (2002) *Fulfilling the Promises: Proposals for a Framework for Services for People with Learning Disabilities*. Cardiff: Welsh Assembly.

Welsh Assembly Government (2002) *Reference Guide for Consent to Examination and Treatment*. Cardiff: Welsh Assembly.

Wilson D, Haire A (1990) Health care screening for people with mental handicap in the community. *British Medical Journal*, **301**, 1379–1381.

Wong JG, Clare ICH, Gunn M, Holland AJ (1999) Capacity to make health care decisions: its importance in clinical practice. *Psychological Medicine*, **29**, 437–446.

Chapter 33

Health promotion

Stewart Piper

INTRODUCTION

It is interesting to note Beattie's (1991) observation that the major health care professions claim increasingly that health promotion underpins practice: interesting because while copious literature on health promotion and nursing is readily accessible in any nursing library, the emphasis tends towards practice and doing. Fundamental questions then, about purpose, fit with practice and scrutiny of the different theoretical approaches and their pertinence for nursing, particularly in relation to specialist areas of practice, remain as much an underdeveloped area now as in 1991.

This whole debate was given fresh impetus in 1992 by The Health of the Nation (HoN), the Government strategy for health in England (DoH 1992). The HoN placed health promotion explicitly on the nursing agenda in general, and on the emergency care agenda in particular, since accidents were one of the five key areas of the strategy. Indeed the HoN (1993 p. 10) also highlighted that:

'Tertiary prevention by Accident and Emergency departments ... will contribute to the overall objective of reducing ill-health, disability and death from accidents.'

Further to this, Targeting Practice (DoH 1993) and Saving Lives: Our healthier nation (DoH 1999), both of which include accident prevention, together with The NHS Plan (DoH 2000), Choosing Health (DoH 2004) and Better information, better choices, better health (DoH 2004) emphasize how health promotion has become more of a health service priority.

Given the above, the intention of this chapter is not to provide an exhaustive account or the final word on health promotion in ED per se, but to emphasize the benefits of a conceptual framework to explore the relationship between health promotion theory and ED nursing practice. Specifically, the mode and focus of intervention and the aims, methods, impact and outcomes of three models that can be operationalized and applied, to a greater or lesser extent, are discussed. The intention is to move the debate beyond any narrow or traditional view of health promotion as simply a form of information or advice giving, and highlight the need for a repertoire of approaches in the modern arena of healthcare and ED nursing.

HEALTH PROMOTION FRAMEWORK

To facilitate conceptual understanding, contextualize and map out the models of health promotion a framework (Fig. 33.1), based on the work of Beattie (1991) and Piper and Brown (1998), is utilized. The framework comprises three models entitled *The Nurse as Behaviour Change Agent, The Nurse as Strategic Practitioner* and *The Nurse as Empowerment Facilitator* that derive from themes and deviant/paradigm cases generated in a qualitative study by the author. The research examined the relationship between hospital nursing practice and health promotion theory and included a small number of ED nurses in the sample group. However, as a deviant/paradigm case *The Nurse as Strategic Practitioner* is not a saturated theme and some of the example indicators of practice in Tables 33.1, 33.2 and 33.3 stem from constructive theorizing to help illuminate the debate. As such, all require the tests of fit and transferability to be applied by the reader.

As can be seen, the combination of a nurse control axis (essentially a power continuum) and a patient focus axis creates three discrete models of health promotion. The former unites *The Nurse as Behaviour Change Agent* and *The Nurse as Strategic Practitioner* models and reflects a 'top-down' nurse-led mode of intervention based on an objective assessment of need and nursing goals. However, they diverge on the individual/patient population axis as the former is concerned with individual action perspectives and

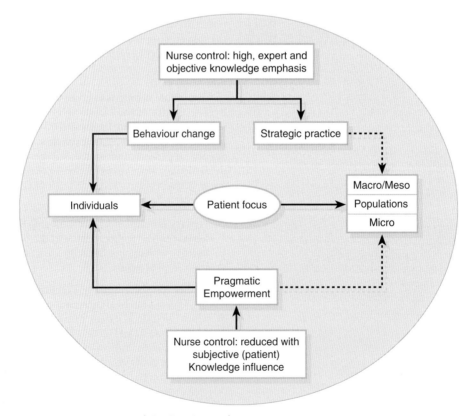

Figure 33.1   Models of health promotion. (After Beattie 1991.)

Table 33.1   The nurse as behaviour change agent

Aims	Methods	Impact	Outcomes
Primary prevention Secondary prevention Tertiary prevention Appropriate use of services	Mass media campaigns Verbal and written instructions on injury/ disease management, complications etc. Supplementary discharge advice Patient teaching Patient information	Change in health-related behaviour Compliance with treatment regimes Self-management by patient Right patient, right place, right time	↓ Accidents ● Mortality ● Morbidity ● Complications ● Relapse

Table 33.2   The nurse as strategic practitioner

Aims	Methods	Impact	Outcomes

Structural change
  (national/local)
 	
Organizational development,
  innovation and policy
  implementation at
  department
  level
	Lobbying:
	● national/local
	Service management e.g. on:
	● Clinical governance
	● Service review
	● Staff rostering
	● Timing of clinics
	● Skill mix and deployment
	  (ENB 199, ALS/ATLS, ENP)
	● Use of protocols
	● Trauma scoring
	● Trauma teams
	● Risk registers
	● Inter-agency and multidisciplinary
	  liaison and training
	● NSFs
	● Collaborative care planning
	● Clinical audit
		↓ Inequalities
		↑ Safety
		Evidence-based practice
		Right staff, right place, right time
		Inter-agency and multidisciplinary
		  collaborative working
		Seamless service
		Support for the vulnerable
			↓ Accidents
			● Mortality
			● Morbidity
			● Injury
			● Disability
			● Complications
			↑ Clinical outcomes
			↑ Patient satisfaction

Table 33.3   The nurse as empowerment facilitator

Aim	Methods	Impact	Outcomes

Empowerment	Humanistic, non-hierarchical
	  patient-centred interaction
	Neutral information provision
	Stages of change model
	Advocacy
	Peer support
		Health agenda determined, directed and
		  validated by patient with support from
		  healthcare workers
		↑ Informed patient decision-making
		↑ Coping strategies
		Support group accessed
			↑ Feelings of control
			Feeling supported

outcomes and the latter with collective health gain. Similarly, when concerned with the former, *The Nurse as Empowerment Facilitator* converges with *The Nurse as Behaviour Change Agent* on the patient focus axis but is polarized on the power continuum when the former is concerned with an individual action perspective. It converges with *The Nurse as Strategic Practitioner* when the focus of intervention is at a population level while remaining divergent in terms of the locus of control.

OPERATIONAL DEFINITIONS

To avoid the debate surrounding the distinction between health education and health promotion, for the purpose of this chapter the definition of Tones is adopted. He states that health promotion:

> 'incorporates all measures deliberately designed to promote health and handle diseases' (Tones 1990 p. 3).

In addition, and consistent with Tones and Green (2004), primary, secondary and tertiary health promotion are defined as follows:

- primary health promotion refers to interventions to prevent new cases of disease or injury;
- secondary health promotion aims to minimize the consequences of disease or injury, prevent them from becoming chronic or irreversible and to restore the patient to their former health status;
- tertiary health promotion aims to maximize health experience within the constraints imposed by a chronic disease (e.g. diabetes, asthma, HIV), injury or concomitant disability, prevent restrictions or further complications and to assist rehabilitation.

THE NURSE AS BEHAVIOUR CHANGE AGENT

The Nurse as Behaviour Change Agent reflects a 'medical model' approach to health promotion and is based on the assumption that individuals make rational, conscious decisions about their health-related behaviour. Primary interventions aim to prevent disease, illness and injury and promote optimum biological functioning by disseminating 'factual' information selectively derived from objective and medically based scientific research to the public. This takes the form of edicts from healthcare professionals, or the ever-present mass media awareness-raising campaigns such as the Clunk Click television campaigns of yesteryear, encouraging the use of cycle helmets, No Smoking Day and Drug Awareness week etc. It is suggested to the public that if they fail to follow a prescribed course of action their 'health' is at risk. The aim is to trigger a 'do-it-yourself' attitude and then behaviour/lifestyle changes consistent with the recommended advice given.

The Nurse as Behaviour Change Agent as a primary health promotion intervention would engage ED nurses in an information-based approach. This could include themed displays in the waiting room on a variety of topics such as accident prevention, first aid, the dangers of alcohol misuse, HIV and sexual health or healthy eating. These must be visually appealing, regularly changed and could reflect national initiatives such as Drinkwise Day or World Aids Day. They should be supported by a wide range of leaflets in display racks, posters strategically placed around the Accident Department and health promotion videos showing in the waiting room if it is suitably equipped. This process can be assisted by contacting local Health Promotion Resource Libraries, who are an important source of information, materials and expertise.

It is important to acknowledge that, while effective at raising awareness about particular health risks when operating as a sole strategy for attitude and behaviour change, the outcomes are likely to be at best uncertain (Naidoo and Wills 2001). In emphasizing the personal controlling of risks and the correcting of individual inadequacies, it is also assumed free choice exists and that lifestyle is the primary cause of ill-health. In isolation such an approach denies that health is a social product, ignores and implicitly condones inequalities and minimal state intervention. For an excellent, albeit old and general (i.e. not related to nursing), critique of such a stance the reader is referred to Mitchell (1982); for a critique related to nursing, but not specific to ED, see Brown and Piper (1997).

The purpose of secondary health promotion, primarily aimed at those discharged home from the accident department, is patient compliance with prescribed treatment regimes. The goal is optimum management of injury and disease by patients to maximize chances of full recovery, and to minimize the risk of complications or relapse. The ED nurse determines the specific behaviour(s) required and supplies the appropriate information, discharge advice, reassurance and patient teaching to achieve this. Obvious examples of daily practice include, for example, advice and information on how to care for a fractured limb in a plaster cast or a sprained ligament or minor head injury, an outline of what potential problems to be alert to and what rehabilitative and preventive actions the patient can take. This is reinforced by an information sheet that the patient and their significant others can take away for reference, and the Accident Department contact telephone number should a problem arise.

Tertiary health promotion essentially adopts the same methods as secondary but it is applied to patients presenting to ED with exacerbations of chronic problems. The issues for consideration are likely to be more complex and more detailed health promotion input may be provided by specialist health care professionals from without the department prior to discharge. The author concedes, however, that the severity of the presenting condition may warrant emergency admission and thus health promotion of the type described above may be problematic, ineffective and inappropriate.

At a simplistic level part of the process of *The Nurse as Behaviour Change Agent* can be likened to an electrical system model (Hills 1979). This undermines the complexity of the nurse–patient interpersonal interaction by reducing it to a mechanistic relationship, but it serves a purpose and can be illustrated as follows:

Input > Coding > Channel > Decoding > Output

The nurse provides the input and the coding and the patient is the decoder. The method is concerned with the sender (ED nurse/expert) validating facts and transmitting knowledge to the receiver (patient), with the latter feeding back information on how the sender's messages have been received.

Ewles and Shipster (1984) take this one step further and refer to intervention of this nature as a three-stage process as follows:

- giving information or advice to a patient about his/ her injury/disease;
- ensuring that the patient understands and remembers that information or advice;
- ensuring that the patient is able to act on the information or advice.

They stress the need to define the objectives and desired outcome for the intervention, to give the information in a structured way emphasizing and repeating the important aspects, and the need to use short words and short sentences to avoid any misunderstanding. If there are any dangers with this crucial facet of ED nursing, it is that the process becomes a 'telling rather than listening' top-down one-way 'didactic model of nurse patient relationships' (Macleod Clark, Wilson-Barnet, Latter 1991) reinforcing the status of the nurse, and engendering patient deference and dependence. The emphasis on professionally determined needs may fail to consider the patients' perception of needs, their social, economic or environmental context or to achieve their participation in care. Examples of the aims, methods, impact and outcomes of *The Nurse as Behaviour Change Agent* are summarized in Table 33.1.

THE NURSE AS STRATEGIC PRACTITIONER

This model of practice fits with what Beattie (1991) refers to as 'Legislative Action for Health'. Here, social factors and social conditions are seen as the major determinants of health status. Social class is considered to be beyond the control of individuals but instrumental in influencing their way of life and thus health status. The poor health experiences and higher accident rates of the lower occupational groups are attributed to these class differentials and concomitant socio-economic inequalities, including the unequal distribution of income, wealth and capital (Townsend & Davidson 1990, Whitehead 1990, Blackburn 1991, Acheson 1998).

Contributions to population (macro) health gain can be achieved by legislative and environmental interventions governing issues such as welfare provision, taxation, the distribution of resources and pollution. The action of industry and persuasive advertising can be monitored and controlled and laws can be enacted. With regard to the latter, and with a particular resonance for ED nurses, Tones and Tilford (2001) report that education to encourage the wearing of front seatbelts was successful to a degree, but that legislation has been much more successful in enforcing their use and has changed the pattern of injury following a road traffic accident, helping to reduce mortality and morbidity.

Although not a feature of patient interaction, *The Nurse as Strategic Practitioner* approach could engage ED nurses in collecting data to construct a profile of the pattern of local accidents, and use this to campaign for traffic-calming measures in residential areas or improved street lighting. This would involve nurses lobbying local policy-makers by submitting written and verbal evidence to appropriate forums (within the boundaries of confidentiality and NMC guidelines) and taking every opportunity to be involved in partnership and multi-agency working. Nationally ED nurses can lobby power-holders through their professional organizations and specialist forums. These can align themselves with other pressure groups to address such issues as poverty and welfare provision, car design, drinking and driving, health and safety laws governing the workplace and advertising bans, e.g. tobacco, or the emphasis placed on the high performance of cars, etc.

More closely related to patients, this frame of reference can be applied from an organizational perspective, and thus what Tones and Tilford (2001) refer to as Meso Level, to an emergency department. The focus is on resource management, clinical governance, quality and standards, education and training issues and collaborative care planning, all of which are concerned with promoting patient population health gain. Resource management could enhance standards of care delivery by effective skill mix (e.g. numbers of nurses on a shift having undergone recognized post-registration training courses) and deployment of senior staff. Standard setting could state the quality levels expected within the department and this could be aligned with promoting evidence-based practice.

Implementation of recognized processes such as trauma scoring, the use of nationally recognized protocols such as those for advanced life support, asthma etc. and appropriate directives from the National Service Frameworks can be closely monitored. The feasibility of service developments and their potential for health gain, such as the establishment of trauma teams, could be explored. These examples of how *The Nurse as Strategic Practitioner* might be adapted and applied by ED nurses are summarized in Table 33.2 in relation to the aims, methods, impact and outcomes of practice.

THE NURSE AS EMPOWERMENT FACILITATOR

Of the previous strategies explored, *The Nurse as Behaviour Change Agent* and *The Nurse as Strategic Practitioner* involve professionally led direct and indirect health promotion respectively and a more traditional demeanour. Neither set out with the purpose of achieving health promotion outcomes in a patient-centred, non-hierarchical, non-coercive way aiming at active participation and thus pragmatic empowerment. *The Nurse as Empowerment Facilitator* seeks to achieve this in two ways: first, and primarily, by enabling and supporting patients to set their own health promotion agendas and by developing scope for personal choice and change following individual patient reflection and clarification of existing health-related behaviours; second, and as a minor role, by seeking to improve health by encouraging and supporting the development of social networks and 'social capital' (Cooper et al. 1999), albeit in the ED context specifically in relation to injury and disease, and by enabling the collective health agenda of like-minded patients and their carers.

This mode of intervention is flagged up because it fits with the developing consumer culture and moves to empower patients' pervading health and social care. Examples of developments in this direction include moves to promote actively an expert patient persona in those with chronic illness (see DoH 2001) and representation for patients via patient advice and liaison services (DoH 2002).

Providing information about the cause and effect of disease may be an important facet of such health promotion, but fundamentally ED nurses would listen rather than just tell. They would strive towards individual patient empowerment through acknowledging and enabling their right to participate actively in decisions on clinical matters, ensuring they were aware of the options open to them and able to exercise informed choice at every opportunity. ED nurses would support patients during this process, act as advocates when required and assist them to acknowledge and draw on their personal resources and strengths to maximize their autonomy. As such, existing power relations between the nurse and the patient would be challenged and equalized and the distance between the two parties reduced.

A model currently popular and compatible with *The Nurse as Empowerment Facilitator* is the Stages of Change (Prochaska & Diclemente 1982). A detailed outline of this work is beyond the scope of this chapter and the reader is referred to the authors' original work for a clear exposition of this process and to Naidoo and Wills (2000). Briefly, however, the cycle has stages through which people who change successfully move, whatever the variety of behaviour. 'Contemplation', the point at which people enter the cycle, represents a form of cognitive dissonance where people become aware of themselves, the nature of their behaviour and its negative consequences and think about the positive consequences of change. At this stage they continue the behaviour, e.g. smoking. 'Action' is when a person has decided to effect change, 'Maintenance' is the point at which there is a belief in the ability to maintain change and 'Relapse', an integral part of the cycle, is where the behaviour and contemplation or pre-contemplation stage is reverted to.

It is of course unrealistic to think that ED nurses would accompany a patient through the entire cycle of change. The process is referred to as it is desirable for ED nurses to have an understanding greater than that alluded to here to enable appropriate supportive intervention in relation to the stage the patient has reached. This would include, for example, referring people who want to stop smoking to smoking-cessation services during the 'contemplation' stage of the cycle.

In addition, ED nurses need to acknowledge the impact of social factors on health, have a knowledge of national and local self-help and support groups and be able to direct appropriate patients towards these. This would necessitate accident departments holding directories of local activity and key contacts. Such groups help reduce isolation, enable patients and/or their relatives and loved ones to use their collective resources to determine their common needs, shape their agenda for 'health' and build support networks. The group members can share experiences, offer coping strategies and draw strength from each other. They can also challenge the medical and nursing professions and lobby for change in both service provision and societal attitudes. Examples of the aims, methods, impact and outcomes of *The Nurse as Empowerment Facilitator* are summarized in Table 33.3.

CONCLUSION

This chapter has endeavoured to combine a brief theoretical discussion on the nature of health promotion with a translation of how the complementary and contradictory models, each with different aims, methods and outcomes relate to ED nursing. It is the author's contention that health promotion is an intrinsic part of holistic ED nursing and that the three models outlined enable legitimate ED health promotion activity, but to varying degrees. Clearly *The Nurse as*

Behaviour Change Agent has considerable and obvious application for individual patients, but equally importantly the collective patient agenda can be addressed by *The Nurse as Strategic Practitioner*, which also delivers valuable indirect health gain. The contribution of the individual and population *Empowerment Facilitation* model to ED nursing is perhaps more limited, but still has a place. The former is important in terms of the absolute right of patients to have control over their own health and health-related decision making where possible and is in line with the developing consumer culture in healthcare. Finally, the author is aware that this chapter may re-label as health promotion, rather than re-shape, elements of existing practice.

References

Acheson D (1998) *Independent Inquiry into Inequalities in Health Report*. London: The Stationery Office.

Beattie A (1991) Knowledge and control in health promotion: a test case for social policy and social theory. In: Gabe J, Calnan M, Bury M (eds). *The Sociology of the Health Service*. Routledge: London.

Blackburn C (1991) *Poverty and Health*. Open University Press: Buckingham.

Brown PA, Piper SM (1997) Nursing and the health of the nation: schism or symbiosis? *Journal of Advanced Nursing*, **25**, 297–310.

Cooper H, Arber S, Fee L, Ginn J (1999) *The Influence of Social Support and Social Capital on Health: a Review and Analysis of British Data*. London: Health Education Authority.

Department of Health (1992) *The Health of the Nation: A Strategy for Health in England*. HMSO: London.

Department of Health (1993) *The Health of the Nation: Key Area Handbook Accidents*. London: HMSO.

Department of Health (1993) *Targeting Practice: The Contribution of Nurses, Midwives and Health Visitors*. The Health of the Nation: London: HMSO.

Department of Health (1999) *Saving Lives: Our Healthier Nation*. London: HMSO.

Department of Health (2000) *The NHS Plan: A Plan for Investment, a Plan for Reform*. London: HMSO.

Department of Health (2001) *The Expert Patient: A New Approach to Chronic Disease Management for the 21st century*. London: Department of Health.

Department of Health (2002) *Patient Advice and Liaison Service*. London: Department of Health.

Department of Health (2004) *Better Information, Better Choices, Better Health: Putting Information at the Centre of Health*. London: Department of Health.

Department of Health (2004) *Choosing Health: Making Healthy Choices Easier*. London: TSO.

Ewles L, Shipster P (1984) *One to One Health Education*. South East Thames Regional Health Authority: London.

Hills P (1979) *Teaching and Learning as a Communication Process*. Croom Helm: London.

Macleod Clark J, Wilson-Barnett J, Latter S (1991) *Health Education in Nursing Project: Results of a National Survey on Senior Nurses' Perceptions of Health Education Practice in Acute Ward Settings*. Department of Nursing Studies, King's College, University of London Education Authority.

Mitchell J (1982) Looking after ourselves: an individual responsibility? *Royal Society of Health Journal*, **4**: 169–173.

Naidoo J, Wills J (2000) *Health Promotion: Foundations for Practice*, 2nd edn. London: Baillière Tindall. Ch. 11.

Naidoo J, Wills J (2001) *Health Studies: An Introduction*. Basingstoke: Palgrave, Ch. 10.

Piper SM, Brown PA (1998) The theory and practice of health education applied to nursing: a bi-polar approach. *Journal of Advanced Nursing*, Feb. 27, 383–389.

Piper SM (2004) An interpretive inquiry testing the relationship between health promotion theory and nursing practice. Unpublished Thesis: APU.

Prochaska JO, Diclemente CC (1982) Transtheoretical therapy: towards a more integrated model of change. psychotherapy, *Theory, Research and Practice*, **19**(3): 276–288.

Tones K (1990) Why theorise? Ideology in Health Education. *Health Education Journal*, **49**(1): 26.

Tones K, Tilford S (2001) *Health Education: Effectiveness, Efficiency and Equity*, 3rd edn. Cheltenham: Nelson Thornes.

Tones K, Green J (2004) *Health Promotion: Planning and Strategies*. London: Sage.

Townsend P, Davidson N (1990) *Inequalities in Health. The Black Report*. Penguin: London.

Whitehead M (1990) *Inequalities in Health. The Health Divide*. Penguin: London.

Chapter 34

Triage

Janet Marsden

CHAPTER CONTENTS

INTRODUCTION

Triage is a system of clinical risk management used in emergency settings (EDs, walk-in centres, minor injury units, general practice) where an undifferentiated and unexpected caseload arrives at a point of care. It is used worldwide to manage the patient flow through these areas safely, when need exceeds the capacity of the service. This chapter will focus on the development of triage roles, types and systems.

THE CONCEPT OF TRIAGE

The word triage originates from the French verb 'trier', meaning 'to sort'. The origins of triage are well documented (Bracken 2003). It was originally used as a means of grading the quality of goods such as coffee beans and wool, and was first adopted for use in a medical context during the Napoleonic wars. For the first time, casualties were treated on the basis of medical need rather than rank or social status. It has been used in every war since, as a means of managing mass casualties. While the term triage is used in both military/disaster triage and emergency departments, it must be recognized that the two processes fulfil very different functions.

Peacetime nursing triage emerged in the United States in the early 1960s, during the war in Vietnam. Highly trained paramedics moved across into civilian hospitals, taking their triage skills with them and adapting the process for use within EDs. It was not until the 1980s that the concept of nurse triage became popular in the UK (Edwards 1999). EDs began introducing schemes around this time, based largely on the experiences of American nursing colleagues.

Emergency department attenders

The unpredictability of workloads within emergency settings and the steadily increasing numbers of attenders are well recognized and documented (Mallet & Woolwich 1990, National Audit Office 2004, Department of Health 2006a). During a 24-hour period a wide spectrum of accidents and emergencies may be seen, sometimes stretching the resources of the department and staff to their limit, and Walk-in Centres and NHS Direct have not been demonstrated to reduce attendance in EDs (Cooke 2005).

Prior to nurse triage, the waiting room was an unknown quantity for the ED staff. It could be full of patients with a diverse range of illnesses and injuries, of varying degrees of severity. There was a risk of a patient's condition deteriorating while waiting to be seen. It is inevitable that with the ever-increasing demands on a finite service, longer waiting times develop for the most vulnerable group of patients; those who are seriously ill and in need of immediate emergency care and treatment. Recognition of all these factors highlights the need for all patients to be assessed on arrival in the ED by a person skilled in triage.

The purpose of triage

The purpose of triage in the emergency care setting is not to reduce the overall waiting time for all patients. Mallet & Woolwich (1990) have shown, in line with other studies, that while the waiting times for the more seriously ill were reduced, overall departmental waiting times steadily increased. The purpose of triage is to 'make the best possible use of the available medical and nursing personnel and facilities' and it is there to assist in determining 'which patients need immediate care ... and which patients can wait' (Potter 1985).

The role and aims of triage

Budassi & Barber (1981) defined the role of triage as 'the process of deciding the priorities for the therapeutic interventions of a given individual or individuals and the place where these interventions should occur'. Therefore, the primary aim of the triage nurse must be the early assessment of patients, in order to determine the priority of care according to the individual's clinical need. There are other aspects of care, however, that nurse triage can meet (Handyside 1996), for instance, more efficient use of the department facilities and resources as patients are allocated to the most appropriate clinical areas within the department and are seen and treated within an

appropriate time. As triage should be a dynamic process, regular reassessment of patients ensures that the appropriateness of the care implemented can be modified as necessary.

The early and appropriate requesting of medical records or relevant previous X-rays will aid clinical assessment and diagnosis. Appropriate first-aid measures can be taken without delay and analgesia appropriate to the patients' level of pain can be given.

The waiting area is now a known quantity and patient flow can be controlled and organized (Ramler & Mohammed 1995). Patients and their relatives have an easily identifiable and reliable source of information for any enquiries. This helps to relieve anxiety and reduce aggression and can increase patient satisfaction with the service (Dolan 1998).

TYPES OF TRIAGE

Non–professional triage

Patients arrive in the ED, register with the receptionist and then sit in the waiting area, without any form of assessment, until they are called to be seen by the clinician. The receptionist will only call a clinician if there appears to be some reason for concern.

In the UK, non-professional triage can still be found functioning in some departments and is more frequently used at certain times, e.g. at night when staff and resources are limited. Mallet & Woolwich (1990) identified this as an area of great concern in their study of nurse triage in an inner-city ED and recommended the provision of a nurse triage service during the night shift. Their concerns are echoed in the findings of a large study of the use of health care assistants (HCAs) in English EDs, which found that HCAs assessed patients on arrival in 28.7% of the 282 departments that responded to the survey (Boyes 1995).

Triage tends to have been recognized as a system which must be undertaken by a competent clinician; however, there are a number of emergency care settings where non-professional triage may be, while not the system of choice, the system which has to be lived with. Walk-in centres and minor injury units may not have levels of professional staff in which a qualified nurse can be allocated to a triage role. Nurses undertaking advanced practice roles are likely to be dealing with existing patients, away from the waiting area and therefore are not aware of the clinical need of those patients walking into the department. Similarly, in general practice, the receptionist is always the first point of contact for the patient and there is little chance of a clinician being present when a patient who needs urgent care walks in. In these circumstances it is imperative that reception staff have a clear set of guidelines to work from to help them to identify those patients for whom urgent professional care must be obtained. Algorithms may be developed which reception staff are able to work through and appropriate training must be given to aid reception staff to undertake this crucial role.

Professional triage

Triage may be undertaken by a range of professionals in emergency care settings such as nurses, medical staff, ambulance paramedics and emergency care practitioners (ECPs). What needs to be common among these clinicians is experience and education. Because triage often uses algorithms to enable reproducible decisions in the care setting, it might be felt that it could be undertaken by anyone working in the setting. The level of decision-making which takes place within the rapid triage encounter requires sound clinical judgement which must be based on professional experience, knowledge and skill. The triage practitioner must be able to interpret, discriminate and evaluate the information he gathers from the patient, relative and carer and must be able to reflect on their decision-making and critically appraise it (Mackway-Jones et al. 2005).

Telephone triage

A major expansion of the triage process has been the recognition and development of telephone triage. As in the case of face-to-face triage, this strategy was first identified in the US (Simenson 2001).

Advice-giving over the telephone has always been a part of the clinician's role, although not one which has been recognized as having a particularly distinct identity. Formalized advice-giving by telephone has the potential to be a valuable tool in many settings – a fact that has been recognized in the development of NHS Direct in England and Wales and NHS 24 in Scotland. Some 6.8 million calls were made to NHS Direct in England in 2005 (Department of Health 2006b).

Telephone triage was first described as a useful emergency care strategy in the UK by Buckles and Carew-McColl in 1991. Various benefits have been attributed to it, including reduced attendance due to explanations and self-care advice, redirection of patients to more appropriate agencies, pre-identification of patient problems, cost-effectiveness, in terms of reduction in workload, and patient empowerment.

Telephone triage has many difficulties. The patient is not visible, so many of the cues which experienced

clinicians take from the patient's appearance and behaviour are not available. The information may be gained from an intermediary such as a relative or neighbour or another health professional who may not know the patient well (Marsden 2000).

Telephone triage must be approached as a distinct role and not undertaken by the member of staff who happens to be passing the telephone when it rings. Early studies of telephone triage suggested that patient assessment in telephone triage was, on the whole, subjective and required careful questioning which was often poor and carried out by unqualified personnel. A designated telephone triage clinician should be the first point of contact for telephone advice or triage in the emergency care setting. Decisions should be as reproducible as those made in face-to-face triage and, therefore, protocols or algorithms need to be developed. A key feature of these must be advice for the patient or carer – advice on self care if the decision is made that this is appropriate, but also advice for the patient or carer about what do to in the interim period between the call and the access to emergency care. This might include advice on basic life support while the ambulance service is directed to the caller

The demarcation line between telephone advice and telephone triage is debatable. But it may be considered that triage occurs when a formalized process of decision-making takes place which allows identification of a clinical priority and allocation to predetermined categories of urgency of need for clinical evaluation and care. Many EDs and walk-in centres no longer offer telephone advice and have a direct transfer to NHS Direct or NHS 24 as appropriate.

What professional triage can become

As stated above, proponents of triage have never claimed that it reduced waiting times in the emergency care setting, merely that it acts as a risk-management tool, prioritizing services in a setting where demand often outstrips capacity. The triage encounter should be a rapid and reproducible assessment which accurately allocates a priority to each patient based on clinical need. A national triage system has been adopted in Portugal, using one of the systems most often used in the UK, the Manchester Triage System, and reports, nationally, that the triage encounter need take no more than 90 seconds (Lipley 2005).

At this initial assessment, opportunities have often been taken for clinicians to 'add in' other aspects of examination and investigation and the triage encounter includes much more than assessment, first aid and prioritization. It is used as a time to administer analgesia, to refer patients to X-ray or other investigations, to give advice about self-care and to initiate patient pathways to other specialities. This vastly increases the time taken to triage each patient and, whereas the triaged patients in the waiting room are a known quantity, the risk is transferred to the queue for triage. The triage assessment has become an 'MOT' rather than the 'pit stop'.

SEE AND TREAT

The premise at the beginning of this chapter is that triage is used to prioritize resources when supply does not meet demand. Where there is sufficient capacity in the emergency care setting, it is clear that prioritization is not required. One of the developments in emergency care in the UK has been the utilization of a 'See and Treat' model in the 'minor' areas of emergency care settings.

The challenge for emergency department in the UK is to provide fast, fair and convenient access to health care in all sectors. There should be minimal wait for care with the right clinicians caring for the right patients at the right time (Windle 2005) and this had been a major challenge for emergency settings. A survey of patient experiences showed that patients prioritized waiting times, especially for less severe conditions, as their main issue of concern (Cooke et al. 2002).

See and Treat is a system of emergency-department organization where patients with minor conditions are seen very quickly after they arrive in an emergency department by a senior clinician. Providing their problem is appropriate, such patients are examined, have definitive treatment and are then discharged (NHS Modernization Agency 2004). This system of care emerged from the need to deal with long waiting times in emergency departments experienced particularly by those with the most minor presentations. It is not new, however, as Redmond described such a service development in 1983 (Redmond & Buxton 1993).

Key concepts in See and Treat

- On arrival, patients are seen, treated and referred or discharged by one practitioner.
- The first person to see the patients, usually a nurse or doctor, is able to make autonomous clinical decisions about treatment, investigations and discharge.
- Other, more seriously ill patients or those requiring in-depth assessment or treatment should be streamed to, and dealt with in, the appropriate area.

- Triage of walk-in patients is unnecessary when See and Treat is in operation and patients are seen shortly after arrival.
- Dedicated staff allocated to separate areas and only withdrawn in exceptional circumstances.
- The system should operate with enough people to allow effective consultations without a queue developing. For instance, one doctor and one nurse has been shown to be effective for an arrival rate of up to 10 walk-in patients per hour.
- Staff development should be undertaken to ensure that all staff involved in See and Treat are able to make the system work effectively (NHS Modernization Agency 2004).

There is no doubt that streaming in the emergency department and the use of See and Treat models has had a major effect on patient throughput (Shrimpling 2002) and has been endorsed by both the RCN Emergency Care Association and British Association for Emergency Medicine (BAEM). However, See and Treat is not without criticism, including the problems of the most senior clinicians dealing with the least serious presentations, thus potentially leaving the small number of seriously ill or injured patients being cared for by less experienced and less well supervised staff, the burn-out or boredom of senior clinicians dealing with interminable minor problems (Leaman 2003, Windle & Mackway Jones 2003) and the lack of adequate evaluation and evidence on which to roll out such programmes (Wardrope & Driscoll 2003).

It is clear though that where See and Treat services work optimally, where there is little or no queue and where there are always enough clinicians to manage the patient at the point of entry, triage is not necessary.

In many emergency departments though, while this may be a true picture on occasion, it is not likely to be the case all the time, with high patient attendance and sub-optimal staffing being the norm in most EDs. There is no doubt that waiting time is reduced using a See and Treat model in many cases but, while waiting times may be reduced, they still exist and where there is any wait at all to be seen by a clinician the waiting room becomes an unknown quantity and clinicians are back to the situation pre-triage where there was no knowledge of who was waiting and a major clinical risk-management issue. Just because a patient walks into the emergency department, it cannot be assumed that his problem is minor.

In any such situation, triage is not only necessary but essential in order to evaluate and prioritize waiting patients and manage the clinical risk. Many departments have implemented a policy of restarting triage when the queue for See and Treat reaches a critical point. The critical point should be determined centrally, after a careful analysis of case mix and workload predictions, and may be anything from 15 to perhaps 45 minutes and beyond. The decision to take the risk of not assessing patients who walk into the department for this length of time is one of 'acceptable' risk and the validity of the acceptability of the risk will only be indicated by the lack of critical incidents associated with it over time. The issues around stopping and restarting triage are clear though – when the wait for See and Treat has increased, who will be made available to begin to triage patients when taking a clinician away from an area will inevitably lead to further delays? This must be balanced though against the clinical governance issues involved here, and flexibility needs to be built into streaming systems to allow them to function safely when their performance is suboptimal due to problems with workload or staffing.

See and Treat is a strategy for use with those patients with minor conditions. For those patients who do not fall into this category, triage is an essential first part of the prioritization and risk management process.

PATIENT ASSESSMENT

Triage, as stated earlier, should be a rapid, relatively superficial assessment taking no longer than a few minutes. Its purpose is to elicit information from the patient in order to determine their presenting problem. While in some cases this may be a quite straightforward process, e.g. a patient presenting with a clear history of simple uncomplicated trauma to an extremity, a significant proportion of attenders to the ED present with a more complex history involving various contributing factors which pre-empted their current illness or injury. It is the latter presentation that calls on the skills of the triage nurse.

Various assessment tools have been developed which will aid the nurse in decision-making and encourage standardization of patients' assessments and subsequent collation of information. SOAP is an assessment tool devised in the US in 1969 (Lee & Fraser 1981). An 'I' for 'implementation' has been added after SOAP and an 'E' to emphasize the need for continual evaluation (Blythin 1988a,b). Blythin's SOAPE became one of the first and most extensively used triage tools in the UK.

One of the potential problems with using this tool for the less experienced nurse is that by working systematically through the acronym, the nurse becomes caught up with the S – subjective assessment – and fails to reach the A, the actual assessment. Although S is the first letter, A and O are crucial elements of the tool. It is the objective assessment (O) which is often the best indicator of a patient's urgency for need of care. There is a rapid absorption of data which combines with a mental comparison with previous cases as the general appearance of the patient is assimilated by the triage nurse from the moment he comes into view. Along with a triage first impression (A), the objective assessment is often the critical factor when making a triage decision. It needs to be understood that the documentation of a triage decision, using any of the assessment tools devised, is secondary to the process of making that decision.

Other assessment tools have included the mnemonic PQRST (Budassi & Barber 1981). They also suggest a tool involving the use of the five senses – looking, listening, smelling, touching and thinking – to evaluate a patient's chief complaint (see Boxes 34.1, 34.2 and 34.3).

Box 34.1 The SOAP model of triage

S   Subjective assessment–The patient's evaluation of their illness or injury

O   Objective assessment–An evaluation based on observable and measurable data

A   Assessment–The clinical impression

P   Plan of care

Box 34.2 PQRST model of triage assessment

P–Provokes– What makes the pain better or worse?

Q–Quality– What does it feel like? Suggestions may be offered to encourage a description, such as, 'burning, stabbing, crushing'

R–Radiates– Where is the pain? Where does it go? Is it in one spot? Show me where it is

S–Severity– Give the pain a score out of ten

T–Time– How long have you had it? When did it start? When did it end?

Box 34.3	Systematic assessment model of triage
EYES	List all the things that you can see
EARS	What is the patient saying and *not* saying? Listen for breath sounds, audible wheeze
NOSE	Smell for ketones, alcohol, incontinence, infection
HANDS	Take the pulse, feel the skin temperature, assess capillary perfusion. Touch 'where it hurts'
BRAIN	Use an assessment tool to aid your triage decision, for example, SOAPE or PQRST

DECISION–MAKING STRATEGIES

There are many theories of decision-making and a number of strategies used in the decision-making process. Unstructured triage methods may involve the triage clinician coming to a decision about a triage category with very little structure on which to base the decision.

Symptom clustering is a method used to assist in determining the clinical need of the patient. Using existing knowledge and experience, the nurse groups together symptoms and aims to identify the severity of the patient's condition. In this manner, 'chest pain' can be more easily associated with a cardiac condition if the symptom cluster includes nausea, shortness of breath on exertion, grey or clammy pallor, radiation of pain to the jaw or left arm, 'crushing' type pain or a 'tight band' across the chest. Conversely, a symptom cluster which includes increased pain on coughing and deep inspiration, shortness of breath on talking, and a productive cough would be more indicative of a respiratory or pulmonary condition (Rund & Rausch 1981).

'Clinical portraits' or pattern recognition is a strategy very commonly used by clinicians (Alfaro-LeFevre 2004). There are some illnesses and injuries that are so easily recognizable and that present so often in the ED that a very clear 'clinical portrait' can be recognized. A symptom cluster narrows the options to a recognized injury or disease process in a particular system. Clinicians interpret the information they gain from the patient and compare it with previous cases. The very fast processing of information undertaken along with years of experience of different presentations and groups of symptoms is recognizable in expert practitioners. This is a technique which develops with experience and may appear to be intuitive.

Benner's (1984) model of skill acquisition looks at the way in which expertise in an area develops through an individual's experience. The novice, proficient or competent practitioner tends to use conscious decision-making where the expert is able to utilize pattern recognition.

Repetitive hypothesizing is a technique also employed by clinicians to test their diagnostic reasoning. By gathering data to prove or refute a particular hypothesis, a decision can be made.

It has been suggested that if the triage categories are clear and unequivocal, the role of the triage nurse can be carried out by any nurse, novice or expert, after the minimum training (Burgess 1992). The presence of a series of signs or symptoms will inherently warrant a particular priority, usually through the adherence to a written protocol in the form of flow charts, algorithms or simply lists of conditions in pre-designated priority categories.

Expertise is needed, however, as it is the experienced practitioner who is able to differentiate, for example, between cardiac and pleuritic chest pain; who understands that not all presentations of myocardial infarction are classical; who has an evidence base that tells them that women present with MI in different ways to men and is able to use all this knowledge to accurately allocate a triage category in a very rapid manner.

It should be recognized that the ability to ask the 'minimum of questions with the maximum of value' (Rund & Rausch 1981) comes with experience in the clinical area.

Priority setting

A reliable system of establishing priorities of care is the linchpin which determines the effectiveness of nurse triage. There may be circumstances whereby there are few data on which to determine a priority. Poor communication due to language difficulties is not uncommon, and the age or condition of the patient may also hinder the triage nurse in making an initial assessment.

DOCUMENTATION

The accurate documentation of nurse triage findings cannot be overemphasized. Estrada (1979) argued that it is a 'professional judgement made by a professional nurse' deserving of careful documentation. It is a means of communication and becomes an integral part of the patient's permanent medical record. As such, it also becomes a legal document for which the triage nurse becomes accountable and responsible. Indeed, the principle of personal accountability is fundamental to nursing practice. Documentation should be generated for all patients presenting to the emergency setting. If the patient leaves the department without waiting to see the doctor, it may be the only record of his attendance (Southard 1989).

When documenting the triage findings, a diagnosis should not be made. The purpose of nurse triage, as previously discussed, is not to establish a diagnosis. The initial assessment made by the triage nurse is no substitute for a full clinical examination, as diagnostic investigations may need to be carried out prior to any definitive diagnosis being made. In quieter departments, if the size of the caseload allows, other clinical information may be added: past medical history, allergies, medication, etc. These data may be used to initiate patient care plans and structured around the nursing model being used in the department. Duplications of information should be avoided, however, as the patient will be asked similar questions by the doctor or nurse practitioner (Jenkins 1996).

It must be recognized that there is little point in a triage episode which delays the patient being examined by a clinician and it should be kept as short as possible.

AUDIT

As triage is a fundamental cornerstone of clinical risk management in the emergency care setting, inaccurate triage is as much of a problem for the department as no triage, as there is no guarantee of safe clinical priorities and this would soon become a governance issue.

Triage systems must be both reproducible, so that every clinician will come to the same triage decision about the same patient, and auditable and continuous audit should be carried out to ensure that the quality of triage is consistent and that practitioners who are less than accurate are identified so that support mechanisms can be put in place. Initial training of staff in triage methodology does not guarantee ongoing competence. Mentoring after initial training is required and an assessment of competence should be carried out. Audit ensures ongoing competence and underpins the quality agenda. Areas that need to be examined include completeness of the documentation and accuracy of the decisions made.

Without complete documentation, the decision made may still be accurate, but there is no way of proving how and on what basis the decision was made. It might then have been a random decision which just happens to be correct.

A simple method of audit is to take a number of randomly generated triage episodes for each practitioner and examine them.

- Completeness of the episode can be expressed as a simple proportion
- Accuracy can be expressed as a simple proportion
- Feedback is given to the practitioner

- Causes of inaccuracy are fed back to the practitioner.

The auditor should be an expert triage practitioner who is fully conversant with the triage method used in a particular department. Unless clinicians within the area are experienced triage practitioners and undertake triage regularly, it is not appropriate for them to audit the practice of those who do.

To ensure consistency of audit, a sample, perhaps 10% of episodes assessed, should be assessed independently by a second expert practitioner. Any differences in perception or decision would be moderated by discussion between the two.

Continuous audit can be time-consuming but is more effective than a set audit period where the triage practitioners know that their work is going to be scrutinized and may perform to a different standard than usual.

A NATIONAL TRIAGE SCALE

The issue of uniformity and triage practice has been the subject of considerable discussion and debate. Following similar initiatives in Australia and Canada, a joint working party with members from both the Royal College of Nursing (RCN) ED Association and the British Association for ED Medicine (BAEM) led to the development of a standard five-point triage scale (Crouch & Marrow 1996). The scale was defined in terms of the maximum time the patient should wait before definitive clinical intervention.

Triage categories are linked to 'time to clinician' targets and, while the scale has been modified as reforms in emergency care and system redesign have led to 98% of patients being discharged from the emergency department within a window of four hours, in general, the categories still apply to all patients attending the emergency care setting.

The categories are colour-coded, in rainbow fashion, from red for the patient needing immediate attention to blue for those patients who have a non-urgent problem

TRIAGE SYSTEMS

A number of triage systems are in place throughout the world and some of these are discussed here.

Manchester Triage System

The Manchester Triage System (MTS) was first published in 1996 and was the result of the recognition by clinicians in emergency department in Manchester, UK, that triage over the health economy was a muddle. A group of around 20 senior emergency physicians and nurses spent a considerable amount of time formulating a solution which would be used in all emergency departments across the city. It was never envisaged that the system would be used outside the city. However, it seemed to appear at a time when triage was identified as an absolute necessity in most emergency departments and MTS became the triage system of choice in at least 90% of the UK's EDs. It appears that the system is generic enough and timely enough to have caught the imagination of EDs across the world. MTS has become the national triage system of Portugal and Holland and is used extensively in a number of European countries and beyond. It is now used, translated into many languages, to triage tens of millions of emergency department attenders each year.

This triage method aims to give a clinical priority to each patient. It was recognized very early on in the group's deliberations that the length of the triage consultation means that any attempt to diagnose at triage is fraught with difficulty and doomed to fail. Even if diagnosis were possible, it is not necessarily linked to the patient's clinical priority, as other issues, such as the level of pain, will change the triage priority. It was also recognized by the group that the triage practitioner tends to look for a symptom and then hypothesize around a particular presentation or diagnosis, seeking symptoms and signs which give them permission to allocate the patient a higher triage priority, rather than assuming the worst and then eliminating signs and symptoms and moving down to a lower priority – a much safer way of working.

The key feature of the MTS is that it is reductive. The worst scenario and highest triage category is used until the patient can definitely be removed from that category (Mackway-Jones et al. 2005).

The triage practitioner is required to choose from a range of 50 presentational flow charts and seek a limited number of signs and symptoms at each level of priority. The signs and symptoms that discriminate between the different priorities are called discriminators and the assessment is carried out by finding the highest level at which the answer given to a discriminator question is positive.

Presentational flow charts are consistent in their approach so that whether the triage practitioner chooses the 'Unwell Adult' chart or the 'Diarrhoea and Vomiting' chart with which to assess a patient, the same priority will apply.

A number of general discriminators apply to every chart

- Life threat (vital ABC functions)
- Haemorrhage

- Pain
- Conscious level
- Temperature
- Acuteness.

From the perspective of the patient, pain is a major factor in determining priority and the use of this as a general discriminator in every chart recognized the priority placed on pain by the patient. The MTS has been criticized for giving pain this level of priority, the concern being that patients will exaggerate their pain in order to achieve a higher priority for care; however, this is not borne out in practice. Pain should be part of every triage assessment as it is the most frequent symptom which prompts a patient to attend any emergency care setting. Ignoring pain is to ignore what is often most important to the patient. The use of a pain tool with behavioural characteristics such as that in the MTS allows the clinician to amend a pain score based on whether behaviour matches the patient's perceived pain, and this may be a move upwards as well as downwards. The use of appropriate analgesia at triage enables pain to be managed early in the patient encounter, and dynamic triage should ensure that a triage priority can be amended if required as pain is controlled.

One of the key tenets of the MTS is that clinical priority should not be confused with management. Different patients will be managed differently in different emergency settings. It may be appropriate to manage, for example, children, quickly, but this decision should not effect a change in clinical priority. The priority is decided by their presentation and the management by the needs and particular circumstances of the department.

There has been some criticism of the MTS triage model since its inception, based on the lack of evidence for its claim to fitness for purpose and its lack of evaluation. While consensus may be the weakest form of evidence, where it is the only evidence it has credibility. Since its introduction, research has emerged to validate the system and a number of publications are available.

Each presentation is based on the best available evidence and has been updated in the second edition as clinical guidelines have changed. A national training strategy is in place for those units who use this method of triage.

Another use of MTS

MTS has now been validated by research and by its use throughout the world. Changes in emergency care practice have led to the recognition that it can be used as part of the streaming process in a concept known as the presentation priority matrix (Mackway-Jones et al. 2005). As the emergency care 'village' becomes more of a reality, the emergency department may not be the most appropriate place for the presenting patient to receive care.

Presentations and discriminators can be mapped against disposition for each emergency care setting: for example, Chest Pain priority 1 will always go to the resuscitation area.

An eye problem may always go to an Emergency Eye Centre where there is one, but may be seen in the general ED where there is no specialist eye provision. Torso injury at level 4 or 5 might be appropriately streamed to the minor injury unit.

Each emergency 'Village' can create a matrix of presentations and dispositions for their local health economy in discussion with all those involved in emergency care provision, including the ambulance service, who can then also work to ensure that patients get the best care in the best place at an appropriate time.

Disposition will, of course, be influenced by what services are available at a particular time. For instance, the minor injury unit or primary care centre may be closed in the evenings, by the current pressures on these services and by the patient's choice.

The Australasian Triage Scale (ATS)

This was developed in Australia from a comprehensive review of the Australian National Triage Scale and was released in 2001. The five categories are based on time to doctor, although this is being debated as nurse clinician roles are ever developing. The category 1 patient is immediate and the category 5 should be seen within 2 hours.

All patients presenting to an ED should be triaged on arrival by a specifically trained and experienced registered nurse. The triage assessment and ATS code allocated must be recorded. The triage assessment involves a combination of the presenting problem and general appearance of the patient and may be combined with pertinent physiological observations. Vital signs are only measured at triage to estimate urgency or if time permits.

Clinical descriptors are listed for each triage category based on available research evidence and expert consensus. The list is not exhaustive or absolute and is considered to be indicative only. Physiological measurements should not be used as the only indicator for allocating to a triage category (ACEM 2005).

During revision of the National Triage Scale, it was recognized that there were many problems associated with inconsistency of application of the scale and also with education for the triage role and, in 2002, the Commonwealth funded the development of a Triage Education Resource Book. The content of the book was developed with the assistance from professional organizations that represent emergency department nurses and the Australasian College for Emergency Medicine and this is used as the basis for triage training (ACEM 2005).

Canada Triage and Acuity scale

The Canada Triage and Acuity Scale was developed, based on the National Triage Scale in Australia. Its use became official policy in Canada in 1997 (Zimmermann 2006). Categories are time-based and congruent with the ATS.

The Canadian ED triage and acuity scale is based on establishing a relationship between a group of sentinel events which are defined by the ICD9CM diagnosis at discharge from the ED, or from an in-patient data base, and the 'usual' way patients with these conditions present.

Re-evaluation of patients is built into the system and nurses are encouraged to upgrade the triage level of patients with lower triage scores if the time objective has not been met. Reassessment is also recommended, at different intervals for different categories of patients; level 4 patients should be reassessed every hour and level 5 every 2 hours.

The Canadian Association of Emergency Physicians state that:

1. All patients should be assessed, at least visually, within 10 minutes of arrival.
2. Full patient assessments should not be done in the triage area unless there are no other patients waiting. Only information required to assign a triage level should be recorded.
3. A primary survey (rapid assessment) should be used when there are 2 or more patients waiting to be triaged, and only after all patients have had some assessment done should level IV and V patients have a more complete assessment done by a triage or treatment nurse.
4. Priority for care may change following a more complete assessment or as patient's signs and symptoms change. There should be documentation of the initial triage as well as any changes. The initial triage level is still used for administrative purposes.
5. Level I and II patients should be in a treatment area and have the complete primary nursing assessment done immediately.

Lists of 'usual' presenting complaints and case scenarios are available to the triage nurse but are, again, not considered to be absolute. Triage personnel are encouraged to use their experience and instincts to 'up triage' priority, even if the patient does not seem to fit exactly with the facts or definitions on the triage scale, and the triage practitioner is asked to consider 'If they look sick then they probably are'. The CAEP strongly suggest that the triager's instinct should not be used to lower the triage level assignment when the facts suggest there may be a problem, but to take the more serious possibilities first and have someone find the proof that nothing is wrong (CAEP 2006).

The Emergency Severity Index Triage Scale

This was developed in the US in the late 1990s. Acuity and complexity are summarized on a 5-point scale where 1 is the highest acuity. It is based on acuity and on the likely resource consumption required to achieve a disposition and add what the patient needs on to when they need it (Zimmermann 2006). Resources include radiography, medications and laboratory tests and resource determination is the triage nurse's best guess based on experience of what the patient is likely to need. After the most life-threatening presentations are dealt with, patients needing 2 or more resources are Emergency Severity Index (ESI) 3, one resource is ESI4 and none is ESI5. Vital signs are used to make a triage decision about patients at ESI level 3 and above.

CONCLUSION

Emergency care continues to develop and care settings and organizations continually strive to meet the needs of patients and the demands of purchasers of services and central government. What is clear is that emergency care is dealing with infinite demand in a context of finite resources. Strategies such as Streaming and See and Treat aim to address some of the problems of a demand-led service, and where the resources match the service needs, where every patient in a minor stream can be met at the door and treated immediately, triage in the minor areas of emergency care settings is not required. The moment that that definitive management is delayed and a queue develops, risk is generated where patients with unknown problems are waiting for assessment.

Triage in other areas of emergency department must follow the same pattern. Where each patient can be treated immediately, triage is not required; however, for almost all of the time, a robust triage system will be needed to discriminate between those patients who need immediate and life-saving intervention and those who have a lower clinical priority.

Triage, when undertaken correctly as a rapid assessment and prioritization strategy, is the gold-standard risk-management tool in emergency care throughout the world. Experience and continuous education along with continuous audit lead to expert clinicians who can triage effectively and manage the work of the emergency care setting in the way that the patients deserve.

References

Alfaro-LeFevre R (2004) *Critical Thinking and Clinical Judgment: A Practical Approach*. Philadelphia: Elsevier Science.

Australasian College for Emergency Medicine (2005) *Guidelines on the Implementation of the Australasian Triage Scale in Emergency Departments*. Sydney: Australasian College for Emergency Medicine.

Buckles E, Carew-McColl M (1991) Triage by telephone. *Nursing Times*, **87**(6), 26–28.

Benner P (1984) *From Novice to Expert: Excellence and Power in Clinical Nursing Practice*. Menlow Park, CA: Addison-Wesley.

Blythin P (1988a) Triage – a nursing care system. In: Wright B, ed. *Managing and Practice in Emergency Nursing*. London: Chapman and Hall.

Blythin P (1988b) Triage in the UK. *Nursing*, **3**(31), 16–20.

Boyes A (1995) Health care assistants: delegation of tasks. *Emergency Nurse*, **3**(2), 6–9.

Bracken J (2003) Triage. In: Newbery L, ed. *Sheehy's Emergency Nursing: Principles and Practice*, 5th edn. St Louis: Mosby.

Budassi S, Barber JM (1981) *Emergency Nursing Principles and Practice*. St Louis: CV Mosby.

Burgess K (1992) A dynamic role that improves the service – combining triage and nurse practitioner roles in A&E. *Professional Nurse*, **7**(5), 301–303.

Canadian Association of Emergency Physicians (2006) *CTAS Implementation Guidelines*. Ottowa: CTAS.

Cooke MW, Wilson S, Pearson S (2002) The effect of a separate stream for minor injuries on accident and emergency department waiting times. *Emergency Medicine Journal*, **19**(1), 28–30.

Cooke M (2005) *Towards Faster Treatment: Reducing Attendance and Waits at Emergency Departments*. London: Department of Health.

Crouch R, Marrow J (1996) Towards a UK triage scale. *Emergency Nurse*, **4**(3), 4–5.

Department of Health (2002) *See and Treat*. London: Department of Health.

Department of Health (2006) *Hospital Activity Statistics*. London: Department of Health.

Department of Health (2006b) *Chief Executive's Report to the NHS*. London: Department of Health.

Dolan B (1998) A dynamic process (Editorial). *Emergency Nurse*, **6**(4), 1.

Edwards B (1999) What's wrong with triage? *Emergency Nurse*, **7**(4), 19–23.

Estrada EG (1979) Advanced triage by an RN. *Journal of Emergency Nursing*, **5**(6), 15–18.

Jenkins A (1996) *Nurse's Notes In: History Taking, Examination and Record Keeping in Emergency Medicine* (ed. HR Guly). Oxford: Oxford University Press.

Handyside G (1996) *Triage in Emergency Practice*. St Louis: Mosby.

Leaman AM (2003) See and Treat: a management driven method of achieving targets or a tool for better patient care? One size does not fit all. *Emergency Medicine Journal*, **20**(2), 118.

Lee G, Fraser S (1981) ED Nursing SOAP Notes. *Journal of Emergency Nursing*, **7**(5), 216–218.

Lipley N (2005) Foreign Exchange. *Emergency Nurse*, **13**(7), 5.

Mackway-Jones K, Marsden J, Windle J (2005) *Emergency Triage*, 2nd edn. Oxford: Blackwell Publishing.

Mallet J, Woolwich C (1990) Triage in accident and emergency departments. *Journal of Advanced Nursing*, **15**, 1443–1451.

Marsden J (2000) *Telephone Triage in an Ophthalmic A&E Department*. London: Whurr Publishers Ltd.

National Audit Office (2004) *Improving Emergency Care in England*. London: NAO.

NHS Modernization Agency (2004) *Making See and Treat Work for Patients and Staff*. London: NHS Modernization Agency.

Potter D Ov (ed.) (1985) *Emergencies Nurses Reference Library*. Pennsylvania: Springhouse Corporation.

Ramler CL, Mohammed N (1995) Triage. In: Kitt S, Selfridge-Thomas J, Proehl JA, Kaiser J. eds. *Emergency Nursing: A Physiological and Clinical Perspective*, 2nd edn. Philadelphia: WB Saunders.

Redmond AD, Buxton N (1993) Consultant triage of minor cases in an accident and emergency department. *Archives of Emergency Medicine*, **10**, 328–330.

Rund DA, Rausch TS (1981) *Triage*. St Louis: CV Mosby.

Shrimpling M (2002) Redesigning triage to reduce waiting times. *Emergency Nurse*, **10**(2), 34–37.

Simenson SM (2001) *Telephone Health Assessment: Guidelines for Practice*, 2nd edn. St Louis: Mosby.

Southard R (1989) COBRA legislation: complying with ED provisions. *Journal of Emergency Nursing*, **15**(1), 23–32.

Wardrope J, Driscoll P (2003) Turbulent times. *Emergency Medicine Journal*, **20**(2), 116.

Windle J (2005) To triage or not to triage…. *Emergency Nurse*, **13**(2), 11.

Windle J, Mackway Jones K (2003) Don't throw triage out with the bathwater. *Emergency Medicine Journal*, **20**(2), 119–120.

Zimmermann P (2006) Canada triage and acuity. In: Zimmermann P, Herr R, eds. *Triage Nursing Secrets*. St Louis: Mosby-Elsevier.

Zimmermann P (2006) The Emergency Severity Index Triage Scale. In: Zimmermann P, Herr R, eds. *Triage Nursing Secrets*. St Louis: Mosby-Elsevier.

PART **8**

Professional issues in ED

Chapter 35

Leadership

Lynda Holt & Andrew Cook

INTRODUCTION

This chapter takes a broad look at leadership, a principle of organizational development which has been debated and studied for over 50 years. During this time the theories have changed considerably (Huczynski & Buchanan 2003); however, one thing has remained consistent, human behaviour is a fundamental part of leadership. It is also clear that in an increasingly political healthcare environment strong clinical leadership is essential for effective patient care, and for nurses' well-being. This chapter will look at some aspects of leadership behaviour and identify the key components of effective clinical leadership as well as some of the principles of clinical supervision.

WHAT IS LEADERSHIP?

Leadership is a much debated term with many conflicting theories and conflicting definitions. Most people recognize a good leader, but it is often harder to identify why that individual is a good leader. It does, however, differ from management in that specific status or organizational position is not necessary for an individual to be a leader. So, if position is not the key factor, what is? Skills are important, but not necessarily the ones that may be expected. For example, management skills, attention to detail, organization, intelligence and planning are not consistent among great leaders (Owen 2005). The same inconsistencies exist when considering styles of leadership. Where consensus does exist it is around a collection of behaviours which together can create a leader; these include honesty and integrity, the ability to motivate others, vision, decisiveness, confidence and intuition. In short, leadership is the ability to influence others without threat or coercion (Huczynski & Buchanan 2003).

In healthcare, the profile and priority given to effective leadership has grown slowly (McDaniel & Wolf 1992), but its importance continues to increase, along with the evidence base showing how powerful effective leadership can be. Effective leadership should not be confused with good management; the two often co-exist, but can also come from two different sources, as the behaviours demonstrated by leaders are not absolutely necessary for effective management.

Management can be seen as the organizational and technical tasks that have to be achieved in order to ensure the fluid delivery of services. Management is head-driven, rational and pragmatic. Leadership can be seen as the inspiration of others, the skills employed, often subtly, to galvanize a group of staff to commit to deliver a quality service. Leadership is heart-driven, emotive and enthusing. The most effective environments have both, and both leaders and managers are most effective when able to use a range of behaviours and skill from each domain, depending on circumstances.

CLINICAL LEADERSHIP

Leadership skills are essential in any clinical environment, and the nature of ED work is such that priorities and pace can change dramatically over a very short period, with a potential for staff to feel threatened by the perceived chaos. To maintain a safe, effective service to patients the clinical leader needs to foster an environment where care delivery has some structure, staff have guidance and security, therefore trust can develop (Cook 1996). These rapidly changing high-pressured clinical areas are the very environments where leadership and management are mostly likely to intertwine. It is not uncommon for the management role to become dominant, resulting in both perceived leaders and their clinical staff feeling disempowered and demoralized with their work. For clinical leadership to be successful, and not just clinical management, an overarching environment where individuals feel empowered and able to develop relies on access to information, power, opportunity and resources (Upenieks 2003). It is only when individuals feel empowered that they can truly lead change, take risks and create the innovation needed to develop clinical care.

The challenge for those leading care on a day-to-day basis in emergency care environments can seem daunting alongside the practical tasks of managing the workload, but often what is required is conscious application of principles used every day. Stanley (2006) discusses the value of congruent leadership as a basis for developing clinical care. Stanley (2006) describes clinical leaders as individuals who are experts in their field, positive clinical role models and good communicators. They are followed because they can translate what they believe about nursing into good clinical care. This is in fact a simple phenomenon; congruent leaders are successful because their values and beliefs and their actions match up; as a result they are credible.

Effective clinical leaders can adapt congruence theory to enhance their current practice. It creates a bridge between the necessary management role and the desired leadership role. The most important component in creating congruence is passion; this comes from trusting, valuing and believing in what you are doing (Thompson 2000).

Congruent leadership can be summed up as leading from the heart, trusting your instincts, and valuing your knowledge and beliefs (Box 35.1).

Step 1 How you feel   It is no accident this is step one, and in the clinical environment nurses do this all the time; they get a feel for when a patient is 'going off' or when they should be wary or feel threatened by some patients and not others displaying similar behaviour. This can be explained as intuition, sixth sense, or tacit or expert knowledge (Benner 1984), and the key is to trust these feelings and act in congruence with them: they are based on both experience and intrinsic beliefs. Leadership behaviour will appear natural and confident, fostering trust and motivation to comply, as opposed to ignoring 'feelings', which can have the reverse effect on leadership behaviour, leaving the leader and the followers feeling anxious and lacking in confidence.

Step 2 Walk the talk   This is about personal congruence, the leader's values and purpose, but most of all their ability to take responsibility for their own thoughts, behaviours and actions, whatever the

Box 35.1   Seven steps to congruent leadership
1.   How you feel
2.   Walk the talk
3.   Constantly interact
4.   Build trust
5.   Lead by example
6.   Resolve conflict
7.   Select followers

outcome. So when things do not go to plan, for example blood results get lost, the leader takes responsibility for the appropriate delegation of that task, discusses the incident with those involved, and does not just pass on blame but follows through with any necessary action to prevent a repeat.

Step 3 Constantly interact Most information in the clinical environment is gained through face-to-face interaction and observation; a leader remote from this cannot lead with passion and congruence. It is also worth remembering that individuals' experiences are different, and therefore their understanding and interpretation of situations may be different too. Interaction ensures the leader understands the reality for others in the clinical area they are leading.

Step 4 Build trust This comes from demonstrated consistency in the leader's behaviour, from equity towards all staff and integrity. Being a role model in the clinical area helps to build trust.

Step 5 Lead by example Again the leader's behaviour determines their success; the role should be carried out with passion, purpose and commitment, instilling confidence and enhancing motivation in followers.

Step 6 Resolve conflict Conflict should not be left to fester, it grows and poisons. Most clinical teams rely heavily on each other to be effective, therefore the leader needs to step in and address conflict rapidly even when it is uncomfortable to do so.

Step 7 Select followers A clinical team is no different to any other team, it needs complementary skills and differing personalities to work, so when selecting new members consideration should be given to what the team needs rather than selecting those in the leader's mould. People with genuine passion for their role usually have a natural energy which spills into the team. They are worth looking out for even if they do not yet have all the skills needed.

Garbett (1995) described leaders as people who have a vision; they make things happen, and at the same time they strengthen and support their followers, inspiring them to trust the leader. These appear to be the core qualities needed to lead the clinical team in ED.

Developing personal leadership behaviour

There are four key components to leadership behaviour:

1. Self-awareness
2. Positivity
3. Focus
4. Influence.

Self-awareness

Personal effectiveness stems from self-awareness. It is only through true understanding of her/his strengths, likes and dislikes that a leader can find an authentic set of leadership behaviours. Through self-awareness the leader can understand what makes her/his feel strong or vulnerable, where she/he feels effective and where she/he is less sure, and what she/he is confident about. It is also through self-awareness that a leader can examine her/his expectations, and beliefs about herself/himself. Many individuals are far better at criticizing themselves than celebrating their strengths; this is probably the single most effective way of undermining self-confidence. Often this internal criticism is based on long-held beliefs and expectations which have no genuine validity. Once the leader becomes aware of this behaviour he/she is better placed to reverse it and replace negative internal dialogue with positive comments and praise for what is good. Box 35.2 offers some areas for self-examination to enhance self-awareness.

It is only with self-awareness that a leader can really understand the impact of her/his behaviour on others, as well as what expertise she/he needs from other team members to enhance the team. It is also worth remembering that behaviours individuals dislike in themselves they usually dislike in others,

---

Box 35.2 Enhancing self-awareness

Know what you like
- Passion
- Experience
- Fun
- Talents
- Needs

Passion
- What gets you going?
- What do you really love?
- What makes you laugh?

What do you need?
- To show yourself affection
- To be happy
- To really get satisfied

Self-sabotage
- What you do to yourself
- Beliefs and values
- Fear
- Criticism
- Blame

so a self-aware leader will be able to head off potential conflict by understanding where those feelings come from. An effective leader is someone who not only understands herself/himself well but is also willing to challenge her/his make-up and change their viewpoint (Welford 2002). The dogmatic leader may appear strong and purposeful but will often close their minds to alternatives that may actually be better.

Positivity

Leaders are positive – in their attitudes, their direction and their responses. Being positive is not down to chance or personality, it is learned behaviour. Being positive is about creating solutions and learning to be lucky. Being lucky is an attitude, a way of behaving, and a way of seeing the world. Fundamentally, individuals create their own luck, and appearing lucky to others is often down to sheer hard work and creating enough opportunities (Box 35.3).

Effective leaders create opportunities, they take risks and they act. They believe outcomes will be positive, and convey a positive and passionate image to others. Positivity as described here is all about attitude and a personal belief system applied to life. It does not mean leaders should gloss over difficult issues, as this can equally alienate staff. Being able to recognize when a situation is genuinely challenging, and being prepared to acknowledge and discuss this with staff, makes the leader credible and 'in touch'. Being able to convey a way forward and potential resolution where staff feel involved, supported and engaged is genuine leadership.

Focus

Focus is an ability to look beyond what is immediately obvious, beyond personal need, and to focus on the overall aim, on what the individual is trying to achieve. This necessitates vision and the ability to create direction, not just provide effective crisis management or reactionary direction as is often seen in clinical environments. When truly focused a leader needs to be both decisive and proactive to ensure action.

This is the ability of the leader to see a finished product, which may be as simple as prioritizing and organizing the nursing work to ensure all demands are met. In terms of clinical leadership, however, focus is often the ability to take an external directive, e.g. the National Health Service (NHS) Plan (Department of Health 2000), and find creative ways of achieving care standards while keeping the activity acceptable to the nurses delivering care.

Vision is the ability to see a way forward to the desired outcome. Selling that vision with enthusiasm, realism and commitment creates followers. It is important to remember that vision is a fluid concept and open to change. Opinions and ideas of followers can help to mould a vision to ensure success; the effective leader will set the destination and involve the team in planning the route.

Influence

This is perhaps the most fundamental skill of leaders; without the ability to influence others a leader may have no followers. All of the above components depend on the ability to influence others, but your ability to influence relies on understanding the impact you make (Box 35.4).

Having a vision that others want to be part of is important, but it is more important to have the ability to sell that vision to others. This is easier if the individual is seen as positive, credible and having integrity.

Communication

Becoming a clinical leader is a time of great personal vulnerability. The leader's knowledge, ability to organize and sustain direction, and skills in supporting others will all come under scrutiny before followers decide to adopt the leader's vision. Effective communication is fundamental to gaining acceptance as a leader. Most ED nurses have experienced a shift where the nurse in charge keeps information about patient progress to him or herself and does not keep staff informed of activity. This results in a withdrawal from the situation; nurses continue to function under direction, but they have no ownership of the activity

---

Box 35.3   Being lucky

Perspective	How you look at situations
Choice	How you respond to situations
Responsibility	Take responsibility for yourself
Persistence	Sticking at something is often the only difference

---

Box 35.4   Having influence

- Communication
- Empowering others
- Team building
- Political savvy

and offer little support to the leader. Conversely, where communication is good and ideas are welcomed from other nurses, staff work as a team, supporting each other and the leader (Haire 1998, Kacperek 1997). The success relies on the ability to communicate effectively with other staff members. This means the leader is able to give direction and feedback to staff, but also can receive feedback, air ideas and develop strategy (Box 35.5).

Empowerment

Empowerment of individuals or a team can be a lengthy process; it is sometimes difficult to imagine this taking place in a busy ED when decision-making is necessarily rapid. The clinical leader needs to work periodically with nurses on an individual basis. She/he needs to understand and appreciate the nurse's contribution, give constructive feedback and invest in the nurse's individual development. This way when rapid decisions do need to be made, the followers are more likely to trust their leader and accept and support the action proposed.

Empowerment does not mean a lack of managerial control. The clinical leader must set boundaries on what are acceptable standards and behaviours and what are unacceptable. These must be communicated to others in the clinical environment and should remain constant. This way the team is free to participate in decision-making within a preset structure. For most people, boundaries provide a sense of stability and security. This can be particularly important when trying to maintain a departmental direction and vision (Senior 1999). Leadership, however, is as much about risk-taking as it is about control. The effective leader will allow her team to make decisions that may be inappropriate or less than efficient (Bowles & Bowles 1999). The risk that should be considered, balanced and judged is whether the

consequences of the staff making the wrong decision will be catastrophic. If this is likely then the leader would be foolish not to make a decision and pass it on; if it will not be then it may be worth allowing others to make the choice and let them glory in their success or learn from their lesson, depending on how things turn out. It might be easier as a leader to just take control and make the decisions; there is little risk of things going wrong, particularly in a busy ED. This fails, however, to empower the team. This lack of empowerment and overly controlling approach can lead to disenfranchisement of staff from the organizational process of their department, simply turning up at work to do their job; or worse the team become so disempowered that staff become unable to make even the most basic and simple of decisions. Every leader must remember that if there is constant downward management there will be constant upward referral. This does nothing to develop the skills of others and is exhausting for the leader. The challenge for the leader is one of balance; in order to empower and develop staff they must feel trusted, capable and supported. In order to achieve this the leader must feel comfortable with the degree of risk he/she is taking.

Team–building

The ability to build and sustain a team is fundamental to being an effective leader. Part of the role of the leader is to draw people together, create common goals and encourage a sense of collaboration. This way a team can be formed that will face challenges together. This is best demonstrated by a well-run resuscitation – the team comes together, each member has a role, and a comprehensive package of care is given.

These teams last only for a short while. In building a team which is expected to work closely for a sustained period, such as a project group within a

---

Box 35.5 Effective communication

- Listening – not waiting to speak, really listening to what is being said and not said
- Talking – conveying ideas, direction, discussing issues
- Body language – these are perhaps the biggest communication cues
- Confidence – a message delivered with confidence and conviction is much stronger and more motivating
- Credibility – act with self-awareness, within personal values, and consistently
- Time – be careful to allow enough time for important conversations, and not too much for corridor conversation. Remember the impact that urgency has on messages delivered and heard
- Trust – this is fostered through communication action and credibility

department, the leader must have an understanding of group dynamics. An effective team is one where there is diversity among the team members and the collective qualities those individuals bring offer a richness to the breadth of skills the team has at its disposal to achieve its goals. Effective leaders will look at their team and understand the differences between the individuals, celebrate these differences, and use them to the benefit of the service and the patients.

There are a number of systems available to analyse the personality profiles of individuals. It can be helpful to undertake such analysis in order to appreciate where the strengths lie within a team. By understanding this, the allocation of tasks can be made based upon people's strengths, so ensuring the best outcome. The effective leader, however, will also use such understanding to identify where an individual's weaknesses lie and sometimes allocate tasks to stretch and develop skills. This can be an uncomfortable experience for the individual that may result in resistance to the leader. The leader must, therefore, ensure that such development is backed up with support, reassurance and positive feedback.

A crucial factor in team-building is the function of the leader. To be successful, this person must remain part of the team, giving direction and support to the other team members. The leader must be secure enough in her/his own knowledge to encourage and utilize the abilities and knowledge of other team members without being threatened. Dean (1995) believes it is important for leaders to recognize their own limitations, but recognition is not sufficient. Declaration of one's own limitations can often encourage loyalty and affiliation to the leader by the followers. This must be undertaken positively and with care and judgement. Listening effectively to the views and opinions of others, while acknowledging one's own short-comings, can lead to better decisions and a stronger team (Caplin-Davies 2000).

Political savvy

As a professional group, nurses are often less aware of how to manage organizational politics than other professional groups in healthcare (Nelson & Gordon 2006). This can have a detrimental effect on leadership ability. The principles of influence are the same regardless of the target audience, so whether the Chief Executive, Director of Nursing or Health Care Assistant is the person to be influenced, the following principles apply.

Clinical leaders should use charm in the same way many medical colleagues do; it will engage others, make them want to talk, and more importantly listen

---

> **Box 35.6 How to charm**
>
> - Smile
> - Make others feel comfortable
> - Remember names, or personal details
> - Ask about people
> - Involve others in conversation and activity
> - Welcome others' views without agreeing
> - Give praise
> - Be consistent

---

to others' views (Box 35.6). As trust grows they will provide the clinical leader with information which increases their political intelligence, but also trust the leaders views and ideas, give the benefit of the doubt because that leader is a known and trusted entity, and as credibility grows other professionals and Trust directors will want to work with the leader who has charmed them because they now know her, trust her/his and rate her/his. That alone makes the clinical leader's job a whole lot easier.

Clinical leaders should see organizational meetings as an opportunity, not an ordeal to be avoided with the slightest excuse. They are where issues discussed and decisions are made and if the clinical leader is not there her opinion is lost: worse, her/his power of influence is diminished. Instead clinical leaders should be political, plan for the meeting, read the agenda, and decide in advance what subjects impact on their clinical area. Prior to the meeting identify natural allies, and discuss issues beforehand, identify critics and have answers for their criticisms. On the day of the meeting arrive early, try to sit facing the chair person as it is easier to get heard, and watch listeners as well as speakers, as they often give away much information about their stance on the discussion. The clinical leader should have prepared what she/he wants to say, and be clear and concise, avoiding any complex clinical analogies, which may lose the attention of non-clinicians. Finally the leader should stay on message responding, not reacting, to others comments. It is often worth practising this technique on meetings with little risk first, but it quickly becomes a habit. Other professional groups have practised in this way for a long while, and nurse leaders are disadvantaged if they do not engage in this process.

Leadership is fundamentally about influence; it is worth thinking about the impact clinical leaders make as individuals to ensure it is the impact they want to make.

CLINICAL SUPERVISION

The importance of clinical supervision was emphasized in the light of serious concerns identified by the Allitt Inquiry (1991). The Health Service Ombudsman at that time repeatedly raised concerns about a number of flaws identified in the delivery of nursing care, including the quality of record-keeping. Clinical supervision offered a potential solution to some of the difficulties being encountered by the nursing profession on an individual and organizational basis. Some areas of nursing, such as psychiatry, have used supervision for many years; however, in acute nursing the concept has been underdeveloped.

The King's Fund (1994) has described clinical supervision as a formal arrangement in which nurses can discuss work with another professional colleague. It has been promoted as a support mechanism for nurses, a tool for professional development and a method of quality control.

Principles to support clinical supervision

The NMC (2002) supports the concept of clinical supervision, as had the UKCC. It has stopped short of identifying any particular model of delivery to allow for local adaptation, but it does stipulate a set of guiding principles which should be used (Box 35.7).

For its introduction to be successful in any clinical environment, it is essential for participants to share a common understanding of their interpretation of clinical supervision. One approach to this is for emergency nurses to explore the many activities and skills in nursing work, including:

- caring
- curing
- supporting
- empowering
- teaching.

These activities all involve interaction with others, such as patients and their relatives or friends, and are not without personal risk. In emergency care, the patient's stay is relatively short and the onus is on the nurse to develop a therapeutic relationship quickly, but how do nurses maintain this relationship when someone is off sick, the shift is busy or the relative has complained about the ever-increasing waiting times?

Types of supervision

Clinical supervision must be clearly separated from issues relating to pay, promotion or discipline. Only then can a trusting relationship be fostered. Several ways of addressing supervision have emerged. These include:

- one-to-one supervision with an expert from a nursing or related background
- one-to-one supervision within a peer group
- group or network supervision
- action learning sets.

Peer supervision means the supervisor and supervisee are involved in similar clinical work, and possibly face similar challenges. The advantages are increased awareness, potentially greater trust and a relationship which is less threatening to the supervisee. The disadvantage is that without effort and commitment from both parties, the activity can become purely one of support and not development. Group and network supervision have been developed in some areas of healthcare, particularly in community settings. This involves a group of similar professionals

---

Box 35.7   NMC principles of clinical supervision

- Clinical supervision supports practice, enabling you to maintain and improve standards of care
- Clinical supervision is a practice-focused professional relationship, involving a practitioner reflecting on practice guided by a skilled supervisor
- The process of clinical supervision should be developed by practitioners and managers according to local circumstances. Ground rules should be agreed so that you and your supervisor approach clinical supervision openly, confidently and are both aware of what is involved

- Every practitioner should have access to clinical supervision. Each supervisor should supervise a realistic number of practitioners
- Preparation for supervisors should be flexible and sensitive to local circumstances. The principles and relevance of clinical supervision should be included in pre-registration and post-registration education programmes
- Evaluation of clinical supervision is needed to assess how it influences care and practice standards
- Evaluation systems should be determined locally (NMC 2002)

sharing experiences and developing their practice using one another. For this to be successful, a large degree of trust and commitment is needed from participants. It does have disadvantages in that some members of the group can remain non-participative or dominate activity. It is perhaps organizationally easier to facilitate than one-to-one supervision. Whichever method of supervision is adopted, it is essential that the clinical supervisor remains clinically challenging. The success of clinical supervision relies on its perceived value to the department (Jones 2006); therefore agreeing the aims and process before implementation is imperative. Bishop (1994) provides three overall aims which act as a bedrock for supervision activities:

- to facilitate professional expertise
- to improve patient care
- to safeguard standards of care.

To achieve these objectives, clinical supervision should be seen as a continuum along with mentorship and preceptorship. A mentor helps to develop clinical competence by guiding a nurse through learning a new skill, such as cannulation. A preceptor helps the nurse gain confidence in that role. A clinical supervisor aids professional development from acquisition of new skills. But for clinical supervision to be successful it is important to consider the impact of the nurse as a whole and not as a technician.

The philosophical approach to clinical supervision does not have to be complicated. Proctor (1986) suggested a simple tripartite approach to supervision (Fig. 35.1). The formative role is one of education, supplementing the supervisee's knowledge and facilitating growth. The restorative aspect relies on support, exploring anxieties or critical incidents and allowing the supervisee to resolve stress. The normative function is one of quality control, looking at actual practice and challenging methods to maintain high standards of patient care.

The success of clinical supervision relies on its perceived value to the department and staff commitment. The activities of clinical supervision revolve around the provision of regular space for reflection on the content and process of work (Fig. 35.2). Its functions are to develop the understanding and skills of the supervisee, to ensure quality nursing care and to provide space to explore and express distress about work. Done effectively this results in the supervisee feeling valued and validated both as a person and as a nurse, as she/he is able to receive feedback and therefore gain new perspectives on her/his work. This empowers the nurse to plan and utilize personal resources and become proactive and innovative. Clinical supervision should not be a forum for self-congratulation or self-destruction, nor should it be personal therapy. The supervisor can facilitate this by observation of practice, encouraging retrospective reflection and participation in evaluating outcomes.

Getting clinical supervision

Clinical supervision is not without personal risk, because the nurse is being asked to expose anxieties or perceived areas of weakness to a close colleague. Trust and confidentiality are therefore pivotal to a successful relationship. The nurse has a responsibility to seek supervision actively by going into a meeting with identified areas for support. She/he must ask for help in these areas and not rely on the supervisor to work it out. For supervision to succeed, the nurse needs to be able to share her/his feelings and be open to feedback, monitoring any tendencies to defend

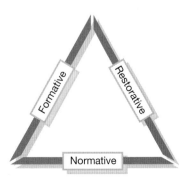

Figure 35.1   Functions of clinical supervision.

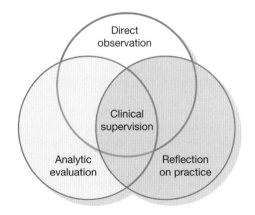

Figure 35.2   Activities of a supervisor.

practice, but also monitoring what feedback is useful. Perhaps most important to the success of the relationship is the ability to be creative about clinical practice.

Self-awareness helps to minimize the impact of any blocks the nurse may have towards supervision, such as negative past experiences, inhibition, misunderstandings or relationship problems such as personality clashes. Much of this can be overcome if the nurse being supervised has a choice of who acts as supervisor. In making this choice it is important that the supervisee chooses a supervisor based on that person's ability to challenge and develop nursing practice and not because of popularity with the supervisee. This person is most likely to be another nurse from the same or a similar speciality. The supervisor needs to apply clinical knowledge in a manner that promotes innovation, is constructive and creative, and facilitates the professional growth of the supervisee. It is not enough to be more senior or more experienced; the supervisor also needs advanced skills in listening, giving positive and negative feedback, facilitating reflection and defusing distress.

Before clinical supervision is established in a department, its ground rules should be identified and agreed by participants (Simms 1993); for example, it should be agreed that any unacceptable breach of the Code of Professional Conduct (NMC 2004) may need to be taken outside the supervisory relationship (Box 35.8).

In addition to these, some practical considerations such as the frequency and length of meetings, criteria for supervisors and termination routes if sessions become destructive should all be agreed. A robust audit tool is useful to measure quantitative data about activity such as the frequency and duration of supervision sessions. Evidence of its value to nurses is largely subjective, but potential benefits are outlined in Box 35.9.

There remains much debate about the real value of clinical supervision. Shanley & Stevenson (2006)

Box 35.9   Potential benefits of clinical supervision

Benefits to the nurse
- Offers support and aids in confidence building
- Invests in staff and acknowledges the value of nurses and nursing
- Helps to develop nursing practice
- Allows nurse to review practice creatively and critically
- Can aid objective setting at Individual Performance Reviews (IPR) and reveal deficits
- Allows practice to change
- Promotes critical reflection on and in practice
- Develops individual accountability
- Aids personal and professional growth
- Helps link theory and practice
- Increases self-awareness

Benefits to the manager
- Helps monitor/maintain standards
- Promotes innovation
- Facilitates professionally accountable practitioners
- Links with organizational audit
- Challenges poor practice
- Strengthens collegiate relationships
- Maximizes training resources
- Creates a dynamic, changing environment
- Improves communication systems

---

argue that it is potentially hazardous in its current form, and models need to become more sophisticated if they are to be successful. Despite the ongoing concern in acute and primary care, clinical supervision has been successful in mental health nursing for many years.

Clinical supervision is a complex activity; it facilitates the development of clinical practice and supports the provision of quality patient care. Perhaps most importantly, clinical supervision provides a forum for innovation and creativity to flourish. Its implementation has been hampered by misunderstanding of its function, not aided by the inference of its title 'supervision'. It is, however, a real opportunity for nurses to develop their nursing practice further, challenge professional boundaries and celebrate the value of nursing.

CONCLUSION

This chapter has identified a range of clinical leadership and supervision issues which emergency nurses should consider when developing themselves and their practice. In an increasingly complex emergency

---

Box 35.8   Ground rules and responsibilities for clinical supervision

- Commitment to confidentiality
- Open and honest learning
- Sharing best practice
- Seeking research for evidence-based practice
- Facilitating new learning opportunities
- Relevance to clinical practice

(RCN 2002)

service, support for and by those responsible for developing services is needed in order to recruit, retain and value that most precious commodity – the staff. The chapter highlights the importance of effective clinical leadership, both for those working within the ED environment and for their benefit within the organization. The chapter reinforces the need for clinical leaders to become more aware of professional and organizational politics, in order to get the best results for their clinical environment, those working in it and their patients. Finally, the chapter identifies that leaders exist at all levels within an organization, and because leadership is learned behaviour anyone can become a leader with a bit of self-awareness, willingness to stand out from the crowd, and the ability to influence others.

References

Benner P (1984) *From Novice to Expert: Excellence and Power in Clinical Nursing Practice.* Menlo Park: Addison-Wesley.

Bishop V (1994) Clinical supervision for an accountable profession. *Nursing Times,* **90**(39), 35–37.

Bowles N, Bowles A (1999) Transformational leadership. *Nursing Times Learning Curve,* **3**(8), 2–4.

Caplin-Davies P (2000) Nurse manager – change thyself. *Nursing Management,* **6**(9) 16–20.

Cook A (1996) Effective clinical leadership in A&E. *Emergency Nurse,* **4**(3), 24–25.

Dean D (1995) Leadership: the hidden dangers. *Nursing Standard,* **10**(13), 54–55.

Department of Health (2000) *The NHS Plan.* London: The Stationery Office.

Garbett R (1995) Leading questions. *Nursing Times,* **91**(27), 26–27.

Haire J (1998) Communication and trauma management. *Emergency Nurse,* **6**(5), 24–30.

Huczynski A, Buchanan D (2003) *Organisational Behaviour: An Introductory Text.* 5th edn. London: Prentice Hall.

Jones A (2006) Clinical supervision: what do we know and what do we need to know? A review and commentary. *Journal of Nursing Management,* **14**(8), 577–585.

Kacperek L (1997) Non-verbal communication – the importance of listening. *British Journal of Nursing,* **6**(5), 275–279.

King's Fund (1994) *Clinical Supervision: An Executive Summary.* London: King's Fund Centre.

McDaniel C, Wolf GA (1992) Transformational leadership in nursing service: a test of theory. *Journal of Nursing Administration,* **22**(2), 60–65.

Nelson S, Gordon S (2006) Moving beyond the virtue script in nursing. In: Nelson S, Gordon S, eds. *The Complexities of Care: Nursing Reconsidered.* Ithaca, N.Y.: Cornell University Press.

Nursing and Midwifery Council (2002) *Supporting Nurses and Midwives Through Life-long Learning.* London: Nursing and Midwifery Council.

Nursing and Midwifery Council (2004) *Code of Professional Conduct: Standards, for Conduct, Performance and Ethics.* London: Nursing and Midwifery Council.

Owen J (2005) *How to Lead.* Edinburgh: Pearson Education Ltd.

Proctor B (1986) Supervision: a co-operative exercise in accountability. In: Marken M, Payne M, eds. *Enabling and Ensuring.* Leicester: Leicester Youth Bureau and Council for Education and Training in Youth and Community Work.

Royal College of Nursing (2002) *Ground Rules and Responsibilities for Clinical Supervision.* London: RCN.

Senior K (1999) ENP scheme: highlighting the barriers. *Emergency Nurse,* **6**(9), 28–32.

Shanley MJ, Stevenson C (2006) Clinical supervision revisited. *Journal of Nursing Management,* **14**(8), 586–592.

Simms J (1993) Supervision. In: Wright H, Giddey M, eds. *Mental Health Nursing.* London: Chapman & Hall.

Stanley D (2006) Recognizing and defining clinical leaders. *British Journal of Nursing,* **15**(2): 108–111.

The Allitt Inquiry (1991) *Independent Inquiry Relating to Deaths and Injuries on the Children's Ward at Grantham and Kesteven General Hospital During the Period February to April 1991.* London: HMSO.

Thompson CM (2000) *A Congruent Life.* San Francisco: Jossey Bass Publications.

Upenieks V (2003) Nurse leaders' perceptions of what compromises successful leadership in today's inpatient environment. *Nursing Administration Quarterly,* **27**(2): 140–152.

Welford C (2002) Transformational leadership – matching theory to practice. *Nursing Management,* **9**(4), 7–11.

Chapter **36**

Clinical decision-making

Emma Tippins

INTRODUCTION

Appropriate clinical decision-making is an intrinsic and frequently complex process at the heart of clinical practice (Ellis 1997), with some situations being more complex than others as they involve more unknowns and uncertainties (Cioffi and Markham 1997, Cioffi 1998). This process should not, therefore, be underestimated. The assessment, evaluation and subsequent changes made to a patient's care are intrinsically involved. The assessment process and the effective use of assessment information through appropriate decision-making are essential to improve outcomes of care (Aitken 2003). Within the patient assessment the nurse should, through a systematic approach, support clinical findings with hard scientific fact.

Requesting tests and the analysis of data complete this process. Simply put, if a nurse omits to request a relevant test there will be no scientific evidence to support the initial working diagnosis. Bochund and Calandra (2003) identified that requesting relevant tests during the initial assessment significantly reduced morbidity and mortality rates.

Within the modern protocol-driven emergency department (ED) a working diagnosis is essential to provide an efficient and structured patient experience through the department, concluding in their discharge or referral to a specialist service.

This chapter focuses on the importance of applying the key skills of critical thinking and clinical decision-making to everyday practice and the ways of facilitating nurses into the acquisition of these key skills. The chapter commences with an overview of emergency nursing and the importance of applying critical thinking to the assessment process. The focus will then be divided between the application of the nursing process within emergency nursing, how nurses construct their thought processes in relation to initial and continual patient assessments, and how the application of the key skills of critical thinking and clinical decision-making within their everyday practice will benefit both patient and nurse.

When assessing a patient the ED nurse must decide what data to collect: this is dependent on the nurse's initial clinical findings. In an age of clinical resource management and target-focused quantitative care it is essential that appropriate tests are ordered, to reduce an unnecessary workload resulting in wasted laboratory test time, to reduce false positives, and to facilitate a proficient cost-effective qualitative service. The importance of these initial data cannot be overemphasized, as analysis of these data will form the pathophysiological basis from which the medical diagnosis is made.

In order to understand the processes involved in clinical decision-making it is essential to consider the context in which decision-making activities are being performed. The Emergency Department (ED) is the portal for over 12.7 million annual visits in England in 2003, of which 20% were admitted (National Audit Office 2004). In the United States of America (USA) there are over 100 million annual visits nationally, accounting for 40% of hospital admissions (McCraig 1999). These millions of patients attend with any number of clinical presentations and complaints requiring the assistance of every medical speciality. The role of the emergency nurse is unique in this respect, as in no other clinical setting is the nurse called upon to assess and identify the needs of such a wide range of potential patient conditions.

INITIAL ASSESSMENT

The ED is the interface between patients and emergency care. Within this setting a patient's first contact with a healthcare professional will usually be with a nurse; the process of initial assessment. Nursing triage is a dynamic decision-making process that will prioritize an individual's need for treatment on arrival to an ED. An efficient triage system aims to identify and expedite time-critical treatment for patients with life-threatening conditions, and ensure every patient requiring emergency treatment is prioritized according to their clinical need. The ethos of triage systems relates to the ability of a professional to detect critical illness, which has to be balanced with resource implications of 'over triage' (a triage category of higher acuity is allocated). A decision that underestimates a person's level of clinical urgency may delay time-critical interventions; furthermore, prolonged triage processes may contribute to adverse

patient outcomes (Geraci & Geraci 1994, Travers 1999).

In this context, the triage nurse's ability to take an accurate patient history, conduct a brief physical assessment, and rapidly determine clinical urgency are crucial to the provision of safe and efficient emergency care (Travers 1999). These responsibilities require triage nurses to justify their clinical decisions with evidence from clinical research, and to be accountable for decisions they make within the clinical environment. The legal significance of undertaking an assessment relates to whether the nurse has sufficient knowledge to perform the assessment competently: if the patient care is compromised a tort of negligence could be issued (Dimond 2004).

It has been identified that many factors impact on the nurse's ability to make accurate decisions; for example, an unpredictable workload, poor professional continuity in relation to communication, and inexperience of the initial nursing assessor, or subsequent nursing staff (O'Neill & LeGrove 2003, Tippins 2005). This has been exacerbated by demographic changes, such as an ageing population and the subsequent associated chronic pathologies, which have placed an enormous strain on primary care services (Dolan & Holt 2000), and secondly on the subjective clinical decision-making of the triage nurse (Cooke & Jinks 1999). If there is a failure to recognize deterioration in a patient's condition and intervention is delayed, the condition of these patients can potentially become critical. The care provided during the ED stay for critically ill patients has been shown to significantly impact on the progression of organ failure and mortality (Church 2003, Rivers et al. 2002). It is, therefore, essential that the care provided in the ED reflects the severity of the condition of the patient, the focal point being that accurate and dynamic patient assessment is imperative.

CONTINUED ASSESSMENT

The continued assessment and monitoring of patients is imperative in order that subtle changes in their condition can be recognized and intervention instigated and evaluated. Physiological monitoring and the identification of deterioration in patients' conditions are an essential part of the role of the ED nurse; however, it remains uncertain whether this translates into the clinical setting. Patients who are critically ill are more likely to be recognized as such at initial assessment than if they deteriorate following that assessment (Cooke & Jinks 1999, Tippins 2005). For example, a patient who presents to the ED with a blood pressure of 89/38, pulse of 127 and respiratory rate of 31 is likely to be allocated a high clinical priority. In contrast, if the same patient presented an hour earlier with a blood pressure of 109/72, pulse of 98 and a respiratory rate of 24, they may not be allocated as high a priority on initial assessment, and their subsequent deterioration an hour later (after their first set of observations) will not necessarily result in a reallocation of priority (Cooke & Jinks 1999, Tippins 2005).

This phenomenon can be explained by a failure in the reassessment process and priority reallocation necessary to reflect the patient's changing physical condition. The introduction of education programmes, such as The Acute Life Threatening Events, Recognition and Treatment (ALERT) course, and tools such as the Modified Early Warning Score (MEWS), may be of benefit to assist staff in identifying patients who are deteriorating or are at risk of doing so. At the very least they ensure a structured approach to patient assessment and the regular and accurate recording of basic physiological observations, a crucial first step in recognizing patients at risk. Other possible explanations for the delay in recognizing patient deterioration could be external factors such as workload pressures or breakdown of communication (Dafurn et al. 1994, O'Neill & LeGrove 2003). The inexperience of staff in dealing with critically ill patients, the impact of teamwork and complacency when faced with certain conditions have also been shown to have an impact on clinical decision-making and, therefore, the care of critically ill patients (Bakalis & Watson 2005, Tippins 2005).

CLINICAL DECISION-MAKING

In emergency care, nurses make multiple decisions rapidly in highly complex environments in order to deliver expert individualized care. Emergency care is different from other areas of nursing, as many patients are critically ill and frequently highly unstable. As a result their rapidly changing condition demands intelligent and decisive decision-making from nurses in short time frames. Despite this there remains minimal research on the clinical decision-making skills of emergency nurses. Consequently much of the content and structure of nurses' decision-making remains unclear (Fonteyn & Ritter 2000).

Clinical decision-making can be defined as the process nurses use to gather patient information, evaluate that information and make a judgement that results in the provision of patient care (White et al. 1992). This process involves collecting information with the use of both scientific and intuitive assessment skills. This information is then interpreted through the use of

knowledge and past experiences (Cioffi 2000a, Evans 2005).

There are many theories on how to teach these essential and dynamic skills; however, learning or the acquisition of new knowledge does not necessarily guarantee the clinical application of expert practice (Tippett 2004) or critical thinking. Many theories of teaching and learning the art of critical thinking and expert clinical decision-making exist; behaviourist, cognitive, and humanistic being the commonly used three (Sheehy & McCarthy 1998). The behaviourist theory relates to reactionary learning whereby the learning occurs when an unmet need causes the learner to embrace the learning process, unfortunately the inclination to learn is often stimulated due to the learner feeling inadequate due to uncertainty and a lack of confidence. The cognitive theory relates to the interaction between the learner and their immediate environment, i.e. learning through experience and professional stimulation. The humanistic theory relates to adult-based learning where the focus is clearly on the learner to ascertain new knowledge through the process of self-discovery. A teacher who has understanding will present organized subject matter which is relevant to the learner's need and will, therefore, propagate learning. The expert practitioner perceives the situation as a whole, uses past concrete situations as paradigms and moves to the accurate region of the problem without wasteful consideration of a large number of irrelevant options.

NURSING PROCESS

The nursing process is a tool used by nurses to assist with decision-making and to predict and evaluate the results of nursing actions (Reeves & Paul 2002). The deliberate intellectual activity of the nursing process guides the professional practice of nursing in providing care in a systematic manner. The nursing process has evolved over recent years to incorporate five or six phases or stages (Box 36.1 and Fig. 36.1) (Lindberg et al. 1994, Oermann 1996, Wilkinson 2001, Reeves & Paul 2002);

Movement between these phases is unusually linear; there is free movement among the phases during clinical practice. Once an assessment begins the nurse should begin to formulate some diagnoses and eliminate others. As more information is gathered, through physical and technological findings, the practitioner should begin to narrow the possibilities. The worst possible diagnosis should be paramount in the practitioner's hypotheses, as this must be addressed and eliminated before moving on. By using a systematic approach patient problems can be identified and

---

Box 36.1 The nursing process

Assessment
- Assessment collection of subjective and objective clinical data to provide a rationale for care

Nursing/working diagnosis
- Analysis of physical presentation confirmed by scientific fact (data collection results)

Planning/outcome identification
- Plan of care and realistic goals discussed with patient

Implementation
- Performing interventions, reassess plan following each intervention to determine initial response

Evaluation
- Have expected outcomes been achieved? Determine patient's level of clinical need and regularity of subsequent assessment

---

acted upon in the most effective way to ensure the best possible outcome for the patient. Examples of a systematic approach are those adopted by the Resuscitation Council (2006) on the Advanced Life Support (ALS) course with the ABC mnemonic (airway, breathing and circulation) and ABCDE (airway, breathing, circulation, disability and environment), taught by the American College of Surgeons (2004) in the Advanced Trauma Life Support (ATLS) course.

An obvious nursing diagnosis, such as difficulty in breathing in the patient with acute exacerbation of asthma, may be developed while data collection is still ongoing. In this situation implementation of life-saving actions, such as administration of oxygen therapy and bronchodilators, in which the desired outcome is obvious, may have begun before the assessment, diagnosis, outcome identification, and planning phases can be verbalized. Throughout the phases, reassessment can lead to immediate changes in any of the previous phases. Reassessment and the further collection and analysis of data is a continuous, ongoing dynamic process and should not be confused with evaluation, which measures outcomes. Reassessment may lead to a change in the working diagnosis, which in turn could lead to a change in outcome identification, planning, implementation and evaluation as the process continues.

In order to demonstrate the nursing process a clinical scenario will be presented and discussed to demonstrate the practice from both a unilateral and a critical thinking perspective (Box 36.2 and Fig. 36.2).

The nurse assessing the patient in a one-dimensional way will focus only on the patient's presenting complaint, and in this case attempt to establish a cause for the collapse. The nurse demonstrating critical thinking, however, will take into account all available information gained from the assessment and utilize it in order to establish a working diagnosis. In this example the one-dimensional process disregards the fact that the patient is pregnant. The dynamic model will take this information into account and process it along with all other available information, considering the bigger picture. With the use of critical thinking a working diagnosis/hypothesis will be formulated: hyperemesis; and appropriate scientific fact sought to either confirm or refute it. When the evaluation phase is reached, the nurse in the one-dimensional example may not have established a cause for the patient's collapse and, as a result, may have to go back to previous phases. In contrast, the critical thinker may have confirmed a working diagnosis, established a subsequent care plan and moved on.

The current demands placed on clinicians require the ED practitioner to be proactive and dynamic in their utilization of the nursing process. They need to know which stages can be safely omitted, combined or delayed, and also which situations warrant a rigorous, comprehensive approach (Alfaro-LeFevre 2004). There is, therefore, a clear need to implement a tool or structure to the diagnostic process directly aimed at ED nurses to facilitate the application of critical thinking. Novice practitioners frequently require a clear-cut approach to patient assessment; this can be achieved by applying the DEAD mnemonic as an aide-memoire or self-questioning analytical tool. This approach is outlined in Box 36.3 (Evan & Tippins 2007).

By utilizing this structured framework, those less experienced in critical thinking will have a clear systematic outline to assist them in the organization of their thought process. This, in turn, could facilitate development of critical thinking and decision-making skills.

CRITICAL THINKING

The clinical scenarios outlined in Box 36.4 will be discussed to demonstrate the critical thinking and clinical decision-making involved in the initial and continuing assessment process.

Data The data the initial assessor will require are based on the patient's presenting complaint and medical history. The initial nursing or working diagnosis in this case would be an acute coronary syndrome (ACS). The nurse should be quick to ascertain the

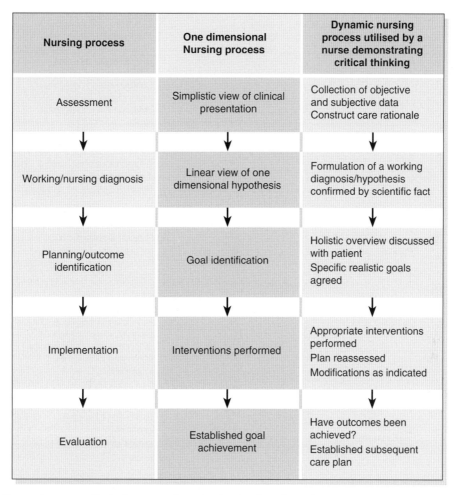

Nursing process	One dimensional Nursing process	Dynamic nursing process utilised by a nurse demonstrating critical thinking
Assessment	Simplistic view of clinical presentation	Collection of objective and subjective data Construct care rationale
Working/nursing diagnosis	Linear view of one dimensional hypothesis	Formulation of a working diagnosis/hypothesis confirmed by scientific fact
Planning/outcome identification	Goal identification	Holistic overview discussed with patient Specific realistic goals agreed
Implementation	Interventions performed	Appropriate interventions performed Plan reassessed Modifications as indicated
Evaluation	Established goal achievement	Have outcomes been achieved? Established subsequent care plan

Figure 36.1   The nursing process illustrating a one-dimensional and a dynamic nursing process.

Box 36.2   Scenario 1

A 28-year-old female attends the ED at 08.30 via the ambulance service as a result of a collapse while on a bus. She is alert and oriented and able to recall the events prior to the collapse, and has not sustained any obvious injuries. The patient states that she has not eaten breakfast as she has been feeling nauseous and has been vomiting for the past 48 hours. The patient also adds that she is 13 weeks pregnant.

---

nature of the patient's pulse. A radial pulse can reflect the onset of physiological shock or the presence of life-threatening arrhythmias, including complete heart block, atrial fibrillation and tachycardias. The nursing diagnosis and need for immediate intervention can be either validated or negated by the

recording of an ECG which would reflect the pathological changes associated with acute ST segment elevated myocardial infarction (STEMI). The data recording at this point should include the requesting of blood tests, particularly as other co-existing pathologies may be exacerbating this presentation, such as anaemia.

Emotions   The assessor's gut reaction in this case should be to consider the working diagnosis of STEMI. Comparing the current presentation with previously experienced situations should alert the nurse to the potential severity of the condition, the process of pattern recognition and experiential learning (Cioffi 2001, Tippins 2005, Muir 2004).

Advantages   The advantages involved in this situation would be an early door to treatment time, which has been shown to dramatically improve morbidity

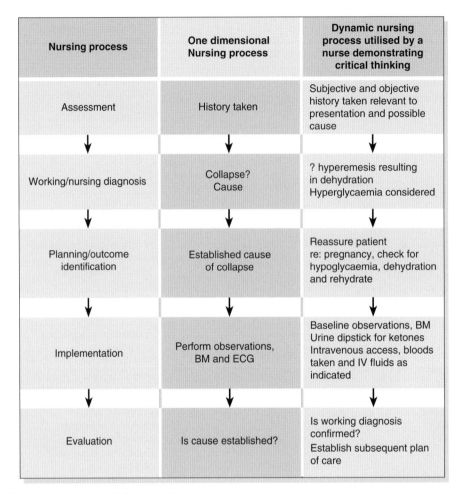

Nursing process	One dimensional Nursing process	Dynamic nursing process utilised by a nurse demonstrating critical thinking
Assessment	History taken	Subjective and objective history taken relevant to presentation and possible cause
↓	↓	↓
Working/nursing diagnosis	Collapse? Cause	? hyperemesis resulting in dehydration Hyperglycaemia considered
↓	↓	↓
Planning/outcome identification	Established cause of collapse	Reassure patient re: pregnancy, check for hypoglycaemia, dehydration and rehydrate
↓	↓	↓
Implementation	Perform observations, BM and ECG	Baseline observations, BM Urine dipstick for ketones Intravenous access, bloods taken and IV fluids as indicated
↓	↓	↓
Evaluation	Is cause established?	Is working diagnosis confirmed? Establish subsequent plan of care

Figure 36.2 The nursing process applied to scenario 1.

and mortality rates. The rapid diagnosis and treatment of life-threatening pathologies such as ACS is essential (Department of Health 2000a).

Disadvantages (differential diagnosis). The priority in this case is to confirm or dispel STEMI. The assessor also needs to consider other possible diagnoses, for example a dissecting aneurism, which would be a contraindication to therapy. This possibility would result in the assessor returning to the data collection phase of the process in order to negate a potential aneurysm via further data collection.

Based on the clinical presentation the nurse will apply the DEAD mnemonic to aid critical thinking and decision-making.

Data What facts does the nurse have? This patient is presenting with the classical clinical signs of a respiratory infection. The fact that he smokes initially

reinforces the nurse's first impression. The patient discussed having chest pain; the nurse should ascertain the nature of this pain, and ask whether it increases on inspiration, for example. The data needed to justify the nursing diagnosis will include the patient's respiratory rate, rhythm and depth. Oxygen saturation and a sample of the sputum should be requested. The nurse should look for clinical manifestations of chronic related pathophysiological changes associated with smoking; these include peripheral and potential central cyanosis and nail bed changes. Radial pulse and capillary refill time should be ascertained; the patient's blood pressure should be noted. An ECG should be recorded, as much respiratory-related pathology coincides with cardiac pathology. The patient's temperature should also be recorded. By recording and requesting data the nurse is validating the working diagnosis and negating other or coexisting pathologies.

Box 36.3 The DEAD mnemonic

D: relates to Data (scientific facts) – this should be based on what facts the nurse has and what other data the nurse can collect to validate or negate them.
E: Emotions – intuition or gut feelings/reactions, what are your instincts telling you, how can you consolidate or negate these.
A: Advantages – what advantage to others would result from actions the nurse takes, i.e. would an action instigated at the initial assessment improve the patient's prognosis, an example being the dispensing of an anti-platelet drug to a patient experiencing an acute coronary syndrome. The practitioner should also consider that a test requested when the patient presents may hasten their visit and result in an increasingly proficient service.
D: Disadvantages (differential diagnoses) – what could go wrong, in the worst case scenario what could this be, how I can rule this out?

Box 36.4 Scenario 2

A 76-year-old woman is admitted to the emergency department via the ambulance service complaining of a sudden onset of left-sided chest pain which commenced two hours previously. The pain radiates through to the centre of her chest; she also complains of a vague discomfort in her left arm. On examination, she has severe pain in her chest and back, she is pale and drowsy.

Vital signs reported: BP 110/60 mmHg, and a weak radial pulse.

Emotions Intuition and previous experience (experiential learning) have instigated this plan of care; the nurse is now applying critical thinking to the intuitive process to provide hard facts to justify gut reactions.

Advantages The nursing goal is to provide the patient with a quick efficient service. From the initial clinical signs and vital sign data collection the nurse has established this is not a life-threatening presentation. Within many departments the nurse will be able to request a chest X-ray, which will save time if requested early on.

Disadvantages The clinical decision-making process must include a quick analysis of the patient's presentation; this should include 'what is the worst case scenario?' Has the assessor negated immediate life-threatening pathologies? The ongoing process of excluding differential diagnoses now begins and the nurse may still think of other possible rule-out tests that could be requested.

PAST EXPERIENCES

In decision-making involving complexity, studies have shown that decision-making strategies are dependent on the individual's experiences (Cioffi & Markham 1997, Cioffi 1998, Tippins 2004). Nurses use past experiences to assist in decision-making by comparing the current situation to previously experienced situations held in their memory (pattern recognition). This can manifest itself in a variety of forms, including recognizing a similarity between the present patient's condition/situation and a group of patients previously cared for with this presenting condition/situation, to describing quite specifically identified characteristics (Cioffi & Markham 1997, Grossman & Wheeler 1997, Cioffi 1998, Cioffi 2001). For example, a nurse who has previously cared for a patient with meningococcal meningitis may identify a future patient with the condition by recognizing a specific sign or symptom witnessed in the first instance, such as the petechial rash. Benner (1984) discusses the differences between a novice and an expert and proposes that they can be attributed to the know-how that is acquired through experience.

Furthermore, past experiences with patients' symptoms and their probable outcomes is a factor that will determine the action a nurse will take in response to a patient's presentation (Radwin 1998). A recommendation for practice, therefore, must be to provide teaching to staff on conditions and situations common, but infrequently experienced, within the ED. This could facilitate the development of pattern-recognition skills, and improve response to critical care events. This could also address the retention of knowledge and skills gained in continuing professional development courses (Department of Health 2002b).

The use of reflection to assist in personal debriefing has an impact on the management of future practices when patients present with similar conditions (Tippins 2005, Evans 2005). By reflecting both on and in practice, with the use of critical thinking, best outcomes can be hypothetically discussed. This will result in modifications in an individual's clinical practice, and ultimately a positive impact on the care of future patients. Reflective practice has become an integral part of daily nursing life (Johns & Freshwater 1998). The need to reflect, critically analyse, develop and, where possible, improve is the constant aim of the nursing profession in the twenty first century.

INTUITION

Generally it is accepted that hard facts or science is the base from which nursing practice is delivered, and that intuition or logic do not directly influence clinical practice. In contrast the reality is very different, the rationalist paradigm of knowledge is logic, and the empiricist paradigm is science. Interestingly empirical knowledge is less certain than logic; it is tentative, responsive to new evidence and better research, and always open to re-testing. The primary aim of applying theory in practice is to improve the patient's quality of care. Experts are able to generate better hypotheses due to a larger database of knowledge from which to pull ideas. This expert knowledge may also be assembled from intuition. Robinson (2000) identifies that clinical decision-making is the foundation of how an expert clinician can utilize their experientially based knowledge base to draw conclusions when assessing each new encounter.

Nurses' experience plays a major role in the development of critical observations, skills and subsequent intuition (Benner & Tanner 1987). When confronted with situations in which clinical judgements are characteristically uncertain, the nurse will rely upon the use of intuition to assist with their clinical decision-making (Benner & Tanner 1987). It has been argued that intuition actually accelerates the analytical process which leads to a nursing intervention (King & Appleton 1997). The use of intuition and systematic processes of decision-making has predominantly been believed to have occurred only in the more experienced and expert nurses (Benner & Tanner 1987, Watkins 1998, Rew 2000). Intuitive aspects of decision-making may, however, commence in nurses at an early point in their career and strengthen or lessen with time depending on their experiences and developing

expertise (King & Appleton 1997, Sirkka et al. 1998, King & MacLeod Clark 2002).

Emergency nurses often have to deal with patients with life-threatening conditions, and sometimes reach a critical stage of perceiving a change in a patient's condition signifying that the patient may soon deteriorate. This use of intuitive judgement has been shown to be useful in the recognition of patient deterioration (Fisher & Fonteyn 1995, Cioffi & Markham 1997, Cioffi 2000b, Tippins 2005). When used to identify deterioration this feeling is associated with knowing the patient (Cioffi 2000b), for which continuity of care is necessary (Grossman & Wheeler 1997).

CONCLUSION

The ultimate aim of emergency education is learning how to apply knowledge and understanding within the clinical setting. In order to achieve satisfactory outcomes the nurse must use elements from both the rationalist and empirical paradigms. The characteristics associated with advanced nursing practice centre on the practitioner utilizing the process of lateral thinking. Experts within the field of clinical decision-making suggest that in the absence of critical thinking, change and subsequent progress within the nursing profession would not have occurred. The ability of the nurse to reflect upon their role within the assessment process enables them to develop key analytical skills, which are essential within the role of emergency practitioners. Once the practitioner is able to demonstrate critical thinking they are able to construct more in-depth hypotheses. Emergency nurses play a pivotal role within the patient's journey by instigating the plan of care through the validation of the working diagnosis or hypothesis. Their role is, therefore, unique and paramount to the patient's subsequent care and clinical outcome.

References

Aitken LM (2003) Critical care nurses' use of decision-making strategies. *Journal of Clinical Nursing*, **12**, 476–483.

Alfaro-LeFevre R (2004) *Critical Thinking and Clinical Judgment: A practical approach*. Philadelphia: Elsevier Science.

American College of Surgeons (2004) *Advanced Trauma Life Support*, 7th edn. Chicago: American College of Surgeons.

Bakalis NA, Watson R (2005) Nurses' decision-making in clinical practice. *Nursing Standard*, **19**(23), 33–39.

Benner P (1984) *From novice to expert: Excellence and power in Clinical Nursing Practice*. California: Addison-Wesley Publications.

Benner P, Tanner C (1987) Clinical judgment: how expert nurses use intuition. *American Journal of Nursing*, **87**, 23–31.

Bochund PY, Calandra T (2003) Science, medicine and the future: Pathogenesis of sepsis: new concepts and implications for future treatment. *British Medical Journal*, **326**:262–266.

Church A (2003) Critical care and emergency medicine. *Critical Care Clinics*, **19**(2), 271–278.

Cioffi J, Markham R (1997) Clinical decision making: managing case complexity. *Journal of Advanced Nursing*, **25**:265–272.

Cioffi J (1998) Decision making by emergency nurses in triage assessment. *Accident and Emergency Nursing*, **6**, 184–191.

Cioffi J (2000a) Recognition of patients who require emergency assistance: a descriptive study. *Heart and Lung*, **29**(4), 262–268.

Cioffi J (2000b) Nurses' experiences of making decisions to call emergency assistance to their patients. *Journal of Advanced Nursing*, **32**(1), 108–114.

Cioffi J (2001) A study of the use of past experiences in clinical decision making in emergency situations. *International Journal of Nursing Studies*, **38**, 591–599.

Cooke MW, Jinks S (1999) Does the Manchester triage system detect the critically ill? *Journal of Accident and Emergency Medicine*, **16**, 179–181.

Daffurn K, Lee A, Hillman KM, Bishop GF, Bauman A (1994) Do nurses know when to summon emergency assistance? *Intensive and Critical Care Nursing*, **10**(2), 115–120.

Department of Health (2000a) *National Service Framework for Coronary Heart Disease*. London: Department of Health.

Department of Health (2000b) *Comprehensive Critical Care – A Review of Adult Critical Care Services*. London, Department of Health.

Dimond B (2004) *Legal Aspects of Nursing*, 4th edn. London: Longman.

Dolan B, Holt, L (2000) Preface. In: Dolan B, Holt L, eds. *Accident and Emergency Theory into Practice*. London, Baillière Tindall.

Ellis P (1997) Processes used by nurses to make decisions in the clinical practice setting. *Nurse Education Today*, **17**, 325–332.

Evans C (2005) Clinical decision making theories: patient assessment in A&E. *Emergency Nurse*, **13**(5), 16–19.

Evans C, Tippins E (2007) Foundation & Emergency Care, Maidenhead, Mcgraw-Hill.

Fisher A, Fonteyn N (1995) An exploration of an innovative methodological approach for examining nurses' heuristic use in clinical practice. *Scholarly Inquiry for Nursing Practice: An International Journal*, **9**, 263–276.

Fonteyn M, Ritter B (2000) Clinical reasoning in nursing. In: Higgs J, Jones M, eds. *Clinical Reasoning in the Health Professions*. Oxford: Butterworth Heinemann.

Geraci EB, Geraci TA (1994) An observational study of the emergency triage role in a managed care facility. *Journal of Emergency Nursing*, **20**, 189–203.

Grossman SC, Wheeler K (1997) Predicting patients' deterioration and recovery. *Clinical Nursing Research*, **6**, 45–58.

Johns C, Freshwater D (1998) *Transforming Nursing Through Reflective Practice*. Oxford: Blackwell Science.

King L, Appleton J (1997) Intuition: a critical review of the research and rhetoric. *Journal of Advanced Nursing*, **26**, 194–202.

King L, MacLeod Clark J (2002) Intuition and the development of expertise in surgical ward and intensive care nurses. *Journal of Advanced Nursing*, **37**(4), 322–329.

Lindberg JB, Hunter ML, Kruszewski AZ (1994) *Introduction to Nursing: Concepts, Issues and Opportunities*, 2nd edn. Philadelphia: Lippincott.

McCraig LF (1999) National Hospital Ambulatory Medical Survey: emergency department summary. *Advance Data*, **320**(1), 36.

Muir N (2004) Clinical decision-making: theory and practice. *Nursing Standard*, **18**(36), 47–52.

National Audit Office (2004) *Improving Emergency Care in England*. London: The Stationery Office.

Oermann MH (1996) *Professional Nursing Practice: A Conceptual Approach*, 2nd edn. Philadelphia: Lippincott.

O'Neill D, LeGrove A (2003) Monitoring critically ill patients in accident and emergency. *Nursing Times*, **99**(45), 32–35.

Radwin LE (1998) Empirically generated attributes of experience in nursing. *Journal of Advanced Nursing*, **28**, 590–595.

Reeves JS, Paul C (2002) Nursing theory in clinical practice. In: George JB ed. *Nursing Theories: The Base for Professional Nursing Practice*. New Jersey: Prentice Hall.

Resuscitation Council (2004) *Advanced Life Support Course Provider Manual*, 5th edn. London: Resuscitation Council (UK).

Rew L (2000) Acknowledging intuition in clinical decision-making. *Journal of Holistic Nursing*, **18**, 94–108.

Rivers E, Nguyen H, Bryant MD et al. (2002) Critical care and emergency medicine. *Current Opinion in Critical Care*, **8**(6), 600–606.

Robinson D (2000) *Clinical Decision-Making: A Case Study Approach*, 2nd edn. Philadelphia: Lippincott.

Sheehy C, McCarthy M (1998) *Advanced Practice Nursing Emphasizing Common Roles*. Philadelphia: Davis Company.

Sirkka L, Salantera S, Callister LC, Harisson S, Kappeli S, MacLeod M (1998) Decision-making of nurses practising in intensive care in Canada, Finland, Northern Ireland, Switzerland and the United States. *Heart and Lung: The Journal of Acute and Critical Care*, **27**, 133–142.

Tippett J (2004) Nurses acquisition and retention of knowledge after trauma training. *Accident and Emergency Nursing*, **12**, 39–46.

Tippins E (2005) How emergency department nurses identify and respond to critical illness. *Emergency Nurse*, **13**(3), 24–33.

Travers D (1999) Triage: how long does it take? How long should it take? *Journal of Emergency Nursing*, **25**, 238–241.

Watkins MP (1998) Decision-making phenomena described by expert nurses working in urban community health settings. *Journal of Professional Nursing*, **14**, 22–33.

White J, Nativo DG, Kobert SN et al. (1992) Content and process in clinical decision making by nurse practitioners. *Image*, **24**, 153–158.

Wilkinson JM (2001) *Nursing Process: A Critical Thinking Approach*, 3rd edn. New Jersey: Prentice-Hall.

Chapter **37**

Ethical issues

Rosie Wilkinson

INTRODUCTION

Perceptions of ethics are as varied as the mores that inform individual behaviour. Some people see ethics as an esoteric abstraction that belongs firmly in the ivory towers of academe; others see it as an ethereal subject that parliamentarians manipulate in matters of political controversy. There are elements of truth in both these perspectives; ethics is, however, much more than this. Nurses and healthcare professionals are involved in decision-making every day and these decisions may have an ethical component to them. The practice of health care requires not only scientific and practical knowledge but also the ability to make judgements regarding a course of action or plan of care. The ability to make these judgements requires reasoning skills from differing approaches.

Unlike many words, the nature and essence of ethics cannot be succinctly reflected in a single definition. Taking this further, Sparkes (1992) questioned the usefulness of dictionaries and argued that the best which can be offered for ethics is a semantic interpretation; this is given as 'the philosophical study of moral conduct and reasoning'. More simply put, ethics is that branch of philosophy which deals with matters of right and wrong. Knowledge of ethical principles may provide a framework for reasoned thought but cannot provide universal answers.

Sparkes's interpretation gives direction and focus to the essential themes of ethics. In essence, it is concerned with the way in which reason can clarify situations that have a moral dimension. This last point gives a prima facie rationale for placing ethics at the centre of the nursing equation, since the focus of that profession is steeped with issues that demand ethical enquiry and a moral response. Mirroring the vibrancy ethical analysis can offer nursing, Tschudin

(1993) asserts that 'ethics is not only at the heart of nursing; it is the heart of nursing. Ethics is about what is right and good. Nursing and caring are synonymous, and the way in which care is carried out is ethically decisive. How a patient is addressed, cared for and treated must be right not only by ordinary standards of care, but also by ethical principles'.

The purpose of this chapter is to use philosophical reasoning to examine some areas of moral concern that frequently confront practitioners not only in accident and emergency departments but in all emergency care settings. These areas will provide a philosophical adjunct to the legal issues that are covered in Chapter 38, e.g. a duty of care, and consent. The reason for this is to conduct an ethical examination of concepts central to healthcare law in this country. The lines between law and ethics have become blurred over the years and to consider ethics in isolation could potentially distort practice. In an increasing litigious society it is apparent that subjects such as informed consent, access to care, confidentiality, rights, postcode prescribing, withholding and withdrawing care are more open to public scrutiny and possible legal challenge.

This exercise will also usefully show that what may be legal may not be moral and what may be moral may not be legal. History abounds with examples that support this position; it was once illegal for women to have the vote or for gay men to give physical expression to their sexuality. A pressing example from the contemporary arena is euthanasia; proponents argue it is both a moral and a humane concept that liberates an individual's self-governance about the manner and time of death – it has, however, no legal standing. Advanced directives which do give an indication of an individuals' care wishes may, however, need to be heeded.

Given that nurses have a legally enforced duty of care towards patients within the emergency care setting its seems fitting that a chapter dealing with ethics should begin by considering the notion of 'duty' as a central theme in the development of a school of ethical analysis called 'deontology'. During this process, strong parallels will be drawn between deontology, duty as a traditional motivational force in nursing and, also, the Nursing and Midwifery Council (NMC) *Code of Professional Conduct* (NMC 2004)

DUTY AS A MORAL ENDEAVOUR

The historical dimensions of nursing are engulfed by the notion of duty; this tradition is succinctly entwined in the most central of nursing edicts, 'a duty of care'. Within contemporary nursing there remains

a strong allegiance to this theme. This approach is based upon the intrinsic and inalienable relationship that exists between 'rights' and 'duties'. Broadly speaking, once a duty of care has been established, the patient has a right to be cared for and the nurse must facilitate care giving – this is both a legal and moral theme.

The NMC *Code of Professional Conduct* encourages high standards during professional endeavours and expects all practitioners to operate within its framework and guidelines. In the edition published in November 2004 the *Code of Professional Conduct* underwent a name change and has become the NMC *Code of Professional Conduct: Standards for Performance and Ethics*. The principle that nursing practice is inextricably linked with ethics cannot be ignored.

The Nursing and Midwifery Council is the organization set up by Parliament to protect the public by ensuring that nurses and midwives provide high standards of care to their patients and clients. It is the regulatory body responsible for identifying the standards of these professions and requiring members of the professions to practise and conduct themselves within the standards and framework provided by the code. Honesty and ethics are included in the list of the NMC's core values.

Statements made in the code of professional conduct serve to reinforce notions of duty and the statements made within the code provide motivational guidelines for nursing actions. Basing actions upon duties, rules or motives has a long history in ethics and is known as deontology. Kendrick (1993) made the following comment about this method of moral thinking: 'This school of ethical analysis maintains that being moral entails acting from a sense of moral duty, respecting others' rights and honouring one's obligations.'

This interpretation clearly aligns itself with the themes of the NMC *Code of Professional Conduct* and the onus which it places upon registered practitioners. The person most closely associated with deontology is the philosopher Immanuel Kant; he was a prolific writer and fervently advocated that people had intrinsic worth and value. Furthermore, he argued that an essential part of being human was the ability to use reason in deliberating over the moral worth of an action. For Kant, this ability invariably found itself rooted in a sense of duty.

There are many attractive elements of Kantian ethics. In particular, it places a great deal of emphasis upon respect amongst persons and encourages a fervent sense of individual duty. Tschudin (1986) summarized these themes by stating 'a right action is only so if it is done out of a sense of duty, and the only good thing without qualification is a person's good will: the will to do what one knows is right'.

Kant devised a complex moral theory, consisting of three formulations, that he called the categorical imperative. Their precise interpretation and mutual relations are a matter of controversy. Kendrick (1993) simplified the different formulations as follows:

- An action is only moral if you are willing for it to be applied to everyone, yourself included, as a universal law.
- For an action to be moral it must never lead to people being seen just as 'means to an end' but always as 'ends' in their own right.
- In wishing to be moral, individuals must act as members of a community where everybody is seen as having intrinsic worth (ends in their own right).

The essence of the categorical imperative can be readily applied to the duty-based nature of nursing; this will now be discussed with particular relevance to practice in emergency care.

APPLYING THE IMPERATIVE TO PRACTICE

The first part of the imperative indicates that all people have intrinsic worth and should attribute respect to each other; for example, most societies would agree that it is intrinsically wrong to murder another person. The implications of Kant's theory are that persons wishing to undertake such acts should be willing to accept the same being done to themselves – as if they were governed by a universal law that related to that given activity. Expressed simply, the first principle is a moral edict that requires us to ask: 'Would I like this act to be done either to myself or to those close to me?' If the answer is 'no' then Kant would have serious reservations about the moral worth of the motives underpinning the action.

These themes are often introduced to the novice nurse who is asked to care from a basis of duty. While this may initially seem a little simplistic, it can act as a strong image for mental reinforcement and maintaining standards during the delivery of care throughout a nurse's career.

The second of Kant's principles further emphasizes the notion of equal respect amongst persons and resolutely argues that individuals should never be seen or treated solely as means to an end. This does not mean that people cannot work together or help each other – the key theme is that this should involve some degree of mutual reciprocity.

An example of this is the staff nurse who needs to attain the skills of suturing. Obviously, to be able to perform this task safely and competently requires the cooperation of a willing patient. While a patient may be used as a means to an end – the end being the nurse suturing competently – this does not echo the full essence of this part of the imperative. Suturing an open wound also offers some therapeutic worth to the patient; thus the process has benefited the nurse through the acquisition of a skill and the patient through the closure of a wound. Kant did not object to individuals being used as a means to an end as long as they are also valued as ends in their own right.

The essence of the second principle in the imperative does not just apply to the nurse/patient relationship but extends to all interaction within the professional milieu. Not only are nurses required to respect patients as being of equal worth, but this must also govern the professional ethos in dealing with colleagues. This duty to enact the principle of respect for persons is a cogent thread throughout the Code of Professional Conduct, and is alluded to in the first clause (NMC 2004).

- 'As a registered nurse, midwife or specialist community public health nurse, you must respect the patient or client as an individual.'
  Paragraphs 2.1–2.5 elaborate further on the importance of respect, e.g.:
- 2.1 'You must recognize and respect the role of patients and clients as partners in their care and the contribution they can make to it. This involves identifying their preferences regarding care and respecting these within the limits of professional practice, existing legislation, resources and the goals of therapeutic relationship.'
- 2.2 'You are personally accountable for ensuring that you promote and protect the interests and dignity of patients and clients, irrespective of gender, age, race, ability, sexuality, economic status, lifestyle, culture and religious or political beliefs.'

Such themes are vitally important given that recent years have seen the blurring of roles between doctors and nurses. If practitioners from both professions are to have shared working practices, it must be through mutual respect and the fervent desire to embellish the care that is offered to patients. Such notions offer the opportunity to embrace the themes of shared governance and create an organizational milieu where all concerned can achieve their potential. Such themes were given sharp focus for nursing by the introduction of the *Scope of Professional Practice* (UKCC 1992) and the associated concept of advanced practice (Kendrick 1997).

Respect is a central element in Kantian thinking and the word appears frequently throughout the NMC *Code of Professional Conduct* (NMC). A strong emphasis upon respect emerges from the third and final part of the imperative; its essential message is that persons form a community where each member has equal worth as a moral decision-maker. Nurses meet colleagues or patients who may have very different values or beliefs from their own. Sometimes these differences are informed by cultural or religious diversity. Kantian ethics suggests that the key issue is to respect the freedom of other individuals to hold moral perspectives and to act upon them – this is part of what it means to treat others as ends.

If this is applied to the professional setting, it asks that all people have equal authority to express and defend their respective positions. Once again, it can be suggested that this theme runs throughout the NMC *Code of Professional Conduct*. However, the first clause in paragraph 2.1 specifically supports this notion:

- 'recognize and respect the role of patients and clients as partners in their care and the contribution they can make to it.'

The fourth clause deals with working cooperatively with others in the team; paragraph 4.1 states:

- You are expected to work co-operatively within teams and to respect the skills expertise and contributions of your colleagues. You must treat them fairly and without discrimination.

To this point it has been seen that duty-based approaches to ethical thinking and analysis have a long history in moral theory. This has been supported with reference to deontology and the philosopher most closely associated with it, Immanuel Kant. Moreover, clear links have been drawn between the deontological approach and the duty-based themes that run throughout nursing.

The NMC *Code of Professional Conduct* provides a series of guidelines and principles that inform a practitioner's professional obligations and preserve the traditional emphasis upon duty-based care-giving. However, while it may be suggested that principles of duty provide indications that can help give directions about professional conduct, there are problems with such approaches that demand clarification and analysis.

DUTY AS A MORAL PROBLEM

A glaring problem with duty-based approaches to morality and Kantian ethics in particular is that they tend to portray certain maxims as absolute, universal and all-encompassing. There are many examples from the real world which highlight an unquestioning bond to duty-based dictums; for example, certain religions require their members not to accept whole blood products during medical treatments. There is much room for debate about whether or not a principle/duty can ever be thought to be ubiquitous and applied as a categorical tenet.

Within nursing there are certain rules which are perceived, as has already been discussed, as absolute; principal among these is the duty of care. However, sometimes the maxims within a duty of care can be at variance with each other. Consider the following principles:

- a duty to do good (beneficence)
- a duty to do no harm (non-maleficence).

At first glance these principles seem closely related. However, further analysis does reveal distinct differences between the two themes. Nurses always try to ensure that their actions promote good and preserve the best interests of the patient. This leads nurses to an interesting and penetrating question: 'Can we say that nursing actions always promote good results for patients?' It is very doubtful that nurses can say 'yes' to this question; to a large extent this is because harm is an intrinsic part of some nursing actions.

The simplest example of this is when a nurse gives an intramuscular injection. Every time the syringe is introduced, it causes pain which, even to a very small degree, can be equated with harm. Many other nursing interventions carry the same ethos: antibiotics may cause an irritating rash; aspirin can cause gastric erosion; and diamorphine or other opiate derivatives can cause chronic constipation. Some of the more advanced nursing practices, e.g. intubation or cannulation, carry a host of risks that can, if realized, greatly harm the patient. Given the amount of harm which can result from some of our actions, the nurse needs to ask if the principle of non-maleficence is appropriate and applicable as a universal tenet in nursing.

Harris (1985) has argued that health care professionals do not have any special obligations, but are subject to the same sort of duties as any other person in society. All individuals have a duty to respect persons or to do no harm however it has been seen that the NMC *Code of Professional Conduct* (2004) identifies certain obligations as part of the professional role.

ABOVE ALL, DO NO HARM

Believing the absolute notion that nursing actions will never do any harm is impractical because it can never be totally achieved within the professional role. Some of the 'harm' which can be induced by nursing actions has already been seen. This theme has been explored and analysed by Illich (1975), with particular reference to the medical profession, but may be applied with equal resonance to nursing, especially now that advanced practice involves nurses performing tasks that formerly fell under the sole auspices of medics.

Illich (1975) used the word 'iatrogenesis' to describe the harmful results and illnesses that can result from the intervention of doctors. For example, Illich (1975) claimed that 'it has been established that one out of every five patients admitted to a typical research hospital acquires an iatrogenic disease, sometimes trivial, usually requiring special treatment, and in one case in thirty leading to death. Half of these episodes resulted from complications of drug therapy; amazingly, one in ten comes from diagnostic procedures. Despite good intentions and claims to public service, with a similar record of performance a military officer would be relieved of his command and a restaurant or amusement centre would be closed by police'.

Illich (1975) has been criticized for not placing enough emphasis upon the amount of good which medicine achieves. This is a valid criticism and it leads to the centre of the debate about absolute duties as all-encompassing principles. It can be stated with a degree of certainty that the primary intention of practitioners is to promote beneficence and to strive to achieve non-maleficence. However, to place these two themes in the language of absolute duties is no more than an exercise in rhetoric and cannot be upheld in the 'real' world of delivering care.

The key issue is not to insist that health professionals abide unquestioningly by a duty to do good and a duty to do no harm – clearly the two duties are not always reconcilable as consummate themes. The essential worth of the two principles is found in balancing them both together, not viewing them as isolated absolutes. Returning to the example of the intramuscular injection, while the initial result may be pain or harm, this is usually outweighed by the amount of good that results from the therapeutic worth of the injected drug. This serves to highlight that the balance between beneficence and non-maleficence can help practitioners to reflect upon the worth of an action.

The essential problem with this is that the consequences of an action cannot always be forecast beforehand – crystal ball gazing is a poor basis for moral analysis. Despite this drawback, trying to weigh the moral worth of an action against the harm which it may produce at least asks for a degree of questioning, reflection and analysis; this is surely more acceptable than a passive acceptance of absolute, but conflicting, duties.

Practitioners at the 'cutting edge' of health care delivery have always had an intuitive awareness of the precarious balance between beneficence and non-maleficence. Unfortunately, the power relationship between doctors and nurses has usually resulted in the nurse handing issues of a moral nature over to the doctor, who then tries to deal with them through the value-free objectivity of a 'clinical decision'. Contemporary practice challenges such themes; 'teamwork' and parity in the decision-making process demand input from all interested parties; this is further supported by Kendrick (1997), who states 'in the UK, doctors need to stop seeing situations that are ethically relevant as something to be subsumed under the broad notion of a 'clinical decision'. In essence, this should mean shared governance with other practitioners – after all, ethics belongs to us all and is not the sole domain of medics.'

This section has presented an argument which highlights the inadequacies of duty-based principles as moral panaceas which can be applied and invoked for all ethical 'ills'. Emerging from this is a clear theme that moral duties can rarely stand as absolute and isolated 'ends'. Moral duties, whatever their nature, remain rhetorical unless they give clear and non-conflicting directions for the pathways of practice.

Chapter 38 gives a focused overview of the legal themes that inform a 'duty of care'. In comparison, this section has given an adjunct to the legal scenario and shown that using duty-based approaches to moral reasoning is often self-limiting. Taking this further, duty has been considered here in relation to such themes as: duty as a traditional force in nursing, the NMC *Code of Professional Conduct* (NMC 2004), the nurse/patient relationship, interprofessional relationships and, finally, the moral conflict that results when duties conflict. However, and this is vital, while nurses may liberally question the philosophical foundation of duty-based methods of ethical analysis, our legal requirement to fulfil a duty of care to patients, once established, remains absolute (Jones 1997).

It has been seen that the duties of beneficence and non-maleficence must have value as means to an end if they are to have meaning and essence for practitioners. This can be said with equal efficacy about the principles embodied in the NMC *Code of Professional Conduct* (2004). In essence, they provide the starting point for discussion, analysis and professional discernment but they are not categorical absolutes. Chadwick & Tadd (1992) pursue this line of enquiry and note 'a code of conduct or ethics should perhaps be seen, not as the last word on ethics, but as a stimulus to moral thinking'. Such themes are vital when considering the moral milieu of nursing practice in emergency care settings. What is also essential is an understanding of the ethical issues that engulf the notion of consent. In Chapter 38, consent is considered within a legal framework; the next part of this chapter will explore the moral dimensions of that concept.

CONSENT AS AN ETHICAL PROCESS

Informed consent, by its very nature, demands that nurses give patients all the information needed to make an informed decision. This theme is reflected by Gillon (1985), who argued that consent can be defined as 'a voluntary and un-coerced decision made by a sufficiently competent or autonomous person, on the basis of adequate information and deliberation, to accept rather than reject some proposed course of action that will affect him or her'.

However, a key issue is: how do nurses define 'adequate information'? For example, how many nurses would divulge to a male patient, brought into A&E with acute urinary retention, the remote possibility that catheterization may result in a perforated urethra? Intrinsic to this notion is a complex and controversial question: how much information should be given to patients before an informed consent can be given to the treatment or intervention offered? (Kendrick 1994).

Broadly speaking, there are two opposing perspectives towards this question. Kendrick (1991) argues that 'at one end of the spectrum there are those who believe that the patient should have access to every conceivable issue involved in their treatment or care. This is based on the understanding that a patient who is privy to both negative and positive aspects of their treatment or care will be able to make an informed and valid consent. In contrast to this perspective is the paternalistic view that a nurse has the necessary insight and professional knowledge to judge when the giving of certain information would be harmful to the patient'.

Both of these positions contain elements which make a valid argument and deserve further examination. This demands an exploration of the key ethical principles which support the notion of a full and informed consent.

The myth of self-governance

In its most basic form, autonomy is concerned with an individual's level of self-government. Faulder (1985) broadened this to offer an interpretation which can be directly applied to nursing practice: 'the

individual's freedom to decide her or his goals and to act according to these goals'. However, the idea of absolute autonomy is something of a myth – nobody can be fully independent and self-governing. Consider the term 'autonomous nurse'; it is facile to think of an individual's practice as something which is free of constraints. Nurses have to work within a framework which is influenced by a Code of Professional Conduct (UKCC 1992a), the organizational milieu and the needs of patients; thus, total autonomy is not reconcilable with the limitations of the real world. These themes are reflected by Henry & Pashley (1990), who state 'full autonomy is an ideal notion and we can only approximate to it. It is obvious that, in reality, some situations, states and circumstances will diminish a person's autonomy, such as the ability to control his or her actions, or both, through being restricted in some way, for example, illness, psychological impairment, physical or mental disability'. Ardagh (2004) offers the practical example of resuscitation where the patient's competence is impaired, as he or she is unable to receive information, undertake rational deliberation or express a decision free from coercion.

However, despite many practical difficulties, nurses must always strive to eliminate barriers which may hinder a patient's autonomy and freedom of choice.

Freedom to choose

There is a close relationship between autonomy and informed consent, the former being concerned with freedom and choice, the latter being the key which unlocks and enables their expression. Taking this further, it would be extremely difficult for patients to take an active part in decisions relating to care if they did not have the necessary information on which to make choices.

If autonomy is respected in practice, then patients should feel uninhibited about identifying their own needs and actively deciding how these should be met. However, a problem with discussing autonomy is that it can create an impression that all patients want to take part in such a full and dynamic role. A missing element here is that patients are, by definition, sick and often vulnerable; this may be particularly relevant to the patients you meet in emergency care – especially given the often shocking nature of sudden illness or trauma. This may conjure up different images for different people. Some patients may see it as a place of safety where their illness or trauma will be addressed, while others see it as a reflection of their own mortality and hear the ringing of the death knell.

For patients who see the emergency department as a symbol of fear, it may be inappropriate to expect them to take an active role in the decision-making process. This is not paternalism; if, after the choice has been offered, patients express no wish to take an active role in their care then it should be accepted as an expression of autonomy. Kendrick (1991) supports this notion and states 'the patient should be given the freedom to say to the nurse that he wishes to surrender any role within the decision-making process. This agreement may be temporary or permanent in nature. What must be emphasized here, is that when a patient gives the nurse responsibility for decisions he does not relinquish autonomy, but gives acknowledgement of it'.

Such approaches indicate the patient's right to freely decide what may or may not be done to his body. Indeed, irrespective of ethical considerations, performing an act without the patient's permission may, as is discussed in Chapter 38, constitute negligence in legal terms. All of this reflects an ethico-legal emphasis which is intended to protect the vulnerable status of patients. Such themes, however, frequently place practitioners in emergency care in very precarious positions; perhaps the most telling example of this is when an unconscious person is brought into the department after taking an overdose. Practitioners do not usually have the benefit of time and must act quickly if life is to be preserved. This is frequently when the maxim 'act first, ask questions later' comes into its own. What happens, however, when a patient is semi-conscious and gives the expressed desire to be left to die? There is no time to get a psychiatrist's opinion, no time to think about the patient's level of competence – just a real dilemma that needs an immediate decision. This is where ethics finds its most cutting edge.

The legal grounds for acting without the patient's consent could well be based on urgency and necessity – remembering also that failing to act holds the risk of being accused of negligence (see Ch. 38). It is an unfortunate aspect of contemporary practice that practitioners may be 'damned if they do and damned if they don't'. Proponents of a literal and absolute interpretation of autonomy (self-governance) may argue that, irrespective of legal defences, health care professionals never have a sufficient moral mandate to override the expressed wish of a patient to be left to die; Brown et al. (1992) offered a brief and cogent comment on such themes: 'we cannot solve the dilemmas by saying that we should always do what the patient wishes'.

Such sober insights give buoyancy to the essential elements of moral reasoning in health care; ethics is not about providing panaceas for all the moral ills of practice. It can, however, offer a focused means of reaching rational decisions about the issues that confront practitioners in emergency departments.

CONCLUSION

This chapter has critically explored two major ethical themes that continually challenge practitioners in emergency care: duty and consent. Within these broad concepts, a host of other issues have also been considered that often cause moral concern. It would be impossible, in a chapter of this size, to do justice to all the dilemmas that confront practitioners in emergency care; such an endeavour would command a book in its own right. However, it is hoped that this chapter has charged the reader with enough creative energy to read further and explore other areas that confront one's own practice.

References

Ardagh M (2004) Ethics of resuscitation. In: Cameron P, Jelinek G, Kelly AM, Murray L, Brown AFT, Heyworth J, eds. *Textbook of Adult Emergency Medicine*, 2nd edn. Edinburgh: Churchill Livingstone.

Brown JM, Kitson A, McKnight TJ (1992) *Challenges in Caring: Explorations in Nursing and Ethics*. London: Chapman and Hall.

Chadwick RF, Tadd W (1992) *Ethics and Nursing Practice: A Case Study Approach*. Basingstoke: Macmillan.

Faulder C (1985) *Whose Body is it?: The Troubling Issues of Informed Consent*. London: Virago.

Gillon R (1985) Autonomy and consent. In: Lockwood M, ed. *Moral Dilemmas in Modern Medicine*. Oxford: Oxford University Press.

Harris J (1985) *The Value of Life*. London: Routledge.

Henry C, Pashley G (1990) *Health Ethics*. Lancaster: Quay Books.

Illich I (1975) *Medical Nemesis: the Expropriation of Health*. London: Calder and Boyers.

Jones G (1997) Liability in A&E nursing. *Emergency Nurse*, **5**(5), 18–20.

Kendrick KD (1991) Partners in passing: ethical aspects of nursing the dying person. *International Journal of Advances in Health and Nursing Care*, **1**(1), 11–27.

Kendrick KD (1993) Ethics and nursing practice. *British Journal of Nursing*, **2**(18), 920–926.

Kendrick KD (1994) Freedom to choose: the ethics of consent. *Professional Nurse*, **9**(11), 739–742.

Kendrick KD (1997) What is advanced nursing? (Editorial) *Professional Nurse*, **12**(10), 689.

Kendrick KD (1998) Ethical issues in critical care. In: Tadd W, ed. *Nursing Ethics: a European Perspective.* Basingstoke: Macmillan.

Nursing and Midwifery Council (2004) *Code of Professional Conduct: Standards for Conduct, Performance and Ethics.* London: NMC.

Sparkes AW (1992) *Talking Philosophy: A Workbook.* London: Routledge.

Tschudin V (1986) *Ethics in Nursing: The Caring Relationship.* London: Heinemann Nursing.

Tschudin V (1993) *Ethics: Aspects of Nursing Care.* London: Scutari Press.

UKCC (1992) *The Scope of Professional Practice.* London: UKCC.

Chapter **38**

Law

Nicola Meeres

INTRODUCTION

This chapter considers the main areas of law relevant to the emergency department (ED). It highlights the key areas where a knowledge of law is essential and discusses some of the legal dilemmas that may arise. Attendance, assessment, treatment and care, consent to treatment, detention of patients, confidentiality, the police, the press and staff health and safety are considered.

AN OUTLINE OF LAW IN THE UK

Although the UK is one state, it is made up of four countries whose laws have developed separately. England and Wales have identical legal systems and whilst the law in Northern Ireland has developed along similar lines, Scottish law has not. Some law is specific to each country; for example the absence of an Abortion Act in Northern Ireland. In this chapter, the law stated applies to England and Wales: where marked differences exist in Northern Ireland and Scotland, these will be mentioned. Otherwise, the reader can assume that the law is broadly applicable across the whole of the UK.

Statute law is created either by Acts of Parliament or through a system of delegated legislation. Statutory Instruments, or Rules, form part of delegated legislation and they empower statutory bodies to expand or amend law for enactment by the Secretary of State. Delegated legislation is becoming increasingly important due to the pressures on parliamentary time.

Case law has developed through the judicial system as judges make decisions on the interpretation of law within the court setting. Once an outcome has been reached then a precedent is set for all other judges to follow in similar circumstances. Decisions made are binding on all courts below that where the precedent was set. For example, decisions made by the House of Lords are binding on all lower courts in the UK, but the House of Lords can overturn its own decisions and The European Court of Justice can set precedent for member states. Case law is of particular relevance to health care (Montgomery 2002).

Department of Health circulars and the Nursing and Midwifery Council (NMC) *Code of Professional Conduct* (NMC 2004) are not legally binding but they are recommended practice. The NMC was established under the Nursing and Midwifery Order (2001) and came into being on 1 April 2002 and has authority to prepare rules that carry the weight of law. The code of professional conduct standards for conduct, performance and ethics (NMC 2004) is issued for 'guidance and advice', laying a moral responsibility rather than a statutory duty on members of the profession. A marked failure to abide by the Code could, in turn, lead to the NMC using its disciplinary function, with legal implications of removal of the nurse's name from the register.

CLASSIFICATION OF LAW

Law is divided into civil and criminal law. Criminal law is concerned with the relationship between the state and individuals. Criminal offences are committed against the state and are punishable by the state, for example drug offences and theft. Civil law is concerned with the rights and duties of individuals towards each other. Legal action is taken by a private citizen rather than the state, and a successful outcome results in an award of monetary compensation only, e.g. a patient suing a hospital for damages following some harm that has resulted from treatment or the lack thereof. Some civil wrongs can also be crimes, e.g. assault and battery, and gross negligence which could become manslaughter.

The concept of a legal defence is an important one as it is a legally recognized reason for the act committed not to have been a criminal or civil wrong. The most widely met example of this is the giving of consent as a defence against assault and battery. Probably two of the most relevant areas of civil law for emergency nursing are negligence, as this relates to the standard of care given to the patient, and the law on assault and battery, as this is relevant to the patients' rights.

Negligence

For negligence of any kind to be proved, it must be shown that the following components exist (Martin 2005):

- that the defendant (nurse) owed a duty of care to the plaintiff (patient) (established in the case of *Donohue* v. *Stevenson* [1932])
- that the defendant was in breach of that duty (*Bolam* v. *Friern Hospital Management Committee* [1957])
- harm to the plaintiff, which was reasonably foreseeable, resulted directly from the breach of duty of care (*Barnett* v. *Kensington & Chelsea Hospital Management Committee* [1969]).

The Bolam case (Pannett 1997) laid down the principle of how to judge the standard of care that must be given as that of the 'reasonably skilled and experienced doctor as accepted by a responsible body of medical men skilled in that particular art' (*Bolam* v. *Friern Hospital Management Committee* 1957). The Wilsher case (*Wilsher* v. *Essex* AHA 1988) made it clear that the standard of care required was that of the post held not of the post-holder (*Tingle & Crabb* 2002). These precedents are applicable to all health care workers (Box 38.1).

Clinical documentation can be pivotal in cases of negligence (National Audit Office 2001, Green 1999). The approach that the law tends to take to record-keeping is that if it has not been recorded, it has not been done. ED nurses should be scrupulous in the documentation of their actions to reduce the risk of legal difficulties should a case be brought against them or their colleagues.

Box 38.1 Negligence checklist. (Carson & Montgomery 1989)

1. Did the nurse have a duty of care? If 'yes', continue. If 'no', there can be no liability
2. Was there a breach in the appropriate standard of care? If 'yes' continue. If 'no', there can be no liability
3. Did the breach of the standard cause the losses? If 'yes' continue. If 'no', there can be no liability
4. Are the losses of a kind recognized by law? If 'yes' continue. If 'no', there can be no liability
5. Were the losses too remote? If 'yes' continue. If 'no', there can be no liability
6. Did the patient contribute to the happening or extent of his or her losses? If 'yes' there has been contributory negligence and the damages will be proportionately reduced.

Assault and battery

The civil wrong of trespass can be committed to land, goods or the person. This last category is also known as assault and battery. Assault is an attempt or threat to apply unlawful force to the person of another, whereby that other person is put in fear of immediate violence or at least bodily contact. Battery is the actual application of force, however slight, to the person of another against his or her will.

There are a number of important defences against a legal action for trespass to the body (Box 38.2). Success in suing for trespass is not high and a number of patients have a better outcome using the law on negligence, e.g. in relation to inadequate information given in order to gain consent (Brazier 2003).

ATTENDANCE

There is a clear legal duty on the hospital running an emergency service to see and treat all those who attend. Purely by virtue of their coming within its doors, the hospital accepts responsibility, even without formally admitting them. A failure to treat those who present themselves could be negligence (Young 1999).

Many people who attend ED are under the influence of alcohol and/or drugs and can be both difficult and disruptive. Healthcare professionals have an obligation to undertake clinical assessment before any decision not to treat is made, even in circumstances where a patient is uncooperative. For example, a hypoglycaemic patient will present as aggressive and uncooperative, often appearing drunk; left untreated hypoglycaemia is life-threatening. The onus is on the nurse to ensure sufficient history or investigation has taken place to determine whether there is a clinical cause for behaviour. Once such assessment has taken place and the outcome been documented, removal or refusal to treat can be ordered with the support of security staff or the police when appropriate.

In such situations, security staff are allowed to use reasonable force to protect themselves, prevent injury or damage to property and to use reasonable force to contain uncooperative persons until the police arrive. Theoretically this situation could possibly give rise to a claim of assault and battery against security staff and/or the police; however, where reasonable force as opposed to excessive force can be identified, this is unlikely to happen or to be upheld.

The situation would be different if those causing these difficulties were not there as patients, but as friends or relatives, or if the patient had already been seen and treated. In this case, the individuals can be asked to leave; a failure to do so would mean they were then trespassing on hospital property and can be evicted.

It is imperative that all incidents of this nature should be accurately and thoroughly documented.

ASSESSMENT

Most emergency departments have a system of assessing the urgency of patients' conditions on arrival. The criteria used to allocate patients to certain treatment groups largely rely on some degree of diagnosis. For the nurse, the crucial issue of undertaking patient assessment is whether he has sufficient knowledge to make an assessment competently, act on this assessment and to know his own limitations. Assessing a patient as less critically ill than in fact is the case, with a subsequent delay in treatment, could result in negligence.

The NMC's *Code of Professional Conduct* (2004) makes a nurse undertaking such roles personally accountable for his practice, that is, answerable for all acts and omissions and for the maintenance of his/her professional knowledge and competence. However, the NMC *Code of Professional Conduct* (2004) Clause 6.2 also states that the nurse must 'acknowledge the limits of her/his professional competence and only undertake practice and accept responsibilities for those activities in which she is competent'.

If the nurse is required to carry out patient assessment, the manager must provide the necessary training and carry the legal responsibility of delegating appropriately, as there can be negligence in delegation. In addition, where patient assessment is seen as part of the nurse's role, the employer will be vicariously liable for any negligence of the employee. This employer liability arises from the old law of master and servant relationship, where the employer has to carry this legal responsibility by reason of having a contract with the employee. Vicarious liability may also exist with agency staff, but its extent may depend on the exact nature of the contract.

Under Section 2 of the Limitation Act (1980), a case for negligence must be commenced within three years

---

Box 38.2 Legal defences to a civil action for assault and battery

- Consent
- Urgency and necessity
- Acting under a statutory power, e.g., the Mental Health Act
- Patients' 'best interests'

of the date of the cause of the action or when the effects become apparent to the plaintiff (Pannett 1997). It may be considerably longer before the case comes to court. Section 14 of the Act also requires that the injury is significant and relates this to the plaintiff's knowledge of the injury. The lengthy timescale underlines the importance of record-keeping for nursing and medical staff.

TREATMENT AND CARE

A vitally important question is: what is the standard of care that is expected and must be reached in the emergency department in order to avoid legal repercussions? From a number of legal cases relating to medical care, it is clear that the standard must be safe care and one which is accepted as proper by a responsible body of medical opinion (Mason & McCall-Smith 2002). Reasonable, rather than excellent, skill is considered sufficient. The standard in the emergency department will be that considered acceptable and reasonable in the conditions and circumstances in which nursing care is given.

The standard must relate to the speciality to which it is applied. Thus, nurses new to emergency department work must be aware that inexperience can never be an excuse for negligence. This was stated very clearly in *Wilsher* v. *Essex* AHA (1988), when inexperience in the work of the neonatal intensive care unit was put forward as a reason for the doctor's mistake in taking the wrong blood from baby Wilsher and subsequently prescribing the wrong level of oxygen (Tingle & Crabb 2002). Both appeal judges were emphatic that the standard of care must be that of the post held, not of the post-holder. The lesson to be learned from this is that adequate training and supervision are vital until the nurse is competent in the skills required.

The legal significance of the above applies to both the varied nature of the work as well as the range of skills of the workforce. For example, a number of people present to an emergency department with mental health problems; ideally these people should be cared for by Community Psychiatric Nurses (CPNs), but in reality most emergency departments do not employ CPNs directly. The general/adult trained nurses therefore have to manage these patients to the best of their ability. In these circumstances, the standard is probably not that of the CPN, but of a nurse experienced in dealing with the range of circumstances presented by those with mental health problems in this particular setting.

The importance of multidisciplinary teamwork is recognized in most patient care settings and is particularly relevant to emergency departments where a number of different professionals work together. Traditionally doctors had overall legal responsibility for the patient, but care roles have become blurred and this is no longer the case. Patients are now solely managed by other health professionals, who take responsibility for their care. Nurses should ensure that they are adequately trained and are working within parameters agreed with the organization, which the organization would then be vicariously liable for. In order to safeguard the different members of the team, care must be taken in delegating tasks to members, whether it is across professional boundaries or from more senior members of the nursing team to those more junior.

Three checks can be made in order to avoid negligence (Young 1991):

- the extent of the nurse's knowledge
- the level of skill in the task delegated either through asking about past experience or through direct observation
- through teaching and supervision over a period.

NURSE'S PRESCRIBING POWERS

Many emergency nurses are either supplementary or independent prescribers. An independent prescriber takes responsibility for the clinical assessment of the patient, establishing a diagnosis and the clinical management required, as well as prescribing where necessary (Department of Health 2004). A supplementary prescriber works with an independent prescriber to implement an agreed patient-specific clinical management plan.

Recent legislation in the form of a Statutory Instrument has extended nurse's prescribing powers (HMSO 2005). The changes, which came into force on the 1st May 2006 in England, allow qualified nurse independent prescribers to prescribe any licensed medicine for any medical condition within their competence, including some controlled drugs. This is a significant change, as independent prescribers can now prescribe from the British National Formulary based on their clinical competence rather than from the nurses' formulary. Both independent prescribers and supplementary prescribers are now able to prescribe opiates in some circumstances.

DEATH AND ORGAN DONATION

There are a number of legal issues surrounding death in the emergency department: the first is the legal definition of death. Although this still stands as the total stoppage of circulation of blood and cessation of animal and vital body functions, the concept of brainstem death is now accepted by the courts. There will not, therefore, be a legal difficulty in turning off a life-support system once brainstem death has been diagnosed. In situations where death has not occurred but prognosis and quality of life are so poor that to continue with treatment seems to have no useful purpose, the law accepts decisions not to do so. Appropriately qualified healthcare professionals can verify that death has taken place; however, brainstem death can only be certified by a doctor.

Organ donation can create legal as well as ethical dilemmas in an emergency department (Wilkinson 2000, Sweet 1996). The Human Tissue Act (2004) makes consent a fundamental principle. If the deceased has not given consent before death, then the consent of a nominated representative is required; in the absence of this, then it will be the consent of a 'qualifying relative' that is needed. These 'qualifying relatives' relationships are ranked in order when consent is being sought to use tissue or organs for scheduled purposes (see Box 38.3).

PATIENT PROPERTY

The same rules apply for the care of property in the emergency department as in a ward, but the clinical condition of some patients demands the nurse to become 'bailiff' for the property of those unable to take this responsibility themselves (Dimond 2004). The task of checking property soon after arrival in these cases is important, due to the open nature of the environment and the high risk of theft. Preferably, two people should together check, list, sign and ensure valuables are locked away safely. When death occurs, valuables should not be given to relatives, but again the proper hospital procedures should be followed.

In an emergency, such as cardiac arrests, clothing may have to be cut off, but this should only be done

---

> **Box 38.3 Qualifying relatives to give consent (in descending order)**
>
> - Spouse or partner
> - Parent or child
> - Brother or sister
> - Grandparent or grandchild
> - Child of a brother or sister
> - Stepfather or stepmother
> - Half brother or half sister
> - Friend of long standing

---

as a last resort. If clothes are heavily contaminated by blood or parasites and need to be destroyed, the patient's permission should be sought where possible and documentation of items destroyed should be made. Additionally, where there is a possibility of legal action, for instance, following criminal activity, resulting in alleged stabbings, gunshot wounds or sexual assault, care must be taken to cut and bag clothing, in ways that will enable forensic examiners to undertake their role to the satisfaction of the courts.

CONSENT TO TREATMENT

For treatment to be given, a patient's consent must be gained in order to avoid being sued for assault and battery. For this consent to be legally effective, the patient must be able to understand and come to a decision about what is involved. Under common law, the patient has the right to give or withdraw consent for treatment or a procedure at any time.

Consent can be given in writing, orally or be assumed from the patient's actions, e.g. from the fact that the patient voluntarily attends the emergency department. However, Cable et al. (2003) argue that the nurse must not assume that a patient is giving consent by virtue of his or her voluntary attendance. Listening to each patient's responses and observing his or her non-verbal behaviour is an essential part of the process of ensuring that legally valid consent is also informed consent. Dimond (2005) cautions that where there is a dispute, written consent is the preferred evidence that consent was given. However, the signature on the consent form should not be seen as the consent itself, but evidence that, following a process of communication between the health professional and the patient which was understood by the patient, consent was given to the proposed intervention. The Department of Health (2001), as part of its implementation of the NHS Plan (Department of Health 2000), has also been keen to promote best process in securing informed consent following recommendations that emerged from the Bristol Royal Infirmary Inquiry Report (Department of Health 2001).

Written consent is usually reserved for those treatments or investigations carrying a marked risk and is usually obtained by the person undertaking the procedure or by the doctor. The nurse may be able to help clarify a patient's lack of understanding or assist the patient in finding out the information required, but the nurse must ensure that he or she is competent to undertake this role and that any information is accurate.

For most nursing actions, consent will be gained orally and this is better practice professionally than assuming consent. Oral consent should be recorded in the clinical record. It is not an unusual occurrence for patients to be brought into the department who are either unable or unwilling to give consent to treatment. As shown in Box 38.2, there are a number of legal 'defences' or reasons that treatment can be given, apart from consent, without there being a case for assault and battery.

When a patient cannot give a valid consent due to a lack of understanding, treatment that is urgent and necessary can still be given. Thus the unconscious, semiconscious or mentally confused patient can be treated on this basis.

Under the Mental Capacity Act (2005), everything that is done for or on behalf of a person who lacks capacity must be in that person's best interests.

Nonetheless, in law, the health professionals' care for patients in the absence of consent is part of their duty to care for them out of necessity in an emergency and they would have to defend any subsequent action for trespass to the person on that basis (Young 1991). Those suffering the effects of alcohol or drugs could also be included in this category.

Under the Police Reform Act (2002), where the police believe that for a medical reason a person is incapable of giving valid consent to having a blood specimen taken, following involvement in a road traffic accident, the police may now request that a blood specimen be taken by the medical practitioner and stored. However, if the medical practitioner in charge of the patient believes that this would be prejudicial to the proper care and treatment of the patient, then the request can be objected to and it will not be carried out.

With a child it is usual, if the child is under 16, for the consent of the parents or guardian to be sought. In the case of unmarried parents, only the mother's consent is legally binding unless the father has legal guardianship. If the situation is too urgent to await the arrival of a parent, the child can give consent if she has sufficient understanding, or the urgency and necessity rule can be used. The Children Act (Department of Health 1989) also makes it clear that the child's wishes are paramount and no court direction overrides the child's right of refusal to be examined provided she has sufficient understanding. A 'Gillick competent' minor is deemed to have sufficient understanding and intelligence to enable him to understand fully what is proposed (Gillick v. W. Norfolk & Wisbech Area Health Authority [1985]).

'Gillick competence' relates to the particular child and the particular treatment: there have been cases where a 17 year old has been found to be insufficiently competent to refuse medical treatment, while in other cases much younger children have been deemed sufficiently competent. It is for the health practitioner to decide whether an individual child is 'Gillick competent' (NHS Confidentiality Guidelines).

Predicaments can arise in any of these situations when relatives either take a different view from the patient or claim that the patient, if mentally capable, would have refused consent. The often-quoted example is of the unconscious patient who is a Jehovah's Witness and requires a blood transfusion. The emergency department team can still proceed on the basis that, as this is an unforeseen emergency, it would be impossible to know the patient's wishes if faced with possible death.

Relatives may also expect to be in the position of giving consent on behalf of an adult patient unable to do so. There is no legal basis for asking relatives for their consent in these circumstances. They may be consulted about the patient's preferences, but the decision to proceed with treatment will be a medical one on the basis of urgency and necessity. The NMC (2004) under Clause 3.8 also supports the notion of proceeding if it is in the patient's 'best interests', stating 'In emergencies where treatment is necessary to preserve life, you may provide care without patients' consent, if they are unable to give it, provided you can demonstrate that you are acting in their best interests'. This guidance does, however, create an ethical dilemma for healthcare practitioners but, in terms of the law, both a decision to treat and a decision not to treat based on evidence of the patient's beliefs would be acceptable.

Health carers also face a difficulty when caring for a patient who is still conscious but is refusing treatment following a drug overdose. The Mental Health Act (1983) may appear to provide a treatment pathway by placing the patient under the emergency section of the Act and then giving treatment against her will, but it would be wrong to assume that all those attempting suicide are mentally disordered under the terms of the Act. It is also unlikely the Act could be applied, as assessment of the patient's mental state could be impaired by the drugs taken. Castledine (1994) has argued that an apparently irrational refusal can still be a competent one and the decision whether to treat or not may then become an ethical one. Proceeding against the patient's will lays the carers open to an action for assault and battery; however, in reality, the likelihood of a patient's bringing and pursuing any such action through the courts is low. Abiding by the patient's wishes, on the other hand, whilst legally correct, places a responsibility on the healthcare practitioner to ensure that the patient understands the potential outcome of no treatment; the healthcare practitioner then has to make a professional decision based on what they perceive the patient's state of mind to be.

In many of these predicaments, the legal difficulty may be one of balancing patients' rights against a possible accusation of negligence in failing to act. Whatever is decided, both arguments should be considered and, if they are particularly contentious, a written record should be made of how the decision was reached.

DETENTION OF PATIENTS

As well as times when it is legally acceptable to treat without the patient's consent, there are also occasions when individuals can be detained against their will (Young 1989). Of relevance to the health care worker in the ED are the following. Patients may be detained under Section 4 of the Mental Health Act (1983). Admission to hospital for assessment in cases of emergency lasts for 72 hours. The grounds for using this order are an urgent necessity that the patient should be admitted and detained for assessment and that compliance with the normal procedure would involve undesirable delay. The recommendation of only one medical practitioner is required. There will be arrangements made for an on-call psychiatrist to attend the ED.

The only other section likely to be met is Section 136. This order can be invoked by the police on finding a person in a public place who appears to be suffering from a mental disorder and in immediate need of care or control. Such a person has to be taken to a designated place of safety; ideally this would be attached to a mental health unit, but in some localities this would be an emergency department. Some patients may be mentally confused due to physical illness, e.g. hypoxia following heart failure. The patient can be detained in the short term for emergency treatment, the law accepting the necessity for this. A failure to do so could be deemed negligence.

Much rarer is the situation of an individual with a certain infectious disease potentially dangerous to others who refuses to stay for treatment. An order made by a magistrate or sheriff can be issued to detain the person, who will then be rapidly transferred to an appropriate unit.

The police may detain a person in the emergency department. For example, the patient may have been injured at the time of arrest. In this case it is the police's responsibility to detain, never the nurse's. Even if the police request the nurse to assist them in preventing the patient leaving the department, he

should refuse to become involved. The fact that someone is a detained prisoner does not lessen her right to treatment, confidentiality or refusal to consent to procedures.

CONFIDENTIALITY, THE POLICE AND THE PRESS

Patient information is generally held under legal and ethical obligations of confidentiality (Department of Health 2003). Professionally, nurses are required to treat information about patients as confidential and use it only for the purposes for which it was given and to protect information from improper disclosure at all times: NMC *Code of Professional Conduct* (2004). Both the Data Protection Act (1998) and the Human Rights Act (1998) seek to preserve and protect the privacy and confidentiality of the individual. The Freedom of Information Act (2000) gives a general right of access to all types of information held by public authorities. However, there are a number of situations where disclosure of information without the patient's consent can be made. These include the following:

- orders from the court before or during legal proceedings
- public interest
- statutory obligation such as
  - infectious diseases regulations
  - notification of registration of births and stillbirths
  - Police and Criminal Evidence Act 1984
  - Health and Social Care Act 2001
  - Prevention of Terrorism Act 2005.

If the nurse has to give evidence in court, privilege on the basis of professional position cannot be claimed and the nurse will have to give the information required. The courts can also order the release of medical and nursing notes prior to the court case. The public interest would cover situations where serious harm is feared to the patient or another person, or in a child protection situation (Dimond 2005). Most departments will have clearly laid down guidelines to follow if symptoms point to child-protection concerns. The disastrous consequences of not taking action have been well publicized, as has the distress caused to both child and parents when action has been taken on grounds that are later found to be unsubstantiated. A team approach is usually seen as essential.

Under the Prevention of Terrorism Act (2005) it is an offence for any person having information which he or she believes may be of material assistance in preventing terrorism or apprehending terrorists to fail, without reasonable cause, to give that information to the police.

While nurses have an obligation to provide police with a statement regarding their own actions and observations, they do not have to provide a statement regarding the patient's medical condition. This can be referred on to the clinician in charge of the patient's care. While inter-agency cooperation is important, healthcare professionals should not feel pressurized into providing statements immediately. In most circumstances, it is quite acceptable to arrange a mutually agreeable time for statements. This enables the health professional to organize their thoughts and seek advice about confidentiality and disclosure if needed.

While there is a need for valid sharing of information between health professionals to ensure the safe care of patients, the Caldicott principles (NHS Executive 1997) should be followed (Box 38.4).

The healthcare worker in the ED is sure to have a certain amount of contact with the police and, possibly, the press. It is important to be aware of the respective rights of patients, hospital employees and police in these circumstances. The police have a number of powers regarding search and arrest and these will apply to a hospital in the same way as to a private dwelling because hospitals are Crown property, not public property. Police can enter premises without a search warrant if the person they wish to search for is suspected of an arrestable offence. An intimate search of body orifices can be authorized if the person concerned is likely to have concealed an item to injure herself or others, or for drugs. Police are entitled to use reasonable force in carrying out an intimate search.

In relation to arrest, police may arrest without a warrant if they suspect that an arrestable offence has been, is being or is about to be committed. Examples of an arrestable offence are unlawful possession of drugs, rape and most offences of violence (English &

Card 2003). If the police suspect that an individual who is currently a patient in the ED has committed a serious offence, the staff should not hinder the police in their work, but should ensure the medical condition of the individual is not jeopardized.

A final situation where patient confidentiality may be put at risk is through press enquiries. Most hospitals will have strict rules on which staff are allowed to talk to the press. It is wise for staff always to refer these enquiries to the appropriate senior member of staff.

STAFF HEALTH AND SAFETY

Both verbal abuse and physical violence against staff are not unusual occurrences in the ED department. Police attendance at such incidents can be requested and the nurses involved will need to make statements to the police. However, quite often no charges will be brought against the individual.

The law can be relevant in a number of ways. First, violent actions could be the crime of assault, battery or causing grievous bodily harm. However, the police are often unable to charge a person on the basis of these crimes as there is often some doubt as to whether the person intended to commit the crime. Proving intention is necessary for a successful prosecution. If the patient is mentally ill, drunk or under the influence of drugs, they could claim that they could not form the necessary intention. Increasingly, however, courts take a poor view of acts of violence carried out under the influence of drink or drugs which offenders have taken to deprive themselves of their self-control or their knowledge of what they were doing. There are moves to try and bring nurses into line with the police, inasmuch as when a police officer is assaulted, it is automatically a criminal offence.

For most criminal charges, not only is self-induced intoxication no defence but, if the offender claims that she/he only did it because of intoxication, the prosecution are absolved from proving any mental element and need simply prove that the act was done. It is thus easier to obtain a conviction (Montague 1996). It also underlines the need for clear, contemporaneous notes to be taken by staff and witnesses in case of legal action being taken. If injuries are sustained, the statement will provide evidence of the event and the nurse may be able to claim from the Criminal Injuries Compensation Board even in the absence of a successful prosecution.

Assault and battery are also civil wrongs. This means the nurse could sue the individual through the civil courts for damages. In this context, intention does not have to be proved, so evidence of the

---

Box 38.4 Caldicott principles

- Justify the purpose
- Do not use patient identifiable information unless it is absolutely necessary
- Use the minimum necessary patient identifiable information
- Access to patient identifiable information should be on a strict need to know basis
- Everyone should be aware of their responsibilities
- Understand and comply with the law

incident would lead to a successful legal action. It is rare, however, for nurses to take this route. Finally, the nurse could complain to the employer that there has been a failure to provide a safe working environment, under common law, the Occupiers Liability Act (1957) and the Health and Safety at Work etc. Act (1974). However, the employer only has to take reasonable steps to ensure the health, safety and welfare of the employees. It is difficult for the employer to create a totally safe environment in emergency departments, because of the nature of the work undertaken and the open access of the department to the public. If the employee considers further measures should be taken, she should consult the health and safety representative of her trade union or professional body.

Other health and safety issues in the emergency department are very similar to those elsewhere, e.g. infection risks, moving and handling patients and fire hazards. European Union Directives, laid out in a number of UK Health and Safety Regulations (1992),

have resulted in the broadening of the requirements and improved protection of staff in the area of safety. The provision of training and adequate equipment are key elements of any statutory requirements. Health and Safety issues are examined in detail in Chapter 39.

CONCLUSION

In the medico legal sense, the emergency department has been described as the most dangerous part of a hospital (Knight 1992). It is important, therefore, for emergency nurses to have a working knowledge of the law if they are to prevent legal problems arising in the first place. This chapter has introduced the main areas of law of relevance in emergency care and discussed the implications for emergency care practitioners. Like practice, however, the law is constantly evolving and it is in the nurse's interest to keep abreast of these developments.

References

Barnett v. Kensington & Chelsea Hospital Management Committee (1969) 1 QB 428.

Bolam v. Friern Hospital Management Committee (1957) 1WLR 582.

Brazier M (2003) Medicine, Patients and the Law, 3rd edn. Harmondsworth: Penguin Books.

Cable S, Lumsdaine J, Semple M (2003) Informed consent. Nursing Standard, 18(12), 47–53.

Carson D, Montgomery J (1989) Nursing and the Law. Basingstoke: Macmillan.

Castledine G (1994) Ethics and the law in ED. Emergency Nurse, 2(1), 25.

Data Protection Act (1998). London: HMSO

Department of Health (2000) NHS Plan. London: Department of Health

Department of Health (2001) Learning from Bristol: The Report of the Inquiry into Children's Heart Surgery at Bristol Royal Infirmary 1984–1995. Command Paper CM (5207). London: HMSO.

Department of Health (2001) Reference Guide to Consent for Examination and Treatment. London: Department of Health.

Department of Health (2003) NHS Code of Conduct. London: Department of Health

Department of Health (2004) Medicines Pharmacy and Industry Group. London: Department of Health.

Dimond B (2004) Legal Aspects of Nursing. Hemel Hempstead: Prentice Hall.

Dimond B (2005) Legal aspects of trauma nursing. In: RA O'Shea ed. Principles and Practice of Trauma Nursing. Edinburgh: Elsevier Churchill Livingstone.

Donohue v. Stevenson (1932) AC 562.

English J, Card R (2003) Butterworth's Police Law. London: Lexis Nexis.

Freedom of Information Act (2000). London: HMSO

Green C (1999) The nurse and professional negligence. Nursing Times, 95(8), 57–59.

Health and Safety at Work etc. Act (1974) London: HMSO.

Human Rights Act (1998) London: The Stationery Office Limited.

Health and Safety (General Provisions) Regulations (1992). London: HMSO.

Human Tissue Act (2004). London: HMSO.

Knight B (1992) Legal Aspects of Medical Practice, 5th edn. Edinburgh: Churchill Livingstone.

Limitation Act (1980). London: HMSO.

Martin J (2005) Clinical negligence and compensation. Nursing Standard, 19(35), 35–39.

Mason JK, McCall-Smith RA (2002) Law and Medical Ethics, 6th edn. London: Lexis Nexis.

Mental Health Act (1983). London: HMSO.

Mental Capacity Act (2005). London: The Stationery Office Limited.

Medicines for Human Use (Prescribing) (Misc Amendments) Order (2005), Statutory Instrument 2005 No. (1507).

Montague A (1996) Legal Problems in Emergency Medicine. Oxford: Oxford University Press.

Montgomery J (2002) Health Care Law, 2nd edn. Oxford: Oxford University Press

Morgan J (1998) How medical negligence is established. Emergency Nurse, 6(5), 15–19.

National Audit Office (2001) Handling Clinical Negligence Claims in England. London: National Audit Office

NHS Executive (1997) *Caldicott Committee: Report on the Review of Patient-identifiable Information*. London: Department of Health.

Nursing and Midwifery Council (2004) *Code of Professional Conduct: Standards for Conduct, Performance and Ethics*. London: Nursing and Midwifery Council

Occupiers Liability Act (1957) London: HMSO.

Pannett AJ (1997) *Law of Torts*, 7th edn. London: Prentice Hall.

Police and Criminal Evidence Act (1984). London: HMSO.

Police Reform Act (2002) London: The Stationery Office Limited.

Prevention of Terrorism Act (2005) London: The Stationery Office Limited.

Sweet A (1996) Organ donation in ED. *Emergency Nurse*, **3**(4), 6–9.

The Children Act (1989). London: HMSO.

The Nursing and Midwifery Order (2001) Statutory Instrument 2002 No. 253. London: The Stationery Office Ltd.

Tingle JH, Cribb A eds. (2002) *Nursing Law and Ethics*. Oxford: Blackwell Science.

Wilkinson R (2000) Organ donation: the debate. *Nursing Standard*, **14**(28), 41–42.

Wilsher v. *Essex AHA* (1988) 1 All ER 871

Young AP (1989) *Legal Problems in Nursing Practice*, 2nd edn. London: Chapman and Hall.

Young AP (1991) *Law and Professional Conduct in Nursing*. London: Scutari Press.

Young AP (1999) *Law Accident & Emergency Theory into Practice*. Baillière Tindall

Chapter **39**

Health and safety

Sheelagh Brewer

INTRODUCTION

It seems incongruous that a service set up to provide emergency care sometimes causes harm to the staff involved in delivering that care. In 2003, the National Audit Office carried out a survey on health and safety risks to staff in the NHS in England (NAO 2003a). They reported that there were 135 172 staff accidents in 2001–2, with wide variations between similar trusts in the number of accidents per 1000 staff. They also highlighted that there is significant under-reporting, so the true figure is likely to be much higher. This is the situation despite the complex set of statutes and regulations, some based on European legislation, designed to provide a safe environment for employees and others, such as patients, visitors, contractors' employees and agency staff. This chapter considers various aspects of accidents at work, describes the main legal responsibilities of employers and employees, and also how this legislation is applied to hazards found in emergency departments.

PREVENTING ACCIDENTS

The Health and Safety Executive (1993) use the term 'accident' to refer to any unplanned event that results in injury or ill health of people, or damage or loss to property, plant, materials or the environment, or a loss of business opportunity. Before any action can be taken to prevent accidents, the causes must be identified. Causes can be divided into unsafe conditions (e.g. wet floors, trailing cables, insufficient manual handling aids, faulty equipment) or unsafe acts (e.g. nurses' failure to wear protective equipment or ignoring safety instructions). Unsafe acts arise from lack of training or nurses' attitudes towards their own safety (Lynch and Cole 2006). Workplaces should be regularly inspected to check that hazards do not exist and, although trade union safety representatives have this as part of their role, it should be a cooperative process between staff, managers and safety representatives. Local policies should encourage nurses to report hazards before accidents occur so that preventive action may be taken. In fact there is a specific duty contained within the Management of Health and Safety at Work Regulations (Health & Safety Executive 2003) which requires employees to report to their employer details of any work situation that might represent a serious and imminent danger.

If an accident does occur, accurate records are needed. From the employer's point of view there is a duty to report certain types of accidents defined within the Reporting of Injury, Diseases and Dangerous Occurrence Regulations (RIDDOR) (1995) to the Health and Safety Executive. Failure to do so is a criminal offence. The employer needs information about an accident so the event can be investigated to prevent its recurrence and risk assessments can be reviewed. Employees are obliged to report accidents and it is in their interests to accurately complete accident forms and accident books to protect themselves in the event of future loss of income or long-term effects of injury or disease.

It has always been difficult to arrive at the true costs of accidents and yet this information could provide an incentive to tackling the problem of workplace accidents, by providing a measurement against which financial loss can be judged. The National Audit Office (2003a) survey of health and safety in hospitals estimated that accidents cost the NHS £173 million in England alone. This is a crude estimate and does not include staff replacement costs, medical treatment costs or court compensation, so the true costs are likely to be much higher. The cost of an accident is directly related to the outcome of that accident, but this can be difficult to predict, as, for example, a needlestick injury may or may not result in a nurse contracting a blood-borne virus such as hepatitis C. The total cost of accidents must include the cost of maintaining a safe environment. A relationship exists between underlying safety control and accident occurrence.

Implementing safety control will involve some cost, such as staff communication and training, physical protection (alarm systems), publicity campaigns, time spent in risk assessment, inspecting the workplace for hazards and maintenance of equipment. These costs will be offset by the direct and indirect costs resulting from accidents and ill health, such as occupational sick pay, equipment damage, disruption in patient care, damage to the environment, costs of replacement staff and costs of litigation. The management responsibility is to decide how much to spend on controlling the causes of accidents in order to minimize their financial impact.

LEGISLATION

The health service was not covered by any health and safety legislation until 1974 when the Health & Safety at Work etc. Act was passed. This is still the major legislative power and any new regulations come under its framework. The Health & Safety at Work etc. Act (1974) specifies the duties of the employer with the general requirement to 'ensure, so far as is reasonably practicable, the health, safety & welfare at work of all his Employees' (Section 2(1)). The Act then specifies the particular areas where this duty applies (see Box 39.1).

Box 39.1   Duties of employer in the Health & Safety at Work etc. Act 1974

- The provision of plant and systems of work that are without risk to health and safety. In addition, the equipment must be maintained so it remains safe. This could include systems of handling and moving patients, infection control procedures or extraction systems to remove hazardous fumes
- Making arrangements in the use, handling, storage and transport of articles and substances so that the risk is minimized. The safe disposal of clinical waste including sharps would be covered by this requirement
- Providing information, instruction, training and supervision so that employees are kept safe at work.

General training on health and safety must be provided along with specific training on particular hazards of handling of loads and fire procedures
- Providing and maintaining a safe place of work so that there is adequate heating, lighting, ventilation and fire exits
- Provision of adequate welfare facilities. Welfare is a very broad area but could include access to occupational health services, vaccination against hepatitis B, facilities for changing, showers and toilets and a smoke-free working environment

Another section of the Health & Safety at Work etc. Act (1974) defines the duty of the employer to non-employees, including patients, visitors and contractors' employees, to ensure these people are also protected from harm whilst they are on the premises. Systems of work must be developed to protect these groups. Floor cleaning is an example of the need to ensure that staff and others are prevented from walking on wet, slippery floors by the use of coned areas and warning signs.

The approach to health and safety legislation is to involve both employers and employees. The Health & Safety at Work etc. Act (1974) specifies that all employees must take reasonable care for the health and safety of themselves and others who may be affected by their acts or omissions and cooperate with the employer to enable compliance with statutory requirements. If the employer provides any protective equipment, such as gloves, goggles or aprons, the employee must wear it. This presumes the employer has defined the need for the equipment and has trained staff in the correct use.

The Health & Safety at Work etc. Act (1974) is a wide-ranging piece of legislation and one that permits further regulations to be developed which refer to specific aspects of health and safety. In 1992, six new sets of regulations were enacted which were based on EC Directives (Health & Safety Executive 1992a–e), but during that period, 1974–1995, other regulations included:

- Safety Representatives & Safety Committees Regulations (1977), which define the rights and functions of trade union appointed safety representatives and the arrangements for safety committees
- Health & Safety (First-Aid) Regulations (1981), which provide a framework for the provision of first aid arrangements for employees. Even in emergency departments procedures need to be defined for staff who suffer an accident
- Reporting of Injuries, Diseases & Dangerous Occurrences Regulations (1995), which specify the duty on the employer to report to the Health & Safety Executive certain categories of injuries, dangerous occurrences and designated diseases.

In the case of disease, the nature of the work is specified. Hepatitis B is a reportable disease for anyone who comes into contact with blood, blood products or body secretions. The regulations specify the type of dangerous occurrences that must be reported, whether or not anyone has been injured. Similarly, the specific types of injury are defined along with a broad category of any injury that results in absence from work for 3 days or more. The other reportable major injuries are outlined in Box 39.2. Any incidents where staff have a needlestick injury where the sharp was known to be contaminated with infected blood must be reported to the Health and Safety Executive under RIDDOR.

Control of Substances Hazardous to Health Regulations (2002)

The Control of Substances Hazardous to Health (COSHH) Regulations (2002) were implemented in response to concerns about the effect on health of exposure to hazardous substances and replaced and revoked the earlier COSHH Regulations (1988). Dangerous substances must be categorized in terms of hazard and risk. A hazardous substance is one that has the potential to cause harm. The risk is the likelihood that it will cause harm in the actual circumstances where it is used. The regulations require the employer to carry out an assessment of the risk and subsequently to establish a safe system of work. The definition of a hazardous substance is any solid,

---

Box 39.2   Reportable major injuries under RIDDOR (1995)

- Fracture other than to fingers, thumbs or toes
- Amputation
- Dislocation of the shoulder, hip, knee or spine
- Loss of sight (temporary or permanent)
- Chemical or hot metal burn to the eye or any penetrating injury to the eye
- Injury resulting from an electric shock or electrical burn leading to unconsciousness or requiring resuscitation or admittance to hospital for more than 24 hours

- Any other injury leading to hypothermia, heat-induced illness or unconsciousness or requiring admittance to hospital for more than 24 hours
- Acute illness requiring medical treatment or loss of consciousness arising from absorption of any substance by inhalation, ingestion or through the skin
- Acute illness requiring medical treatment where there is reason to believe that this resulted from exposure to a biological agent or its toxins or infected material

liquid, gas, fume, vapour or microorganism that can endanger health by being absorbed or injected through the skin or mucous membranes, inhaled or digested. One exclusion is substances administered as part of a medical treatment, although the impact on the healthcare worker would need to be assessed, for instance, during the preparation of cytotoxic drugs.

Once the assessment has been carried out, steps must be taken to prevent or at least control exposure. Prevention is the ideal solution to the problem but there will be circumstances where this is not reasonably practicable. Glutaraldehyde used to be the most effective cold disinfectant available but increasingly has been substituted by other safer chemicals or even cold sterilization (Royal College of Nursing 2000a,b). The more commonly used alternatives include disinfectants based on peracetic acid, chlorine dioxide and hypochlorous acid (also referred to as superoxidized saline) (Medical Devices Agency 2002). The regulations require the control measures to be properly used and maintained and for employees and non-employees to be informed, instructed and trained in what the risks are and how to control them.

Where nurses have been exposed to risk there is a requirement to carry out health surveillance. Health surveillance is needed to protect the health of individuals by detecting adverse changes attributed to exposure to hazardous substances at the earliest possible stage. This will help in assessing the effectiveness of control measures. Where health surveillance is carried out, the employees' health records must be kept for 30 years.

Within emergency departments and fracture clinics there are three main areas of risk where COSHH assessments should be carried out. The first is chemical exposure, including drugs and plaster of Paris dust. The assessment and subsequent control measures should consider storage, local ventilation, waste disposal, need for personal protective equipment, training and air monitoring. Special attention should be paid to the type of environment and the potential for patients, accompanying relatives and children to gain unauthorized access to materials such as antiseptics.

The second group of substances comprises the disinfectants such as phenolics, hypochlorites, glutaraldehyde alcohol mixtures and idophors. Many of these can be irritant to the skin and eyes. The third group of hazards involves the microbiological hazards from contact with body fluids such as blood, vomit and urine. Every patient must be regarded as a potential biohazard and it is impossible to identify all those who are seropositive to HIV or hepatitis B.

Clear infection control procedures must be adhered to by nurses and routine barrier methods used to prevent contamination by blood or body fluids. The RCN (2006) gives clear guidance on universal precautions as part of its campaign on MRSA. Chlorine-releasing disinfecting agents used in spillages of urine can be used as an example of the application of COSHH. The indiscriminate use of powdered or granular products designed to disinfect and contain spills of body fluids can lead to ill effects in staff and patients through exposure to chlorine. The use of such a substance must be controlled so it does not become a greater danger than the risk of infection. A COSHH assessment in this instance would consider both microbiological and chemical hazards. It would take into account the urgency of any situation, the nature of the spillage, the quantities that might be spilt and the degree of ventilation. With this information a system of work may be defined to cover storage, handling and use of any disinfecting agent, the procedure for dissolving or diluting it before use and the need for any personal protection for the user.

LEGISLATION SINCE 1992

Health and safety is an issue which has featured prominently in European legislation. Article 118A of the Single European Act 1986 (EU 1986) states that member states shall pay particular attention to encouraging improvements especially in the working environment as regards the health and safety of workers and shall set as their objective the harmonization of conditions in this area, whilst maintaining the improvements made.

Directly arising out of this article was a Framework Directive (EC Directive 1989) on health and safety, with a number of so called 'daughter directives' covering manual handling, personal protective equipment, work equipment, the workplace, temporary workers and display-screen equipment. Once these directives were agreed, European Union member states were required to include the provisions of the directives into their own law by 1992. In the UK, this resulted in a set of regulations often referred to as 'the six pack', comprising:

- the Management of Health & Safety at Work Regulations 1992 (Health & Safety Commission 1992)
- the Display Screen Equipment Regulations 1992 (Health & Safety Executive 1992a)
- the Manual Handling Operations Regulations 1992 (Health & Safety Executive 1992b)
- the Personal Protective Equipment Regulations 1992 (Health & Safety Executive 1992c)

- the Work Equipment Regulations 1992 (Health & Safety Executive 1992d) (replaced by the Provision and Use of Work Equipment Regulations 1998 and the Lifting Equipment Regulations 1998)
- the Workplace Regulations 1992 (Health & Safety Executive 1992e).

Although all of these have relevance in emergency departments, the first two are considered in more detail.

The Management of Health & Safety at Work Regulations (1992)

These regulations build on and make more explicit the duties of employers and employees defined in the Health & Safety at Work Act (1974). The main requirement is the need to carry out a risk assessment for every hazard in the workplace (see Box 39.3). All of the activities and processes carried out within the emergency service should be subjected to the process of risk assessment.

Risk assessment

Nursing staff should be involved in risk assessment because they are familiar with the environment, the procedures and equipment used. Risk assessment is the starting point for total risk management. The aim is to identify where things could go wrong and what the effect would be. Risk may arise from physical hazards, e.g. unsafe flooring, poor lighting, no alarm systems, or working practices, e.g. failure to dispose of sharps safely, failure to wear gloves, failure to alter bed heights when moving patients. Risk assessment then identifies:

- probability of exposure to risk
- frequency of exposure to risk
- maximum probable effect which could range from minor injury to fatal injury
- number of persons at risk.

Some risk assessment procedures apply numerical values to these items, which are multiplied together to produce an overall risk score. This can be used to introduce greater objectivity and to look at relative risks from hazards, but in some cases it may be misleading. With manual handling, for example, an uncooperative patient will have an impact on the assessment. A skilled assessor, sensitive to all the variables, may produce a more useful assessment than the application of numerical values.

The process of risk assessment should result in a decision as to whether the risk is acceptable or not. If not, further work is required to control the risk. Elimination is the ideal solution but may not be always possible. Other methods of control are:

- to substitute a less hazardous process or substance
- to use engineering methods such as ventilation systems
- to redefine systems of work
- to provide personal protective equipment
- to immunize staff where possible
- to define emergency procedures.

The results of the risk assessment must be written and all staff affected must be informed about the risks and about the preventive measures or controls to be used (Clough 1998).

There are specific requirements relating to pregnant employees which were incorporated as a result of the EU Pregnant Workers Directive (1992). The risk assessment must cover any risks to the health and safety of a new or expectant mother from physical, biological or chemical agents. Where the risk cannot be avoided, the employer must alter the individual's working conditions or hours of work. If it is not reasonable to do so or if it would not avoid the risk, the employer must offer suitable alternative employment or suspend the employee from work. Furthermore, if the employee works nights and medical evidence states that this is a health risk, the employer must provide other employment or suspend her from work.

In addition to the requirement to carry out risk assessment, the Management of Health & Safety at Work Regulations (2003) contain other important duties. If the assessment identifies that nurses will

---

> **Box 39.3   Some possible hazards in the workplace**
>
> - Chemical hazards, e.g. glutaraldehyde and formaldehyde
> - Biological hazards, e.g. blood-borne and airborne infections
> - Electrical hazards
> - Manual handling
> - Physical hazards, e.g. violence
> - Psychological hazards, e.g. stress
> - Equipment, e.g. autoclaves, sharp instruments, computers
> - Ionizing radiation, e.g. diagnostic X-rays
> - Hot and cold working conditions
> - Poor lighting
> - Fire
> - Workplace layout and design

be exposed to risk, it may be necessary to provide health surveillance. This is needed where there is an identifiable disease related to the work and where the techniques exist to detect indications of the disease. Under these regulations the employer must appoint one or more competent persons to provide health and safety assistance. This could be one person or a team depending on the size of the organization. They may be appointed from existing employees or brought in on a consultancy basis. In any event they must have adequate time and resources to carry out their functions.

The employer must take account of employers' capabilities, training and knowledge experience when allocating work. Training on health and safety must be given in working practices and systems introducing new equipment. The training must be repeated periodically and carried out during the employees' working hours. Specific reference is made to temporary staff. Where agency or bank staff are used, essential information must be provided about the workplace and about any particular risks to health and safety. These regulations clearly define what is needed to develop an organizational safety culture and provide the framework within which departmental approaches are developed.

Employees' duties

The duty of the employee to cooperate includes the use of equipment, dangerous substances, transport equipment, means of production or safety device and the need to operate these in accordance with training and instruction received. Additional duties are specified; each employee must inform the employer of any work situation which represents a serious and immediate danger to health and safety and any shortcoming in the protection arrangements for health and safety believed to exist by the employee.

This duty can be considered in the light of provisions within the Employment Rights Act (1996), which gives employment protection to employees in relation to health and safety. Employees and safety representatives have the right not to have action short of dismissal or be dismissed in the following circumstances:

- where they have been designated by the employer to carry out activities to prevent or reduce risks to health and safety and have done so or are proposing to do so
- where the employee is a safety representative and is acting in that capacity
- where the employee left the workplace because of serious and imminent danger

- where the employee took steps to, or proposed to take appropriate steps to, protect himself or others from the danger. The protection applies regardless of length of service.

Nurses are able to combine their responsibilities in the NMC Code of Professional Conduct (2004) with health and safety regulations to take action to secure a safe working environment. Staff are an expensive resource and staffing costs are now closely monitored and reduced wherever possible. If a nurse believes staffing levels are insufficient to provide safe standards of practice, she has a responsibility to report this. It is also likely that such staffing levels would pose a risk to the health and safety of other staff and so the nurse would be compelled under health and safety legislation to report this also.

Manual handling operations regulations 1992

The impact of manual handling on the health of nurses has long been recognized, but these are the first set of regulations to address the problem specifically. In health care, 50% of all accidents reported to the Health and Safety Executive are related to manual handling and, of these, 70% are as a result of patient handling (Royal College of Nursing 1996). The National Audit Office Survey (2003a) noted that although the number of ill-health early retirements due to musculo-skeletal conditions has reduced, the proportion of this type of pension award has remained fairly constant at around 40%. In 2002 the Department of Health launched a national campaign 'Back in Work' which included some back facts such as that 5% of NHS staff surveyed had more than 20 days off work in a year due to back pain and 24% of NHS staff regularly experience back pain.

The Manual Handling Operations Regulations (Health & Safety Executive 1992b) require the employer to avoid the need for employees to undertake any manual handling operations at work which involve a risk of injury. This is qualified by the phrase 'so far as is reasonably practicable' and where this applies the employer must carry out an assessment to reduce the risk to the lowest level reasonably practicable. The approach in the risk assessment is based on ergonomic principles of optimizing the fit between the nurse and her work.

The guidance to the regulations identifies four factors for the assessment:

- the task
- the load
- the environment
- individual capability.

These factors are interrelated and may not be considered in isolation. What is required is a completely new attitude to the manual handling of patients which starts from an approach that no nurse should be required to manually lift any patients and that systems of work must be developed which enable this to happen. In 1996, the Royal College of Nursing revised its code of practice for patient handling. The aim is to eliminate hazardous manual handling in all but exceptional or life-threatening situations.

Examples of the risk factors under the four headings are summarized in Box 39.4. Once the risk factors have been identified, the next stage is to take steps to eliminate or reduce the risk. Possible control measures are summarized in Box 39.5.

The assessment will take place at two levels. First, the workplace itself must be assessed by the department manager in conjunction with any specialist help. This assessment will take into account departmental accident and absence statistics, layout, availability of handling aids and training of staff. Once completed, the risk-reducing actions are likely to have been identified and action plans developed.

The particular needs of the nature of the work make a difference to the assessment. In emergency areas, it would be appropriate to develop generic assessments for many of the transfers which take place, e.g. trolley to bed, wheelchair to bed. In emergency situations, an on-the-spot assessment is needed by skilled staff to judge whether the generic assessment is relevant. The risk assessment must be written and should be available to staff who need the information. If circumstances change so that the assessment is no longer valid, it must be updated. The next level of assessment is in relation to individual patients. In wards or in the community, a manual handling assessment would be incorporated into the patient care plan. Within emergency departments,

---

Box 39.4   Risk factors in lifting patients

Patients
- Weight
- Cooperation
- Dependency
- Consciousness level
- Condition
- Pain
- Comprehension
- Behavioural problems

Task
- Frequency
- Repetition
- Job rotation
- Holding loads away from trunk, reaching upwards long distances
- Restrictions by uniform twisting/stooping
- Awkward posture
- Urgency of task

Environment
- Space to move freely
- Floor slippery, uneven, lightly adequate
- Other tripping hazards, equipment available, equipment in good repair

Employee
- Training
- Danger to pregnant staff
- Danger to those with health problems, stress levels

Box 39.5   Control factors when lifting patients

Patient
- Use mechanical equipment
- Involve patient
- Explain to patient
- Consider patient's dignity
- Consider any attachments to patient

Task
- Sufficient number of staff
- Improved design of task
- Rest breaks for staff
- Decreased distances for moving patient, improved equipment
- Adjustable heights on equipment

Environment
- Use of ranges for easier movement
- Harmonize heights of work surfaces, location of equipment
- Improve lighting, temperature, noise levels
- Improve tidiness and cleanliness

Employee
- Improve individual technique
- Report unsafe systems
- Provide training
- Consider individual situations, e.g. pregnancy
- Increase level of supervision to eliminate poor practice

a system should exist which would enable an initial manual handling assessment to be carried out; this would need updating as the patient's condition and treatment are known.

The duties of the employee under these regulations are to make full and proper use of the systems provided by the employer. Nursing staff have a responsibility for their own actions and their own competence. Where training on manual handling is available the nurse should attend. If the training is not provided, the nurse should be requesting that she has the opportunity to receive this training.

INFECTION CONTROL

Infection control is particularly important within emergency departments because the status of each patient arriving in the department will not be known and treatment may be necessary before there is any indication that the patient may present a risk. Specific local infection control policies are needed in relation to cleaning the workplace, use of disinfectants, hand washing, dealing with laundry, protective clothing, disposal of waste and transport of specimens.

Contact with patient's blood/body fluids now carries with it the risk of occupational exposure to blood-borne infections such as HIV or hepatitis B or hepatitis C. Health care workers need to follow standard precautions to prevent contamination by blood/body fluids. These precautions include covering any abrasions to exposed skin, wearing disposable powder-free latex gloves and plastic aprons, thorough hand washing between procedures, and wearing eye protection if there is any risk of blood splashes or flying contaminated debris.

Accidental inoculation with infected blood presents a real risk to the nurse although for most incidents there will be no harm to the nurse. However, sharps injury is a major cause of transmission of blood-borne viruses from patient to nurse. In 2005 the Health Protection Agency reported that there had been nine hepatitis C sero-conversions following significant exposure over a seven-year period 2006. Extreme care is needed with the use and disposal of sharps. Risk assessment must be carried out and safer systems of work implemented. There are now technological solutions, with a wide range of safety-engineered devices which can significantly reduce the risk of a needlestick injury.

In the event of a needlestick injury, the immediate action is to make the puncture wound bleed by gentle squeezing of the area. Wash thoroughly with soap and water and apply a waterproof dressing. If the source patient is known, a record should be kept with the name of the patient. In any event, contact should be made with occupational health and an accident form completed. Procedures should be defined for spillages of blood and body fluids using sodium dichloroisocyanurate granules or paper towels with 10 000 ppm sodium hypochlorite solution. Household gloves and plastic apron should be worn and these disposed of with the spillage as clinical waste.

HIV/AIDS

HIV is infectious, not contagious, and the most likely method of transmission to emergency department staff would be through inoculation of infected blood by a sharps injury or exposure of mucous membranes to blood. This reinforces the need for staff to adhere to the universal precautions. All patients attending an emergency department should be approached in the same way as far as infection control is concerned. If it becomes clear that the patient is HIV antibody-positive and there is extensive haemorrhage or severe diarrhoea, the need for isolation must be considered. If a nurse suffers a needlestick injury, blood samples for storage and possible testing for HIV antibodies must not be taken from the injured nurse or the source patient without informed consent and pre-test counselling.

Hepatitis B

Hepatitis B has been known to be a problem to health-care staff for over 20 years, and recently other strains of hepatitis have been identified. Hepatitis B is a stable virus, resistant to common antiseptics, and is therefore highly infectious. Hypochlorite, glutaraldehyde, chlorine and autoclaving at 134 °C for a minimum of three minutes are known to destroy the virus (Royal College of Nursing 2000).

In emergency departments it is most unlikely that there will be any indication that a patient is infected with hepatitis B. It is advisable that all staff are vaccinated with the hepatitis B vaccine in accordance with Department of Health guidance (UK Health Departments 1993). This guidance specifies that anyone who is HBeAg-positive must not be involved in exposure-prone procedures. These are defined as those where there is a risk that injury to the worker may result in the exposure of the patient's open tissues to the blood of the worker. These procedures include those where the worker's gloved hands may be in contact with sharp instruments, needle tips and sharp tissues, such as spicules of bone or teeth, inside a patient's open body cavity, wound or confined anatomical space where the hands or fingertips may not be completely visible at all times.

Staff who are hepatitis B surface antigen (HBsAg) positive but not HBeAg-positive will not be a risk to patients and need not be barred from any area of work. It must be emphasized that good routine infection-control procedures are the key to preventing transmission of blood-borne viruses.

The risk of transmission to a healthcare worker from an infected patient following such an injury has been shown to be around 1 in 3 when a source patient is infected with hepatitis B virus and is 'e' antigen positive, around 1 in 30 when the patient is infected with hepatitis C virus and around 1 in 300 when the patient is infected with HIV (UK Health Departments 1998).

WORKING TIME DIRECTIVE

It is clear that the organization of work in emergency departments, which normally provide a 24-hour service, is a factor that can have an impact on the health of staff. Working time had not been covered specifically by health and safety legislation until the European Directive on Working Time was agreed in (1993EC). The UK introduced regulations to implement the directive in 1998, the Working Time Regulations, which were revised in 2004 to extend the provisions to junior doctors. The average working week for junior doctors must now not exceed 56 hours per week and this will reduce to 48 hours in 2009. The basic provisions of the directive are outlined in Box 39.6.

All workers are entitled to four weeks paid annual leave. The implementation of the Working Time Directive (EC Directive 93/104/EC 1993) is likely to mean that working patterns and hours of work will be the subject of negotiation between employers and their employees, but the key purpose is to ensure that the arrangements do not have a detrimental effect on the health of staff.

FRAMEWORK FOR MAINTAINING A SAFE ENVIRONMENT

Health and safety is covered by extensive legislation aimed at producing working environments that are safe for both nurses and patients. The legislation must be translated into practical policies which are known and understood. The main employer must have an overall safety policy but particular areas should have departmental policies which address problems in those areas. In emergency departments, specific policies may be needed for manual handling, dealing with violence and aggressive behaviour, disposal of clinical waste and infection control. Each member of staff, whether clinical or not, should be clear about her responsibility for health and safety.

Procedures should be defined in the event of any accident taking place, from immediate first aid to the reporting procedures. The policy should specify the consultative arrangements which may exist. Normally this would be a safety committee with management and trade union safety representatives, along with specialist support such as occupational health safety adviser, infection control and radiation protection adviser. Safety problems which cannot be resolved within the department should be addressed by the safety committee.

Violence

In 2003, the National Audit Office carried out a survey examining the impact of violence and aggression in the NHS. This report demonstrated a rising incidence of violence and aggression and made wide-ranging

---

Box 39.6   Basic provisions of Working Time Directive

- Entitlement to a rest break of 11 consecutive hours per 24-hour period
- Entitlement to an uninterrupted rest period of at least 24 hours per 7-day period. These provisions may be varied for health care workers provided that equivalent compensatory periods of rest are arranged
- Weekly working time including overtime must not exceed 48 hours. This can be averaged out over a period of 17 weeks or longer by agreement
- Normal hours of night work may not exceed an average of 8 hours in any 24-hour period. This can be
- averaged out over a period of time as agreed through collective bargaining
- Night workers are entitled to a free health assessment prior to starting night work and then at regular intervals
- Night workers suffering from health problems recognized as being connected with the fact that they perform night work are to be transferred to day work wherever possible
- Records of night workers are to be maintained and provided to competent authorities on request

recommendations (National Audit Office 2003b) (se also Chapter 11: Violence and Aggression).

Following this survey, the NHS Security Management Service (SMS) was established and given the operational and policy remit for security in the NHS (England) in 2003. It has developed a strategy which is being implemented. The key elements are:

- A national syllabus on conflict resolution. It is intended that all front line NHS staff should have the opportunity to attend this training.
- A national system for reporting physical assaults to the SMS
- The appointment of local security management specialists in every trust with a programme of professional training
- The establishment of a Legal Protection Unit which will advise and support trusts in pursuing private prosecutions of offenders where the police and / or the Crown Prosecution Service take no action. (Security Management Service 2003).

In a Royal College of Nursing Survey (2006) on nurses' working environment, nearly eight in ten nurses working in emergency departments report having been assaulted in the previous 12 months and 95% reported experiencing verbal abuse at some time in their career. Violence is a complex problem with a range of causes but clearly this is a significant risk in emergency departments with the potential for interaction with those whose behaviour is influenced by drugs or alcohol. The application of the risk-control approach is appropriate and action is needed to prevent as many incidents as possible by the use of technology such as CCTV, alarm systems, security staff and managing the environment. It is unlikely that all incidents can be prevented, so systems are needed for supporting staff, reporting to the police and ensuring that there is a clear message to the public that violent and aggressive behaviour will not be tolerated.

Stress

The Health and Safety Executive (HSE 2005) reported that nurses, particularly in the public sector, are one of the occupation groups with highest prevalence rates of work-related stress. The management of stress should be approached in the same way as any other health and safety hazard: identify the hazards, assess the risk, implement control measures and review. HSE has developed a set of six Stress Management Standards to identify and tackle work-related stress. There are six dimensions which, if not properly managed, may become sources of workplace stress. These dimensions are:

- Demands – such as workload, working patterns and the working environment
- Control – the extent to which individuals can control the way they do their work
- Support – level of support from the organization, line managers and colleagues in terms of encouragement, resources
- Relationships – such as promoting positive working to avoid conflict and dealing with unacceptable behaviour
- Roles – understanding roles within the organization and avoidance of role conflict
- Change – management and communication of organizational changes.

The Royal College of Nursing (2006) incorporated these scales into a survey of nurses' working environment and found that nurses working in emergency departments scored most negatively compared to other groups, indicating that working in this speciality can result in workplace stress. The survey also used a measure of psychological wellbeing, and nurses working in emergency have poorer psychological health scores than those working in other areas of hospitals.

CONCLUSION

Professional competence must now include a positive attitude to health, safety and welfare. High standards of care can only be provided in an environment which is not going to cause harm to the nurse or the patient. Health and safety legislation is developing and is driven by European Directives. Nurses need a good basic knowledge of the statutory requirements and a thorough understanding of how these apply to their own workplace. This has been recognized within the Knowledge and Skills Framework (KSF) which supports Agenda for Change, as health, safety and security constitute one of the core dimensions to be included in every KSF job outline. Principles of health and safety should be incorporated in the culture of the department and not be considered as a separate issue. Managers should be regularly reviewing policies, setting performance standards and reviewing progress. All staff must take responsibility for identifying hazards and taking appropriate action. The majority of accidents are foreseeable and therefore preventable. Accident prevention will reduce costs, both direct and indirect, and will lead to a healthier, more productive workforce.

References

Clough J (1998) Assessing and controlling risk. *Nursing Standard*, **12**(31), 49–54.

Control of Substances Hazardous to Health Regulations (1988) London: HMSO.

Control of Substances Hazardous to Health Regulations (2002) London: HMSO.

Department of Health (2002) *Back in Work.* London: Department of Health.

EC Directive 89/391/EEC (1989) *Council Directive of the 12th June 1989 on the Introduction of Measures to Encourage Improvements in the Safety and Health of Workers at Work.* Luxembourg: EC.

EC Directive 92/85 EEC (1992) *Pregnant Workers Directive.* Luxembourg: EC.

EC Directive 93/104/EC (1993) *Concerning Certain Aspects of the Organisation of Working Time.* Luxembourg: EC.

Employment Rights Act (1996) London: HMSO.

European Union (1986) *Single European Act.* Luxembourg: EC.

Health Protection Agency (2006) *Eye of the Needle – Surveillance of Significant Occupational Exposure to Blood Borne Viruses in Healthcare Workers.* London HPA.

Health & Safety Commission (1992) *Workplace Health, Safety and Welfare Approved Code of Practice and Guidance L24.* London: HMSO.

Health & Safety Executive (1992a) *Display Screen Equipment Work Guidance on Regulations L26.* London: HMSO.

Health & Safety Executive (1992b) *Manual Handling Operations Regulations Guidance on Regulations L23.* London: HMSO.

Health & Safety Executive (1992c) *Personal Protective Equipment at Work Guidance on Regulations L25.* London: HMSO.

Health & Safety Executive (1992d) *Work Equipment Guidance on Regulations L22.* London: HMSO.

Health & Safety Executive (1992e) *Workplace Guidance on Regulations.* London: HMSO.

Health & Safety Executive (1993) *The Costs of Accidents at Work.* Health & Safety series booklet HS(G) 96. London, HMSO.

Health and Safety Executive (2003) *Health and Safety at Work Regulations 1999* (The management regulations), HSC13 (rev1). London: H&SE.

Health and Safety Executive (2005) *Working Together to Reduce Stress at Work.* London: H&SE.

Health and Safety at Work etc. Act (1974) London: HMSO.

Health and Safety (First Aid) Regulations (1981) London: HMSO.

Lynch A, Cole E (2006) Human factors in emergency care: the need for team resource management. *Emergency Nurse,* **14**(2), 32–35.

Medical Devices Agency (2002) *Decontamination of Endoscopes.* London: Medical Devices Agency.

National Audit Office (2003a) *A Safer Place to Work: Improving the Management of Health and Safety Risks to Staff in NHS Trusts.* London: The Stationery Office.

National Audit Office (2003b) *A Safer Place to Work: Protecting NHS Hospital and Ambulance Staff from Violence and Aggression.* London: The Stationery Office.

Nursing and Midwifery Council (2004) *The NMC Code of Professional Conduct: Standards for Conduct, Performance and Ethics.* London: NMC.

Reporting of Injuries, Diseases and Dangerous Occurrences Regulations (1995) London: HMSO.

Royal College of Nursing (2006) *At Breaking Point? A Survey of the Wellbeing and Working Lives of Nurses in 2005.* London: RCN.

Royal College of Nursing (2000a) *Universal Precautions Poster.* London: RCN.

Royal College of Nursing (2000b) *Is There an Alternative to Gluteraldehyde?* London: RCN.

Royal College of Nursing (1996) *Code of Practice for the Handling of Patients,* 2nd edn. London: RCN.

Safety Representatives and Safety Committees Regulations (1977) London: HMSO.

Security Management Service (2003) *A Professional Approach to Managing Security.* London: Department of Health.

The Control of Substances Hazardous to Health, Guidance for the Initial Assessment in Hospitals (1994) London: HMSO.

The Management of Health and Safety at Work Regulations (1992) London: HMSO.

UK Health Departments (1998) *Guidance for Clinical Health Care Workers: Protection Against Infection with Blood-borne Viruses.* London: HMSO.

UK Health Departments (1993) *Protecting Health Care Workers & Patients from Hepatitis B.* London: HMSO.

Working Time Regulations (1998) (SI 1998 No. 1833). London: The Stationery Office.

Appendix

Normal values

HAEMATOLOGY

Haemoglobin
   Male — 13.5–17.7 g/dL
   Female — 11.5–16.5 g/dL
Mean corpuscular haemoglobin (MCH) — 27–32 pg
Mean corpuscular haemoglobin concentration (MCHC) — 32–36 g/dL
Mean corpuscular volume (MCV) — 80–96 fL
Packed cell volume (PCV)
   Male — 0.40–0.54 L/L
   Female — 0.37–0.47 L/L
White blood count (WBC) — $4-11 \times 10^9$/L
   Basophil granulocytes — $<0.01-0.1 \times 10^9$/L
   Eosinophil granulocytes — $0.04-0.4 \times 10^9$/L
   Lymphocytes — $1.5-4.0 \times 10^9$/L
   Monocytes — $0.2-0.8 \times 10^9$/L
   Neutrophil granulocytes — $2.0-7.5 \times 10^9$/L
Total blood volume — 60–80 ml/kg
Plasma volume — 40–50 ml/kg
Platelet count — $150-400 \times 10^9$/L
Serum B_{12} — 160–925 ng/L (150–675 pmol/L)
Serum folate — 2.9–18 µg/L (3.6–63 nmol/L)
Red cell folate — 149–640 µg/L
Red cell mass
   Male — 25–35 ml/kg
   Female — 20–30 ml/kg
Reticulocyte count — 0.5–2.5% of red cells ($50-100 \times 10^9$/L)
Erythrocyte sedimentation rate (ESR) — <20 mm in 1 hour
Plasma viscosity — 1.5–1.72 mPa.s

Coagulation

Bleeding time (Ivy method)	3–9 min
Activated partial thromboplastin time (APTT)	23–31 s
Prothrombin time	12–16 s
International Normalized Ratio (INR)	1.0–1.3
D-dimer	<500 ng/ml

BIOCHEMISTRY (SERUM/PLASMA)

Alanine aminotransferase (ALT)	5–40 U/L
Albumin	35–50 g/L
Alkaline phosphatase	39–117 U/L
Amylase	25–125 U/L
Angiotensin-converting enzyme	10–70 U/L
α_1-antitrypsin	1.1–2.1 g/L
Aspartate aminotransferase (AST)	12–40 U/L
Bicarbonate	22–30 mmol/L
Bilirubin	<17 µmol/L (0.3–1.5 mg/dL)
Caeruloplasmin	1.5–2.9 µmol/L
Calcium	2.20–2.67 mmol/L (8.5–10.5 mg/dL)
Chloride	98–106 mmol/L
Complement	
C3	0.75–1.65 g/L
C4	0.20–0.60 g/L
Copper	11–20 µmol/L (100–200 mg/dL)
C-reactive protein	<10 mg/L
Creatinine	79–118 µmol/L (0.6–1.5 mg/dL)
Creatine kinase (CPK)	
Female	24–170 U/L
Male	24–195 U/L
CK-MB fraction	<25 U/L (<60% of total activity)
Ferritin	
Female	6–110 µg/L
Male	20–260 µg/L
Post menopausal	12–230 µg/L
α-fetoprotein	<10k U/L
Glucose (fasting)	4.5–5.6 mmol/L (70–110 mg/dL)
Fructosamine up to	285 µmol/L
γ-glutamyl transpeptidase (γ-GT)	
Male	11–58 U/L
Female	7–32 U/L
Glycosylated (glycated) haemoglobin (HbA$_{10}$)	3.7–5.1%
Hydroxybutyric dehydrogenase (HBD)	72–182 U/L
Immunoglobulins (11 years and over)	
IgA	0.8–4 g/L
IgG	5.5–16.5 g/L
IgM	0.4–2.0 g/L
Iron	13–32 µmol/L (50–150 µg/dL)
Iron binding capacity (total) (TIBC)	42–80 µmol/L (250–410 µg/dL)
Lactate dehydrogenase	240–480 U/L
Magnesium	0.7–1.1 mmol/L
β_2- microglobulin	1.0–3.0 mg/L
Osmolality	275–295 mOsm/kg
Phosphate	0.8–1.5 mmol/L
Potassium	3.5–5.0 mmol/L
Prostate-specific antigen (PSA) up to	4.0 µg/L
Protein (total)	62–77 g/L
Sodium	135–146 mmol/L
Urate	0.18–0.42 mmol/L (3.0–7.0 mg/dL)
Urea	2.5–6.7 mmol/L (8–25 mg/dL)
Vitamin A	0.5–2.01 µmol/L
Vitamin D	
25-hydroxy	37–200 mmol/L (0.15–0.80 ng/L)
1.25-dihydroxy	60–108 pmol/L (0.24–0.45 pg/L)
Zinc	11–24 µmol/L

Lipids and lipoproteins

Cholesterol	3.5–6.5 mmol/L (ideal <5.2 mmol/L)
HDL cholesterol	
Male	0.8–1.8 mmol/L
Female	1.0–2.3 mmol/L
LDL cholesterol	<4.0 mmol/L
Lipids (total)	4.0–10.0 g/L
Lipoproteins	
VLDL	0.128–0.645 mmol/L
LDL	1.55–4.4 mmol/L
HDL	
Male	0.70–2.1 mmol/L
Female	0.50–1.70 mmol/L
Phospholipid	2.9–5.2 mmol/L
Triglycerides	
Male	0.70–2.1 mmol/L
Female	0.50–1.70 mmol/L

Blood gases (arterial)

P_aco_2	4.8–6.1 kPa (36–46 mmHg)
P_ao_2	10–13.3 kPa (75–100 mmHg)
[H+]	35–45 mmol/L
pH	7.35–7.45
Bicarbonate	22–26 mmol/L

Urine values

Calcium	7.5 mmol daily or less (<300 mg daily)
Copper	0.2–1.0 µmol daily
Creatinine	0.13–0.22 mmol per kilogram body weight, daily
5-hydroxyindole acetic acid (5HIAA)	<75 µmol daily; amounts lower in females than males
Protein (quantitative)	<0.15 g per 24 hours
Sodium	60–80 mmol per 24 hours

Index

Page numbers for figures have suffix **f**, those for tables have suffix **t**